18th Edition

The Reference Manual of the

Official Documents

of the American Occupational Therapy Association, Inc.

The American
Occupational Therapy
Association, Inc.

AOTA Vision Statement

The American Occupational Therapy Association advances occupational therapy as the pre-eminent profession in promoting the health, productivity, and quality of life of individuals and society through the therapeutic application of occupation.

AOTA Mission Statement

The American Occupational Therapy Association advances the quality, availability, use, and support of occupational therapy through standard-setting, advocacy, education, and research on behalf of its members and the public.

AOTA *Centennial Vision*

We envision that occupational therapy is a powerful, widely recognized, science-driven, and evidence-based profession with a globally connected and diverse workforce meeting society's occupational needs.

AOTA Staff

Frederick P. Somers, *Executive Director*
Christopher M. Bluhm, *Chief Operating Officer*

Chris Davis, *Director, AOTA Press*
Caroline Polk, *Managing Editor,* AJOT *and Test Prep*
Ashley Hofmann, *Development/Production Editor*
Victoria Davis, *Production/Digital Editor*

Beth Ledford, *Director, Marketing*
Amanda Fogle, *Marketing Specialist*
Jennifer Folden, *Marketing Specialist*

The American Occupational Therapy Association, Inc.
4720 Montgomery Lane
Bethesda, MD 20814
Phone: 301-652-AOTA (2682)
TDD: 800-377-8555
Fax: 301-652-7711
www.aota.org

Disclaimers

This publication is designed to provide accurate and authoritative information in regard to the subject matter covered. It is sold or distributed with the understanding that the publisher is not engaged in rendering legal, accounting, or other professional service. If legal advice or other expert assistance is required, the services of a competent professional person should be sought.
—*From the Declaration of Principles jointly adopted by the American Bar Association and a Committee of Publishers and Associations*

It is the objective of the American Occupational Therapy Association to be a forum for free expression and interchange of ideas. The opinions expressed by the contributors to this work are their own and not necessarily those of the American Occupational Therapy Association.

ISBN-13: 978-1-56900-347-3

Printing by Automated Graphic Systems, Inc., White Plains, MD

Reference citation: American Occupational Therapy Association. (2013). *The reference manual of the official documents of the American Occupational Therapy Association, Inc.* (18th ed.). Bethesda, MD: Author.

However, the preferred citation for individual chapters is their original citation from the *American Journal of Occupational Therapy.*

For permissions inquiries, visit www.copyright.com.

Contents

*Articles in **bold** are new to this edition.*

Introduction

The Reference Manual of the Official Documents of the American Occupational Therapy Association, Inc. (AOTA) was first published in 1980 and had been fully revised biennially in even-numbered years, with an addendum produced in alternate years. In 2006, AOTA Press began publishing a fully revised edition of the *Reference Manual* annually.

The 18th edition of this important work contains the following material:

- Part I contains AOTA's current official documents, which have been "constructed by the Association and approved by the Association for the use of the Association and its membership" (AOTA, 2007).

- Part II contains Societal Statements.

- Part III contains information about the American Occupational Therapy Foundation (AOTF).

- Part IV contains historical information on past official documents.

Types of official and other documents (AOTA, 2004) include the following:

I. Types of Official Documents

A. **Concept Papers**—Provide a thoughtful discussion of an issue or topic, synthesizing varying perspectives to assist members to more thoroughly understand the issue or topic. These documents are developed in response to a particular issue, concern, or need and can be written for internal or external use.

B. **Guidelines**—Provide descriptions, examples, or recommendations of procedures pertaining to the education and practice of occupational therapy. The Occupational Therapy Practice Guidelines Series has a separate development process and is not included in the official document development or adoption process.

C. **Position Papers**—Present the official stance of the Association on a substantive issue or subject. They are developed in response to a particular issue, concern, or need of the Association and may be written for internal or external use.

D. **Roles Papers**—Present a guide to the major roles common in the profession of occupational therapy. The roles listed in these documents are those frequently held by occupational therapists and occupational therapy assistants and are not all-inclusive.

E. **Specialized Knowledge and Skills Papers**—Provide a detailed outline of the specialized knowledge and skills needed for competent practice. Rationale for the development of this type of document is to provide a structure for acquiring competency in an area where there are specialized evaluation and intervention processes.

F. **Standards**—Include a general description of the topic and define the minimum requirements for performance and quality.

G. **Statements**—Describe and clarify an aspect or issue related to education or practice and are linked to the fundamental concepts of occupational therapy.

II. Other Types of Documents

Other association documents that are included in this publication are

- **Societal statements**—Written in the form of public announcements, these statements identify a societal issue of concern; state how the issue affects the participation of individuals, families, groups, or communities in society; and may offer action to be taken by individuals, groups, or communities.

- **AOTF information**—Although AOTF is separate from AOTA, this information has been included at reader request.

The documents contained in this manual have been developed by the combined efforts of many AOTA volunteers and staff. Authorship and citations for where these documents have been published in the *American Journal of Occupational Therapy* can be found at the end of each document. For additional information, visit www.aota.org and http://ajot.aotapress.net. Official documents are also included in the ECRI Institute Online Directory (www.ecri.org), and Practice Guidelines are abstracted in the National Guideline Clearinghouse (www.guideline.gov).

References

American Occupational Therapy Association. (2009). *COE and COP standard operating procedures—Official documents (Attachment A).* (Available from American Occupational Therapy Association, 4720 Montgomery Lane, Bethesda, MD 20824-1220)

American Occupational Therapy Association. (2007). *Definition of official documents.* (Adopted by the AOTA Representative Assembly during its 2006 online meeting)

Categories of Occupational Therapy Personnel

Code: RA Motion 7/94, 4/95, 2003M54, 2006C379
Effective: 7/94
Revised: 4/95, 4/96, 4/98, 4/99, 4/01, 6/03, 4/06
BPPC Reviewed: 10/01, 1/02, 1/03, 1/06
Rescinded:

PURPOSE: To establish policy assuring that Association documents use consistent terminology when referring to individuals who provide or support the delivery of occupational therapy services.

It Shall Be the Policy of the Association That

The following terms are used as defined herein in all Association documents and publications:

1. **Occupational Therapy Personnel:** Individuals who work in an occupational therapy program/ department/unit to ensure the delivery of occupational therapy services to consumers. Occupational therapy personnel may include occupational therapist (OT), occupational therapy assistant (OTA), occupational therapy student (OTS), occupational therapy assistant student (OTAS), and aide.

2. **Occupational Therapist (OT):** Any individual initially certified to practice as an OT or licensed or regulated by a state, commonwealth, district, or territory of the United States to practice as an occupational therapist and who has not had that certification, license, or regulation revoked due to disciplinary action.

3. **Occupational Therapy Assistant (OTA):** Any individual initially certified to practice as an OTA or licensed or regulated by a state, commonwealth, district, or territory of the United States to practice as an OTA and who has not had that certification, license, or regulation revoked due to disciplinary action.

4. **Occupational Therapy Student (OTS):** Any individual who is enrolled in an occupational therapy educational program that is accredited or pending accreditation by ACOTE.®

5. **Occupational Therapy Assistant Student (OTAS):** An individual who is enrolled in an occupational therapy assistant educational program that is accredited or pending accreditation by ACOTE.®

6. **Occupational Therapy Practitioner:** An individual initially certified to practice as an OT or OTA or licensed or regulated by a state, district, commonwealth, or territory of the United States to practice as an OT or OTA and who has not had that certification, license, or regulation revoked due to disciplinary action.

7. **Aide:** A person who is not licensed or regulated and who provides supportive services to OTs and OTAs. An aide shall function under the guidance and responsibility of the licensed or regulated OT and may be supervised by the OT or an OTA for specifically selected routine tasks for which the aide has been trained and has demonstrated competence. The aide is not a primary service provider of occupational therapy in a practice setting and does not provide skilled occupational therapy services.

PART I

Official Documents

Incorporation Papers and Bylaws

The

Articles of Incorporation
Of
The American Occupational Therapy
Association

******

Composite Articles of Incorporation of The American Occupational Therapy Association
as amended*

We, The Undersigned, All being persons of full age, and all being citizens of the United States desiring to form a corporation, pursuant to Sub-Chapter 3, of Chapter 18, of the Code of Law for the District of Columbia, do hereby make, sign and acknowledge this Certificate as follows:

FIRST: The name of the corporation is to be "The American Occupational Therapy Association."**

SECOND: The term of existence of the corporation shall be perpetual.

THIRD: The purpose or purposes which it will hereafter pursue are to *advance the therapeutic value of occupation; to research the effects of occupation upon human beings and to disseminate that research;* to promote the use of occupational therapy and to advance the standards of education and training in this field; *to educate consumers about the effect of occupation upon their well-being;* and to engage in such other activities as may be considered to be advantageous to the profession, its members, and the consumers of occupational therapy services. [Italicized portions adopted by Executive Board 1/16/76.]

FOURTH: *The Corporation is to have members.*

FIFTH: *The Corporation is to be divided into classes of members. The designation of each class of members, the qualifications, rights, and limitations of the members of each class and conferring, limiting, or denying the right to vote are as follows:*

a. Members: The classes of members are (1) occupational therapist, (2) occupational therapy assistant, (3) occupational therapy student, (4) organizational, and (5) associate. The Bylaws may designate other classes of members.

b. Qualifications, Rights, and Limitations: The qualifications, rights, and limitations of the members of each class shall be provided in the Bylaws

c. Voting: Members are entitled to vote for Association officers and bylaw changes; members shall have such other voting rights as are provided in the Bylaws. Associate members and Organizational members shall not be entitled to vote for Association Officers and bylaw changes.

SIXTH: All corporate powers shall be exercised by and under the authority of the board of directors except as provided in this Sixth Article. The number of trustees, directors, or managers of the corporation shall be not less than five (5) or more than fifty (50), and shall be known as the Board of Directors. The manner of election or appointment of such directors shall be provided in the Bylaws. There shall be a designated body of the board known as the Representative Assembly which shall be directly responsible for the establishment of professional standards and policies.

SEVENTH: The territory in which its operations are principally to be conducted is the United States of America, the territories, possessions, and dependencies thereof and the District of Columbia, but the operations of the corporation shall not be limited to such territory.

EIGHTH: The location of the principal office of the corporation shall be fixed by the Bylaws of the corporation.

NINTH: The time for holding its annual meeting shall be fixed by the Bylaws of the corporation.

TENTH: *In the event this corporation shall be dissolved for any reason, any remaining assets shall be distributed for purposes within the scope of Internal Revenue code 501(c) (6) or any amendment thereto, and in accordance with the corporate statutes of the District of Columbia.*

ELEVENTH: The address, including street and number, of its registered office in the District of Columbia is 918-16th St N.W., Washington, DC 20006, and the name of its registered agent at such address is C.T. Corporation System.

TWELFTH: The names and places of residence of the persons to be its directors until its first annual meeting are as follows:
William R. Dunton, Jr., MD, of Sheppard and Enoch Pratt Hospital of Towson, Maryland; Susan C. Johnson, of 350 West 85th Street, New York City, New York; Eleanor Clarke Slagle, of the Hotel Alexandria, Chicago, Illinois; Susan E. Tracy, of Jamaica Plain, Massachusetts; and George Edward Barton, of Consolation House, Clifton Springs, New York.

IN WITNESS WHEREOF: We have made signed and acknowledged this certificate in duplicate.
Date, Clifton Springs, Ontario County, New York, this fifteenth day of March, A.D. 1917.
William R. Dunton, Jr.
Susan C. Johnson
Eleanor Clarke Slagle
George Edward Barton
Isabel G. Newton
T.B. Kidner

STATE OF NEW YORK
COUNTY OF ONTARIO: SS
On the fifteenth day of March, 1917, before me personally came William R. Dunton, Jr., Susan C. Johnson, Eleanor Clarke Slagle, George Edward Barton, Isabel G. Newton, and T.B. Kidner, to me known and known to me to be the same persons described in and who executed the foregoing certificate the same.
James A. Rolfe,
Notary Public.

(NOTARIAL SEAL)

* A resolution recommending that the corporation accept the jurisdiction of the District of Columbia Nonprofit Corporation Act (29 D.C. Code Chapter 10 then) was adopted at a meeting of the Executive Board on January 16, 1976. The formal Statement of Election to Accept was filed and certified on August 30, 1976. Italicized items were filed as part of that Statement to amend existing article number three, and to add new provisions with information required to be included in the Articles under Chapter 10 (now Chapter 5).

The 1981 amendment added the organizational category of membership without vote in Article 5, and corrected the word "The" in Article one.

The 1990 amendment added the Associate category of membership without vote in Article 5 and provides for other classes of membership to be designated in the Bylaws.

This compilation represents a re-numbered composite of all official amendments or documents affecting incorporation from March 1917 through May 1990.

The 2003 amendments removed "registered" and "certified" in Members in Article 5 and changed from "Executive Board" to "Board of Directors" in Article 6.

The 2013 amendments add by name the Representative Assembly as a designated body of the board, responsible for the establishment of professional standards and policies. This change was made to incorporate AOTA's then existing organizational structure into the framework of the 2012 changes in the DC nonprofit corporate law.

** Name changed from National Society for the Promotion of Occupational Therapy, Inc. Jan. 27, 1923

CERTIFICATE OF INCORPORATION

OF THE

NATIONAL SOCIETY FOR THE PROMOTION OF OCCUPATIONAL THERAPY, INC.

We, The Undersigned, All being persons of full age, and all being citizens of the United States, desiring to form a corporation, pursuant to Sub-Chapter 3 of Chapter 18, of the Code of Law for the District of Columbia, do hereby make, sign and acknowledge this Certificate as follows:

FIRST: The name of the Corporation is to be "THE NATIONAL SOCIETY FOR THE PROMOTION OF OCCUPATIONAL THERAPY, INC."

SECOND: The particular objects for which the corporation is formed are as follows: The advancement of occupation as a therapeutic measure; for the study of the effect of occupation upon the human being; and for the scientific dispensation of this knowledge.

THIRD: The territory in which its operations are to be principally conducted is the United States of America.

FOURTH: Its principal business office is to be located in the Village of Clifton Springs, County of Ontario and State of New York.

FIFTH: The number of its directors is to be five.

SIXTH: The names and places of residence of the persons to be its directors until its first annual meeting are as follows:

William R. Dunton, Jr., M.D. of Sheppard and Enoch Pratt Hospital of Towson, Maryland.

Susan C. Johnson, of 350 West 85th Street, New York City, New York.

Eleanor Clarke Slagle, of the Hotel Alexandria, Chicago, Illinois.

George Edward Barton, of Consolation House, Clifton Springs, New York.

SEVENTH: The time for holding its annual meeting is on the first Monday of September in each year.

IN WITNESS WHEREOF: We have made, signed and acknowledged this certificate in duplicate.

Dated, Clifton Springs, Ontario County, New York, this fifteenth day of March, A.D. 1917.

William R. Dunton, Jr.
Susan C. Johnson
Eleanor Clarke Slagle
George Edward Barton
Isabel G. Newton
T. B. Kidner

STATE OF NEW YORK

COUNTY OF ONTARIO: SS

On this fifteenth day of March, 1917, before me personally came William R. Dunton, Jr., Susan C. Johnson, Eleanor Clarke Siagle, George Edward Barton, Isabel G. Newton and T. B. Kidner, to me known and known to me to be the same persons described in and who executed the foregoing certificate and they severally duly acknowledged to me that they executed the same.

James A. Rolfe,

Notary Public

(NOTARIAL SEAL)

The

Official Bylaws
of
The American Occupational
Therapy Association, Inc.

2013

******

Table of Contents
Bylaws

Bylaws Revisions (4-27-13)

The American Occupational Therapy Association, Inc.

Bylaws
Table of Contents

i

ARTICLE I.

Name

Section 1.   Name

The name of the organization shall be The American Occupational Therapy Association, Inc., hereinafter referred to as the Association.

Section 2.   Purpose

The Association is organized under the District of Columbia (D.C.) Nonprofit Corporation Act.

ARTICLE II.

Noninurement

Section 1.   Noninurement

No part of the net earnings of the Association shall inure to the use or benefit of any individual. The Association shall not engage in any activities that are prohibited by the Internal Revenue Code, Section 501(c) (6).

ARTICLE III.

Members

Section 1.   Membership Classes

There shall be six (6) classes of membership.

A.   Occupational Therapist (OT): Any individual initially certified to practice as an OT or licensed or regulated by a state, commonwealth, district, or territory of the United States to practice as an occupational therapist and who has not had that certification, license, or regulation revoked due to disciplinary action shall be eligible to be an Occupational Therapist Member.

B.   Occupational Therapist New Practitioner and Occupational Therapy Assistant New Practitioner: Any individual who has graduated with an occupational therapy degree from an occupational therapy or occupational therapy assistant entry level educational program that is accredited by the Accreditation Council for Occupational Therapy Education (ACOTE®) and that is located in the United States, or in a state, commonwealth, district, or territory of the United States in the past 24 months.

1

C. Occupational Therapy Assistant (OTA): Any individual initially certified to practice as an OTA or licensed or regulated by a state, commonwealth, district, or territory of the United States to practice as an occupational therapy assistant and who has not had that certification, license, or regulation revoked due to disciplinary action shall be eligible to be an Occupational Therapy Assistant Member.

D. Occupational Therapy Student (OTS) and Occupational Therapy Assistant Student (OTAS): Any individual enrolled in an entry level occupational therapy educational program that is accredited, or pending accreditation by the Accreditation Council for Occupational Therapy Education (ACOTE®) and that is located in the United States, or in a state, commonwealth, district, or territory of the United States, shall be eligible to be a Student Member.

E. Organizational: An organization, institution, or agency interested in occupational therapy may be an Organizational Member.

F. Associate: An individual interested in occupational therapy that does not satisfy the requirements of subsections A, B, C, or D of this section may be an Associate Member.

Section 2. **Voting Rights and Privileges of Members**

A. Occupational Therapist, Occupational Therapy Assistant, and OT/OTA New Practitioner Members:

 1. Shall be entitled to vote

  a. for Officers of the Association, Board Directors, and Delegate and Alternate Delegate to the World Federation of Occupational Therapists (WFOT);

  b. for Representative(s);

  c. for Chairpersons-Elect of the Commission on Education (COE), Commission on Practice (COP), Ethics Commission (EC), Commission on Continuing Competence and Professional Development (CCCPD), Special Interest Sections Council (SISC), Chairperson of the Volunteer Leadership Development Committee (VLDC), and for the OTA Representative and OTA Representative-Elect to the Assembly;

  d. at Annual Business Meetings and special meetings of the Association; and

2

e.   for Association Bylaws.

2.   May submit resolutions and motions to the Agenda Committee of the Assembly.

3.   May serve on Association commissions/committees and run for offices of the Association.

4.   Shall be eligible to receive other privileges as designated by the Board.

5.   May have voice in all appropriate forums in accordance with established practice.

6.   May seek review of the Associations actions pursuant to the procedures set forth in Article XV.

7.   May inspect and copy records of the Association upon delivering a signed notice to the secretary of the Association at the Association headquarters at least 21 calendar days before the date a member wishes to inspect the records during reasonable business hours at the office of the Association. The Association shall keep and members shall have the right to inspect and copy the records required by and under the terms of the D.C. law applicable to nonprofit corporations.

B.   Student Members:

1.   Shall be entitled to vote

     a.   for Officers of the Association, Board Directors, and Delegate and Alternate Delegate to the WFOT;

     b.   at Annual Business Meetings or special meetings of the Association;

     c.   for Chairpersons-Elect of the COE, COP, EC, CCCPD, SISC, Chairperson of the VLDC and for Representatives, the OTA Representative and OTA Representative-Elect to the Assembly;

     d.   for Chairperson and Officers of the ASD and Student Member Representative to the Assembly; and

     e.   for Association Bylaws.

2.   May submit resolutions and motions to the Agenda Committee of the Assembly.

3

3.   May serve on Association commissions/committees.

4.   Shall be eligible to be an officer or member of ASD.

5.   Shall be entitled to receive other privileges as designated by the Board.

6.   May seek review of the Associations actions pursuant to the procedures set forth in Article XV.

7.   May inspect and copy records of the Association upon delivering a signed notice to the secretary of the Association at least 21 days before the date a member wishes to inspect the records during reasonable business hours at office of the Association. The Association shall keep and members shall have the right to inspect and copy the records required by and under the terms of the D.C. law applicable to nonprofit corporations.

C.   Organizational and Associate Members:

Shall be entitled to receive privileges as designated by the Board.

Section 3.   **Dues and Good Standing**

A.   Dues and fees, if any, for all classes of membership shall be established by the Board.

B.   A member shall be in good standing if he or she currently meets the qualifications for the class of membership, has paid all applicable dues, and membership has not been terminated pursuant to Section 4.

Section 4.   **Termination of Membership**

A.   Any member whose dues are still in arrears 30 days after payment is due shall automatically be removed from membership. Membership shall automatically be reinstated by payment of dues in arrears.

B.   Members of any classification may have their membership revoked or suspended for cause. Cause may include violation of the AOTA *Occupational Therapy Code of Ethics and Ethics Standards* (Code and Ethics Standards).

C.   For any cause other than nonpayment of dues, a vote for revocation or suspension shall occur only after the member has been notified of the complaint for revocation and has been given reasonable opportunity for defense pursuant to the *Enforcement Procedures for the Occupational Therapy Code of Ethics and Ethics Standards*.

4

ARTICLE IV.

Meetings of the Membership of the Association

Section 1.   **Meeting Location**

A.   Annual or special meetings of the membership need not be held in a geographic location. Alternatively, the meeting may be held by means of the internet or other electronic communications technology in a fashion such that the members have the opportunity to read or hear the proceedings substantially concurrently (although not necessarily simultaneous) with their occurrence, vote on matters submitted to the members, and pose questions and make comments.

B.   The President shall be the chairperson at all membership meetings, and in the absence of the President it shall be the Vice President.

Section 2.   **Annual Business Meeting**

A.   The regular meeting of the membership, the Annual Business Meeting, shall be held within each calendar year.

B.   An official publication of the Association shall list the place, day, and hour of the Annual Business Meeting at least 90 days before the meeting date.

C.   The record date for determining members entitled to notice of and to vote at an annual meeting shall be 30 days prior to the meeting or action requiring a determination by the members.

Section 3.   **Special Meetings**

A.   The President, a majority of voting members of the Board, two thirds of the Assembly with respect to a matter within the scope of its Purpose as set forth in Article VII, Section 1, or 10% of the members of the Association may call a special meeting.

B.   Members shall be notified by mail, electronic, or telephonic transmission of the place, day, hour, and purpose of the special meeting at least 21 days before the meeting.

C.   At a special meeting, the only business conducted shall be the matters stated in the meeting notification.

D.   The record date for determining members entitled to demand a special meeting shall be the date the first member signs a demand for the special

5

meeting.

E.   The record date for determining members entitled to give notice of and to vote at a special meeting is the day the first notice is given to members, and the record date shall not be more than 30 days before the meeting or action requiring a determination by the members.

Section 4.   Quorum for Annual and Special Meetings

A quorum shall be 100 members.

Section 5.   Voting

A.   Mail, electronic, or telephonic transmission may be used by OT, OTA, and student members for voting.

B.   At any annual or special meeting of the members, there shall be no voting by proxy.

C.   The Board in conformance with the law applicable to non-profit corporations in D.C. shall determine the process for counting and recording the vote except as otherwise provided in Article IX of these Bylaws.

D.   Any action that may be taken at any annual, special, or regular meeting of the members may be taken without a meeting by ballot in accordance with D.C. Law. Elections by ballots shall be conducted by ballot in accordance with Article IX.

E.   An action is approved by the membership if the votes cast favoring the action exceed the votes cast opposing the action, unless the Articles, Bylaws, or D.C. law requires a greater or lesser number of affirmative votes for the specific matter that is the subject of the vote.

ARTICLE V.

Board of Directors

Section 1.   Purpose

The Board of Directors, herein called the Board, shall govern the affairs of the Association in accordance with all duly vested statutory, corporate, and Bylaws powers. Each member of the Board shall have a fiduciary duty when discharging duties as a director to act in good faith and in a manner reasonably believed to be in the best interest of the Association and otherwise in accordance with standards of conduct under D.C. law for directors in non-profit associations.

6

Section 2.   **Composition**

A.   Voting Members

    1.   Officers of the Association: President, Vice President, Secretary, and Treasurer

    2.   Six Directors (at least one of whom must be an OTA and at least one of whom must be an OT)

    3.   Speaker of the Assembly

B.   Nonvoting Members

    1.   President-Elect

    2.   Public Advisor

    3.   Consumer Advisor

    4.   AOTA Executive Director

    5.   President, American Occupational Therapy Foundation (AOTF)

    6.   An additional person designated by AOTF from their board of directors

Section 3.   **Term and Qualifications of Board Directors**

A.   Term of Office

    1.   A Director shall serve a 3-year term, or until a successor has been elected but in no event shall a Director serve in excess of 5 consecutive years without being appointed or elected to a new term.

    2.   A Director shall only be eligible to serve another elected term after the expiration of 2 intervening years.

    3.   A vacancy on the Board may be filled until the next scheduled election by a vote of a majority of the Directors remaining in office, even if they constitute less than a quorum.

    4.   Directors may only be removed for cause by the members of the Board as provided in Article XII or by a vote of the membership. Notice of a meeting at which removal of a Director is being considered shall state that the purpose, or one of the purposes, of the meeting is removal of the Director(s).

7

B.   Qualifications

    1.   A Director shall have been initially certified with at least 5 years of experience as an OT or OTA at the time of nomination.

    2.   A Director shall have the qualifications necessary to execute the duties of the office held as outlined by the Volunteer Leadership Development Committee (VLDC).

Section 4.   Appointment, Term, and Qualifications of Appointed Participants

A.   Appointment

The Consumer Advisor and Public Advisor are appointed by the President.

B.   Term of Office

The Consumer Advisor and Public Advisor shall serve a 3-year term that coincides with the term of the President.

C.   Qualifications

    1.   Consumer Advisor

        a.   Knowledge of the profession of occupational therapy through personal experience.

        b.   Experience serving on boards, committees, or other bodies.

    2.   Public Advisor

        a.   Knowledge of the profession of occupational therapy through professional experience in health care reimbursement, regulatory, or policy arenas.

        b.   Experience serving on boards, committees, or other bodies.

Section 5.   Functions

The Board shall perform such functions as are necessary to fulfill the purpose of the Board of Directors set forth in this Article at Section 1, including the functions set forth below.

A.   Establish the policies and procedures of the Board and the Association with the exception of the procedures that govern the Assembly.

B. Develop and approve the Strategic Plan of the Association.

C. Review and approve the Association budget for each fiscal year.

D. Manage the Association headquarters through appointment of the Executive Director as Chief Executive Officer of the Association.

E. Approve investment policies of the Association and review compliance therewith.

F. Unless otherwise provided, act as, or appoint, the appeal body of the Association for matters for which such appeals are provided under these Bylaws.

G. Determine location of the principal office of the Association.

H. Declare and take action during an emergency.

I. Create committees of the Board and advisory committees and entities.

Section 6.   Meetings

A. Regular Meetings

    1. The Board shall have at least one regular meeting a year.

    2. The time and place of a regular meeting shall be designated at least 30 days before the meeting date by mail, electronic, or telephonic transmission to Board members.

    3. The Board may invite any person to a Board meeting to advance the business of the Board.

    4. The Board may permit any or all Directors to participate in regular or special meetings by, or conduct the meetings through, the use of any means of communication by which all Directors participating may simultaneously hear each other during the meeting.

B. Special Meetings

    1. Special meetings of the Board may be called by the President or any three members to address specific issues.

    2. Board members shall be notified by mail, electronic, or telephonic transmission of the date, time, place, and purpose of the meeting at least 1 week before the date.

    3. Only business as stated in the call may be transacted at the special

9

meeting.

4.   Urgent business may be transacted by voting members of the Board via conference call on notice that is appropriate under the circumstances.

C.   Quorum

A majority of all voting members, including at least two officers, shall constitute a quorum.

D.   Voting

1.   If a quorum is present when a vote is taken, the affirmative vote of a majority of the Directors present shall be an act of the Directors unless a greater vote is required by the Articles of Incorporation, Bylaws, or law for the specific matter before the Board.

2.   Action may be taken without a meeting if each Director signs consent in the form of a record describing the action to be taken.

3.   Actions taken at a Board meeting approving a transaction and contract where a board member or officer has an actual or potential conflict of interest shall be valid if the interested Director disclosed the conflict to the Board prior to the vote and if the transaction or contract would not be void or voidable under D.C. Code § 29-406.70(a) (1) or (a) (2). That a contract or transaction meets the fairness requirement of D.C. Code § 29-406.70(a) (3) shall not be sufficient basis to validate a Board action in which a board member had a conflict of interest.

Section 7.   Committees of the Board

The Board shall have the authority to establish committees consisting of board members as necessary to carry out the purposes of the Association provided that the Board may not delegate overall responsibility for conduct of the business of the Association. The Board shall also have authority to establish advisory committees that may consist of Board and/or non-Board members. Advisory committees cannot exercise any power of the Board.

Section 8.   Organizational Advisors

The following entities shall act in an advisory capacity to the Board to provide information regarding strategic planning and budgeting with respect to matters within the expertise of the specific Organizational Advisor: Accreditation Council for Occupational Therapy Education (ACOTE®) Chairperson, American Occupational Therapy Political Action Committee (AOTPAC) Chairperson, Affiliated State Association Presidents

10

(ASAP) Chairperson, Assembly of Student Delegates (ASD) Chairperson, World Federation of Occupational Therapists (WFOT) Delegate, OT Program Directors' Education Council (OTPDEC) Chairperson, and OTA Program Directors' Education Council (OTAPDEC) Chairperson.

Section 9.   Standing Advisory Committees

The following committees shall be standing advisory committees of the Board.

A.   Finance and Audit Committee

Purpose: To assist the Board in its oversight of
   a. Integrity in financial statements;
   b. Compliance with legal and regulatory requirements as well as Association conflict of interest policies; and
   c. Selection of a qualified independent auditor.

The Treasurer shall serve as the Chairperson of the Finance and Audit Committee for a 3-year term.

B.   Bylaws, Policies, and Procedures Committee (BPPC)

Purpose: To review Association governance documents and recommend changes to appropriate body(ies) for consideration. The Board shall appoint the Chairperson of BPPC for a 3-year term.

C.   VLDC

Purpose: To promote member participation and engagement, volunteer leadership development, and participation initiatives of the Association. The VLDC will identify and recruit diverse and qualified candidates for service to the Association through routine elections and appointments, recipients of awards, and other leadership activities.

D.   SISC

Purpose: To coordinate and facilitate activities of the Special Interest Sections with standing and advisory commissions and committees of the Association.

E.   ASD

Purpose: To provide an opportunity for student members to have input into decision making and actions of the Association; to promote participation, professional growth, and leadership development of students; and to enhance students' knowledge of the structure of the Association.

11

Unless otherwise stated above, the Chairpersons of the Standing Advisory Committees shall be elected by the membership for a 3-year term and shall hold only one position in the Association at a time.

The Board may set forth in standard operating procedures (SOPs) the procedures for selection and approval of the members of the standing advisory committee, the term of the members, and any other matters relating to operation of the committees.

Section 10. Associated Advisory Council of the Board

ACOTE®

Purpose: To accredit occupational therapy educational programs and occupational therapy assistant educational programs. ACOTE® establishes, approves, and administers educational standards to evaluate occupational therapy and occupational therapy assistant educational programs. ACOTE® shall have complete autonomy in establishing standards for educational programs; developing and implementing policies, rules, and procedures for conducting accreditation reviews; and making accreditation decisions.

ARTICLE VI.

Officers of the Association

Section 1. Officers

The Officers shall be the President, Vice President, Secretary, and Treasurer.

Section 2. Officer Qualifications

A. Officers shall have been initially certified with at least 10 years of experience as an OT or OTA at the time of nomination.

B. An officer shall have the qualifications necessary to execute duties of the office held as stated in Association documents.

C. An officer shall be a member in good standing of the Association and of a state affiliate at the time of nomination and throughout the term of office.

Section 3. Duties

A. President

1. Shall be the chief elected officer of the Association and represent the Association to the public.

2. Shall be an ex officio member of all committees of the Association except the VLDC and the EC.

3. Shall preside at all meetings of the Association membership.

4. Shall preside at Board meetings as Chairperson of the Board.

5. Shall appoint ad hoc committee chairpersons.

6. Shall appoint a member of the Board to serve as liaison to ASD.

7. Shall appoint liaisons to external national organizations.

8. Shall perform all other duties incident to the office of President.

B. President-Elect

1. Shall prepare for duties of the President.

2. Shall perform assignments made by the President.

C. Vice President

1. Shall fulfill presidential duties in the absence of the President.

2. Shall perform all other duties incident to the office of Vice President.

D. Secretary

1. Shall record minutes of the Annual Business Meeting and special meetings of the Association and minutes of Board meetings and be the custodian of such records.

2. Shall serve as a member of the BPPC.

3. Shall call to order an Annual Business Meeting or special meeting of the Association in the absence of the President and Vice President and shall preside over an election by the members present of a chairperson pro tempore.

4. Shall perform all other duties incident to the office of Secretary.

E. Treasurer

1. Shall oversee financial affairs of the Association.

2. Shall serve as chairperson of the Board's Finance and Audit

13

Committee.

3. Shall be bonded at the expense of the Association.

4. Shall have accounts of the Association audited annually by an independent auditor.

5. Shall perform all other duties incident to the office of Treasurer.

ARTICLE VII.

Representative Assembly

Section 1. Purpose

The Representative Assembly, herein called the Assembly, shall be a designated body of the Board directly responsible for the establishment of professional standards and policies. With respect to matters within the scope of its purpose, each member of the Assembly shall have a fiduciary duty when discharging responsibilities as a member of the Assembly to act in good faith and in a manner reasonably believed to be in the best interest of the Association and otherwise in accordance with standards of conduct under the D.C. law for fiduciaries in non-profit associations.

Section 2. Composition

A. Voting Members

1. Elected Representative(s), as determined by proportional representation of the election area(s).

2. A Representative for Internationally Based Practitioners

3. Officials of the Assembly: Speaker, Vice Speaker, and Recorder

4. Officers of the Association: President, Vice President, Secretary, and Treasurer

5. Student member representative

6. OTA Representative

7. Chairpersons of the COE, COP, CCCPD, and EC

8. ASAP Representative

9. Consumer Member

14

B.   Nonvoting Members

      1.   President-Elect

      2.   AOTA Executive Director

      3.   Chairpersons-Elect of the COE, COP, CCCPD, and EC, and OTA Representative-Elect

      4.   Chairpersons of the Agenda and Credentials Review and Accountability Committee (CRAC)

Section 3.   **Election, Term, and Qualifications of Elected Members**

A.   Election

      1.   Representatives of an election area are elected by OT, OTA, and student members within that election area. The election will be conducted by the Association. An election area is defined by state, district, commonwealth, or territory boundaries and there shall be only one election area within the boundaries of each state, district, commonwealth, or territory.

      2.   ASD shall conduct the election for Student Member Representative to the Assembly.

B.   Term of Office

      1.   Representatives shall serve a 3-year term or until successors have been elected.

      2.   Representatives shall not be eligible to serve more than two consecutive terms in the same position.

      3.   The Student Member Representative shall serve a 2-year term.

      4.   The OTA Representative shall serve a 3-year term.

      5.   Vacancies in the Assembly may be filled until the next regular election by a majority vote of the Representative Assembly Leadership Committee (RALC).

C.   Qualifications

      1.   Representatives shall have the qualifications necessary to execute duties of the office held as stated in Association documents.

15

2.   Representatives shall be members in good standing of the Association, and of his/her state election area at the time of nomination and throughout the term of office.

3.   The OTA Representative and OTA Representative-Elect shall be members in good standing of the Association, and of a state affiliate at the time of nomination and throughout the term of office.

4.   Representatives, the OTA Representative, and the OTA Representative- Elect shall maintain any election area regulatory requirements necessary to identify themselves as an OT or OTA throughout the term of office.

5.   The Student Representative shall be a voting member in good standing of the Association, and of his/her state election area and must be enrolled in an accredited occupational therapy educational program with at least 6 months remaining in his/her program (coursework, fieldwork, and thesis) following induction into office.

Section 4.   **Appointment, Term, and Qualifications of Consumer Member**

A.   Appointment

The Consumer Member is appointed by the Speaker.

B.   Term of Office

The Consumer Member shall serve a 3-year term that coincides with the term of the Speaker.

C.   Qualifications

1.   Knowledge of the profession of occupational therapy through personal experience.

2.   Experience serving on boards, committees, or other bodies.

Section 5.   **Functions**

A.   Formulate and approve Association policies relating to the specific purposes of the Assembly as set forth in Section 1 above.

B.   Exercise powers and functions necessary to carry out duties of the Assembly's associated advisory commissions and committees.

C.   Elect a Chairperson for each of the following Committees: Agenda and

16

CRAC.

Section 6.   **Meetings**

A.   Regular Meetings

    1.   At least one meeting of the Assembly shall be held annually.

    2.   The time and place of the meeting shall be designated by mail, electronic, or telephonic transmission to Representatives at least 30 days before the meeting date and shall be published in an official publication of the Association.

    3.   The Assembly may invite any person to an Assembly meeting to advance business of the Assembly.

B.   Special Meetings

    1.   Special meetings may be called by one third of the Assembly members, the Speaker of the Assembly, the Board, or the President of the Association.

    2.   Special meetings of the Assembly may be held by electronic means including, but not limited to, electronic or other Internet communication systems, telephone, or video conferences.

    3.   The time, place, and purpose of the meeting shall be designated by mail, electronic, or telephonic transmission to Representatives at least 21 days before the meeting date and shall be published in an official publication of the Association.

    4.   Only business stated in the notice may be transacted at the special meeting.

C.   Conduct of the Meeting

All meetings are open to Association members, except when the Assembly is in Executive Session.

D.   Quorum

A majority of voting members shall constitute a quorum at any meeting of the Assembly.

E.   Voting

    1.   If a quorum is present when a vote is taken, the affirmative vote of a majority of the Representatives present shall be an act of the

17

Assembly unless a greater vote is required by the Articles of Incorporation, Bylaws, or by law for the specific matter before the Assembly.

2. The Assembly meetings need not be held in a geographic location. Alternatively, the meeting may be held by means of the internet or other electronic communications technology in a fashion such that Representatives have the opportunity to read or hear the proceedings substantially concurrently (although not necessarily simultaneous) with their occurrence, vote on matters submitted to the Representatives, and pose questions and make comments.

Section 7.   Advisory Commissions and Committees of the Assembly

The Assembly shall have the authority to establish advisory commissions and committees as necessary to carry out the purposes of the Assembly. The Assembly shall establish membership criteria for all such commissions and committees. The Assembly shall have the following:

A. COE

    Purpose: To promote the quality of education for OTs and OTAs relative to educator, student, and consumer needs.

B. COP

    Purpose: To promote and guide best practice in, and standards for, occupational therapy relative to practitioner and consumer needs.

C. EC

    Purpose: To serve Association members and the public through development, review, interpretation, and education of the Code and Ethics Standards and to provide the process whereby they are enforced.

D. CCCPD

    Purpose: To promote continuing competence and professional development of practitioners in accordance with the Association's standards.

E. Agenda Committee

    Purpose: To facilitate business of the Assembly.

18

F.   CRAC

Purpose: To ensure that Representatives from each election area, committee/commission chairpersons and chairpersons-elect, officers, officials, Representative for Internationally Based Practitioners, ASAP Representative, ASD Representative, OTA Representative and Representative-Elect, and Agenda and CRAC Chairpersons meet the qualifications to be members of the Assembly.

G.   Representative Assembly Coordinating Committee (RACC)

Purpose: To coordinate activities and manage integrated projects of the COE, COP, EC, and CCCPD.

Members of the RACC shall be the chairpersons of the COE, COP, EC and CCCPD; and the Speaker as Ex Officio. The Vice Speaker shall be the Chairperson of the RACC.

H.   RALC

Purpose: To plan, manage, and expedite work of the Assembly.

Members of the RALC shall be the Speaker, Vice Speaker, Agenda Chairperson, CRAC Chairperson, and Recorder. The Speaker shall be the Chairperson of the RALC.

Unless otherwise stated above, Chairpersons of the Advisory Commissions and Committees of the Assembly shall be elected by the membership for a 3-year term and shall hold only one position in the Association at a time.

The Chairpersons of the Agenda Committee and CRAC are elected by the Assembly for a 3-year term and shall hold only one position in the Association at a time.

ARTICLE VIII.

Officials of the Representative Assembly

Section 1.   Officials

The officials shall be the Speaker, Vice Speaker, and Recorder.

Section 2.   Election

A.   The officials shall be elected by voting members of the Assembly.

B.   The VLDC shall prepare a slate, preferably of at least two qualified candidates, for each position and shall conduct the election.

19

30

C.   When a Representative is elected as an official, the person shall vacate the position of Representative.

Section 3.   Qualifications

A.   A candidate shall have the qualifications necessary to execute duties of the position held as stated in Association documents.

B.   A candidate shall be a member in good standing of the Association, and an election area affiliate at the time of nomination and throughout the term of office.

C.   A candidate shall be or have been a duly elected Representative, current commission or committee chairperson, or a current official seeking election.

D.   A candidate shall have served at least 2 full years in the Assembly within 5 years of the election.

Section 4.   Duties

A.   Speaker

    1.   Shall preside at Assembly meetings.

    2.   Shall have the same voting rights as other voting members of the Assembly but may abstain from voting to maintain impartiality as the presiding officer unless it would affect the outcome.

    3.   Shall be an ex officio member of all committees of the Assembly except those associated with the EC.

    4.   Shall appoint ad hoc chairpersons and members of ad hoc committees of the Assembly.

    5.   Shall perform all other duties incident to the office of Speaker.

    6.   Shall serve as a member of the Board.

B.   Vice Speaker

    1.   Shall fulfill duties of the Speaker in the absence of the Speaker.

    2.   Shall serve as Chairperson to the RACC.

C.   Recorder

1.   Shall take minutes of the meetings of the Assembly.

2.   Shall be the custodian of such records.

ARTICLE IX.

Nominations and Elections of the Association

Section 1.   **Nominations**

A.   Any member of the Association may submit nominations to the VLDC for:

1.   Officers and Officers-Elect of the Association,

2.   Board Directors,

3.   Delegate and Alternate Delegate to the WFOT,

4.   Representative of an election area in which the individual member is a voting member,

5.   OTA Representative-Elect,

6.   Chairpersons-Elect of COE, COP, CCCPD, SISC, and EC, and Chairperson of VLDC.

B.   Any member of ASD may submit nominations to the VLDC for ASD officers.

C.   Any member of the Assembly may submit nominations to the VLDC for Officials of the Assembly.

D.   The call for nominations for the positions provided for in this Section shall be placed in an official publication of the Association 45 days before preparation of the ballot.

Section 2.   **Eligibility**

All candidates for elected and appointed positions must be members of AOTA with the exception of public and consumer members of the Board and Assembly. An individual elected or appointed to a position may not serve in any other position at the same time unless designated in a SOP or job description (JD) or appointed to a smaller group of the body to which he or she was elected.

Section 3.   **Slate**

The VLDC shall prepare a slate, preferably of at least two qualified candidates, for all

21

elected positions to be filled.

Section 4.   **Ballot for Elections of the Association**

A.   Preparation

        1.   The VLDC shall prepare a ballot for the election of positions listed in Section 1.A of this Article.

        2.   The Ballot: shall:
           a.   set forth the name of the candidates,
           b.   provide the opportunity to vote for, or withhold a vote for each candidate for election, and
           c.   indicate the number of responses needed to meet quorum requirements.

        3.   Ballots shall be delivered by mail, electronic, telephonic, or facsimile transmission to each member of the Association entitled to vote in the election.

        4.   Ballots shall state the deadline date for receipt of the ballot and the address or location to which the ballot shall be returned.

        5.   Ballots must have a method of authenticating the eligibility of each voter (e.g., a member number).

B.   Deadline

        1.   The deadline for receipt of all marked ballots by the agent authorized to receive and count ballots shall be at least 45 days before the Annual Business Meeting.

        2.   The election shall be closed on the deadline date and no ballots received thereafter shall be counted.

C.   Vote

        1.   The election of a candidate shall be by plurality vote of those ballots cast by members entitled to vote in the election at a meeting at which a quorum is present.

        2.   Approval by ballot in an election is valid only when the number of votes cast by ballot equals or exceeds the quorum required to be present at a meeting where the election voting would take place.

22

D.   Tie Vote

    1.   In the event of a tie vote the ballots shall be recounted.

    2.   In the event that the result is still tied, the election for that position shall be conducted again.

E.   Contested Vote

    1.   In the event that a vote is contested and the vote tally is separated by no more than 5% of ballots counted, the ballots shall be recounted.

    2.   Results of the recount shall be binding.

F.   Invalid Election

The VLDC shall have the authority to determine grounds for declaring an invalid election subject to approval of the Board.

ARTICLE X.

Election Area Affiliates

Section 1.   Boundaries

An Affiliate represents members located within an individual state, commonwealth, the District of Columbia, or Puerto Rico.

Section 2.   Purpose

An Affiliate is a professional organization of OTs, OTAs, and students that has been recognized by the Association. The purpose of the affiliation is to foster communication and collaboration between the Association and Affiliates.

Section 3.   Recognition

An organization becomes an Affiliate of the Association through the process described in the *Affiliation Principles for AOTA and State Associations*. Continued recognition is dependent on compliance with the *Affiliation Principles for AOTA and State Associations*.

Section 4.   Termination

Termination (disaffiliation) of an Affiliate can occur for the reasons and through the process described in the *Affiliation Principles for AOTA and State Associations*.

23

Section 5. **Appeal Process**

The election area affiliate shall have notice and opportunity to appeal.

Section 6. **Affiliated State Association Presidents (ASAP)**

The Presidents of the election area affiliates will be the voice and resource representing state affiliate members to the Association; advising the Board and the Assembly; and providing a forum for communicating, networking, training, and mentoring state affiliate leadership.

ARTICLE XI.

World Federation of Occupational Therapists—Delegates

Section 1. **Delegates**

The Association shall have a Delegate and an Alternate Delegate as representatives to the World Federation of Occupational Therapists, hereinafter referred to as WFOT.

Section 2. **Election and Term of Office**

A.   The Delegate and Alternate Delegate to WFOT shall be elected by OT, OTA, and student members of the Association.

B.   The Delegate and Alternate Delegate shall serve an initial term of 4 years or until successors are elected. The Delegate and Alternate Delegate shall be eligible for reelection to successive terms of 2 years for a maximum of 8 years served.

Section 3. **Qualifications**

A.   Shall be an OT member of the Association with a minimum of 5 years of experience.

B.   Shall be an individual member of WFOT for at least 3 years prior to running for office.

Section 4. **Duties**

A.   Delegate

        1.   Shall be instructed by the Board on the agenda to come before the WFOT council and shall represent the Association to WFOT.

        2.   Shall represent WFOT to the Association.

24

3.   Shall serve as an Organizational Advisor to the Board.

B.   Alternate Delegate

1.   Shall serve in the Assembly with voice and vote as the Internationally Based Practitioners' Representative.

2.   Shall assume duties of the Delegate in the absence of the Delegate.

ARTICLE XII.

Administrative Procedures for All Elected or Appointed Positions

Section 1.   Resignation

A.   Elected or appointed officials of the Association shall submit a written resignation to the appropriate Association official as provided in the Administrative SOP.

B.   The Association shall act upon such requests, including notifying appropriate committees concerning the vacancy.

Section 2.   Censure

Elected and appointed officials may be subject to censure as the term is defined in Policy 1.14.1 of the Official Policies of the Association. Motions for censure of an elected or appointed official may be made by any member of the committee, body or other entity in which the elected or appointed official holds a position. The determination of such motion shall be made by the committee, body or other entity in which the elected or appointed official holds a position in accordance with a fundamentally fair process set forth in the disciplinary procedures in the Administrative SOP.

Section 3.   Removal

Elected and appointed officials shall only be removed for cause. Grounds for removal for cause of an elected or appointed official are: (1) those set forth in Policy 1.15 of the Official Policies of the Association, and/or (2) violation of the Code and Ethics Standards. Motions for removal of an elected or appointed official may be made by any member of the committee, body, or other entity in which the elected or appointed official holds a position. The determination of such motion shall be made by the committee, body, or other entity in which the elected or appointed official holds a position in accordance with a fundamentally fair process set forth in the disciplinary procedures in the Administrative SOP.

Section 4.   Appeal

The decision to remove an elected or appointed official may be appealed in accordance

25

with due process as set forth in the Administrative SOP.

Section 5. Vacancies

Unless otherwise provided, in the case of vacancy in any office, except the President, the vacancy shall be filled by appointment by the presiding officer of the Board or Assembly until the next regular election. In the case of a vacancy in the office of the President, the Vice President shall serve.

Section 6. Assumption of Office

With the exception of ASD officers, all elected and appointed officials assume office on July 1.

ARTICLE XIII.

Fiscal Year

The fiscal year of the Association shall be determined by the Board.

ARTICLE XIV.

Dissolution Clause

Should the corporation be dissolved for any reason, the remaining assets shall be distributed for purposes within the scope of the Internal Revenue Code, Section 501(c)(6), or any amendment thereto, and in accordance with the corporate statutes of the District of Columbia (D.C.).

ARTICLE XV.

Petition to Challenge Association Action

Members shall have the right to submit a written objection to an action of the Association taken by the membership, Board, or Assembly to the extent that the member is or may be affected by such action.

Any member seeking to challenge Association action shall do so in conformance with the procedure set forth in this Article, unless there is another designated procedure set forth in the official documents of the Association that specifically addresses the action which the member seeks to challenge. Any challenge to Association action covered by this Article shall be in the form of a written Petition addressed to the Board setting forth the specific action challenged, the grounds for the challenge, and requested action. The Petition must be filed within 90 days of the action challenged and shall be delivered to the Secretary at the Association's headquarters. The Board shall submit the Petition to an ad hoc committee of the Board to investigate the matter, to determine the merits of the Petition, and to make a recommendation to the President as to the appropriate disposition.

26

The President shall provide the Association's response to the Petition in writing to the Petitioner in not more than 90 days from the date the Petition was received by the Secretary and shall include a concise statement of the reasons for the disposition. The ad hoc committee of the Board shall process the Petition in accordance with the procedure set forth in the Administrative SOP specifically designated for Challenges to Association Action.

ARTICLE XVI.

Amendments to Bylaws

Section 1. **Procedure**

A.   BPPC shall announce a call for amendments in an official publication to all OT, OTA, and student members.

B.   OT, OTA, and student members shall have 60 days from the date of publication to submit suggestions to the BPPC.

C.   BPPC shall present to the Board a report containing proposed Amendments to and comments on the Bylaws

D.   The Board shall consider and approve at its regular meetings any proposed Bylaws amendments.

E.   Proposed Bylaws amendments shall be presented to OT, OTA, and student members at the Annual Business Meeting for adoption.

Section 2. **Technical Corrections**

The BPPC is authorized to correct Article and Section designations, punctuation, and cross-references and to make such other technical and conforming changes to the Bylaws and other governing documents of the Association as may be necessary to reflect the intent of vote of the membership in approving the Bylaws and amendments.

Section 3. **Effective Date**

Amendments to the Bylaws shall become effective immediately upon adoption by vote of the membership or at such other time designated by the membership in connection with the adoption of the Bylaws.

ARTICLE XVII.

Indemnification

Any present or former Board member, officer, employee, official, or agent of the Association, or other such persons so designated at the discretion of the Board, or the legal representative of such person, shall be indemnified (including advances against expenses) by the Association against all judgments, fines, settlements, and other reasonable costs, expenses, and counsel fees paid or incurred in connection with any action, suit, or proceeding to which any person or his or her legal representative may be made a party by reason of his or her being or having been such a Board member, officer, employee, official, or agent, to the greatest extent permitted by law. No indemnification or advance against expenses shall be approved by the Board or paid by the Association until after receipt from legal counsel of an opinion concerning the legality of the proposed indemnification or advance.

28

The
Glossary
of the
American Occupational Therapy
Association
2010
******

Absence

Failure to attend or appear when expected; the state of being away or not present (e.g., the Treasurer is not present for the Association Annual Business Meeting).

Accreditation

The process by which an agency or organization evaluates and recognizes a program of study or an institution as meeting certain predetermined qualifications or standards. It applies only to institutions and their programs of study or their services.

ACOTE®

Accreditation Council for Occupational Therapy Education

Ad Hoc

A special body (e.g., committee, task force, task group, body) not established by the Bylaws. An ad hoc body is appointed for a specific purpose and assigned a specific task that is not an ongoing function in the Association.

Advisory

Having the function of giving advice, usually with the implication that the advice given need not be followed.

Affiliate

A professional organization representing OTs, OTAs, and students that is recognized by the Association.

Agenda (plural for Agendum)

A list of things to be done, especially the program for a meeting (e.g., the order of business of the Assembly meeting).

Amendments

Changes to the Bylaws that are neither revisions nor technical corrections.

Annual Business Meeting

The scheduled gathering of Association members that must occur at least one time per year.

Annual Conference

A meeting of persons from across the country to discuss or consult on various topics or issues (e.g., the Annual Conference of the Association).

AOTF

American Occupational Therapy Foundation

Appeal

Make an earnest request (e.g., an officer pleads against removal from office).

Approval

This is synonymous with ratification.

Articles of Incorporation

The original statements that provided the framework for the development and organization of the Association.

ASAP

Affiliated State Association Presidents

Assembly

A group of people meeting as a deliberative or lawmaking body.

BPPC Reviewed: 9/7/03, 1/05, 1/07, 1/08, 9/10
Adopted RA: 11/03, 5/05, 4/07, 11/10

ASD
Assembly of Student Delegates

Associated Body of the Board
A body that operates at "arm's length" according to specific legal or regulatory requirements to achieve its stated purpose.

Association
An organized body of people who have some interest, activity, or purpose in common (e.g., The American Occupational Therapy Association, Inc.).

Association headquarters
The headquarters of the Association, which houses the staff who are responsible for carrying out activities as assigned by the Board or Assembly.

Award
An honor that is conferred on designated individuals (e.g., Slagle Lectureship, Award of Merit).

Ballot
A written, printed, or electronic document used to cast or register a vote.

Board
A group of people chosen to make executive or managerial decisions for an organization.

Board
The Board of Directors

Body
An organized group of individuals that has an official function.

Boundaries
A border or limit (e.g., the border that defines an election area or state association).

Budget
An estimate of expected income and expenses, an itemized allotment of funds for a given year (e.g., a yearly allotment of Association funds for a committee).

Bylaw
A rule adopted by an organization for the governance of its members and the regulation of its affairs (e.g., the Bylaws of The American Occupational Therapy Association, Inc.).

BPPC
Bylaws, Policies, and Procedures Committee

Censure
A formal expression of strong disapproval that is public.

Certification
The process by which a nongovernmental agency or association grants recognition to an individual who has met certain predetermined qualifications specified by that agency or association.

Chairperson
The presiding officer

BPPC Reviewed: 9/7/03, 1/05, 1/07, 1/08, 9/10
Adopted RA: 11/03, 5/05, 4/07, 11/10

Commission
A group of people authorized or directed to carry out a duty or task. A commission is responsible for a broad area of information relevant to the Association.

CCCPD
Commission on Continuing Competence and Professional Development

Code of Ethics and Ethics Standards
An official document that serves as a "public statement of principles used to promote and maintain high standards of conduct with the profession." (Preamble to the AOTA *Occupational Therapy Code of Ethics and Ethics Standards 2010*)

COE
Commission on Education

COP
Commission on Practice

Committee
A body of one or more persons, elected or appointed by the Board or Assembly, to consider, investigate, or take action on certain matters or subjects.

Communication
The means of sending or giving messages, orders, and so forth, including telephone, telegraph, radio, books, films, and e-mail.

Component
An element or part of something larger in structure and organization (e.g., a subcommittee is a component of a committee).

Council
An appointed or elected body of people with an administrative, advisory, or representative function.

Credentials
Evidence of authority, status, rights, entitlement, or privileges, usually in written form (e.g., written notice of election of a person as a representative from an election area).

CRAC
Credentials Review and Accountability Committee

Delegate
Somebody chosen to represent or given the authority to act on behalf of another person, group, or organization (e.g., at a meeting or conference).

Dissolution
The breaking up or undoing of an Assembly or organization (e.g., the dissolution of The American Occupational Therapy Association, Inc.).

Duty
Something that one is expected or required to do by moral or legal obligation (e.g., conduct the meeting).

BPPC Reviewed: 9/7/03, 1/05, 1/07, 1/08, 9/10
Adopted RA: 11/03, 5/05, 4/07, 11/10

Edit
To alter, adapt, or refine, especially to bring about conformity to a standard or to suit a particular purpose.

Education
The act or process of importing or acquiring general knowledge and of developing the powers of reasoning and judgment.

Election
The selection of a person or persons for office by vote (e.g., choosing a President, Secretary, etc.).

Election Area
A geographic area that is defined as eligible for representation in the Assembly.

Emergency, Association
An emergency that would alter the Association's ability to effectively conduct business may be declared by the Executive Director, President, or Vice President.

Emergency, National
An emergency declared by the President of the United States or Congress that results in restriction of travel, expenditures or collections, or personal activity, and a temporary policy or procedure is required to meet the situation.

Ethics
A body of moral principles or values.

EC
Ethics Commission

Executive Director
The person having administrative or managerial authority (e.g., of the headquarters of the Association).

Executive Session
A meeting or portion of a meeting at which the proceedings are secret and only members, special invitees, and designated staff may be present. In the Association, Executive Session is used primarily to discuss information and issues that involve privileged data affecting individual member and personnel matters of the Association, or matters that may be the subject of litigation and/or are subject to attorney–client privilege. The purpose is to protect confidentiality, not to deprive members of their right to know (e.g., the Assembly is in Executive Session to hear the case of a member charged with unethical behavior).

Fee
A sum paid or charged for a privilege (e.g., the fee for membership in the Association).

Fiscal
Pertaining to financial matters in general.

Formation
How the group is organized to do business (e.g., Assembly business is conducted in formal session).

Function
What the group is charged to do (e.g., the Assembly is charged to make policy for the Association).

BPPC Reviewed: 9/7/03, 1/05, 1/07, 1/08, 9/10
Adopted RA: 11/03, 5/05, 4/07, 11/10

Good Standing

A statement that identifies that a member has met and maintained the qualifications to belong to the Association.

Job Description

Regular procedures or actions that are taken by an individual to accomplish an activity, charge, or item of business. Job descriptions are recorded in written form.

Legislative

Involved in writing and passing laws or regulations.

Liaison

The contact maintained between bodies to ensure concerted action. An individual serving in this position is not an official member of the body to which he or she is serving as a liaison.

Logo (short for logotype)

A trademark or company name or device (e.g., the name, "The American Occupational Therapy Association, Inc.").

Meetings

The sequence of events an Association body experiences to conduct business, from the initial call to order to adjournment. Meeting agendas generally include approval of prior minutes, reports, and old and new business. A meeting may be made up of several sessions.

Members

Persons or organizations that meet and maintain the qualifications to belong to and compose the Association.

Motion

A formal proposal by a member in an official meeting for a certain action. The proposed action may be of a substantive nature, or it may express a certain view or direct that a particular investigation be conducted and the findings be reported for possible further action.

NBCOT®

National Board for Certification in Occupational Therapy®

Nominate

To propose someone as a proper or suitable person for appointment or election to an office.

Noninurement

Not to accrue to the advantage or benefit of an individual(s); specifically monies earned by or for the Association cannot be given to or taken by individuals for their own use.

Occupational Therapist

Any individual initially certified to practice as an OT or licensed or regulated by a state, commonwealth, district, or territory of the United States to practice as an OT and who has not had that certification, license, or regulation revoked due to disciplinary action shall be eligible to be an Occupational Therapist Member.

OT

Occupational Therapist

BPPC Reviewed: 9/7/03, 1/05, 1/07, 1/08, 9/10
Adopted RA: 11/03, 5/05, 4/07, 11/10

Occupational Therapy Assistant

Any individual initially certified to practice as an OTA or licensed or regulated by a state, commonwealth, district, or territory of the United States to practice as an OTA and who has not had that certification, license, or regulation revoked due to disciplinary action shall be eligible to be an Occupational Therapy Assistant Member.

OTA

Occupational Therapy Assistant

Officer

One who holds a position of authority or command and serves in a designated capacity in the Association and Board (e.g., President, Treasurer).

Official Document

Those documents constructed by the Association and approved by the Association for the use of the Association and its members.

Organizational Advisors

Critical governance bodies within the organization that advise the Board and promote active collaboration and effective dialogue between the Board, appropriate bodies of the Board, the Assembly, and AOTA.

Organizational Member

Institutions or agencies that are interested in the profession or practice of occupational therapy (e.g., another professional health care organization).

OTFC

OTs in Foreign Countries

Parliamentary

In accordance with the rules governing deliberative bodies.

Personnel

A body of persons employed in any work, undertaking, or service (e.g., the Association staff).

Policy

A definite course or method of action selected to guide and determine present and future decisions.

Postprofessional Program

An educational curriculum in occupational therapy that offers courses designed to enhance knowledge and skills beyond the basic entry level for persons who are already OTs.

Practice

Action or process of performing or doing something, the exercise or pursuit of a profession or occupation (e.g., delivering occupational therapy services to a client).

President

The highest executive officer elected to preside over an organized body.

President-Elect

A person who has been duly elected to the presidency but whose term of office as President has not begun.

BPPC Reviewed: 9/7/03, 1/05, 1/07, 1/08, 9/10
Adopted RA: 11/03, 5/05, 4/07, 11/10

Principal Office
The main or central place of business

Privileges
Those things or activities that a member is permitted to do by virtue of being a member of the Association (e.g., seek services that are provided).

Procedure
A particular way or series of steps followed to accomplish something or a way of acting; an established way of doing things.

Professional Education
An educational curriculum in occupational therapy that offers courses designed to provide education for entry-level performance of the OT.

Proportional Representation
The means of determining the number of representatives on the basis of percentage.

Pro Tem (Pro Tempore)
Temporarily; for the time being (e.g., a person who acts as a Chairperson for a group for a meeting).

Publications
Those publications that are designated as belonging to or representing the views of The American Occupational Therapy Association, Inc.

Purpose
A summary statement of the goals and/or objectives of the group.

Qualifications
An accomplishment, experience, or skill that fits a person for some function, office, or the like (e.g., has served on a committee).

Quorum
A quorum is the number of voting members who must be present in order that business can be legally transacted. The quorum refers to the number of such members present, not to the number actually voting on a particular question.

RA
Representative Assembly

RACC
Representative Assembly Coordinating Council

RALT
Representative Assembly Leadership Team

Recognition
The act of showing appreciation, achievement, service, merit, and so forth, as by some reward, public honor, or the like (e.g., Award of Merit, Slagle Lectureship).

Recorder
A person who sets down something in writing or other permanent form (e.g., the person who prepares and keeps the minutes of the Assembly).

BPPC Reviewed: 9/7/03, 1/05, 1/07, 1/08, 9/10
Adopted RA: 11/03, 5/05, 4/07, 11/10

Removal
The act of taking away the title and duties of a position.

Representative
An individual who votes or speaks on behalf of others.

Representative Assembly
The body composed of representatives from identified constituencies (election areas) whose function is to legislate and establish policy for the Association.

Reprimand
Formal expression of disapproval that is privately communicated.

Resignation
The act of giving up or renouncing one's office or position (e.g., the Secretary notifies the President that he or she will no longer perform the duties of Secretary).

Resolution
A complex motion that is a formal statement of an expression of opinion put before an Assembly or decision adopted by an Assembly (e.g., a resolution submitted to and passed by the Assembly).

Revision
Changes of the Bylaws that are so extensive and general that they are scattered throughout the Bylaws and should be effected through the substitution of an entirely new set of Bylaws (Robert's Rules of Order, p. 575). Revisions include roles and responsibilities of individuals, functions of the bodies, relationships between bodies, election of individuals to bodies, and number of voting members.

Rights
Those things to which a member has just claim by virtue of being a member of the Association (e.g., access to member pages on the Web site).

Robert's Rules
The rules contained in the current edition of *Robert's Rules of Order, Newly Revised,* shall govern the Association in all cases in which they are applicable and in which they are not inconsistent with the Bylaws and any special rules of order the Association may adopt.

SCB
Specialty Certification Board

Seated
A position from which authority is exercised; also, the approval a person receives from the group authorizing participation in the conduct of business.

Secretary
An officer who is in charge of the records, correspondence, minutes of Board meetings and Annual Business Meetings, and related affairs of an organization, company, or Association.

Session
A portion of a meeting, from the Call to Order to a Recess.

Slate
A list of candidates, officers, and so forth to be considered for nomination, appointment, election, and the like.

BPPC Reviewed: 9/7/03, 1/05, 1/07, 1/08, 9/10
Adopted RA: 11/03, 5/05, 4/07, 11/10

Speaker

The presiding officer of a legislative assembly (e.g., Speaker of the Assembly).

Special Interest Section

A group of members recognized by the Assembly as having a mutual interest in a practical area of practice in occupational therapy.

SISs

Special Interest Sections

SISC

Special Interest Sections Council

Standard

Something considered by an authority as a basis of comparison, as an approved model.

Standard Operating Procedure

Regular procedures or actions that are taken by a group to accomplish an activity, charge, or item of business. Standard operating procedures are recorded in written form and are referred to as SOPs.

Standing Committee

A permanent committee established in the Bylaws dealing with a designated subject (e.g., fees, personnel, recognitions). A committee is responsible for a specific area of information relevant to the Association.

State Affiliate

See Affiliate

Steering Committee

A selected group of persons charged to function as an organizing unit to conduct certain business for a larger group. The function of the Steering Committee is to expedite the work of a larger group.

Strategic Plan

A document outlining the goals and activities that the Association members have agreed to strive to achieve and to which resources will be assigned.

Student

Any person who is enrolled in an occupational therapy education program that is accredited or approved by the Association for the first technical or professional degree.

Substantive Change

A change of an essential part, or constituent, or relating to what is essential.

Technical Education

An educational curriculum in occupational therapy that offers courses designed to provide education for entry-level performance of the OTA.

Term (of Office)

A period of time to which limits have been set (e.g., selected for a term of 2 years).

Tracking

Following the course or progress of or keeping informed about (e.g., the secretary is charged to monitor the progress of motions and charges so that tasks are assigned and completed and reports are filed).

BPPC Reviewed: 9/7/03, 1/05, 1/07, 1/08, 9/10
Adopted RA: 11/03, 5/05, 4/07, 11/10

Treasurer

An officer who is charged with overseeing the financial affairs of the Association.

Vacancy

An unoccupied position or office (e.g., the Presidency is vacant due to the resignation of the President).

Vice President

The officer next in rank to the President who succeeds to the Presidency on the resignation, removal, death, or disability of the President. The Vice President may act for the President in the absence or on the command of the President.

Vice Speaker

The officer who is next in rank to the Speaker and succeeds to the position of Speaker on the resignation, removal, death, or disability of the Speaker. The Vice Speaker may act for the Speaker in the absence or on the command of the Speaker.

Vote

A formal expression of preference for a candidate for office, proposed resolution, motion of an issue, or Bylaws change.

WFOT

World Federation of Occupational Therapists

BPPC Reviewed: 9/7/03, 1/05, 1/07, 1/08, 9/10
Adopted RA: 11/03, 5/05, 4/07, 11/10

Accreditation

2011 Accreditation Council for Occupational Therapy Education (ACOTE®) Standards

(Adopted December 4, 2011; effective July 31, 2013)

Standard Number	Accreditation Standards for a Doctoral-Degree-Level Educational Program for the Occupational Therapist	Accreditation Standards for a Master's-Degree-Level Educational Program for the Occupational Therapist	Accreditation Standards for an Associate-Degree-Level Educational Program for the Occupational Therapy Assistant
	PREAMBLE		
	The rapidly changing and dynamic nature of contemporary health and human services delivery systems provides challenging opportunities for the occupational therapist to use knowledge and skills in a practice area as a direct care provider, consultant, educator, manager, leader, researcher, and advocate for the profession and the consumer.	The rapidly changing and dynamic nature of contemporary health and human services delivery systems requires the occupational therapist to possess basic skills as a direct care provider, consultant, educator, manager, researcher, and advocate for the profession and the consumer.	The rapidly changing and dynamic nature of contemporary health and human services delivery systems requires the occupational therapy assistant to possess basic skills as a direct care provider, educator, and advocate for the profession and the consumer.
	A graduate from an ACOTE-accredited doctoral-degree-level occupational therapy program must • Have acquired, as a foundation for professional study, a breadth and depth of knowledge in the liberal arts and sciences and an understanding of issues related to diversity. • Be educated as a generalist with a broad exposure to the delivery models and systems used in settings where occupational therapy is currently practiced and where it is emerging as a service.	A graduate from an ACOTE-accredited master's-degree-level occupational therapy program must • Have acquired, as a foundation for professional study, a breadth and depth of knowledge in the liberal arts and sciences and an understanding of issues related to diversity. • Be educated as a generalist with a broad exposure to the delivery models and systems used in settings where occupational therapy is currently practiced and where it is emerging as a service.	A graduate from an ACOTE-accredited associate-degree-level occupational therapy assistant program must • Have acquired an educational foundation in the liberal arts and sciences, including a focus on issues related to diversity. • Be educated as a generalist with a broad exposure to the delivery models and systems used in settings where occupational therapy is currently practiced and where it is emerging as a service.

(Continued)

Standard Number	Accreditation Standards for a Doctoral-Degree-Level Educational Program for the Occupational Therapist	Accreditation Standards for a Master's-Degree-Level Educational Program for the Occupational Therapist	Accreditation Standards for an Associate-Degree-Level Educational Program for the Occupational Therapy Assistant
	• Have achieved entry-level competence through a combination of academic and field-work education.	• Have achieved entry-level competence through a combination of academic and field-work education.	• Have achieved entry-level competence through a combination of academic and field-work education.
	• Be prepared to articulate and apply occupational therapy theory and evidence-based evaluations and interventions to achieve expected outcomes as related to occupation.	• Be prepared to articulate and apply occupational therapy theory and evidence-based evaluations and interventions to achieve expected outcomes as related to occupation.	• Be prepared to articulate and apply occupational therapy principles and intervention tools to achieve expected outcomes as related to occupation.
	• Be prepared to articulate and apply therapeutic use of occupations with individuals or groups for the purpose of participation in roles and situations in home, school, workplace, community, and other settings.	• Be prepared to articulate and apply therapeutic use of occupations with individuals or groups for the purpose of participation in roles and situations in home, school, workplace, community, and other settings.	• Be prepared to articulate and apply therapeutic use of occupations with individuals or groups for the purpose of participation in roles and situations in home, school, work-place, community, and other settings.
	• Be able to plan and apply occupational therapy interventions to address the physical, cognitive, psychosocial, sensory, and other aspects of performance in a variety of contexts and environments to support engagement in everyday life activities that affect health, well-being, and quality of life.	• Be able to plan and apply occupational therapy interventions to address the physical, cognitive, psychosocial, sensory, and other aspects of performance in a variety of contexts and environments to support engagement in everyday life activities that affect health, well-being, and quality of life.	• Be able to apply occupational therapy interventions to address the physical, cognitive, psychosocial, sensory, and other aspects of performance in a variety of contexts and environments to support engagement in everyday life activities that affect health, well-being, and quality of life.
	• Be prepared to be a lifelong learner and keep current with evidence-based professional practice.	• Be prepared to be a lifelong learner and keep current with evidence-based professional practice.	• Be prepared to be a lifelong learner and keep current with the best practice.
	• Uphold the ethical standards, values, and attitudes of the occupational therapy profession.	• Uphold the ethical standards, values, and attitudes of the occupational therapy profession.	• Uphold the ethical standards, values, and attitudes of the occupational therapy profession.
	• Understand the distinct roles and responsibilities of the occupational therapist and occupational therapy assistant in the supervisory process.	• Understand the distinct roles and responsibilities of the occupational therapist and occupational therapy assistant in the supervisory process.	• Understand the distinct roles and responsibilities of the occupational therapist and occupational therapy assistant in the supervisory process.

(Continued)

Standard Number	Accreditation Standards for a Doctoral-Degree-Level Educational Program for the Occupational Therapist	Accreditation Standards for a Master's-Degree-Level Educational Program for the Occupational Therapist	Accreditation Standards for an Associate-Degree-Level Educational Program for the Occupational Therapy Assistant
	• Be prepared to effectively communicate and work interprofessionally with those who provide care for individuals and/or populations in order to clarify each member's responsibility in executing components of an intervention plan. • Be prepared to advocate as a professional for the occupational therapy services offered and for the recipients of those services. • Be prepared to be an effective consumer of the latest research and knowledge bases that support practice and contribute to the growth and dissemination of research and knowledge. • Demonstrate in-depth knowledge of delivery models, policies, and systems related to the area of practice in settings where occupational therapy is currently practiced and where it is emerging as a service. • Demonstrate thorough knowledge of evidence-based practice. • Demonstrate active involvement in professional development, leadership, and advocacy. • Relate theory to practice and demonstrate synthesis of advanced knowledge in a practice area through completion of a culminating project.	• Be prepared to effectively communicate and work interprofessionally with those who provide care for individuals and/or populations in order to clarify each member's responsibility in executing components of an intervention plan. • Be prepared to advocate as a professional for the occupational therapy services offered and for the recipients of those services. • Be prepared to be an effective consumer of the latest research and knowledge bases that support practice and contribute to the growth and dissemination of research and knowledge.	• Be prepared to effectively communicate and work interprofessionally with those who provide care for individuals and/or populations in order to clarify each member's responsibility in executing components of an intervention plan. • Be prepared to advocate as a professional for the occupational therapy services offered and for the recipients of those services.

(Continued)

55

Standard Number	Accreditation Standards for a Doctoral-Degree-Level Educational Program for the Occupational Therapist	Accreditation Standards for a Master's-Degree-Level Educational Program for the Occupational Therapist	Accreditation Standards for an Associate-Degree-Level Educational Program for the Occupational Therapy Assistant
	• Develop in-depth experience in one or more of the following areas through completion of a doctoral experiential component: clinical practice skills, research skills, administration, leadership, program and policy development, advocacy, education, and theory development.		

SECTION A: GENERAL REQUIREMENTS

A.1.0. SPONSORSHIP AND ACCREDITATION

Standard Number	Doctoral	Master's	Associate
A.1.1.	The sponsoring institution(s) and affiliates, if any, must be accredited by the recognized regional accrediting authority. For programs in countries other than the United States, ACOTE will determine an alternative and equivalent external review process.	The sponsoring institution(s) and affiliates, if any, must be accredited by the recognized regional accrediting authority. For programs in countries other than the United States, ACOTE will determine an alternative and equivalent external review process.	The sponsoring institution(s) and affiliates, if any, must be accredited by a recognized regional or national accrediting authority.
A.1.2.	Sponsoring institution(s) must be authorized under applicable law or other acceptable authority to provide a program of postsecondary education and have appropriate doctoral degree–granting authority.	Sponsoring institution(s) must be authorized under applicable law or other acceptable authority to provide a program of postsecondary education and have appropriate degree-granting authority.	Sponsoring institution(s) must be authorized under applicable law or other acceptable authority to provide a program of postsecondary education and have appropriate degree-granting authority, or the institution must be a program offered within the military services.

(Continued)

Standard Number	Accreditation Standards for a Doctoral-Degree-Level Educational Program for the Occupational Therapist	Accreditation Standards for a Master's-Degree-Level Educational Program for the Occupational Therapist	Accreditation Standards for an Associate-Degree-Level Educational Program for the Occupational Therapy Assistant
A.1.3.	Accredited occupational therapy educational programs may be established only in senior colleges, universities, or medical schools.	Accredited occupational therapy educational programs may be established only in senior colleges, universities, or medical schools.	Accredited occupational therapy assistant educational programs may be established only in community, technical, junior, and senior colleges; universities; medical schools; vocational schools or institutions; or military services.
A.1.4.	The sponsoring institution(s) must assume primary responsibility for appointment of faculty, admission of students, and curriculum planning at all locations where the program is offered. This would include course content, satisfactory completion of the educational program, and granting of the degree. The sponsoring institution(s) must also be responsible for the coordination of classroom teaching and supervised fieldwork practice and for providing assurance that the practice activities assigned to students in a fieldwork setting are appropriate to the program.	The sponsoring institution(s) must assume primary responsibility for appointment of faculty, admission of students, and curriculum planning at all locations where the program is offered. This would include course content, satisfactory completion of the educational program, and granting of the degree. The sponsoring institution(s) must also be responsible for the coordination of classroom teaching and supervised fieldwork practice and for providing assurance that the practice activities assigned to students in a fieldwork setting are appropriate to the program.	The sponsoring institution(s) must assume primary responsibility for appointment of faculty, admission of students, and curriculum planning at all locations where the program is offered. This would include course content, satisfactory completion of the educational program, and granting of the degree. The sponsoring institution(s) must also be responsible for the coordination of classroom teaching and supervised fieldwork practice and for providing assurance that the practice activities assigned to students in a fieldwork setting are appropriate to the program.
A.1.5.	The program must • Inform ACOTE of the transfer of program sponsorship or change of the institution's name within 30 days of the transfer or change.	The program must • Inform ACOTE of the transfer of program sponsorship or change of the institution's name within 30 days of the transfer or change.	The program must • Inform ACOTE of the transfer of program sponsorship or change of the institution's name within 30 days of the transfer or change.

(Continued)

Standard Number	Accreditation Standards for a Doctoral-Degree-Level Educational Program for the Occupational Therapist	Accreditation Standards for a Master's-Degree-Level Educational Program for the Occupational Therapist	Accreditation Standards for an Associate-Degree-Level Educational Program for the Occupational Therapy Assistant
	• Inform ACOTE within 30 days of the date of notification of any adverse accreditation action taken to change the sponsoring institution's accreditation status to probation or withdrawal of accreditation. • Notify and receive ACOTE approval for any significant program changes prior to the admission of students into the new/changed program. • Inform ACOTE within 30 days of the resignation of the program director or appointment of a new or interim program director. • Pay accreditation fees within 90 days of the invoice date. • Submit a Report of Self-Study and other required reports (e.g., Interim Report, Plan of Correction, Progress Report) within the period of time designated by ACOTE. All reports must be complete and contain all requested information. • Agree to a site visit date before the end of the period for which accreditation was previously awarded. • Demonstrate honesty and integrity in all interactions with ACOTE.	• Inform ACOTE within 30 days of the date of notification of any adverse accreditation action taken to change the sponsoring institution's accreditation status to probation or withdrawal of accreditation. • Notify and receive ACOTE approval for any significant program changes prior to the admission of students into the new/changed program. • Inform ACOTE within 30 days of the resignation of the program director or appointment of a new or interim program director. • Pay accreditation fees within 90 days of the invoice date. • Submit a Report of Self-Study and other required reports (e.g., Interim Report, Plan of Correction, Progress Report) within the period of time designated by ACOTE. All reports must be complete and contain all requested information. • Agree to a site visit date before the end of the period for which accreditation was previously awarded. • Demonstrate honesty and integrity in all interactions with ACOTE.	• Inform ACOTE within 30 days of the date of notification of any adverse accreditation action taken to change the sponsoring institution's accreditation status to probation or withdrawal of accreditation. • Notify and receive ACOTE approval for any significant program changes prior to the admission of students into the new/changed program. • Inform ACOTE within 30 days of the resignation of the program director or appointment of a new or interim program director. • Pay accreditation fees within 90 days of the invoice date. • Submit a Report of Self-Study and other required reports (e.g., Interim Report, Plan of Correction, Progress Report) within the period of time designated by ACOTE. All reports must be complete and contain all requested information. • Agree to a site visit date before the end of the period for which accreditation was previously awarded. • Demonstrate honesty and integrity in all interactions with ACOTE.

(Continued)

Standard Number	Accreditation Standards for a Doctoral-Degree-Level Educational Program for the Occupational Therapist	Accreditation Standards for a Master's-Degree-Level Educational Program for the Occupational Therapist	Accreditation Standards for an Associate-Degree-Level Educational Program for the Occupational Therapy Assistant
A.2.0.	**ACADEMIC RESOURCES**		
A.2.1.	The program must identify an individual as the program director who is assigned to the occupational therapy educational program on a full-time basis. The director may be assigned other institutional duties that do not interfere with the management and administration of the program. The institution must document that the program director has sufficient release time to ensure that the needs of the program are being met.	The program must identify an individual as the program director who is assigned to the occupational therapy educational program on a full-time basis. The director may be assigned other institutional duties that do not interfere with the management and administration of the program. The institution must document that the program director has sufficient release time to ensure that the needs of the program are being met.	The program must identify an individual as the program director who is assigned to the occupational therapy educational program on a full-time basis. The director may be assigned other institutional duties that do not interfere with the management and administration of the program. The institution must document that the program director has sufficient release time to ensure that the needs of the program are being met.
A.2.2.	The program director must be an initially certified occupational therapist who is licensed or otherwise regulated according to regulations in the state(s) or jurisdiction(s) in which the program is located. The program director must hold a doctoral degree awarded by an institution that is accredited by a regional accrediting body recognized by the U.S. Department of Education (USDE). The doctoral degree is not limited to a doctorate in occupational therapy.	The program director must be an initially certified occupational therapist who is licensed or otherwise regulated according to regulations in the state(s) or jurisdiction(s) in which the program is located. The program director must hold a doctoral degree awarded by an institution that is accredited by a regional accrediting body recognized by the U.S. Department of Education (USDE). The doctoral degree is not limited to a doctorate in occupational therapy.	The program director must be an initially certified occupational therapist or occupational therapy assistant who is licensed or otherwise regulated according to regulations in the state(s) or jurisdiction(s) in which the program is located. The program director must hold a minimum of a master's degree awarded by an institution that is accredited by a regional or national accrediting body recognized by the U.S. Department of Education (USDE). The master's degree is not limited to a master's degree in occupational therapy.

(Continued)

Standard Number	Accreditation Standards for a Doctoral-Degree-Level Educational Program for the Occupational Therapist	Accreditation Standards for a Master's-Degree-Level Educational Program for the Occupational Therapist	Accreditation Standards for an Associate-Degree-Level Educational Program for the Occupational Therapy Assistant
A.2.3.	The program director must have a minimum of 8 years of documented experience in the field of occupational therapy. This experience must include • Clinical practice as an occupational therapist; • Administrative experience including, but not limited to, program planning and implementation, personnel management, evaluation, and budgeting; • Scholarship (e.g., scholarship of application, scholarship of teaching and learning); and • At least 3 years of experience in a full-time academic appointment with teaching responsibilities at the postbaccalaureate level.	The program director must have a minimum of 8 years of documented experience in the field of occupational therapy. This experience must include • Clinical practice as an occupational therapist; • Administrative experience including, but not limited to, program planning and implementation, personnel management, evaluation, and budgeting; • Scholarship (e.g., scholarship of application, scholarship of teaching and learning); and • At least 3 years of experience in a full-time academic appointment with teaching responsibilities at the postsecondary level.	The program director must have a minimum of 5 years of documented experience in the field of occupational therapy. This experience must include • Clinical practice as an occupational therapist or occupational therapy assistant; • Administrative experience including, but not limited to, program planning and implementation, personnel management, evaluation, and budgeting; • Understanding of and experience with occupational therapy assistants; and • At least 1 year of experience in a full-time academic appointment with teaching responsibilities at the postsecondary level.
A.2.4.	The program director must be responsible for the management and administration of the program, including planning, evaluation, budgeting, selection of faculty and staff, maintenance of accreditation, and commitment to strategies for professional development.	The program director must be responsible for the management and administration of the program, including planning, evaluation, budgeting, selection of faculty and staff, maintenance of accreditation, and commitment to strategies for professional development.	The program director must be responsible for the management and administration of the program, including planning, evaluation, budgeting, selection of faculty and staff, maintenance of accreditation, and commitment to strategies for professional development.

(Continued)

Standard Number	Accreditation Standards for a Doctoral-Degree-Level Educational Program for the Occupational Therapist	Accreditation Standards for a Master's-Degree-Level Educational Program for the Occupational Therapist	Accreditation Standards for an Associate-Degree-Level Educational Program for the Occupational Therapy Assistant
A.2.5.	*(No related Standard)*	*(No related Standard)*	In addition to the program director, the program must have at least one full-time equivalent (FTE) faculty position at each accredited location where the program is offered. This position may be shared by up to three individuals who teach as adjunct faculty. These individuals must have one or more additional responsibilities related to student advisement, supervision, committee work, program planning, evaluation, recruitment, and marketing activities.
A.2.6.	The program director and faculty must possess the academic and experiential qualifications and backgrounds (identified in documented descriptions of roles and responsibilities) that are necessary to meet program objectives and the mission of the institution.	The program director and faculty must possess the academic and experiential qualifications and backgrounds (identified in documented descriptions of roles and responsibilities) that are necessary to meet program objectives and the mission of the institution.	The program director and faculty must possess the academic and experiential qualifications and backgrounds (identified in documented descriptions of roles and responsibilities) that are necessary to meet program objectives and the mission of the institution.
A.2.7.	The program must identify an individual for the role of academic fieldwork coordinator who is specifically responsible for the program's compliance with the fieldwork requirements of Standards Section C.1.0 and is assigned to the occupational therapy educational program as a full-time faculty member as defined by ACOTE. The academic fieldwork coordinator may be assigned other institutional duties that do not interfere with the management and administration	The program must identify an individual for the role of academic fieldwork coordinator who is specifically responsible for the program's compliance with the fieldwork requirements of Standards Section C.1.0 and is assigned to the occupational therapy educational program as a full-time faculty member as defined by ACOTE. The academic fieldwork coordinator may be assigned other institutional duties that do not interfere with the management and administra-	The program must identify an individual for the role of academic fieldwork coordinator who is specifically responsible for the program's compliance with the fieldwork requirements of Standards Section C.1.0 and is assigned to the occupational therapy educational program as a full-time faculty member as defined by ACOTE. The academic fieldwork coordinator may be assigned other institutional duties that do not interfere with the management and administration

(Continued)

Standard Number	Accreditation Standards for a Doctoral-Degree-Level Educational Program for the Occupational Therapist	Accreditation Standards for a Master's-Degree-Level Educational Program for the Occupational Therapist	Accreditation Standards for an Associate-Degree-Level Educational Program for the Occupational Therapy Assistant
	of the fieldwork program. The institution must document that the academic fieldwork coordinator has sufficient release time to ensure that the needs of the fieldwork program are being met.	tion of the fieldwork program. The institution must document that the academic fieldwork coordinator has sufficient release time to ensure that the needs of the fieldwork program are being met.	of the fieldwork program. The institution must document that the academic fieldwork coordinator has sufficient release time to ensure that the needs of the fieldwork program are being met.
	This individual must be a licensed or otherwise regulated occupational therapist. Coordinators must hold a doctoral degree awarded by an institution that is accredited by a USDE-recognized regional accrediting body.	This individual must be a licensed or otherwise regulated occupational therapist. Coordinators must hold a minimum of a master's degree awarded by an institution that is accredited by a USDE-recognized regional accrediting body.	This individual must be a licensed or otherwise regulated occupational therapist or occupational therapy assistant. Coordinators must hold a minimum of a baccalaureate degree awarded by an institution that is accredited by a USDE-recognized regional or national accrediting body.
A.2.8.	Core faculty who are occupational therapists or occupational therapy assistants must be currently licensed or otherwise regulated according to regulations in the state or jurisdiction in which the program is located.	Core faculty who are occupational therapists or occupational therapy assistants must be currently licensed or otherwise regulated according to regulations in the state or jurisdiction in which the program is located.	Core faculty who are occupational therapists or occupational therapy assistants must be currently licensed or otherwise regulated according to regulations in the state or jurisdiction in which the program is located.
	Faculty in residence and teaching at additional locations must be currently licensed or otherwise regulated according to regulations in the state or jurisdiction in which the additional location is located.	Faculty in residence and teaching at additional locations must be currently licensed or otherwise regulated according to regulations in the state or jurisdiction in which the additional location is located.	Faculty in residence and teaching at additional locations must be currently licensed or otherwise regulated according to regulations in the state or jurisdiction in which the additional location is located.

(Continued)

Standard Number	Accreditation Standards for a Doctoral-Degree-Level Educational Program for the Occupational Therapist	Accreditation Standards for a Master's-Degree-Level Educational Program for the Occupational Therapist	Accreditation Standards for an Associate-Degree-Level Educational Program for the Occupational Therapy Assistant
A.2.9.	*(No related Standard)*	*(No related Standard)*	In programs where the program director is an occupational therapy assistant, an occupational therapist must be included on faculty and contribute to the functioning of the program through a variety of mechanisms including, but not limited to, teaching, advising, and committee work. In a program where there are only occupational therapists on faculty who have never practiced as an occupational therapy assistant, the program must demonstrate that an individual who is an occupational therapy assistant or an occupational therapist who has previously practiced as an occupational therapy assistant is involved in the program as an adjunct faculty or teaching assistant.
A.2.10.	All full-time faculty teaching in the program must hold a doctoral degree awarded by an institution that is accredited by a USDE-recognized regional accrediting body. The doctoral degree is not limited to a doctorate in occupational therapy.	The majority of full-time faculty who are occupational therapists or occupational therapy assistants must hold a doctoral degree. All full-time faculty must hold a minimum of a master's degree. All degrees must be awarded by an institution that is accredited by a USDE-recognized regional accrediting body. The degrees are not limited to occupational therapy. For an even number of full-time faculty, at least half must hold doctorates. The program director is counted as a faculty member.	All occupational therapy assistant faculty who are full-time must hold a minimum of a baccalaureate degree awarded by an institution that is accredited by a USDE-recognized regional or national accrediting body.

(Continued)

Standard Number	Accreditation Standards for a Doctoral-Degree-Level Educational Program for the Occupational Therapist	Accreditation Standards for a Master's-Degree-Level Educational Program for the Occupational Therapist	Accreditation Standards for an Associate-Degree-Level Educational Program for the Occupational Therapy Assistant
A.2.11.	The faculty must have documented expertise in their area(s) of teaching responsibility and knowledge of the content delivery method (e.g., distance learning).	The faculty must have documented expertise in their area(s) of teaching responsibility and knowledge of the content delivery method (e.g., distance learning).	The faculty must have documented expertise in their area(s) of teaching responsibility and knowledge of the content delivery method (e.g., distance learning).
A.2.12.	For programs with additional accredited location(s), the program must identify a faculty member who is an occupational therapist as site coordinator at each location who is responsible for ensuring uniform implementation of the program and ongoing communication with the program director.	For programs with additional accredited location(s), the program must identify a faculty member who is an occupational therapist as site coordinator at each location who is responsible for ensuring uniform implementation of the program and ongoing communication with the program director.	For programs with additional accredited location(s), the program must identify a faculty member who is an occupational therapist or occupational therapy assistant as site coordinator at each location who is responsible for ensuring uniform implementation of the program and ongoing communication with the program director.
A.2.13.	The occupational therapy faculty at each accredited location where the program is offered must be sufficient in number and must possess the expertise necessary to ensure appropriate curriculum design, content delivery, and program evaluation. The faculty must include individuals competent to ensure delivery of the broad scope of occupational therapy practice. Multiple adjuncts, part-time faculty, or full-time faculty may be configured to meet this goal. Each accredited additional location must have at least one full-time equivalent (FTE) faculty member.	The occupational therapy faculty at each accredited location where the program is offered must be sufficient in number and must possess the expertise necessary to ensure appropriate curriculum design, content delivery, and program evaluation. The faculty must include individuals competent to ensure delivery of the broad scope of occupational therapy practice. Multiple adjuncts, part-time faculty, or full-time faculty may be configured to meet this goal. Each accredited additional location must have at least one full-time equivalent (FTE) faculty member.	The occupational therapy assistant faculty at each accredited location where the program is offered must be sufficient in number and must possess the expertise necessary to ensure appropriate curriculum design, content delivery, and program evaluation. The faculty must include individuals competent to ensure delivery of the broad scope of occupational therapy practice. Multiple adjuncts, part-time faculty, or full-time faculty may be configured to meet this goal. Each accredited additional location must have at least one full-time equivalent (FTE) faculty member.

(Continued)

Standard Number	Accreditation Standards for a Doctoral-Degree-Level Educational Program for the Occupational Therapist	Accreditation Standards for a Master's-Degree-Level Educational Program for the Occupational Therapist	Accreditation Standards for an Associate-Degree-Level Educational Program for the Occupational Therapy Assistant
A.2.14.	Faculty responsibilities must be consistent with and supportive of the mission of the institution.	Faculty responsibilities must be consistent with and supportive of the mission of the institution.	Faculty responsibilities must be consistent with and supportive of the mission of the institution.
A.2.15.	The faculty–student ratio must permit the achievement of the purpose and stated objectives for laboratory and lecture courses, be compatible with accepted practices of the institution for similar programs, and ensure student and consumer safety.	The faculty–student ratio must permit the achievement of the purpose and stated objectives for laboratory and lecture courses, be compatible with accepted practices of the institution for similar programs, and ensure student and consumer safety.	The faculty–student ratio must permit the achievement of the purpose and stated objectives for laboratory and lecture courses, be compatible with accepted practices of the institution for similar programs, and ensure student and consumer safety.
A.2.16.	Clerical and support staff must be provided to the program, consistent with institutional practice, to meet programmatic and administrative requirements, including support for any portion of the program offered by distance education.	Clerical and support staff must be provided to the program, consistent with institutional practice, to meet programmatic and administrative requirements, including support for any portion of the program offered by distance education.	Clerical and support staff must be provided to the program, consistent with institutional practice, to meet programmatic and administrative requirements, including support for any portion of the program offered by distance education.
A.2.17.	The program must be allocated a budget of regular institutional funds, not including grants, gifts, and other restricted sources, sufficient to implement and maintain the objectives of the program and to fulfill the program's obligation to matriculated and entering students.	The program must be allocated a budget of regular institutional funds, not including grants, gifts, and other restricted sources, sufficient to implement and maintain the objectives of the program and to fulfill the program's obligation to matriculated and entering students.	The program must be allocated a budget of regular institutional funds, not including grants, gifts, and other restricted sources, sufficient to implement and maintain the objectives of the program and to fulfill the program's obligation to matriculated and entering students.
A.2.18.	Classrooms and laboratories must be provided that are consistent with the program's educational objectives, teaching methods, number of students, and safety and health standards of the	Classrooms and laboratories must be provided that are consistent with the program's educational objectives, teaching methods, number of students, and safety and health standards of the	Classrooms and laboratories must be provided that are consistent with the program's educational objectives, teaching methods, number of students, and safety and health standards of the

(Continued)

Standard Number	Accreditation Standards for a Doctoral-Degree-Level Educational Program for the Occupational Therapist	Accreditation Standards for a Master's-Degree-Level Educational Program for the Occupational Therapist	Accreditation Standards for an Associate-Degree-Level Educational Program for the Occupational Therapy Assistant
		institution, and they must allow for efficient operation of the program.	institution, and they must allow for efficient operation of the program.
A.2.19.	If the program offers distance education, it must include • A process through which the program establishes that the student who registers in a distance education course or program is the same student who participates in and completes the program and receives academic credit, • Technology and resources that are adequate to support a distance-learning environment, and • A process to ensure that faculty are adequately trained and skilled to use distance education methodologies.	If the program offers distance education, it must include • A process through which the program establishes that the student who registers in a distance education course or program is the same student who participates in and completes the program and receives academic credit, • Technology and resources that are adequate to support a distance-learning environment, and • A process to ensure that faculty are adequately trained and skilled to use distance education methodologies.	If the program offers distance education, it must include • A process through which the program establishes that the student who registers in a distance education course or program is the same student who participates in and completes the program and receives academic credit, • Technology and resources that are adequate to support a distance-learning environment, and • A process to ensure that faculty are adequately trained and skilled to use distance education methodologies.
A.2.20.	Laboratory space provided by the institution must be assigned to the occupational therapy program on a priority basis. If laboratory space for occupational therapy lab classes is provided by another institution or agency, there must be a written and signed agreement to ensure assignment of space for program use.	Laboratory space provided by the institution must be assigned to the occupational therapy program on a priority basis. If laboratory space for occupational therapy lab classes is provided by another institution or agency, there must be a written and signed agreement to ensure assignment of space for program use.	Laboratory space provided by the institution must be assigned to the occupational therapy assistant program on a priority basis. If laboratory space for occupational therapy assistant lab classes is provided by another institution or agency, there must be a written and signed agreement to ensure assignment of space for program use.
A.2.21.	Adequate space must be provided to store and secure equipment and supplies.	Adequate space must be provided to store and secure equipment and supplies.	Adequate space must be provided to store and secure equipment and supplies.

(Continued)

(Continued)

Standard Number	Accreditation Standards for a Doctoral-Degree-Level Educational Program for the Occupational Therapist	Accreditation Standards for a Master's-Degree-Level Educational Program for the Occupational Therapist	Accreditation Standards for an Associate-Degree-Level Educational Program for the Occupational Therapy Assistant
A.2.22.	The program director and faculty must have office space consistent with institutional practice.	The program director and faculty must have office space consistent with institutional practice.	The program director and faculty must have office space consistent with institutional practice.
A.2.23.	Adequate space must be provided for the private advising of students.	Adequate space must be provided for the private advising of students.	Adequate space must be provided for the private advising of students.
A.2.24.	Appropriate and sufficient equipment and supplies must be provided by the institution for student use and for the didactic, supervised fieldwork, and experiential components of the curriculum.	Appropriate and sufficient equipment and supplies must be provided by the institution for student use and for the didactic and supervised fieldwork components of the curriculum.	Appropriate and sufficient equipment and supplies must be provided by the institution for student use and for the didactic and supervised fieldwork components of the curriculum.
A.2.25.	Students must be given access to and have the opportunity to use the evaluative and treatment methodologies that reflect both current practice and practice in the geographic area served by the program.	Students must be given access to and have the opportunity to use the evaluative and treatment methodologies that reflect both current practice and practice in the geographic area served by the program.	Students must be given access to and have the opportunity to use the evaluative and treatment methodologies that reflect both current practice and practice in the geographic area served by the program.
A.2.26.	Students must have ready access to a supply of current and relevant books, journals, periodicals, computers, software, and other reference materials needed for the practice areas and to meet the requirements of the curriculum. This may include, but is not limited to, libraries, online services, interlibrary loan, and resource centers.	Students must have ready access to a supply of current and relevant books, journals, periodicals, computers, software, and other reference materials needed to meet the requirements of the curriculum. This may include, but is not limited to, libraries, online services, interlibrary loan, and resource centers.	Students must have ready access to a supply of current and relevant books, journals, periodicals, computers, software, and other reference materials needed to meet the requirements of the curriculum. This may include, but is not limited to, libraries, online services, interlibrary loan, and resource centers.

Standard Number	Accreditation Standards for a Doctoral-Degree-Level Educational Program for the Occupational Therapist	Accreditation Standards for a Master's-Degree-Level Educational Program for the Occupational Therapist	Accreditation Standards for an Associate-Degree-Level Educational Program for the Occupational Therapy Assistant
A.2.27.	Instructional aids and technology must be available in sufficient quantity and quality to be consistent with the program objectives and teaching methods.	Instructional aids and technology must be available in sufficient quantity and quality to be consistent with the program objectives and teaching methods.	Instructional aids and technology must be available in sufficient quantity and quality to be consistent with the program objectives and teaching methods.
A.3.0. STUDENTS			
A.3.1.	Admission of students to the occupational therapy program must be made in accordance with the practices of the institution. There must be stated admission criteria that are clearly defined and published and reflective of the demands of the program.	Admission of students to the occupational therapy program must be made in accordance with the practices of the institution. There must be stated admission criteria that are clearly defined and published and reflective of the demands of the program.	Admission of students to the occupational therapy assistant program must be made in accordance with the practices of the institution. There must be stated admission criteria that are clearly defined and published and reflective of the demands of the program.
A.3.2.	Institutions must require that program applicants hold a baccalaureate degree or higher prior to admission to the program.	(No related Standard)	(No related Standard)
A.3.3.	Policies pertaining to standards for admission, advanced placement, transfer of credit, credit for experiential learning (if applicable), and prerequisite educational or work experience requirements must be readily accessible to prospective students and the public.	Policies pertaining to standards for admission, advanced placement, transfer of credit, credit for experiential learning (if applicable), and prerequisite educational or work experience requirements must be readily accessible to prospective students and the public.	Policies pertaining to standards for admission, advanced placement, transfer of credit, credit for experiential learning (if applicable), and prerequisite educational or work experience requirements must be readily accessible to prospective students and the public.
A.3.4.	Programs must document implementation of a mechanism to ensure that students receiving	Programs must document implementation of a mechanism to ensure that students receiving	Programs must document implementation of a mechanism to ensure that students receiving

(Continued)

Standard Number	Accreditation Standards for a Doctoral-Degree-Level Educational Program for the Occupational Therapist	Accreditation Standards for a Master's-Degree-Level Educational Program for the Occupational Therapist	Accreditation Standards for an Associate-Degree-Level Educational Program for the Occupational Therapy Assistant
	credit for previous courses and/or work experience have met the content requirements of the appropriate doctoral Standards.	credit for previous courses and/or work experience have met the content requirements of the appropriate master's Standards.	credit for previous courses and/or work experience have met the content requirements of the appropriate occupational therapy assistant Standards.
A.3.5.	Criteria for successful completion of each segment of the educational program and for graduation must be given in advance to each student.	Criteria for successful completion of each segment of the educational program and for graduation must be given in advance to each student.	Criteria for successful completion of each segment of the educational program and for graduation must be given in advance to each student.
A.3.6.	Evaluation content and methods must be consistent with the curriculum design; objectives; competencies of the didactic, fieldwork, and experiential components of the program.	Evaluation content and methods must be consistent with the curriculum design, objectives, and competencies of the didactic and fieldwork components of the program.	Evaluation content and methods must be consistent with the curriculum design, objectives, and competencies of the didactic and fieldwork components of the program.
A.3.7.	Evaluation must be conducted on a regular basis to provide students and program officials with timely indications of the students' progress and academic standing.	Evaluation must be conducted on a regular basis to provide students and program officials with timely indications of the students' progress and academic standing.	Evaluation must be conducted on a regular basis to provide students and program officials with timely indications of the students' progress and academic standing.
A.3.8.	Students must be informed of and have access to the student support services that are provided to other students in the institution.	Students must be informed of and have access to the student support services that are provided to other students in the institution.	Students must be informed of and have access to the student support services that are provided to other students in the institution.
A.3.9.	Advising related to professional coursework, fieldwork education, and the experiential component of the program must be the responsibility of the occupational therapy faculty.	Advising related to professional coursework and fieldwork education must be the responsibility of the occupational therapy faculty.	Advising related to coursework in the occupational therapy assistant program and fieldwork education must be the responsibility of the occupational therapy assistant faculty.

(Continued)

Standard Number	Accreditation Standards for a Doctoral-Degree-Level Educational Program for the Occupational Therapist	Accreditation Standards for a Master's-Degree-Level Educational Program for the Occupational Therapist	Accreditation Standards for an Associate-Degree-Level Educational Program for the Occupational Therapy Assistant
A.4.0.	**OPERATIONAL POLICIES**		
A.4.1.	All program publications and advertising—including, but not limited to, academic calendars, announcements, catalogs, handbooks, and Web sites—must accurately reflect the program offered.	All program publications and advertising—including, but not limited to, academic calendars, announcements, catalogs, handbooks, and Web sites—must accurately reflect the program offered.	All program publications and advertising—including, but not limited to, academic calendars, announcements, catalogs, handbooks, and Web sites—must accurately reflect the program offered.
A.4.2.	Accurate and current information regarding student and program outcomes must be readily available to the public on the program's Web page. At a minimum, the following data must be reported for the previous 3 years: • Total number of program graduates • Graduation rates. The program must provide the direct link to the National Board for Certification in Occupational Therapy (NBCOT) program data results on the program's home page.	Accurate and current information regarding student and program outcomes must be readily available to the public on the program's Web page. At a minimum, the following data must be reported for the previous 3 years: • Total number of program graduates • Graduation rates. The program must provide the direct link to the National Board for Certification in Occupational Therapy (NBCOT) program data results on the program's home page.	Accurate and current information regarding student and program outcomes must be readily available to the public on the program's Web page. At a minimum, the following data must be reported for the previous 3 years: • Total number of program graduates, • Graduation rates. The program must provide the direct link to the National Board for Certification in Occupational Therapy (NBCOT) program data results on the program's home page.
A.4.3.	The program's accreditation status and the name, address, and telephone number of ACOTE must be published in all of the following materials used by the institution: catalog, Web site, and program-related brochures or flyers available to prospective students. A link to www.acoteonline.org must be provided on the program's home page.	The program's accreditation status and the name, address, and telephone number of ACOTE must be published in all of the following materials used by the institution: catalog, Web site, and program-related brochures or flyers available to prospective students. A link to www.acoteonline.org must be provided on the program's home page.	The program's accreditation status and the name, address, and telephone number of ACOTE must be published in all of the following materials used by the institution: catalog, Web site, and program-related brochures or flyers available to prospective students. A link to www.acoteonline.org must be provided on the program's home page.

(Continued)

Standard Number	Accreditation Standards for a Doctoral-Degree-Level Educational Program for the Occupational Therapist	Accreditation Standards for a Master's-Degree-Level Educational Program for the Occupational Therapist	Accreditation Standards for an Associate-Degree-Level Educational Program for the Occupational Therapy Assistant
A.4.4.	All practices within the institution related to faculty, staff, applicants, and students must be nondiscriminatory.	All practices within the institution related to faculty, staff, applicants, and students must be nondiscriminatory.	All practices within the institution related to faculty, staff, applicants, and students must be nondiscriminatory.
A.4.5.	Graduation requirements, tuition, and fees must be accurately stated, published, and made known to all applicants. When published fees are subject to change, a statement to that effect must be included.	Graduation requirements, tuition, and fees must be accurately stated, published, and made known to all applicants. When published fees are subject to change, a statement to that effect must be included.	Graduation requirements, tuition, and fees must be accurately stated, published, and made known to all applicants. When published fees are subject to change, a statement to that effect must be included.
A.4.6.	The program or sponsoring institution must have a defined and published policy and procedure for processing student and faculty grievances.	The program or sponsoring institution must have a defined and published policy and procedure for processing student and faculty grievances.	The program or sponsoring institution must have a defined and published policy and procedure for processing student and faculty grievances.
A.4.7.	Policies and procedures for handling complaints against the program must be published and made known. The program must maintain a record of student complaints that includes the nature and disposition of each complaint.	Policies and procedures for handling complaints against the program must be published and made known. The program must maintain a record of student complaints that includes the nature and disposition of each complaint.	Policies and procedures for handling complaints against the program must be published and made known. The program must maintain a record of student complaints that includes the nature and disposition of each complaint.
A.4.8.	Policies and processes for student withdrawal and for refunds of tuition and fees must be published and made known to all applicants.	Policies and processes for student withdrawal and for refunds of tuition and fees must be published and made known to all applicants.	Policies and processes for student withdrawal and for refunds of tuition and fees must be published and made known to all applicants.
A.4.9.	Policies and procedures for student probation, suspension, and dismissal must be published and made known.	Policies and procedures for student probation, suspension, and dismissal must be published and made known.	Policies and procedures for student probation, suspension, and dismissal must be published and made known.

(Continued)

Standard Number	Accreditation Standards for a Doctoral-Degree-Level Educational Program for the Occupational Therapist	Accreditation Standards for a Master's-Degree-Level Educational Program for the Occupational Therapist	Accreditation Standards for an Associate-Degree-Level Educational Program for the Occupational Therapy Assistant
A.4.10.	Policies and procedures for human-subject research protocol must be published and made known.	Policies and procedures for human-subject research protocol must be published and made known.	Policies and procedures for human-subject research protocol must be published and made known (if applicable to the program).
A.4.11.	Programs must make available to students written policies and procedures regarding appropriate use of equipment and supplies and for all educational activities that have implications for the health and safety of clients, students, and faculty (including infection control and evacuation procedures).	Programs must make available to students written policies and procedures regarding appropriate use of equipment and supplies and for all educational activities that have implications for the health and safety of clients, students, and faculty (including infection control and evacuation procedures).	Programs must make available to students written policies and procedures regarding appropriate use of equipment and supplies and for all educational activities that have implications for the health and safety of clients, students, and faculty (including infection control and evacuation procedures).
A.4.12.	A program admitting students on the basis of ability to benefit (defined by the USDE as admitting students who do not have either a high school diploma or its equivalent) must publicize its objectives, assessment measures, and means of evaluating the student's ability to benefit.	A program admitting students on the basis of ability to benefit (defined by the USDE as admitting students who do not have either a high school diploma or its equivalent) must publicize its objectives, assessment measures, and means of evaluating the student's ability to benefit.	A program admitting students on the basis of ability to benefit (defined by the USDE as admitting students who do not have either a high school diploma or its equivalent) must publicize its objectives, assessment measures, and means of evaluating the student's ability to benefit.
A.4.13.	Documentation of all progression, retention, graduation, certification, and credentialing requirements must be published and made known to applicants. A statement on the program's Web site about the potential impact of a felony conviction on a graduate's eligibility for certification and credentialing must be provided.	Documentation of all progression, retention, graduation, certification, and credentialing requirements must be published and made known to applicants. A statement on the program's Web site about the potential impact of a felony conviction on a graduate's eligibility for certification and credentialing must be provided.	Documentation of all progression, retention, graduation, certification, and credentialing requirements must be published and made known to applicants. A statement on the program's Web site about the potential impact of a felony conviction on a graduate's eligibility for certification and credentialing must be provided.
A.4.14.	The program must have a documented and published policy to ensure that students complete all	The program must have a documented and published policy to ensure that students complete all	The program must have a documented and published policy to ensure that students

(Continued)

Standard Number	Accreditation Standards for a Doctoral-Degree-Level Educational Program for the Occupational Therapist	Accreditation Standards for a Master's-Degree-Level Educational Program for the Occupational Therapist	Accreditation Standards for an Associate-Degree-Level Educational Program for the Occupational Therapy Assistant
	graduation, fieldwork, and experiential component requirements in a timely manner. This policy must include a statement that all Level II fieldwork and the experiential component of the program must be completed within a time frame established by the program.	graduation and fieldwork requirements in a timely manner. This policy must include a statement that all Level II fieldwork must be completed within a time frame established by the program.	complete all graduation and fieldwork requirements in a timely manner. This policy must include a statement that all Level II fieldwork must be completed within a time frame established by the program.
A.4.15.	Records regarding student admission, enrollment, fieldwork, and achievement must be maintained and kept in a secure setting. Grades and credits for courses must be recorded on students' transcripts and permanently maintained by the sponsoring institution.	Records regarding student admission, enrollment, fieldwork, and achievement must be maintained and kept in a secure setting. Grades and credits for courses must be recorded on students' transcripts and permanently maintained by the sponsoring institution.	Records regarding student admission, enrollment, fieldwork, and achievement must be maintained and kept in a secure setting. Grades and credits for courses must be recorded on students' transcripts and permanently maintained by the sponsoring institution.

A.5.0. STRATEGIC PLAN AND PROGRAM ASSESSMENT

For programs that are offered at more than one location, the program's strategic plan, evaluation plan, and results of ongoing evaluation must address each program location as a component of the overall plan.

Standard Number	Accreditation Standards for a Doctoral-Degree-Level Educational Program for the Occupational Therapist	Accreditation Standards for a Master's-Degree-Level Educational Program for the Occupational Therapist	Accreditation Standards for an Associate-Degree-Level Educational Program for the Occupational Therapy Assistant
A.5.1.	The program must document a current strategic plan that articulates the program's future vision and guides the program development (e.g., faculty recruitment and professional growth, scholarship, changes in the curriculum design, priorities in academic resources, procurement of fieldwork and experiential component sites). A program strategic plan must be for a minimum	The program must document a current strategic plan that articulates the program's future vision and guides the program development (e.g., faculty recruitment and professional growth, scholarship, changes in the curriculum design, priorities in academic resources, procurement of fieldwork sites). A program strategic plan must be for a minimum of a	The program must document a current strategic plan that articulates the program's future vision and guides the program development (e.g., faculty recruitment and professional growth, scholarship, changes in the curriculum design, priorities in academic resources, procurement of fieldwork sites). A program strategic plan must be for a minimum of a

(Continued)

Standard Number	Accreditation Standards for a Doctoral-Degree-Level Educational Program for the Occupational Therapist	Accreditation Standards for a Master's-Degree-Level Educational Program for the Occupational Therapist	Accreditation Standards for an Associate-Degree-Level Educational Program for the Occupational Therapy Assistant
	of a 3-year period and include, but need not be limited to, <ul><li>Evidence that the plan is based on program evaluation and an analysis of external and internal environments.</li><li>Long-term goals that address the vision and mission of both the institution and the program, as well as specific needs of the program.</li><li>Specific measurable action steps with expected timelines by which the program will reach its long-term goals.</li><li>Person(s) responsible for action steps.</li><li>Evidence of periodic updating of action steps and long-term goals as they are met or as circumstances change.</li></ul>	3-year period and include, but need not be limited to, <ul><li>Evidence that the plan is based on program evaluation and an analysis of external and internal environments.</li><li>Long-term goals that address the vision and mission of both the institution and the program, as well as specific needs of the program.</li><li>Specific measurable action steps with expected timelines by which the program will reach its long-term goals.</li><li>Person(s) responsible for action steps.</li><li>Evidence of periodic updating of action steps and long-term goals as they are met or as circumstances change.</li></ul>	3-year period and include, but need not be limited to, <ul><li>Evidence that the plan is based on program evaluation and an analysis of external and internal environments.</li><li>Long-term goals that address the vision and mission of both the institution and the program, as well as specific needs of the program.</li><li>Specific measurable action steps with expected timelines by which the program will reach its long-term goals.</li><li>Person(s) responsible for action steps.</li><li>Evidence of periodic updating of action steps and long-term goals as they are met or as circumstances change.</li></ul>
A.5.2.	The program director and each faculty member who teaches two or more courses must have a current written professional growth and development plan. Each plan must contain the signature of the faculty member and supervisor. At a minimum, the plan must include, but need not be limited to, <ul><li>Goals to enhance the faculty member's ability to fulfill designated responsibilities (e.g., goals related to currency in areas of teaching responsibility, teaching effectiveness, research, scholarly activity).</li></ul>	The program director and each faculty member who teaches two or more courses must have a current written professional growth and development plan. Each plan must contain the signature of the faculty member and supervisor. At a minimum, the plan must include, but need not be limited to, <ul><li>Goals to enhance the faculty member's ability to fulfill designated responsibilities (e.g., goals related to currency in areas of teaching responsibility, teaching effectiveness, research, scholarly activity).</li></ul>	The program director and each faculty member who teaches two or more courses must have a current written professional growth and development plan. Each plan must contain the signature of the faculty member and supervisor. At a minimum, the plan must include, but need not be limited to, <ul><li>Goals to enhance the faculty member's ability to fulfill designated responsibilities (e.g., goals related to currency in areas of teaching responsibility, teaching effectiveness, research, scholarly activity).</li></ul>

(Continued)

Standard Number	Accreditation Standards for a Doctoral-Degree-Level Educational Program for the Occupational Therapist	Accreditation Standards for a Master's-Degree-Level Educational Program for the Occupational Therapist	Accreditation Standards for an Associate-Degree-Level Educational Program for the Occupational Therapy Assistant
	• Specific measurable action steps with expected timelines by which the faculty member will achieve the goals. • Evidence of annual updates of action steps and goals as they are met or as circumstances change. • Identification of the ways in which the faculty member's professional development plan will contribute to attaining the program's strategic goals.	• Specific measurable action steps with expected timelines by which the faculty member will achieve the goals. • Evidence of annual updates of action steps and goals as they are met or as circumstances change. • Identification of the ways in which the faculty member's professional development plan will contribute to attaining the program's strategic goals.	• Specific measurable action steps with expected timelines by which the faculty member will achieve the goals. • Evidence of annual updates of action steps and goals as they are met or as circumstances change. • Identification of the ways in which the faculty member's professional development plan will contribute to attaining the program's strategic goals.
A.5.3.	Programs must routinely secure and document sufficient qualitative and quantitative information to allow for meaningful analysis about the extent to which the program is meeting its stated goals and objectives. This must include, but need not be limited to, • Faculty effectiveness in their assigned teaching responsibilities. • Students' progression through the program. • Student retention rates. • Fieldwork and experiential component performance evaluation. • Student evaluation of fieldwork and the experiential component experience. • Student satisfaction with the program. • Graduates' performance on the NBCOT certification exam.	Programs must routinely secure and document sufficient qualitative and quantitative information to allow for meaningful analysis about the extent to which the program is meeting its stated goals and objectives. This must include, but need not be limited to, • Faculty effectiveness in their assigned teaching responsibilities. • Students' progression through the program. • Student retention rates. • Fieldwork performance evaluation. • Student evaluation of fieldwork experience. • Student satisfaction with the program. • Graduates' performance on the NBCOT certification exam. • Graduates' job placement and performance as determined by employer satisfaction.	Programs must routinely secure and document sufficient qualitative and quantitative information to allow for meaningful analysis about the extent to which the program is meeting its stated goals and objectives. This must include, but need not be limited to, • Faculty effectiveness in their assigned teaching responsibilities. • Students' progression through the program. • Student retention rates. • Fieldwork performance evaluation. • Student evaluation of fieldwork experience. • Student satisfaction with the program. • Graduates' performance on the NBCOT certification exam. • Graduates' job placement and performance as determined by employer satisfaction.

(Continued)

Standard Number	Accreditation Standards for a Doctoral-Degree-Level Educational Program for the Occupational Therapist	Accreditation Standards for a Master's-Degree-Level Educational Program for the Occupational Therapist	Accreditation Standards for an Associate-Degree-Level Educational Program for the Occupational Therapy Assistant
	• Graduates' job placement and performance as determined by employer satisfaction. • Graduates' scholarly activity (e.g., presentations, publications, grants obtained, state and national leadership positions, awards).		
A.5.4.	Programs must routinely and systematically analyze data to determine the extent to which the program is meeting its stated goals and objectives. An annual report summarizing analysis of data and planned action responses must be maintained.	Programs must routinely and systematically analyze data to determine the extent to which the program is meeting its stated goals and objectives. An annual report summarizing analysis of data and planned action responses must be maintained.	Programs must routinely and systematically analyze data to determine the extent to which the program is meeting its stated goals and objectives. An annual report summarizing analysis of data and planned action responses must be maintained.
A.5.5.	The results of ongoing evaluation must be appropriately reflected in the program's strategic plan, curriculum, and other dimensions of the program.	The results of ongoing evaluation must be appropriately reflected in the program's strategic plan, curriculum, and other dimensions of the program.	The results of ongoing evaluation must be appropriately reflected in the program's strategic plan, curriculum, and other dimensions of the program.
A.5.6.	The average pass rate over the 3 most recent calendar years for graduates attempting the national certification exam within 12 months of graduation from the program must be 80% or higher (regardless of the number of attempts). If a program has less than 25 test takers in the 3 most recent calendar years, the program may include test takers from additional years until it reaches 25 or until the 5 most recent calendar years are included in the total.	The average pass rate over the 3 most recent calendar years for graduates attempting the national certification exam within 12 months of graduation from the program must be 80% or higher (regardless of the number of attempts). If a program has less than 25 test takers in the 3 most recent calendar years, the program may include test takers from additional years until it reaches 25 or until the 5 most recent calendar years are included in the total.	The average pass rate over the 3 most recent calendar years for graduates attempting the national certification exam within 12 months of graduation from the program must be 80% or higher (regardless of the number of attempts). If a program has less than 25 test takers in the 3 most recent calendar years, the program may include test takers from additional years until it reaches 25 or until the 5 most recent calendar years are included in the total.

(Continued)

Standard Number	Accreditation Standards for a Doctoral-Degree-Level Educational Program for the Occupational Therapist	Accreditation Standards for a Master's-Degree-Level Educational Program for the Occupational Therapist	Accreditation Standards for an Associate-Degree-Level Educational Program for the Occupational Therapy Assistant
A.6.0.	**CURRICULUM FRAMEWORK** The curriculum framework is a description of the program that includes the program's mission, philosophy, and curriculum design.		
A.6.1.	The curriculum must ensure preparation to practice as a generalist with a broad exposure to current practice settings (e.g., school, hospital, community, long-term care) and emerging practice areas (as defined by the program). The curriculum must prepare students to work with a variety of populations including, but not limited to, children, adolescents, adults, and elderly persons in areas of physical and mental health.	The curriculum must include preparation for practice as a generalist with a broad exposure to current practice settings (e.g., school, hospital, community, long-term care) and emerging practice areas (as defined by the program). The curriculum must prepare students to work with a variety of populations including, but not limited to, children, adolescents, adults, and elderly persons in areas of physical and mental health.	The curriculum must include preparation for practice as a generalist with a broad exposure to current practice settings (e.g., school, hospital, community, long-term care) and emerging practice areas (as defined by the program). The curriculum must prepare students to work with a variety of populations including, but not limited to, children, adolescents, adults, and elderly persons in areas of physical and mental health.
A.6.2.	The curriculum must include course objectives and learning activities demonstrating preparation beyond a generalist level in, but not limited to, practice skills, research skills, administration, professional development, leadership, advocacy, and theory.	*(No related Standard)*	*(No related Standard)*
A.6.3.	The occupational therapy doctoral degree must be awarded after a period of study such that the total time to the degree, including both preprofessional and professional preparation, equals at least 6 FTE academic years. The program must document a system and rationale for ensuring that the length of study of the program is appropriate to the expected learning and competence of the graduate.	The program must document a system and rationale for ensuring that the length of study of the program is appropriate to the expected learning and competence of the graduate.	The program must document a system and rationale for ensuring that the length of study of the program is appropriate to the expected learning and competence of the graduate.

(Continued)

Standard Number	Accreditation Standards for a Doctoral-Degree-Level Educational Program for the Occupational Therapist	Accreditation Standards for a Master's-Degree-Level Educational Program for the Occupational Therapist	Accreditation Standards for an Associate-Degree-Level Educational Program for the Occupational Therapy Assistant
A.6.4.	The curriculum must include application of advanced knowledge to practice through a combination of experiential activities and a culminating project.		
A.6.5.	The statement of philosophy of the occupational therapy program must reflect the current published philosophy of the profession and must include a statement of the program's fundamental beliefs about human beings and how they learn.	The statement of philosophy of the occupational therapy program must reflect the current published philosophy of the profession and must include a statement of the program's fundamental beliefs about human beings and how they learn.	The statement of philosophy of the occupational therapy assistant program must reflect the current published philosophy of the profession and must include a statement of the program's fundamental beliefs about human beings and how they learn.
A.6.6.	The statement of the mission of the occupational therapy program must be consistent with and supportive of the mission of the sponsoring institution. The program's mission statement should explain the unique nature of the program and how it helps fulfill or advance the mission of the sponsoring institution, including religious missions.	The statement of the mission of the occupational therapy program must be consistent with and supportive of the mission of the sponsoring institution. The program's mission statement should explain the unique nature of the program and how it helps fulfill or advance the mission of the sponsoring institution, including religious missions.	The statement of the mission of the occupational therapy assistant program must be consistent with and supportive of the mission of the sponsoring institution. The program's mission statement should explain the unique nature of the program and how it helps fulfill or advance the mission of the sponsoring institution, including religious missions.
A.6.7.	The curriculum design must reflect the mission and philosophy of both the occupational therapy program and the institution and must provide the basis for program planning, implementation, and evaluation. The design must identify curricular threads and educational goals and describe the selection of the content, scope, and sequencing of coursework.	The curriculum design must reflect the mission and philosophy of both the occupational therapy program and the institution and must provide the basis for program planning, implementation, and evaluation. The design must identify curricular threads and educational goals and describe the selection of the content, scope, and sequencing of coursework.	The curriculum design must reflect the mission and philosophy of both the occupational therapy assistant program and the institution and must provide the basis for program planning, implementation, and evaluation. The design must identify curricular threads and educational goals and describe the selection of the content, scope, and sequencing of coursework.

Row A.6.4. note: (No related Standard) appears in the Master's and Associate columns.

(Continued)

Standard Number	Accreditation Standards for a Doctoral-Degree-Level Educational Program for the Occupational Therapist	Accreditation Standards for a Master's-Degree-Level Educational Program for the Occupational Therapist	Accreditation Standards for an Associate-Degree-Level Educational Program for the Occupational Therapy Assistant
A.6.8.	The program must have clearly documented assessment measures by which students are regularly evaluated on their acquisition of knowledge, skills, attitudes, and competencies required for graduation.	The program must have clearly documented assessment measures by which students are regularly evaluated on their acquisition of knowledge, skills, attitudes, and competencies required for graduation.	The program must have clearly documented assessment measures by which students are regularly evaluated on their acquisition of knowledge, skills, attitudes, and competencies required for graduation.
A.6.9.	The program must have written syllabi for each course that include course objectives and learning activities that, in total, reflect all course content required by the Standards. Instructional methods (e.g., presentations, demonstrations, discussion) and materials used to accomplish course objectives must be documented. Programs must also demonstrate the consistency between course syllabi and the curriculum design.	The program must have written syllabi for each course that include course objectives and learning activities that, in total, reflect all course content required by the Standards. Instructional methods (e.g., presentations, demonstrations, discussion) and materials used to accomplish course objectives must be documented. Programs must also demonstrate the consistency between course syllabi and the curriculum design.	The program must have written syllabi for each course that include course objectives and learning activities that, in total, reflect all course content required by the Standards. Instructional methods (e.g., presentations, demonstrations, discussion) and materials used to accomplish course objectives must be documented. Programs must also demonstrate the consistency between course syllabi and the curriculum design.

Section B: CONTENT REQUIREMENTS

The content requirements are written as expected student outcomes. Faculty are responsible for developing learning activities and evaluation methods to document that students meet these outcomes.

Standard Number	Doctoral	Master's	Associate
B.1.0.	FOUNDATIONAL CONTENT REQUIREMENTS

Program content must be based on a broad foundation in the liberal arts and sciences. A strong foundation in the biological, physical, social, and behavioral sciences supports an understanding of occupation across the lifespan. If the content of the Standard is met through prerequisite coursework, the application of foundational content in sciences must also be evident in professional coursework. The student will be able to | FOUNDATIONAL CONTENT REQUIREMENTS

Program content must be based on a broad foundation in the liberal arts and sciences. A strong foundation in the biological, physical, social, and behavioral sciences supports an understanding of occupation across the lifespan. If the content of the Standard is met through prerequisite coursework, the application of foundational content in sciences must also be evident in professional coursework. The student will be able to | FOUNDATIONAL CONTENT REQUIREMENTS

Program content must be based on a broad foundation in the liberal arts and sciences. A strong foundation in the biological, physical, social, and behavioral sciences supports an understanding of occupation across the |

(Continued)

Standard Number	Accreditation Standards for a Doctoral-Degree-Level Educational Program for the Occupational Therapist	Accreditation Standards for a Master's-Degree-Level Educational Program for the Occupational Therapist	Accreditation Standards for an Associate-Degree-Level Educational Program for the Occupational Therapy Assistant
			lifespan. If the content of the Standard is met through prerequisite coursework, the application of foundational content in sciences must also be evident in professional coursework. The student will be able to
B.1.1.	Demonstrate knowledge and understanding of the structure and function of the human body to include the biological and physical sciences. Course content must include, but is not limited to, biology, anatomy, physiology, neuroscience, and kinesiology or biomechanics.	Demonstrate knowledge and understanding of the structure and function of the human body to include the biological and physical sciences. Course content must include, but is not limited to, biology, anatomy, physiology, neuroscience, and kinesiology or biomechanics.	Demonstrate knowledge and understanding of the structure and function of the human body to include the biological and physical sciences. Course content must include, but is not limited to, anatomy, physiology, and biomechanics.
B.1.2.	Demonstrate knowledge and understanding of human development throughout the lifespan (infants, children, adolescents, adults, and older adults). Course content must include, but is not limited to, developmental psychology.	Demonstrate knowledge and understanding of human development throughout the lifespan (infants, children, adolescents, adults, and older adults). Course content must include, but is not limited to, developmental psychology.	Demonstrate knowledge and understanding of human development throughout the lifespan (infants, children, adolescents, adults, and older adults). Course content must include, but is not limited to, developmental psychology.
B.1.3.	Demonstrate knowledge and understanding of the concepts of human behavior to include the behavioral sciences, social sciences, and occupational science. Course content must include, but is not limited to, introductory psychology, abnormal psychology, and introductory sociology or introductory anthropology.	Demonstrate knowledge and understanding of the concepts of human behavior to include the behavioral sciences, social sciences, and occupational science. Course content must include, but is not limited to, introductory psychology, abnormal psychology, and introductory sociology or introductory anthropology.	Demonstrate knowledge and understanding of the concepts of human behavior to include the behavioral and social sciences (e.g., principles of psychology, sociology, abnormal psychology) and occupational science.

(Continued)

(Continued)

Standard Number	Accreditation Standards for a Doctoral-Degree-Level Educational Program for the Occupational Therapist	Accreditation Standards for a Master's-Degree-Level Educational Program for the Occupational Therapist	Accreditation Standards for an Associate-Degree-Level Educational Program for the Occupational Therapy Assistant
B.1.4.	Apply knowledge of the role of sociocultural, socioeconomic, and diversity factors and lifestyle choices in contemporary society to meet the needs of individuals and communities. Course content must include, but is not limited to, introductory psychology, abnormal psychology, and introductory sociology or introductory anthropology.	Demonstrate knowledge and appreciation of the role of sociocultural, socioeconomic, and diversity factors and lifestyle choices in contemporary society. Course content must include, but is not limited to, introductory psychology, abnormal psychology, and introductory sociology or introductory anthropology.	Demonstrate knowledge and appreciation of the role of sociocultural, socioeconomic, and diversity factors and lifestyle choices in contemporary society (e.g., principles of psychology, sociology, and abnormal psychology).
B.1.5.	Demonstrate an understanding of the ethical and practical considerations that affect the health and wellness needs of those who are experiencing or are at risk for social injustice, occupational deprivation, and disparity in the receipt of services.	Demonstrate an understanding of the ethical and practical considerations that affect the health and wellness needs of those who are experiencing or are at risk for social injustice, occupational deprivation, and disparity in the receipt of services.	Articulate the ethical and practical considerations that affect the health and wellness needs of those who are experiencing or are at risk for social injustice, occupational deprivation, and disparity in the receipt of services.
B.1.6.	Demonstrate knowledge of global social issues and prevailing health and welfare needs of populations with or at risk for disabilities and chronic health conditions.	Demonstrate knowledge of global social issues and prevailing health and welfare needs of populations with or at risk for disabilities and chronic health conditions.	Demonstrate knowledge of global social issues and prevailing health and welfare needs of populations with or at risk for disabilities and chronic health conditions.
B.1.7.	Apply quantitative statistics and qualitative analysis to interpret tests, measurements, and other data for the purpose of establishing and/or delivering evidence-based practice.	Demonstrate the ability to use statistics to interpret tests and measurements for the purpose of delivering evidence-based practice.	Articulate the importance of using statistics, tests, and measurements for the purpose of delivering evidence-based practice.
B.1.8.	Demonstrate an understanding of the use of technology to support performance, participation, health and well-being. This technology may	Demonstrate an understanding of the use of technology to support performance, participation, health and well-being. This technology may	Demonstrate an understanding of the use of technology to support performance, participation, health and well-being. This technology may

Standard Number	Accreditation Standards for a Doctoral-Degree-Level Educational Program for the Occupational Therapist	Accreditation Standards for a Master's-Degree-Level Educational Program for the Occupational Therapist	Accreditation Standards for an Associate-Degree-Level Educational Program for the Occupational Therapy Assistant
	include, but is not limited to, electronic documentation systems, distance communication, virtual environments, and telehealth technology.	include, but is not limited to, electronic documentation systems, distance communication, virtual environments, and telehealth technology.	include, but is not limited to, electronic documentation systems, distance communication, virtual environments, and telehealth technology.

B.2.0. BASIC TENETS OF OCCUPATIONAL THERAPY
Coursework must facilitate development of the performance criteria listed below. The student will be able to

Standard Number	Accreditation Standards for a Doctoral-Degree-Level Educational Program for the Occupational Therapist	Accreditation Standards for a Master's-Degree-Level Educational Program for the Occupational Therapist	Accreditation Standards for an Associate-Degree-Level Educational Program for the Occupational Therapy Assistant
B.2.1.	Explain the history and philosophical base of the profession of occupational therapy and its importance in meeting society's current and future occupational needs.	Articulate an understanding of the importance of the history and philosophical base of the profession of occupational therapy.	Articulate an understanding of the importance of the history and philosophical base of the profession of occupational therapy.
B.2.2.	Explain the meaning and dynamics of occupation and activity, including the interaction of areas of occupation, performance skills, performance patterns, activity demands, context(s) and environments, and client factors.	Explain the meaning and dynamics of occupation and activity, including the interaction of areas of occupation, performance skills, performance patterns, activity demands, context(s) and environments, and client factors.	Describe the meaning and dynamics of occupation and activity, including the interaction of areas of occupation, performance skills, performance patterns, activity demands, context(s) and environments, and client factors.
B.2.3.	Articulate to consumers, potential employers, colleagues, third-party payers, regulatory boards, policymakers, other audiences, and the general public both the unique nature of occupation as viewed by the profession of occupational therapy and the value of occupation to support performance, participation, health, and well-being.	Articulate to consumers, potential employers, colleagues, third-party payers, regulatory boards, policymakers, other audiences, and the general public both the unique nature of occupation as viewed by the profession of occupational therapy and the value of occupation to support performance, participation, health, and well-being.	Articulate to consumers, potential employers, colleagues, third-party payers, regulatory boards, policymakers, other audiences, and the general public both the unique nature of occupation as viewed by the profession of occupational therapy and the value of occupation support performance, participation, health, and well-being.

(Continued)

Standard Number	Accreditation Standards for a Doctoral-Degree-Level Educational Program for the Occupational Therapist	Accreditation Standards for a Master's-Degree-Level Educational Program for the Occupational Therapist	Accreditation Standards for an Associate-Degree-Level Educational Program for the Occupational Therapy Assistant
B.2.4.	Articulate the importance of balancing areas of occupation with the achievement of health and wellness for the clients.	Articulate the importance of balancing areas of occupation with the achievement of health and wellness for the clients.	Articulate the importance of balancing areas of occupation with the achievement of health and wellness for the clients.
B.2.5.	Explain the role of occupation in the promotion of health and the prevention of disease and disability for the individual, family, and society.	Explain the role of occupation in the promotion of health and the prevention of disease and disability for the individual, family, and society.	Explain the role of occupation in the promotion of health and the prevention of disease and disability for the individual, family, and society.
B.2.6.	Analyze the effects of heritable diseases, genetic conditions, disability, trauma, and injury to the physical and mental health and occupational performance of the individual.	Analyze the effects of heritable diseases, genetic conditions, disability, trauma, and injury to the physical and mental health and occupational performance of the individual.	Understand the effects of heritable diseases, genetic conditions, disability, trauma, and injury to the physical and mental health and occupational performance of the individual.
B.2.7.	Demonstrate task analysis in areas of occupation, performance skills, performance patterns, activity demands, context(s) and environments, and client factors to formulate an intervention plan.	Demonstrate task analysis in areas of occupation, performance skills, performance patterns, activity demands, context(s) and environments, and client factors to formulate an intervention plan.	Demonstrate task analysis in areas of occupation, performance skills, performance patterns, activity demands, context(s) and environments, and client factors to implement the intervention plan.
B.2.8.	Use sound judgment in regard to safety of self and others and adhere to safety regulations throughout the occupational therapy process as appropriate to the setting and scope of practice.	Use sound judgment in regard to safety of self and others and adhere to safety regulations throughout the occupational therapy process as appropriate to the setting and scope of practice.	Use sound judgment in regard to safety of self and others and adhere to safety regulations throughout the occupational therapy process as appropriate to the setting and scope of practice.
B.2.9.	Express support for the quality of life, well-being, and occupation of the individual, group, or population to promote physical and mental health and	Express support for the quality of life, well-being, and occupation of the individual, group, or population to promote physical and mental health and	Express support for the quality of life, well-being, and occupation of the individual, group, or population to promote physical and mental

(Continued)

Standard Number	Accreditation Standards for a Doctoral-Degree-Level Educational Program for the Occupational Therapist	Accreditation Standards for a Master's-Degree-Level Educational Program for the Occupational Therapist	Accreditation Standards for an Associate-Degree-Level Educational Program for the Occupational Therapy Assistant
	prevention of injury and disease considering the context (e.g., cultural, personal, temporal, virtual) and environment.	prevention of injury and disease considering the context (e.g., cultural, personal, temporal, virtual) and environment.	health and prevention of injury and disease considering the context (e.g., cultural, personal, temporal, virtual) and environment.
B.2.10.	Use clinical reasoning to explain the rationale for and use of compensatory strategies when desired life tasks cannot be performed.	Use clinical reasoning to explain the rationale for and use of compensatory strategies when desired life tasks cannot be performed.	Explain the need for and use of compensatory strategies when desired life tasks cannot be performed.
B.2.11.	Analyze, synthesize, evaluate, and apply models of occupational performance.	Analyze, synthesize, and apply models of occupational performance.	Identify interventions consistent with models of occupational performance.

B.3.0. OCCUPATIONAL THERAPY THEORETICAL PERSPECTIVES
The program must facilitate the development of the performance criteria listed below. The student will be able to

Standard Number	Doctoral-Degree-Level	Master's-Degree-Level	Associate-Degree-Level
B.3.1.	Evaluate and apply theories that underlie the practice of occupational therapy.	Apply theories that underlie the practice of occupational therapy.	Describe basic features of the theories that underlie the practice of occupational therapy.
B.3.2.	Compare, contrast, and integrate a variety of models of practice and frames of reference that are used in occupational therapy.	Compare and contrast models of practice and frames of reference that are used in occupational therapy.	Describe basic features of models of practice and frames of reference that are used in occupational therapy.
B.3.3.	Use theories, models of practice, and frames of reference to guide and inform evaluation and intervention.	Use theories, models of practice, and frames of reference to guide and inform evaluation and intervention.	(No related Standard)

(Continued)

84

Standard Number	Accreditation Standards for a Doctoral-Degree-Level Educational Program for the Occupational Therapist	Accreditation Standards for a Master's-Degree-Level Educational Program for the Occupational Therapist	Accreditation Standards for an Associate-Degree-Level Educational Program for the Occupational Therapy Assistant
B.3.4.	Analyze and discuss how occupational therapy history, occupational therapy theory, and the sociopolitical climate influence and are influenced by practice.	Analyze and discuss how occupational therapy history, occupational therapy theory, and the sociopolitical climate influence practice.	Discuss how occupational therapy history and occupational therapy theory, and the sociopolitical climate influence practice.
B.3.5.	Apply theoretical constructs to evaluation and intervention with various types of clients in a variety of practice contexts and environments, including population-based approaches, to analyze and effect meaningful occupation outcomes.	Apply theoretical constructs to evaluation and intervention with various types of clients in a variety of practice contexts and environments to analyze and effect meaningful occupation outcomes.	*(No related Standard)*
B.3.6.	Articulate the process of theory development in occupational therapy and its desired impact and influence on society.	Discuss the process of theory development and its importance to occupational therapy.	*(No related Standard)*
B.4.0.	**SCREENING, EVALUATION, AND REFERRAL** The process of screening, evaluation, referral, and diagnosis as related to occupational performance and participation must be culturally relevant and based on theoretical perspectives, models of practice, frames of reference, and available evidence. In addition, this process must consider the continuum of need from individuals to populations. The program must facilitate development of the performance criteria listed below. The student will be able to	**SCREENING, EVALUATION, AND REFERRAL** The process of screening, evaluation, and referral as related to occupational performance and participation must be culturally relevant and based on theoretical perspectives, models of practice, frames of reference, and available evidence. In addition, this process must consider the continuum of need from individuals to populations. The program must facilitate development of the performance criteria listed below. The student will be able to	**SCREENING AND EVALUATION** The process of screening and evaluation as related to occupational performance and participation must be conducted under the supervision of and in cooperation with the occupational therapist and must be culturally relevant and based on theoretical perspectives, models of practice, frames of reference, and available evidence. The program must facilitate development of the performance criteria listed below. The student will be able to

(Continued)

Standard Number	Accreditation Standards for a Doctoral-Degree-Level Educational Program for the Occupational Therapist	Accreditation Standards for a Master's-Degree-Level Educational Program for the Occupational Therapist	Accreditation Standards for an Associate-Degree-Level Educational Program for the Occupational Therapy Assistant
B.4.1.	Use standardized and nonstandardized screening and assessment tools to determine the need for occupational therapy intervention. These tools include, but are not limited to, specified screening tools; assessments; skilled observations; occupational histories; consultations with other professionals; and interviews with the client, family, significant others, and community.	Use standardized and nonstandardized screening and assessment tools to determine the need for occupational therapy intervention. These tools include, but are not limited to, specified screening tools; assessments; skilled observations; occupational histories; consultations with other professionals; and interviews with the client, family, significant others, and community.	Gather and share data for the purpose of screening and evaluation using methods including, but not limited to, specified screening tools; assessments; skilled observations; occupational histories; consultations with other professionals; and interviews with the client, family, and significant others.
B.4.2.	Select appropriate assessment tools on the basis of client needs, contextual factors, and psychometric properties of tests. These must be culturally relevant, based on available evidence, and incorporate use of occupation in the assessment process.	Select appropriate assessment tools on the basis of client needs, contextual factors, and psychometric properties of tests. These must be culturally relevant, based on available evidence, and incorporate use of occupation in the assessment process.	Administer selected assessments using appropriate procedures and protocols (including standardized formats) and use occupation for the purpose of assessment.
B.4.3.	Use appropriate procedures and protocols (including standardized formats) when administering assessments.	Use appropriate procedures and protocols (including standardized formats) when administering assessments.	(No related Standard)
B.4.4.	Evaluate client(s)' occupational performance in activities of daily living (ADLs), instrumental activities of daily living (IADLs), education, work, play, rest, sleep, leisure, and social participation. Evaluation of occupational performance using	Evaluate client(s)' occupational performance in activities of daily living (ADLs), instrumental activities of daily living (IADLs), education, work, play, rest, sleep, leisure, and social participation. Evaluation of occupational performance using	Gather and share data for the purpose of evaluating client(s)' occupational performance in activities of daily living (ADLs), instrumental activities of daily living (IADLs), education, work, play, rest, sleep, leisure, and social

(Continued)

Standard Number	Accreditation Standards for a Doctoral-Degree-Level Educational Program for the Occupational Therapist	Accreditation Standards for a Master's-Degree-Level Educational Program for the Occupational Therapist	Accreditation Standards for an Associate-Degree-Level Educational Program for the Occupational Therapy Assistant
	standardized and nonstandardized assessment tools includes • The occupational profile, including participation in activities that are meaningful and necessary for the client to carry out roles in home, work, and community environments. • Client factors, including values, beliefs, spirituality, body functions (e.g., neuromuscular, sensory and pain, visual, perceptual, cognitive, mental) and body structures (e.g., cardiovascular, digestive, nervous, genitourinary, integumentary systems). • Performance patterns (e.g., habits, routines, rituals, roles). • Context (e.g., cultural, personal, temporal, virtual) and environment (e.g., physical, social). • Performance skills, including motor and praxis skills, sensory–perceptual skills, emotional regulation skills, cognitive skills, and communication and social skills.	standardized and nonstandardized assessment tools includes • The occupational profile, including participation in activities that are meaningful and necessary for the client to carry out roles in home, work, and community environments. • Client factors, including values, beliefs, spirituality, body functions (e.g., neuromuscular, sensory and pain, visual, perceptual, cognitive, mental) and body structures (e.g., cardiovascular, digestive, nervous, genitourinary, integumentary systems). • Performance patterns (e.g., habits, routines, rituals, roles). • Context (e.g., cultural, personal, temporal, virtual) and environment (e.g., physical, social). • Performance skills, including motor and praxis skills, sensory–perceptual skills, emotional regulation skills, cognitive skills, and communication and social skills.	participation. Evaluation of occupational performance includes • The occupational profile, including participation in activities that are meaningful and necessary for the client to carry out roles in home, work, and community environments. • Client factors, including values, beliefs, spirituality, body functions (e.g., neuromuscular, sensory and pain, visual, perceptual, cognitive, mental) and body structures (e.g., cardiovascular, digestive, nervous, genitourinary, integumentary systems). • Performance patterns (e.g., habits, routines, rituals, roles). • Context (e.g., cultural, personal, temporal, virtual) and environment (e.g., physical, social). • Performance skills, including motor and praxis skills, sensory–perceptual skills, emotional regulation skills, cognitive skills, and communication and social skills.
B.4.5	Compare and contrast the role of the occupational therapist and occupational therapy assistant in the screening and evaluation process along with the importance of and rationale for supervision and collaborative work between the occupational therapist and occupational therapy assistant in that process.	Compare and contrast the role of the occupational therapist and occupational therapy assistant in the screening and evaluation process along with the importance of and rationale for supervision and collaborative work between the occupational therapist and occupational therapy assistant in that process.	Articulate the role of the occupational therapy assistant and occupational therapist in the screening and evaluation process along with the importance of and rationale for supervision and collaborative work between the occupational therapy assistant and occupational therapist in that process.

(Continued)

Standard Number	Accreditation Standards for a Doctoral-Degree-Level Educational Program for the Occupational Therapist	Accreditation Standards for a Master's-Degree-Level Educational Program for the Occupational Therapist	Accreditation Standards for an Associate-Degree-Level Educational Program for the Occupational Therapy Assistant
B.4.6.	Interpret criterion-referenced and norm-referenced standardized test scores on the basis of an understanding of sampling, normative data, standard and criterion scores, reliability, and validity.	Interpret criterion-referenced and norm-referenced standardized test scores on the basis of an understanding of sampling, normative data, standard and criterion scores, reliability, and validity.	(No related Standard)
B.4.7.	Consider factors that might bias assessment results, such as culture, disability status, and situational variables related to the individual and context.	Consider factors that might bias assessment results, such as culture, disability status, and situational variables related to the individual and context.	(No related Standard)
B.4.8.	Interpret the evaluation data in relation to accepted terminology of the profession, relevant theoretical frameworks, and interdisciplinary knowledge.	Interpret the evaluation data in relation to accepted terminology of the profession and relevant theoretical frameworks.	(No related Standard)
B.4.9.	Evaluate appropriateness and discuss mechanisms for referring clients for additional evaluation to specialists who are internal and external to the profession.	Evaluate appropriateness and discuss mechanisms for referring clients for additional evaluation to specialists who are internal and external to the profession.	Identify when to recommend to the occupational therapist the need for referring clients for additional evaluation.
B.4.10.	Document occupational therapy services to ensure accountability of service provision and to meet standards for reimbursement of services, adhering to the requirements of applicable facility, local, state, federal, and reimbursement agencies. Documentation must effectively communicate the need and rationale for occupational therapy services.	Document occupational therapy services to ensure accountability of service provision and to meet standards for reimbursement of services, adhering to the requirements of applicable facility, local, state, federal, and reimbursement agencies. Documentation must effectively communicate the need and rationale for occupational therapy services.	Document occupational therapy services to ensure accountability of service provision and to meet standards for reimbursement of services, adhering to the requirements of applicable facility, local, state, federal, and reimbursement agencies. Documentation must effectively communicate the need and rationale for occupational therapy services.

(Continued)

(Continued)

Standard Number	Accreditation Standards for a Doctoral-Degree-Level Educational Program for the Occupational Therapist	Accreditation Standards for a Master's-Degree-Level Educational Program for the Occupational Therapist	Accreditation Standards for an Associate-Degree-Level Educational Program for the Occupational Therapy Assistant
B.4.11.	Articulate screening and evaluation processes for all practice areas. Use evidence-based reasoning to analyze, synthesize, evaluate, and diagnose problems related to occupational performance and participation.	*(No related Standard)*	*(No related Standard)*
B.5.0.	**INTERVENTION PLAN: FORMULATION AND IMPLEMENTATION** **The process of formulation and implementation of the therapeutic intervention plan to facilitate occupational performance and participation must be culturally relevant; reflective of current and emerging occupational therapy practice; based on available evidence; and based on theoretical perspectives, models of practice, and frames of reference. In addition, this process must consider the continuum of need from individual-to population-based interventions. The program must facilitate development of the performance criteria listed below. The student will be able to**	**INTERVENTION PLAN: FORMULATION AND IMPLEMENTATION** **The process of formulation and implementation of the therapeutic intervention plan to facilitate occupational performance and participation must be culturally relevant; reflective of current occupational therapy practice; based on available evidence; and based on theoretical perspectives, models of practice, and frames of reference. The program must facilitate development of the performance criteria listed below. The student will be able to**	**INTERVENTION AND IMPLEMENTATION** **The process of intervention to facilitate occupational performance and participation must be done under the supervision of and in cooperation with the occupational therapist and must be culturally relevant, reflective of current occupational therapy practice, and based on available evidence. The program must facilitate development of the performance criteria listed below. The student will be able to**
B.5.1.	Use evaluation findings to diagnose occupational performance and participation based on appropriate theoretical approaches, models of practice, frames of reference, and interdisciplinary knowledge. Develop occupation-based intervention	Use evaluation findings based on appropriate theoretical approaches, models of practice, and frames of reference to develop occupation-based intervention plans and strategies (including goals and methods to achieve them) on the	Assist with the development of occupation-based intervention plans and strategies (including goals and methods to achieve them) on the basis of the stated needs of the client as well as data gathered during the evaluation

Standard Number	Accreditation Standards for a Doctoral-Degree-Level Educational Program for the Occupational Therapist	Accreditation Standards for a Master's-Degree-Level Educational Program for the Occupational Therapist	Accreditation Standards for an Associate-Degree-Level Educational Program for the Occupational Therapy Assistant
	plans and strategies (including goals and methods to achieve them) on the basis of the stated needs of the client as well as data gathered during the evaluation process in collaboration with the client and others. Intervention plans and strategies must be culturally relevant, reflective of current occupational therapy practice, and based on available evidence. Interventions address the following components: • The occupational profile, including participation in activities that are meaningful and necessary for the client to carry out roles in home, work, and community environments. • Client factors, including values, beliefs, spirituality, body functions (e.g., neuromuscular, sensory and pain, visual, perceptual, cognitive, mental) and body structures (e.g., cardiovascular, digestive, nervous, genitourinary, integumentary systems). • Performance patterns (e.g., habits, routines, rituals, roles). • Context (e.g., cultural, personal, temporal, virtual) and environment (e.g., physical, social). • Performance skills, including motor and praxis skills, sensory–perceptual skills, emotional regulation skills, cognitive skills, and communication and social skills.	basis of the stated needs of the client as well as data gathered during the evaluation process in collaboration with the client and others. Intervention plans and strategies must be culturally relevant, reflective of current occupational therapy practice, and based on available evidence. Interventions address the following components: • The occupational profile, including participation in activities that are meaningful and necessary for the client to carry out roles in home, work, and community environments. • Client factors, including values, beliefs, spirituality, body functions (e.g., neuromuscular, sensory and pain, visual, perceptual, cognitive, mental) and body structures (e.g., cardiovascular, digestive, nervous, genitourinary, integumentary systems). • Performance patterns (e.g., habits, routines, rituals, roles). • Context (e.g., cultural, personal, temporal, virtual) and environment (e.g., physical, social). • Performance skills, including motor and praxis skills, sensory–perceptual skills, emotional regulation skills, cognitive skills, and communication and social skills.	process in collaboration with the client and others. Intervention plans and strategies must be culturally relevant, reflective of current occupational therapy practice, and based on available evidence. Interventions address the following components: • The occupational profile, including participation in activities that are meaningful and necessary for the client to carry out roles in home, work, and community environments. • Client factors, including values, beliefs, spirituality, body functions (e.g., neuromuscular, sensory and pain, visual, perceptual, cognitive, mental) and body structures (e.g., cardiovascular, digestive, nervous, genitourinary, integumentary systems). • Performance patterns (e.g., habits, routines, rituals, roles). • Context (e.g., cultural, personal, temporal, virtual) and environment (e.g., physical, social). • Performance skills, including motor and praxis skills, sensory–perceptual skills, emotional regulation skills, cognitive skills, and communication and social skills.

(Continued)

Standard Number	Accreditation Standards for a Doctoral-Degree-Level Educational Program for the Occupational Therapist	Accreditation Standards for a Master's-Degree-Level Educational Program for the Occupational Therapist	Accreditation Standards for an Associate-Degree-Level Educational Program for the Occupational Therapy Assistant
B.5.2.	Select and provide direct occupational therapy interventions and procedures to enhance safety, health and wellness, and performance in ADLs, IADLs, education, work, play, rest, sleep, leisure, and social participation.	Select and provide direct occupational therapy interventions and procedures to enhance safety, health and wellness, and performance in ADLs, IADLs, education, work, play, rest, sleep, leisure, and social participation.	Select and provide direct occupational therapy interventions and procedures to enhance safety, health and wellness, and performance in ADLs, IADLs, education, work, play, rest, sleep, leisure, and social participation.
B.5.3.	Provide therapeutic use of occupation, exercises, and activities (e.g., occupation-based intervention, purposeful activity, preparatory methods).	Provide therapeutic use of occupation, exercises, and activities (e.g., occupation-based intervention, purposeful activity, preparatory methods).	Provide therapeutic use of occupation, exercises, and activities (e.g., occupation-based intervention, purposeful activity, preparatory methods).
B.5.4.	Design and implement group interventions based on principles of group development and group dynamics across the lifespan.	Design and implement group interventions based on principles of group development and group dynamics across the lifespan.	Implement group interventions based on principles of group development and group dynamics across the lifespan.
B.5.5.	Provide training in self-care, self-management, health management and maintenance, home management, and community and work integration.	Provide training in self-care, self-management, health management and maintenance, home management, and community and work integration.	Provide training in self-care, self-management, health management and maintenance, home management, and community and work integration.
B.5.6.	Provide development, remediation, and compensation for physical, mental, cognitive, perceptual, neuromuscular, behavioral skills, and sensory functions (e.g., vision, tactile, auditory, gustatory, olfactory, pain, temperature, pressure, vestibular, proprioception).	Provide development, remediation, and compensation for physical, mental, cognitive, perceptual, neuromuscular, behavioral skills, and sensory functions (e.g., vision, tactile, auditory, gustatory, olfactory, pain, temperature, pressure, vestibular, proprioception).	Provide development, remediation, and compensation for physical, mental, cognitive, perceptual, neuromuscular, behavioral skills, and sensory functions (e.g., vision, tactile, auditory, gustatory, olfactory, pain, temperature, pressure, vestibular, proprioception).

(Continued)

Standard Number	Accreditation Standards for a Doctoral-Degree-Level Educational Program for the Occupational Therapist	Accreditation Standards for a Master's-Degree-Level Educational Program for the Occupational Therapist	Accreditation Standards for an Associate-Degree-Level Educational Program for the Occupational Therapy Assistant
B.5.7.	Demonstrate therapeutic use of self, including one's personality, insights, perceptions, and judgments, as part of the therapeutic process in both individual and group interaction.	Demonstrate therapeutic use of self, including one's personality, insights, perceptions, and judgments, as part of the therapeutic process in both individual and group interaction.	Demonstrate therapeutic use of self, including one's personality, insights, perceptions, and judgments, as part of the therapeutic process in both individual and group interaction.
B.5.8.	Develop and implement intervention strategies to remediate and/or compensate for cognitive deficits that affect occupational performance.	Develop and implement intervention strategies to remediate and/or compensate for cognitive deficits that affect occupational performance.	Implement intervention strategies to remediate and/or compensate for cognitive deficits that affect occupational performance.
B.5.9.	Evaluate and adapt processes or environments (e.g., home, work, school, community) applying ergonomic principles and principles of environmental modification.	Evaluate and adapt processes or environments (e.g., home, work, school, community) applying ergonomic principles and principles of environmental modification.	Adapt environments (e.g., home, work, school, community) and processes, including the application of ergonomic principles.
B.5.10.	Articulate principles of and be able to design, fabricate, apply, fit, and train in assistive technologies and devices (e.g., electronic aids to daily living, seating and positioning systems) used to enhance occupational performance and foster participation and well-being.	Articulate principles of and be able to design, fabricate, apply, fit, and train in assistive technologies and devices (e.g., electronic aids to daily living, seating and positioning systems) used to enhance occupational performance and foster participation and well-being.	Articulate principles of and demonstrate strategies with assistive technologies and devices (e.g., electronic aids to daily living, seating and positioning systems) used to enhance occupational performance and foster participation and well-being.
B.5.11.	Provide design, fabrication, application, fitting, and training in orthotic devices used to enhance occupational performance and participation. Train in the use of prosthetic devices, based on scientific principles of kinesiology, biomechanics, and physics.	Provide design, fabrication, application, fitting, and training in orthotic devices used to enhance occupational performance and participation. Train in the use of prosthetic devices, based on scientific principles of kinesiology, biomechanics, and physics.	Provide fabrication, application, fitting, and training in orthotic devices used to enhance occupational performance and participation, and training in the use of prosthetic devices.

(Continued)

Standard Number	Accreditation Standards for a Doctoral-Degree-Level Educational Program for the Occupational Therapist	Accreditation Standards for a Master's-Degree-Level Educational Program for the Occupational Therapist	Accreditation Standards for an Associate-Degree-Level Educational Program for the Occupational Therapy Assistant
B.5.12.	Provide recommendations and training in techniques to enhance functional mobility, including physical transfers, wheelchair management, and mobility devices.	Provide recommendations and training in techniques to enhance functional mobility, including physical transfers, wheelchair management, and mobility devices.	Provide training in techniques to enhance functional mobility, including physical transfers, wheelchair management, and mobility devices.
B.5.13.	Provide recommendations and training in techniques to enhance community mobility, including public transportation, community access, and issues related to driver rehabilitation.	Provide recommendations and training in techniques to enhance community mobility, including public transportation, community access, and issues related to driver rehabilitation.	Provide training in techniques to enhance community mobility, including public transportation, community access, and issues related to driver rehabilitation.
B.5.14.	Provide management of feeding, eating, and swallowing to enable performance (including the process of bringing food or fluids from the plate or cup to the mouth, the ability to keep and manipulate food or fluid in the mouth, and swallowing assessment and management) and train others in precautions and techniques while considering client and contextual factors.	Provide management of feeding, eating, and swallowing to enable performance (including the process of bringing food or fluids from the plate or cup to the mouth, the ability to keep and manipulate food or fluid in the mouth, and swallowing assessment and management) and train others in precautions and techniques while considering client and contextual factors.	Enable feeding and eating performance (including the process of bringing food or fluids from the plate or cup to the mouth, the ability to keep and manipulate food or fluid in the mouth, and the initiation of swallowing) and train others in precautions and techniques while considering client and contextual factors.
B.5.15.	Demonstrate safe and effective application of superficial thermal and mechanical modalities as a preparatory measure to manage pain and improve occupational performance, including foundational knowledge, underlying principles, indications, contraindications, and precautions.	Demonstrate safe and effective application of superficial thermal and mechanical modalities as a preparatory measure to manage pain and improve occupational performance, including foundational knowledge, underlying principles, indications, contraindications, and precautions.	Recognize the use of superficial thermal and mechanical modalities as a preparatory measure to improve occupational performance. On the basis of the intervention plan, demonstrate safe and effective administration of superficial thermal and mechanical modalities to achieve established goals while adhering to contraindications and precautions.

(Continued)

Standard Number	Accreditation Standards for a Doctoral-Degree-Level Educational Program for the Occupational Therapist	Accreditation Standards for a Master's-Degree-Level Educational Program for the Occupational Therapist	Accreditation Standards for an Associate-Degree-Level Educational Program for the Occupational Therapy Assistant
B.5.16.	Explain the use of deep thermal and electrotherapeutic modalities as a preparatory measure to improve occupational performance, including indications, contraindications, and precautions.	Explain the use of deep thermal and electrotherapeutic modalities as a preparatory measure to improve occupational performance, including indications, contraindications, and precautions.	(No related Standard)
B.5.17.	Develop and promote the use of appropriate home and community programming to support performance in the client's natural environment and participation in all contexts relevant to the client.	Develop and promote the use of appropriate home and community programming to support performance in the client's natural environment and participation in all contexts relevant to the client.	Promote the use of appropriate home and community programming to support performance in the client's natural environment and participation in all contexts relevant to the client.
B.5.18.	Demonstrate an understanding of health literacy and the ability to educate and train the client, caregiver, family and significant others, and communities to facilitate skills in areas of occupation as well as prevention, health maintenance, health promotion, and safety.	Demonstrate an understanding of health literacy and the ability to educate and train the client, caregiver, family and significant others, and communities to facilitate skills in areas of occupation as well as prevention, health maintenance, health promotion, and safety.	Demonstrate an understanding of health literacy and the ability to educate and train the client, caregiver, and family and significant others to facilitate skills in areas of occupation as well as prevention, health maintenance, health promotion, and safety.
B.5.19.	Apply the principles of the teaching–learning process using educational methods to design experiences to address the needs of the client, family, significant others, communities, colleagues, other health providers, and the public.	Apply the principles of the teaching–learning process using educational methods to design experiences to address the needs of the client, family, significant others, colleagues, other health providers, and the public.	Use the teaching–learning process with the client, family, significant others, colleagues, other health providers, and the public. Collaborate with the occupational therapist and learner to identify appropriate educational methods.
B.5.20.	Effectively interact through written, oral, and nonverbal communication with the client, family, significant others, communities, colleagues, other health providers, and the public in a professionally acceptable manner.	Effectively interact through written, oral, and nonverbal communication with the client, family, significant others, colleagues, other health providers, and the public in a professionally acceptable manner.	Effectively interact through written, oral, and nonverbal communication with the client, family, significant others, colleagues, other health providers, and the public in a professionally acceptable manner.

(Continued)

Standard Number	Accreditation Standards for a Doctoral-Degree-Level Educational Program for the Occupational Therapist	Accreditation Standards for a Master's-Degree-Level Educational Program for the Occupational Therapist	Accreditation Standards for an Associate-Degree-Level Educational Program for the Occupational Therapy Assistant
B.5.21.	Effectively communicate, coordinate, and work interprofessionally with those who provide services to individuals, organizations, and/or populations in order to clarify each member's responsibility in executing components of an intervention plan.	Effectively communicate and work interprofessionally with those who provide services to individuals, organizations, and/or populations in order to clarify each member's responsibility in executing an intervention plan.	Effectively communicate and work interprofessionally with those who provide services to individuals and groups in order to clarify each member's responsibility in executing an intervention plan.
B.5.22.	Refer to specialists (both internal and external to the profession) for consultation and intervention.	Refer to specialists (both internal and external to the profession) for consultation and intervention.	Recognize and communicate the need to refer to specialists (both internal and external to the profession) for consultation and intervention.
B.5.23.	Grade and adapt the environment, tools, materials, occupations, and interventions to reflect the changing needs of the client, the sociocultural context, and technological advances.	Grade and adapt the environment, tools, materials, occupations, and interventions to reflect the changing needs of the client, the sociocultural context, and technological advances.	Grade and adapt the environment, tools, materials, occupations, and interventions to reflect the changing needs of the client and the sociocultural context.
B.5.24.	Select and teach compensatory strategies, such as use of technology and adaptations to the environment, that support performance, participation, and well-being.	Select and teach compensatory strategies, such as use of technology and adaptations to the environment, that support performance, participation, and well-being.	Teach compensatory strategies, such as use of technology and adaptations to the environment, that support performance, participation, and well-being.
B.5.25.	Identify and demonstrate techniques in skills of supervision and collaboration with occupational therapy assistants and other professionals on therapeutic interventions.	Identify and demonstrate techniques in skills of supervision and collaboration with occupational therapy assistants and other professionals on therapeutic interventions.	Demonstrate skills of collaboration with occupational therapists and other professionals on therapeutic interventions.

(Continued)

Standard Number	Accreditation Standards for a Doctoral-Degree-Level Educational Program for the Occupational Therapist	Accreditation Standards for a Master's-Degree-Level Educational Program for the Occupational Therapist	Accreditation Standards for an Associate-Degree-Level Educational Program for the Occupational Therapy Assistant
B.5.26.	Demonstrate use of the consultative process with groups, programs, organizations, or communities.	Understand when and how to use the consultative process with groups, programs, organizations, or communities.	Understand when and how to use the consultative process with specific consumers or consumer groups as directed by an occupational therapist.
B.5.27.	Demonstrate care coordination, case management, and transition services in traditional and emerging practice environments.	Describe the role of the occupational therapist in care coordination, case management, and transition services in traditional and emerging practice environments.	Describe the role of the occupational therapy assistant in care coordination, case management, and transition services in traditional and emerging practice environments.
B.5.28.	Monitor and reassess, in collaboration with the client, caregiver, family, and significant others, the effect of occupational therapy intervention and the need for continued or modified intervention.	Monitor and reassess, in collaboration with the client, caregiver, family, and significant others, the effect of occupational therapy intervention and the need for continued or modified intervention.	Monitor and reassess, in collaboration with the client, caregiver, family, and significant others, the effect of occupational therapy intervention and the need for continued or modified intervention, and communicate the identified needs to the occupational therapist.
B.5.29.	Plan for discharge, in collaboration with the client, by reviewing the needs of the client, caregiver, family, and significant others; available resources; and discharge environment. This process includes, but is not limited to, identification of client's current status within the continuum of care; identification of community, human, and fiscal resources; recommendations for environmental adaptations; and home programming to facilitate the client's progression along the continuum toward outcome goals.	Plan for discharge, in collaboration with the client, by reviewing the needs of the client, caregiver, family, and significant others; available resources; and discharge environment. This process includes, but is not limited to, identification of client's current status within the continuum of care; identification of community, human, and fiscal resources; recommendations for environmental adaptations; and home programming to facilitate the client's progression along the continuum toward outcome goals.	Facilitate discharge planning by reviewing the needs of the client, caregiver, family, and significant others; available resources; and discharge environment, and identify those needs to the occupational therapist, client, and others involved in discharge planning. This process includes, but is not limited to, identification of community, human, and fiscal resources; recommendations for environmental adaptations; and home programming.

(Continued)

Standard Number	Accreditation Standards for a Doctoral-Degree-Level Educational Program for the Occupational Therapist	Accreditation Standards for a Master's-Degree-Level Educational Program for the Occupational Therapist	Accreditation Standards for an Associate-Degree-Level Educational Program for the Occupational Therapy Assistant
B.5.30.	Organize, collect, and analyze data in a systematic manner for evaluation of practice outcomes. Report evaluation results and modify practice as needed to improve client outcomes.	Organize, collect, and analyze data in a systematic manner for evaluation of practice outcomes. Report evaluation results and modify practice as needed to improve client outcomes.	Under the direction of an administrator, manager, or occupational therapist, collect, organize, and report on data for evaluation of client outcomes.
B.5.31.	Terminate occupational therapy services when stated outcomes have been achieved or it has been determined that they cannot be achieved. This process includes developing a summary of occupational therapy outcomes, appropriate recommendations, and referrals and discussion of postdischarge needs with the client and with appropriate others.	Terminate occupational therapy services when stated outcomes have been achieved or it has been determined that they cannot be achieved. This process includes developing a summary of occupational therapy outcomes, appropriate recommendations, and referrals and discussion of post-discharge needs with the client and with appropriate others.	Recommend to the occupational therapist the need for termination of occupational therapy services when stated outcomes have been achieved or it has been determined that they cannot be achieved. Assist with developing a summary of occupational therapy outcomes, recommendations, and referrals.
B.5.32.	Document occupational therapy services to ensure accountability of service provision and to meet standards for reimbursement of services. Documentation must effectively communicate the need and rationale for occupational therapy services and must be appropriate to the context in which the service is delivered.	Document occupational therapy services to ensure accountability of service provision and to meet standards for reimbursement of services. Documentation must effectively communicate the need and rationale for occupational therapy services and must be appropriate to the context in which the service is delivered.	Document occupational therapy services to ensure accountability of service provision and to meet standards for reimbursement of services. Documentation must effectively communicate the need and rationale for occupational therapy services and must be appropriate to the context in which the service is delivered.
B.5.33.	Provide population-based occupational therapy intervention that addresses occupational needs as identified by a community.	*(No related Standard)*	*(No related Standard)*

(Continued)

B.6.0. CONTEXT OF SERVICE DELIVERY

Context of service delivery includes the knowledge and understanding of the various contexts, such as professional, social, cultural, political, economic, and ecological, in which occupational therapy services are provided. The program must facilitate development of the performance criteria listed below. The student will be able to

Standard Number	Accreditation Standards for a Doctoral-Degree-Level Educational Program for the Occupational Therapist	Accreditation Standards for a Master's-Degree-Level Educational Program for the Occupational Therapist	Accreditation Standards for an Associate-Degree-Level Educational Program for the Occupational Therapy Assistant
B.6.1.	Evaluate and address the various contexts of health care, education, community, political, and social systems as they relate to the practice of occupational therapy.	Evaluate and address the various contexts of health care, education, community, political, and social systems as they relate to the practice of occupational therapy.	Describe the contexts of health care, education, community, and social systems as they relate to the practice of occupational therapy.
B.6.2.	Analyze the current policy issues and the social, economic, political, geographic, and demographic factors that influence the various contexts for practice of occupational therapy.	Analyze the current policy issues and the social, economic, political, geographic, and demographic factors that influence the various contexts for practice of occupational therapy.	Identify the potential impact of current policy issues and the social, economic, political, geographic, or demographic factors on the practice of occupational therapy.
B.6.3.	Integrate current social, economic, political, geographic, and demographic factors to promote policy development and the provision of occupational therapy services.	Integrate current social, economic, political, geographic, and demographic factors to promote policy development and the provision of occupational therapy services.	(No related Standard)
B.6.4.	Advocate for changes in service delivery policies, effect changes in the system, and identify opportunities to address societal needs.	Articulate the role and responsibility of the practitioner to advocate for changes in service delivery policies, to effect changes in the system, and to identify opportunities in emerging practice areas.	Identify the role and responsibility of the practitioner to advocate for changes in service delivery policies, to effect changes in the system, and to recognize opportunities in emerging practice areas.

(Continued)

Standard Number	Accreditation Standards for a Doctoral-Degree-Level Educational Program for the Occupational Therapist	Accreditation Standards for a Master's-Degree-Level Educational Program for the Occupational Therapist	Accreditation Standards for an Associate-Degree-Level Educational Program for the Occupational Therapy Assistant
B.6.5.	Analyze the trends in models of service delivery, including, but not limited to, medical, educational, community, and social models, and their potential effect on the practice of occupational therapy.	Analyze the trends in models of service delivery, including, but not limited to, medical, educational, community, and social models, and their potential effect on the practice of occupational therapy.	*(No related Standard)*
B.6.6.	Integrate national and international resources in education, research, practice, and policy development.	Utilize national and international resources in making assessment or intervention choices and appreciate the influence of international occupational therapy contributions to education, research, and practice.	*(No related Standard)*
B.7.0.	**LEADERSHIP AND MANAGEMENT** **Leadership and management skills include principles and applications of leadership and management theory. The program must facilitate development of the performance criteria listed below. The student will be able to**	**MANAGEMENT OF OCCUPATIONAL THERAPY SERVICES** **Management of occupational therapy services includes the application of principles of management and systems in the provision of occupational therapy services to individuals and organizations. The program must facilitate development of the performance criteria listed below. The student will be able to**	**ASSISTANCE WITH MANAGEMENT OF OCCUPATIONAL THERAPY SERVICES** **Assistance with management of occupational therapy services includes the application of principles of management and systems in the provision of occupational therapy services to individuals and organizations. The program must facilitate development of the performance criteria listed below. The student will be able to**
B.7.1.	Identify and evaluate the impact of contextual factors on the management and delivery of occupational therapy services for individuals and populations.	Describe and discuss the impact of contextual factors on the management and delivery of occupational therapy services.	Identify the impact of contextual factors on the management and delivery of occupational therapy services.

(Continued)

Standard Number	Accreditation Standards for a Doctoral-Degree-Level Educational Program for the Occupational Therapist	Accreditation Standards for a Master's-Degree-Level Educational Program for the Occupational Therapist	Accreditation Standards for an Associate-Degree-Level Educational Program for the Occupational Therapy Assistant
B.7.2.	Identify and evaluate the systems and structures that create federal and state legislation and regulations and their implications and effects on practice and policy.	Describe the systems and structures that create federal and state legislation and regulations and their implications and effects on practice.	Identify the systems and structures that create federal and state legislation and regulations and their implications and effects on practice.
B.7.3.	Demonstrate knowledge of applicable national requirements for credentialing and requirements for licensure, certification, or registration under state laws.	Demonstrate knowledge of applicable national requirements for credentialing and requirements for licensure, certification, or registration under state laws.	Demonstrate knowledge of applicable national requirements for credentialing and requirements for licensure, certification, or registration under state laws.
B.7.4.	Demonstrate knowledge of various reimbursement systems (e.g., federal, state, third party, private payer), appeals mechanisms, and documentation requirements that affect society and the practice of occupational therapy.	Demonstrate knowledge of various reimbursement systems (e.g., federal, state, third party, private payer), appeals mechanisms, and documentation requirements that affect the practice of occupational therapy.	Demonstrate knowledge of various reimbursement systems (e.g., federal, state, third party, private payer) and documentation requirements that affect the practice of occupational therapy.
B.7.5.	Demonstrate leadership skills in the ability to plan, develop, organize, and market the delivery of services to include the determination of programmatic needs and service delivery options and formulation and management of staffing for effective service provision.	Demonstrate the ability to plan, develop, organize, and market the delivery of services to include the determination of programmatic needs and service delivery options and formulation and management of staffing for effective service provision.	Demonstrate the ability to participate in the development, marketing, and management of service delivery options.
B.7.6.	Demonstrate leadership skills in the ability to design ongoing processes for quality improvement (e.g., outcome studies analysis) and develop program changes as needed to ensure quality of services and to direct administrative changes.	Demonstrate the ability to design ongoing processes for quality improvement (e.g., outcome studies analysis) and develop program changes as needed to ensure quality of services and to direct administrative changes.	Participate in the documentation of ongoing processes for quality improvement and implement program changes as needed to ensure quality of services.

(Continued)

(Continued)

Standard Number	Accreditation Standards for a Doctoral-Degree-Level Educational Program for the Occupational Therapist	Accreditation Standards for a Master's-Degree-Level Educational Program for the Occupational Therapist	Accreditation Standards for an Associate-Degree-Level Educational Program for the Occupational Therapy Assistant
B.7.7.	Develop strategies for effective, competency-based legal and ethical supervision of occupational therapy and non–occupational therapy personnel.	Develop strategies for effective, competency-based legal and ethical supervision of occupational therapy and non–occupational therapy personnel.	Identify strategies for effective, competency-based legal and ethical supervision of nonprofessional personnel.
B.7.8.	Describe the ongoing professional responsibility for providing fieldwork education and the criteria for becoming a fieldwork educator.	Describe the ongoing professional responsibility for providing fieldwork education and the criteria for becoming a fieldwork educator.	Describe the ongoing professional responsibility for providing fieldwork education and the criteria for becoming a fieldwork educator.
B.7.9.	Demonstrate knowledge of and the ability to write program development plans for provision of occupational therapy services to individuals and populations.	*(No related Standard)*	*(No related Standard)*
B.7.10.	Identify and adapt existing models or develop new service provision models to respond to policy, regulatory agencies, and reimbursement and compliance standards.	*(No related Standard)*	*(No related Standard)*
B.7.11.	Identify and develop strategies to enable occupational therapy to respond to society's changing needs.	*(No related Standard)*	*(No related Standard)*
B.7.12.	Identify and implement strategies to promote staff development that are based on evaluation of the personal and professional abilities and competencies of supervised staff as they relate to job responsibilities.	*(No related Standard)*	*(No related Standard)*

Standard Number	Accreditation Standards for a Doctoral-Degree-Level Educational Program for the Occupational Therapist	Accreditation Standards for a Master's-Degree-Level Educational Program for the Occupational Therapist	Accreditation Standards for an Associate-Degree-Level Educational Program for the Occupational Therapy Assistant
B.8.0. SCHOLARSHIP Promotion of scholarly endeavors will serve to describe and interpret the scope of the profession, establish new knowledge, and interpret and apply this knowledge to practice. The program must facilitate development of the performance criteria listed below. The student will be able to			
B.8.1.	Articulate the importance of how scholarly activities contribute to the development of a body of knowledge relevant to the profession of occupational therapy.	Articulate the importance of how scholarly activities contribute to the development of a body of knowledge relevant to the profession of occupational therapy.	Articulate the importance of how scholarly activities and literature contribute to the development of the profession.
B.8.2.	Effectively locate, understand, critique, and evaluate information, including the quality of evidence.	Effectively locate, understand, critique, and evaluate information, including the quality of evidence.	Effectively locate and understand information, including the quality of the source of information.
B.8.3.	Use scholarly literature to make evidence-based decisions.	Use scholarly literature to make evidence-based decisions.	Use professional literature to make evidence-based practice decisions in collaboration with the occupational therapist.
B.8.4.	Select, apply, and interpret basic descriptive, correlational, and inferential quantitative statistics and code, analyze, and synthesize qualitative data.	Understand and use basic descriptive, correlational, and inferential quantitative statistics and code, analyze, and synthesize qualitative data.	*(No related Standard)*
B.8.5.	Understand and critique the validity of research studies, including their design (both quantitative and qualitative) and methodology.	Understand and critique the validity of research studies, including their design (both quantitative and qualitative) and methodology.	*(No related Standard)*

(Continued)

(Continued)

Standard Number	Accreditation Standards for a Doctoral-Degree-Level Educational Program for the Occupational Therapist	Accreditation Standards for a Master's-Degree-Level Educational Program for the Occupational Therapist	Accreditation Standards for an Associate-Degree-Level Educational Program for the Occupational Therapy Assistant
B.8.6.	Design a scholarly proposal that includes the research question, relevant literature, sample, design, measurement, and data analysis.	Demonstrate the skills necessary to design a scholarly proposal that includes the research question, relevant literature, sample, design, measurement, and data analysis.	*(No related Standard)*
B.8.7.	Implement a scholarly study that evaluates professional practice, service delivery, and/or professional issues (e.g., Scholarship of Integration, Scholarship of Application, Scholarship of Teaching and Learning).	Participate in scholarly activities that evaluate professional practice, service delivery, and/or professional issues (e.g., Scholarship of Integration, Scholarship of Application, Scholarship of Teaching and Learning).	Identify how scholarly activities can be used to evaluate professional practice, service delivery, and/or professional issues (e.g., Scholarship of Integration, Scholarship of Application, Scholarship of Teaching and Learning).
B.8.8.	Write scholarly reports appropriate for presentation or for publication in a peer-reviewed journal. Examples of scholarly reports would include position papers, white papers, and persuasive discussion papers.	Demonstrate skills necessary to write a scholarly report in a format for presentation or publication.	Demonstrate the skills to read and understand a scholarly report.
B.8.9.	Demonstrate an understanding of the process of locating and securing grants and how grants can serve as a fiscal resource for scholarly activities.	Demonstrate an understanding of the process of locating and securing grants and how grants can serve as a fiscal resource for scholarly activities.	*(No related Standard)*
B.8.10.	Complete a culminating project that relates theory to practice and demonstrates synthesis of advanced knowledge in a practice area.	*(No related Standard)*	*(No related Standard)*

B.9.0. PROFESSIONAL ETHICS, VALUES, AND RESPONSIBILITIES

Professional ethics, values, and responsibilities include an understanding and appreciation of ethics and values of the profession of occupational therapy. The program must facilitate development of the performance criteria listed below. The student will be able to

Standard Number	Accreditation Standards for a Doctoral-Degree-Level Educational Program for the Occupational Therapist	Accreditation Standards for a Master's-Degree-Level Educational Program for the Occupational Therapist	Accreditation Standards for an Associate-Degree-Level Educational Program for the Occupational Therapy Assistant
B.9.1.	Demonstrate knowledge and understanding of the American Occupational Therapy Association (AOTA) *Occupational Therapy Code of Ethics and Ethics Standards* and AOTA *Standards of Practice* and use them as a guide for ethical decision making in professional interactions, client interventions, and employment settings.	Demonstrate knowledge and understanding of the American Occupational Therapy Association (AOTA) *Occupational Therapy Code of Ethics and Ethics Standards* and AOTA *Standards of Practice* and use them as a guide for ethical decision making in professional interactions, client interventions, and employment settings.	Demonstrate knowledge and understanding of the American Occupational Therapy Association (AOTA) *Occupational Therapy Code of Ethics and Ethics Standards* and AOTA *Standards of Practice* and use them as a guide for ethical decision making in professional interactions, client interventions, and employment settings.
B.9.2.	Discuss and justify how the role of a professional is enhanced by knowledge of and involvement in international, national, state, and local occupational therapy associations and related professional associations.	Discuss and justify how the role of a professional is enhanced by knowledge of and involvement in international, national, state, and local occupational therapy associations and related professional associations.	Explain and give examples of how the role of a professional is enhanced by knowledge of and involvement in international, national, state, and local occupational therapy associations and related professional associations.
B.9.3.	Promote occupational therapy by educating other professionals, service providers, consumers, third-party payers, regulatory bodies, and the public.	Promote occupational therapy by educating other professionals, service providers, consumers, third-party payers, regulatory bodies, and the public.	Promote occupational therapy by educating other professionals, service providers, consumers, third-party payers, regulatory bodies, and the public.
B.9.4.	Identify and develop strategies for ongoing professional development to ensure that practice is consistent with current and accepted standards.	Discuss strategies for ongoing professional development to ensure that practice is consistent with current and accepted standards.	Discuss strategies for ongoing professional development to ensure that practice is consistent with current and accepted standards.

(Continued)

104

Standard Number	Accreditation Standards for a Doctoral-Degree-Level Educational Program for the Occupational Therapist	Accreditation Standards for a Master's-Degree-Level Educational Program for the Occupational Therapist	Accreditation Standards for an Associate-Degree-Level Educational Program for the Occupational Therapy Assistant
B.9.5.	Discuss professional responsibilities related to liability issues under current models of service provision.	Discuss professional responsibilities related to liability issues under current models of service provision.	Identify professional responsibilities related to liability issues under current models of service provision.
B.9.6.	Discuss and evaluate personal and professional abilities and competencies as they relate to job responsibilities.	Discuss and evaluate personal and professional abilities and competencies as they relate to job responsibilities.	Identify personal and professional abilities and competencies as they relate to job responsibilities.
B.9.7.	Discuss and justify the varied roles of the occupational therapist as a practitioner, educator, researcher, policy developer, program developer, advocate, administrator, consultant, and entrepreneur.	Discuss and justify the varied roles of the occupational therapist as a practitioner, educator, researcher, consultant, and entrepreneur.	Identify and appreciate the varied roles of the occupational therapy assistant as a practitioner, educator, and research assistant.
B.9.8.	Explain and justify the importance of supervisory roles, responsibilities, and collaborative professional relationships between the occupational therapy assistant.	Explain and justify the importance of supervisory roles, responsibilities, and collaborative professional relationships between the occupational therapist and the occupational therapy assistant.	Identify and explain the need for supervisory roles, responsibilities, and collaborative professional relationships between the occupational therapist and the occupational therapy assistant.
B.9.9.	Describe and discuss professional responsibilities and issues when providing service on a contractual basis.	Describe and discuss professional responsibilities and issues when providing service on a contractual basis.	Identify professional responsibilities and issues when providing service on a contractual basis.
B.9.10.	Demonstrate strategies for analyzing issues and making decisions to resolve personal and organizational ethical conflicts.	Demonstrate strategies for analyzing issues and making decisions to resolve personal and organizational ethical conflicts.	Identify strategies for analyzing issues and making decisions to resolve personal and organizational ethical conflicts.

(Continued)

Standard Number	Accreditation Standards for a Doctoral-Degree-Level Educational Program for the Occupational Therapist	Accreditation Standards for a Master's-Degree-Level Educational Program for the Occupational Therapist	Accreditation Standards for an Associate-Degree-Level Educational Program for the Occupational Therapy Assistant
B.9.11.	Demonstrate a variety of informal and formal strategies for resolving ethics disputes in varying practice areas.	Explain the variety of informal and formal systems for resolving ethics disputes that have jurisdiction over occupational therapy practice.	Identify the variety of informal and formal systems for resolving ethics disputes that have jurisdiction over occupational therapy practice.
B.9.12.	Describe and implement strategies to assist the consumer in gaining access to occupational therapy and other health and social services.	Describe and discuss strategies to assist the consumer in gaining access to occupational therapy services.	Identify strategies to assist the consumer in gaining access to occupational therapy services.
B.9.13.	Demonstrate advocacy by participating in and exploring leadership positions in organizations or agencies promoting the profession (e.g., AOTA, state occupational therapy associations, World Federation of Occupational Therapists, advocacy organizations), consumer access and services, and the welfare of the community.	Demonstrate professional advocacy by participating in organizations or agencies promoting the profession (e.g., AOTA, state occupational therapy associations, advocacy organizations).	Demonstrate professional advocacy by participating in organizations or agencies promoting the profession (e.g., AOTA, state occupational therapy associations, advocacy organizations).

SECTION C: FIELDWORK EDUCATION AND DOCTORAL EXPERIENTIAL COMPONENT

C.1.0. FIELDWORK EDUCATION
Fieldwork education is a crucial part of professional preparation and is best integrated as a component of the curriculum design. Fieldwork experiences should be implemented and evaluated for their effectiveness by the educational institution. The experience should provide the student with the opportunity to carry out professional responsibilities under supervision of a qualified occupational therapy practitioner serving as a role model. The academic fieldwork coordinator is responsible for the program's compliance with fieldwork education requirements. The academic fieldwork coordinator will

| C.1.1. | Ensure that the fieldwork program reflects the sequence and scope of content in the curriculum design in collaboration with faculty so that | Ensure that the fieldwork program reflects the sequence and scope of content in the curriculum design in collaboration with faculty so that | Ensure that the fieldwork program reflects the sequence and scope of content in the curriculum design in collaboration with faculty so that |

(Continued)

Standard Number	Accreditation Standards for a Doctoral-Degree-Level Educational Program for the Occupational Therapist	Accreditation Standards for a Master's-Degree-Level Educational Program for the Occupational Therapist	Accreditation Standards for an Associate-Degree-Level Educational Program for the Occupational Therapy Assistant
	fieldwork experiences strengthen the ties between didactic and fieldwork education.	fieldwork experiences strengthen the ties between didactic and fieldwork education.	fieldwork experiences strengthen the ties between didactic and fieldwork education.
C.1.2.	Document the criteria and process for selecting fieldwork sites, to include maintaining memoranda of understanding, complying with all site requirements, maintaining site objectives and site data, and communicating this information to students.	Document the criteria and process for selecting fieldwork sites, to include maintaining memoranda of understanding, complying with all site requirements, maintaining site objectives and site data, and communicating this information to students.	Document the criteria and process for selecting fieldwork sites, to include maintaining memoranda of understanding, complying with all site requirements, maintaining site objectives and site data, and communicating this information to students.
C.1.3.	Demonstrate that academic and fieldwork educators collaborate in establishing fieldwork objectives and communicate with the student and fieldwork educator about progress and performance during fieldwork.	Demonstrate that academic and fieldwork educators collaborate in establishing fieldwork objectives and communicate with the student and fieldwork educator about progress and performance during fieldwork.	Demonstrate that academic and fieldwork educators collaborate in establishing fieldwork objectives and communicate with the student and fieldwork educator about progress and performance during fieldwork.
C.1.4.	Ensure that the ratio of fieldwork educators to students enables proper supervision and the ability to provide frequent assessment of student progress in achieving stated fieldwork objectives.	Ensure that the ratio of fieldwork educators to students enables proper supervision and the ability to provide frequent assessment of student progress in achieving stated fieldwork objectives.	Ensure that the ratio of fieldwork educators to students enables proper supervision and the ability to provide frequent assessment of student progress in achieving stated fieldwork objectives.
C.1.5.	Ensure that fieldwork agreements are sufficient in scope and number to allow completion of graduation requirements in a timely manner in accordance with the policy adopted by the program as required by Standard A.4.14.	Ensure that fieldwork agreements are sufficient in scope and number to allow completion of graduation requirements in a timely manner in accordance with the policy adopted by the program as required by Standard A.4.14.	Ensure that fieldwork agreements are sufficient in scope and number to allow completion of graduation requirements in a timely manner in accordance with the policy adopted by the program as required by Standard A.4.14.

(Continued)

Standard Number	Accreditation Standards for a Doctoral-Degree-Level Educational Program for the Occupational Therapist	Accreditation Standards for a Master's-Degree-Level Educational Program for the Occupational Therapist	Accreditation Standards for an Associate-Degree-Level Educational Program for the Occupational Therapy Assistant
C.1.6.	The program must have evidence of valid memoranda of understanding in effect and signed by both parties at the time the student is completing the Level I or Level II fieldwork experience. (Electronic memoranda of understanding and signatures are acceptable.) Responsibilities of the sponsoring institution(s) and each fieldwork site must be clearly documented in the memorandum of understanding.	The program must have evidence of valid memoranda of understanding in effect and signed by both parties at the time the student is completing the Level I or Level II fieldwork experience. (Electronic memoranda of understanding and signatures are acceptable.) Responsibilities of the sponsoring institution(s) and each fieldwork site must be clearly documented in the memorandum of understanding.	The program must have evidence of valid memoranda of understanding in effect and signed by both parties at the time the student is completing the Level I or Level II fieldwork experience. (Electronic memoranda of understanding and signatures are acceptable.) Responsibilities of the sponsoring institution(s) and each fieldwork site must be clearly documented in the memorandum of understanding.
C.1.7.	Ensure that at least one fieldwork experience (either Level I or Level II) has as its focus psychological and social factors that influence engagement in occupation.	Ensure that at least one fieldwork experience (either Level I or Level II) has as its focus psychological and social factors that influence engagement in occupation.	Ensure that at least one fieldwork experience (either Level I or Level II) has as its focus psychological and social factors that influence engagement in occupation.
The goal of Level I fieldwork is to introduce students to the fieldwork experience, to apply knowledge to practice, and to develop understanding of the needs of clients. The program will			
C.1.8.	Ensure that Level I fieldwork is integral to the program's curriculum design and include experiences designed to enrich didactic coursework through directed observation and participation in selected aspects of the occupational therapy process.	Ensure that Level I fieldwork is integral to the program's curriculum design and include experiences designed to enrich didactic coursework through directed observation and participation in selected aspects of the occupational therapy process.	Ensure that Level I fieldwork is integral to the program's curriculum design and include experiences designed to enrich didactic coursework through directed observation and participation in selected aspects of the occupational therapy process.
C.1.9.	Ensure that qualified personnel supervise Level I fieldwork. Examples may include, but are not limited to, currently licensed or otherwise	Ensure that qualified personnel supervise Level I fieldwork. Examples may include, but are not limited to, currently licensed or otherwise	Ensure that qualified personnel supervise Level I fieldwork. Examples may include, but are not limited to, currently licensed or otherwise

(Continued)

Standard Number	Accreditation Standards for a Doctoral-Degree-Level Educational Program for the Occupational Therapist	Accreditation Standards for a Master's-Degree-Level Educational Program for the Occupational Therapist	Accreditation Standards for an Associate-Degree-Level Educational Program for the Occupational Therapy Assistant
	regulated occupational therapists and occupational therapy assistants, psychologists, physician assistants, teachers, social workers, nurses, and physical therapists.	regulated occupational therapists and occupational therapy assistants, psychologists, physician assistants, teachers, social workers, nurses, and physical therapists.	regulated occupational therapists and occupational therapy assistants, psychologists, physician assistants, teachers, social workers, nurses, and physical therapists.
C.1.10.	Document all Level I fieldwork experiences that are provided to students, including mechanisms for formal evaluation of student performance. Ensure that Level I fieldwork is not substituted for any part of Level II fieldwork.	Document all Level I fieldwork experiences that are provided to students, including mechanisms for formal evaluation of student performance. Ensure that Level I fieldwork is not substituted for any part of Level II fieldwork.	Document all Level I fieldwork experiences that are provided to students, including mechanisms for formal evaluation of student performance. Ensure that Level I fieldwork is not substituted for any part of Level II fieldwork.
	The goal of Level II fieldwork is to develop competent, entry-level, generalist occupational therapists. Level II fieldwork must be integral to the program's curriculum design and must include an in-depth experience in delivering occupational therapy services to clients, focusing on the application of purposeful and meaningful occupation and research, administration, and management of occupational therapy services. It is recommended that the student be exposed to a variety of clients across the lifespan and to a variety of settings. The program will		**The goal of Level II fieldwork is to develop competent, entry-level, generalist occupational therapy assistants. Level II fieldwork must be integral to the program's curriculum design and must include an in-depth experience in delivering occupational therapy services to clients, focusing on the application of purposeful and meaningful occupation. It is recommended that the student be exposed to a variety of clients across the lifespan and to a variety of settings. The program will**
C.1.11.	Ensure that the fieldwork experience is designed to promote clinical reasoning and reflective practice, to transmit the values and beliefs that enable	Ensure that the fieldwork experience is designed to promote clinical reasoning and reflective practice, to transmit the values and beliefs that enable	Ensure that the fieldwork experience is designed to promote clinical reasoning approriate to the occupational therapy assistant role,

(Continued)

Standard Number	Accreditation Standards for a Doctoral-Degree-Level Educational Program for the Occupational Therapist	Accreditation Standards for a Master's-Degree-Level Educational Program for the Occupational Therapist	Accreditation Standards for an Associate-Degree-Level Educational Program for the Occupational Therapy Assistant
	ethical practice, and to develop professionalism and competence in career responsibilities.	ethical practice, and to develop professionalism and competence in career responsibilities.	to transmit the values and beliefs that enable ethical practice, and to develop professionalism and competence in career responsibilities.
C.1.12.	Provide Level II fieldwork in traditional and/or emerging settings, consistent with the curriculum design. In all settings, psychosocial factors influencing engagement in occupation must be understood and integrated for the development of client-centered, meaningful, occupation-based outcomes. The student can complete Level II fieldwork in a minimum of one setting if it is reflective of more than one practice area, or in a maximum of four different settings.	Provide Level II fieldwork in traditional and/or emerging settings, consistent with the curriculum design. In all settings, psychosocial factors influencing engagement in occupation must be understood and integrated for the development of client-centered, meaningful, occupation-based outcomes. The student can complete Level II fieldwork in a minimum of one setting if it is reflective of more than one practice area, or in a maximum of four different settings.	Provide Level II fieldwork in traditional and/or emerging settings, consistent with the curriculum design. In all settings, psychosocial factors influencing engagement in occupation must be understood and integrated for the development of client-centered, meaningful, occupation-based outcomes. The student can complete Level II fieldwork in a minimum of one setting if it is reflective of more than one practice area, or in a maximum of three different settings.
C.1.13.	Require a minimum of 24 weeks' full-time Level II fieldwork. This may be completed on a part-time basis, as defined by the fieldwork placement in accordance with the fieldwork placement's usual and customary personnel policies, as long as it is at least 50% of an FTE at that site.	Require a minimum of 24 weeks' full-time Level II fieldwork. This may be completed on a part-time basis, as defined by the fieldwork placement in accordance with the fieldwork placement's usual and customary personnel policies, as long as it is at least 50% of an FTE at that site.	Require a minimum of 16 weeks' full-time Level II fieldwork. This may be completed on a part-time basis, as defined by the fieldwork placement in accordance with the fieldwork placement's usual and customary personnel policies, as long as it is at least 50% of an FTE at that site.
C.1.14.	Ensure that the student is supervised by a currently licensed or otherwise regulated occupational therapist who has a minimum of 1 year full-time (or its equivalent) of practice experience subsequent to initial certification and who is adequately prepared to serve as a fieldwork	Ensure that the student is supervised by a currently licensed or otherwise regulated occupational therapist who has a minimum of 1 year full-time (or its equivalent) of practice experience subsequent to initial certification and who is adequately prepared to serve as a fieldwork	Ensure that the student is supervised by a currently licensed or otherwise regulated occupational therapist or occupational therapy assistant (under the supervision of an occupational therapist) who has a minimum of 1 year full-time (or its equivalent) of practice experience subsequent

(Continued)

Standard Number	Accreditation Standards for a Doctoral-Degree-Level Educational Program for the Occupational Therapist	Accreditation Standards for a Master's-Degree-Level Educational Program for the Occupational Therapist	Accreditation Standards for an Associate-Degree-Level Educational Program for the Occupational Therapy Assistant
	educator. The supervising therapist may be engaged by the fieldwork site or by the educational program.	educator. The supervising therapist may be engaged by the fieldwork site or by the educational program.	to initial certification and who is adequately prepared to serve as a fieldwork educator. The supervising therapist may be engaged by the fieldwork site or by the educational program.
C.1.15.	Document a mechanism for evaluating the effectiveness of supervision (e.g., student evaluation of fieldwork) and for providing resources for enhancing supervision (e.g., materials on supervisory skills, continuing education opportunities, articles on theory and practice).	Document a mechanism for evaluating the effectiveness of supervision (e.g., student evaluation of fieldwork) and for providing resources for enhancing supervision (e.g., materials on supervisory skills, continuing education opportunities, articles on theory and practice).	Document a mechanism for evaluating the effectiveness of supervision (e.g., student evaluation of fieldwork) and for providing resources for enhancing supervision (e.g., materials on supervisory skills, continuing education opportunities, articles on theory and practice).
C.1.16.	Ensure that supervision provides protection of consumers and opportunities for appropriate role modeling of occupational therapy practice. Initially, supervision should be direct and then decrease to less direct supervision as appropriate for the setting, the severity of the client's condition, and the ability of the student.	Ensure that supervision provides protection of consumers and opportunities for appropriate role modeling of occupational therapy practice. Initially, supervision should be direct and then decrease to less direct supervision as appropriate for the setting, the severity of the client's condition, and the ability of the student.	Ensure that supervision provides protection of consumers and opportunities for appropriate role modeling of occupational therapy practice. Initially, supervision should be direct and then decrease to less direct supervision as appropriate for the setting, the severity of the client's condition, and the ability of the student.
C.1.17.	Ensure that supervision provided in a setting where no occupational therapy services exist includes a documented plan for provision of occupational therapy services and supervision by a currently licensed or otherwise regulated occupational therapist with at least 3 years' full-time or its equivalent of professional experience. Supervision must include a minimum of 8 hours	Ensure that supervision provided in a setting where no occupational therapy services exist includes a documented plan for provision of occupational therapy services and supervision by a currently licensed or otherwise regulated occupational therapist with at least 3 years' full-time or its equivalent of professional experience. Supervision must include a minimum of 8 hours	Ensure that supervision provided in a setting where no occupational therapy services exist includes a documented plan for provision of occupational therapy assistant services and supervision by a currently licensed or otherwise regulated occupational therapist or occupational therapy assistant (under the direction of an occupational therapist) with at least 3 years'

(Continued)

Standard Number	Accreditation Standards for a Doctoral-Degree-Level Educational Program for the Occupational Therapist	Accreditation Standards for a Master's-Degree-Level Educational Program for the Occupational Therapist	Accreditation Standards for an Associate-Degree-Level Educational Program for the Occupational Therapy Assistant
	of direct supervision each week of the fieldwork experience. An occupational therapy supervisor must be available, via a variety of contact measures, to the student during all working hours. An on-site supervisor designee of another profession must be assigned while the occupational therapy supervisor is off site.	of direct supervision each week of the fieldwork experience. An occupational therapy supervisor must be available, via a variety of contact measures, to the student during all working hours. An on-site supervisor designee of another profession must be assigned while the occupational therapy supervisor is off site.	full-time or its equivalent of professional experience. Supervision must include a minimum of 8 hours of direct supervision each week of the fieldwork experience. An occupational therapy supervisor must be available, via a variety of contact measures, to the student during all working hours. An on-site supervisor designee of another profession must be assigned while the occupational therapy supervisor is off site.
C.1.18.	Document mechanisms for requiring formal evaluation of student performance on Level II fieldwork (e.g., the AOTA *Fieldwork Performance Evaluation for the Occupational Therapy Student* or equivalent).	Document mechanisms for requiring formal evaluation of student performance on Level II fieldwork (e.g., the AOTA *Fieldwork Performance Evaluation for the Occupational Therapy Student* or equivalent).	Document mechanisms for requiring formal evaluation of student performance on Level II fieldwork (e.g., the AOTA *Fieldwork Performance Evaluation for the Occupational Therapy Assistant Student* or equivalent).
C.1.19.	Ensure that students attending Level II fieldwork outside the United States are supervised by an occupational therapist who graduated from a program approved by the World Federation of Occupational Therapists and has 1 year of experience in practice.	Ensure that students attending Level II fieldwork outside the United States are supervised by an occupational therapist who graduated from a program approved by the World Federation of Occupational Therapists and has 1 year of experience in practice.	Ensure that students attending Level II fieldwork outside the United States are supervised by an occupational therapist who graduated from a program approved by the World Federation of Occupational Therapists and has 1 year of experience in practice.
C.2.0. **DOCTORAL EXPERIENTIAL COMPONENT** The goal of the doctoral experiential component is to develop occupational therapists with advanced skills (those that are beyond a generalist level). The doctoral experiential component shall be an integral part of the pro-			

(Continued)

Standard Number	Accreditation Standards for a Doctoral-Degree-Level Educational Program for the Occupational Therapist	Accreditation Standards for a Master's-Degree-Level Educational Program for the Occupational Therapist	Accreditation Standards for an Associate-Degree-Level Educational Program for the Occupational Therapy Assistant
	gram's curriculum design and shall include an in-depth experience in one or more of the following: clinical practice skills, research skills, administration, leadership, program and policy development, advocacy, education, or theory development.		
	The student must successfully complete all coursework and Level II fieldwork and pass a competency requirement prior to the commencement of the doctoral experiential component. The specific content and format of the competency requirement is determined by the program. Examples include a written comprehensive exam, oral exam, NBCOT certification exam readiness tool, and the NBCOT practice exams.		
C.2.1.	Ensure that the doctoral experiential component is designed and administered by faculty and provided in setting(s) consistent with the program's curriculum design, including individualized specific objectives and plans for supervision.	*(No related Standard)*	*(No related Standard)*
C.2.2.	Ensure that there is a memorandum of understanding that, at a minimum, includes individualized specific objectives, plans for supervision or mentoring, and responsibilities of all parties.	*(No related Standard)*	*(No related Standard)*
C.2.3.	Require that the length of this doctoral experiential component be a minimum of 16 weeks (640 hours). This may be completed on a part-	*(No related Standard)*	*(No related Standard)*

(Continued)

Standard Number	Accreditation Standards for a Doctoral-Degree-Level Educational Program for the Occupational Therapist	Accreditation Standards for a Master's-Degree-Level Educational Program for the Occupational Therapist	Accreditation Standards for an Associate-Degree-Level Educational Program for the Occupational Therapy Assistant
	time basis and must be consistent with the individualized specific objectives and culminating project. No more than 20% of the 640 hours can be completed outside of the mentored practice setting(s). Prior fieldwork or work experience may not be substituted for this experiential component.		
C.2.4.	Ensure that the student is mentored by an individual with expertise consistent with the student's area of focus. The mentor does not have to be an occupational therapist.	(No related Standard)	(No related Standard)
C.2.5.	Document a formal evaluation mechanism for objective assessment of the student's performance during and at the completion of the doctoral experiential component.	(No related Standard)	(No related Standard)

Glossary

Definitions given below are for the purposes of these documents.

ability to benefit—A phrase that refers to a student who does not have a high school diploma or its recognized equivalent but is eligible to receive funds under the Title IV Higher Education Act programs after taking an independently administered examination and achieving a score, specified by the Secretary of the U.S. Department of Education (USDE), indicating that the student has the ability to benefit from the education being offered.

academic calendar—The official institutional document that lists registration dates, semester/quarter stop and start dates, holidays, graduation dates, and other pertinent events. Generally, the academic year is divided into two major semesters, each approximately 14 to 16 weeks long. A smaller number of institutions have quarters rather than semesters. Quarters are approximately 10 weeks long; there are three major quarters and the summer session.

activity—A term that describes a class of human actions that are goal directed (AOTA, 2008b).

advanced—The stage of being beyond the elementary or introductory.

affiliate—An entity that formally cooperates with a sponsoring institution in implementing the occupational therapy educational program.

areas of occupation—Activities in which people engage: activities of daily living, instrumental activities of daily living, rest and sleep, education, work, play, leisure, and social participation.

assist—To aid, help, or hold an auxiliary position.

body functions—The physiological functions of body systems (including psychological functions).

body structures—Anatomical parts of the body, such as organs, limbs, and their components.

care coordination—The process that links clients with appropriate services and resources.

case management—A system to ensure that individuals receive appropriate health care services.

client—The term used to name the entity that receives occupational therapy services. Clients may include (1) individuals and other persons relevant to the client's life, including family, caregivers, teachers, employers, and others who may also help or be served indirectly; (2) organizations, such as businesses, industries, or agencies; and (3) populations within a community (AOTA, 2008b).

client-centered service delivery—An orientation that honors the desires and priorities of clients in designing and implementing interventions.

client factors—Factors that reside within the client and that may affect performance in areas of occupation. Client factors include body functions and body structures.

clinical reasoning—Complex multifaceted cognitive process used by practitioners to plan, direct, perform, and reflect on intervention.

collaborate—To work together with a mutual sharing of thoughts and ideas.

competent—To have the requisite abilities/qualities and capacity to function in a professional environment.

consumer—The direct and/or indirect recipient of educational and/or practitioner services offered.

context/contextual factors and environment:

> **context**—The variety of interrelated conditions within and surrounding the client that influence performance. Contexts include cultural, personal, temporal, and virtual aspects.

> **environment**—The external physical and social environment that surrounds the client and in which the client's daily life occupations occur.

context of service delivery—The knowledge and understanding of the various contexts in which occupational therapy services are provided.

criterion-referenced—Tests that compare the performance of an individual with that of another group, known as the *norm group.*

culminating project—A project that is completed by a doctoral student that demonstrates the student's ability to relate theory to practice and to synthesize advanced knowledge in a practice area.

curriculum design—An overarching set of assumptions that explains how the curriculum is planned, implemented, and evaluated. Typically, a curriculum design includes educational goals and curriculum threads and provides a clear rationale for the selection of content, the determination of scope of content, and the sequence of the content. A curriculum design is expected to be consistent with the mission and philosophy of the sponsoring institution and the program.

curriculum threads—Curriculum threads, or *themes,* are identified by the program as areas of study and development that follow a path through the curriculum and represent the unique qualities of the program, as demonstrated by the program's graduates. Curriculum threads are typically based on the profession's and program's vision, mission, and philosophy (e.g., occupational needs of society, critical thinking/professional reasoning, diversity/globalization; AOTA, 2008a).

diagnosis—The process of analyzing the cause or nature of a condition, situation, or problem. Diagnosis as stated in Standard B.4.0. refers to the occupational therapist's ability to analyze a problem associated with occupational performance and participation.

distance education—Education that uses one or more of the technologies listed below to deliver instruction to students who are separated from the instructor and to support regular and substantive interaction between the students and the instructor, either synchronously or asynchronously. The technologies may include

- The Internet;

- One-way and two-way transmissions through open broadcast, closed circuit, cable, microwave, broadband lines, fiber optics, satellite, or wireless communications devices;

- Audio conferencing; or

- Video cassettes, DVDs, and CD-ROMs, if the cassettes, DVDs, or CD-ROMs are used in a course.

driver rehabilitation—Specialized evaluation and training to develop mastery of specific skills and techniques to effectively drive a motor vehicle independently and in accordance with state department of motor vehicles regulations.

entry-level occupational therapist—The outcome of the occupational therapy educational and certification process; an individual prepared to begin generalist practice as an occupational therapist with less than 1 year of experience.

entry-level occupational therapy assistant—The outcome of the occupational therapy educational and certification process; an individual prepared to begin generalist practice as an occupational therapy assistant with less than 1 year of experience.

faculty:

> **faculty, core**—Persons who are resident faculty, including the program director, appointed to and employed primarily in the occupational therapy educational program.

> **faculty, full time**—Core faculty members who hold an appointment that is full time, as defined by the institution, and whose job responsibilities include teaching and/or contributing to the delivery of the designed curriculum regardless of the position title (e.g., full-time instructional staff and clinical instructors would be considered faculty).

> **faculty, part time**—Core faculty members who hold an appointment that is considered by that institution to constitute less than full-time service and whose job responsibilities include teaching and/or contributing to the delivery of the designed curriculum regardless of the position title.

> **faculty, adjunct**—Persons who are responsible for teaching at least 50% of a course and are part-time, nonsalaried, non-tenure-track faculty members who are paid for each class they teach.

fieldwork coordinator—Faculty member who is responsible for the development, implementation, management, and evaluation of fieldwork education.

frame of reference—A set of interrelated, internally consistent concepts, definitions, postulates, and principles that provide a systematic description of a practitioner's interaction with clients. A frame of reference is intended to link theory to practice.

full-time equivalent (FTE)—An equivalent position for a full-time faculty member (as defined by the institution). An FTE can be made up of no more than three individuals.

graduation rate—The total number of students who graduated from a program within 150% of the published length of the program, divided by the number of students on the roster who started in the program.

habits—"Automatic behavior that is integrated into more complex patterns that enable people to function on a day-to-day basis" (Neidstadt & Crepeau, 1998).

health literacy—Degree to which individuals have the capacity to obtain, process, and understand basic health information and services needed to make appropriate health decisions (National Network of Libraries of Medicine, 2011).

interprofessional collaborative practice—"Multiple health workers from different professional backgrounds working together with patients, families, careers, and communities to deliver the highest quality of care" (World Health Organization, 2010).

memorandum of understanding (MOU)—A document outlining the terms and details of an agreement between parties, including each parties' requirements and responsibilities. A memorandum of understanding may be signed by any individual who is authorized by the institution to sign fieldwork memoranda of understanding on behalf of the institution.

mentoring—A relationship between two people in which one person (the mentor) is dedicated to the personal and professional growth of the other (the mentee). A mentor has more experience and knowledge than the mentee.

mission—A statement that explains the unique nature of a program or institution and how it helps fulfill or advance the goals of the sponsoring institution, including religious missions.

modalities—Application of a therapeutic agent, usually a physical agent modality.

> **deep thermal modalities**—Modalities such as therapeutic ultrasound and phonophoresis.

electrotherapeutic modalities—Modalities such as biofeedback, neuromuscular electrical stimulation, functional electrical stimulation, transcutaneous electrical nerve stimulation, electrical stimulations for tissue repair, high-voltage galvanic stimulation, and iontophoresis.

mechanical modalities—Modalities such as vasopneumatic devices and continuous passive motion.

superficial thermal—Modalities such as hydrotherapy, whirlpool, cryotherapy, fluidotherapy, hot packs, paraffin, water, and infrared.

model of practice—The set of theories and philosophies that defines the views, beliefs, assumptions, values, and domain of concern of a particular profession or discipline. Models of practice delimit the boundaries of a profession.

occupation—"Activities . . . of everyday life, named, organized and given value and meaning by individuals and a culture. Occupation is everything that people do to occupy themselves, including looking after themselves . . . enjoying life . . . and contributing to the social and economic fabric of their communities" (Law, Polatajko, Baptiste, & Townsend, 1997).

occupational profile—An analysis of a client's occupational history, routines, interests, values, and needs to engage in occupations and occupational roles.

occupational therapy—The art and science of applying occupation as a means to effect positive, measurable change in the health status and functional outcomes of a client by a qualified occupational therapist and/or occupational therapy assistant (as appropriate).

occupational therapy practitioner—An individual who is initially credentialed as an occupational therapist or an occupational therapy assistant.

participation—Active engagement in occupations.

performance patterns—Patterns of behavior related to daily life activities that are habitual or routine. Performance patterns include habits, routines, rituals, and roles.

performance skills—Features of what one does, not what one has, related to observable elements of action that have implicit functional purposes. Performance skills include motor and praxis, sensory–perceptual, emotional regulation, cognitive, and communication and social skills.

philosophy—The underlying belief and value structure for a program that is consistent with the sponsoring institution and which permeates the curriculum and the teaching learning process.

population-based interventions—Interventions focused on promoting the overall health status of the community by preventing disease, injury, disability, and premature death. A population-based health intervention can include assessment of the community's needs, health promotion and public education, disease and disability prevention, monitoring of services, and media interventions. Most interventions are tailored to reach a subset of a population, although some may be targeted toward the population at large. Populations and subsets may be defined by geography, culture, race and ethnicity, socioeconomic status, age, or other characteristics. Many of these characteristics relate to the health of the described population (Keller, Schaffer, Lia-Hoagberg, & Strohschein, 2002).

preparatory methods—Intervention techniques focused on client factors to help a client's function in specific activities.

program director (associate-degree-level occupational therapy assistant)—An initially certified occupational therapist or occupational therapy assistant who is licensed or credentialed according to regulations in the state or jurisdiction in which the program is located. The program director must hold a minimum of a master's degree.

program director (master's-degree-level occupational therapist)—An initially certified occupational therapist who is licensed or credentialed according to regulations in the state or jurisdiction in which the program is located. The program director must hold a doctoral degree.

program director (doctoral-degree-level occupational therapist)—An initially certified occupational therapist who is licensed or credentialed according to regulations in the state or jurisdiction in which the program is located. The program director must hold a doctoral degree.

program evaluation—A continuing system for routinely and systematically analyzing data to determine the extent to which the program is meeting its stated goals and objectives.

purposeful activity—"An activity used in treatment that is goal directed and that the [client] sees as meaningful or purposeful" (Low, 2002).

recognized regional or national accrediting authority—Regional and national accrediting agencies recognized by the USDE and/or the Council for Higher Education Accreditation (CHEA) to accredit postsecondary educational programs/institutions. The purpose of recognition is to ensure that the accrediting agencies are reliable authorities for evaluating quality education or training programs in the institutions they accredit.

Regional accrediting bodies recognized by USDE:

- Accrediting Commission for Community and Junior Colleges, Western Association of Schools and Colleges (ACCJC/WASC)
- Accrediting Commission for Senior Colleges and Universities, Western Association of Schools and Colleges (ACSCU/WASC)
- Commission on Colleges, Southern Association of Colleges and Schools (SACS)
- Commission on Institutions of Higher Education, New England Association of Schools and Colleges (CIHE/NEASC)
- Higher Learning Commission, North Central Association of Colleges and Schools (HLC)
- Middle States Commission on Higher Education, Middle States Association of Colleges and Schools (MSCHE)
- Northwest Commission on Colleges and Universities (NWCCU)

National accrediting bodies recognized by USDE:

- Accrediting Bureau of Health Education Schools (ABHES)
- Accrediting Commission of Career Schools and Colleges (ACCSC)
- Accrediting Council for Continuing Education and Training (ACCET)
- Accrediting Council for Independent Colleges and Schools (ACICS)
- Council on Occupational Education (COE)
- Distance Education and Training Council Accrediting Commission (DETC)

reflective practice—Thoughtful consideration of one's experiences and knowledge when applying such knowledge to practice. Reflective practice includes being coached by professionals.

release time—Period when a person is freed from regular duties, especially teaching, to allow time for other tasks or activities.

retention rate—A measure of the rate at which students persist in their educational program, calculated as the percentage of students on the roster, after the add period, from the beginning of the previous academic year who are again enrolled in the beginning of the subsequent academic year.

scholarship—"A systematic investigation . . . designed to develop or to contribute to generalizable knowledge" (45 CFR § 46). Scholarship is made public, subject to review, and part of the discipline or professional knowledge base (Glassick, Huber, & Maeroff, 1997). It allows others to build on it and further advance the field (AOTA, 2009).

> **scholarship of discovery:** Engagement in activity that leads to the development of "knowledge for its own sake." The Scholarship of Discovery encompasses original research that contributes to expanding the knowledge base of a discipline (Boyer, 1990).

> **scholarship of integration:** Investigations making creative connections both within and across disciplines to integrate, synthesize, interpret, and create new perspectives and theories (Boyer, 1990).

> **scholarship of application:** Practitioners apply the knowledge generated by scholarship of discovery or integration to address real problems at all levels of society (Boyer, 1990). In occupational therapy, an example would be the application of theoretical knowledge to practice interventions or to teaching in the classroom.

> **scholarship of teaching and learning:** "Involves the systematic study of teaching and/or learning and the public sharing and review of such work through presentations, publications, and performances" (McKinney, 2007, p. 10).

skill—The ability to use one's knowledge effectively and readily in execution or performance.

sponsoring institution—The identified legal entity that assumes total responsibility for meeting the minimal standards for ACOTE accreditation.

strategic plan—A comprehensive plan that articulates the program's future vision and guides the program development (e.g., faculty recruitment and professional growth, changes in the curriculum design, priorities in academic resources, procurement of fieldwork sites). A program's strategic plan must include, but need not be limited to,

- Evidence that the plan is based on program evaluation and an analysis of external and internal environments,
- Long-term goals that address the vision and mission of both the institution and program as well as specific needs of the program,
- Specific measurable action steps with expected timelines by which the program will reach its long-term goals,
- Person(s) responsible for action steps, and
- Evidence of periodic updating of action steps and long-term goals as they are met or as circumstances change.

supervise—To direct and inspect the performance of workers or work.

supervision, direct—Supervision that occurs in real time and offers both audio and visual capabilities to ensure opportunities for timely feedback.

supervisor—One who ensures that tasks assigned to others are performed correctly and efficiently.

theory—A set of interrelated concepts used to describe, explain, or predict phenomena.

transfer of credit—A term used in higher education to award a student credit for courses earned in another institution prior to admission to the occupational therapy or occupational therapy assistant program.

References

American Occupational Therapy Association. (2008a). *Occupational therapy model curriculum.* Bethesda MD: Author. Retrieved from www.aota.org/Educate/EdRes/COE/Other-Education-Documents/OT-Model-Curriculum.aspx

American Occupational Therapy Association. (2008b). Occupational therapy practice framework: Domain and process (2nd ed.). *American Journal of Occupational Therapy, 62,* 625–683.

American Occupational Therapy Association. (2009). Scholarship in occupational therapy. *American Journal of Occupational Therapy, 63,* 790–796. http://dx.doi.org/10.5014/ajot.63.6.790

Boyer, E. L. (1990). *Scholarship reconsidered: Priorities of the professoriate.* San Francisco: Jossey-Bass.

Crepeau, E. B., Cohn, E., & Schell, B. (Eds.). (2008). *Willard and Spackman's occupational therapy* (11th ed.). Philadelphia: Lippincott Williams & Wilkins.

Glassick, C. E., Huber, M. T., & Maeroff, G. I. (1997). *Scholarship assessed: Evaluation of the professoriate.* San Francisco: Jossey-Bass.

Interprofessional Education Collaborative Expert Panel. (2011). *Core competencies for interprofessional collaborative practice: Report of an expert panel.* Washington, DC: Interprofessional Education Collaborative.

Keller, L., Schaffer, M., Lia-Hoagberg, B., & Strohschein S. (2002). Assessment, program planning and evaluation in population-based public health practice. *Journal of Public Health Management and Practice, 8*(5), 30–44.

Law, M., Polatajko, H., Baptiste, W., & Townsend, E. (1997). Core concepts of occupational therapy. In E. Townsend (Ed.), *Enabling occupation: An occupational therapy perspective* (pp. 29–56). Ottawa, ON: Canadian Association of Occupational Therapists.

Low, J. (2002). Historical and social foundations for practice. In C. A. Trombly & M. V. Radomski (Eds.), *Occupational therapy for physical dysfunction* (5th ed., pp. 17–30). Philadelphia: Lippincott Williams & Wilkins.

McKinney, K. (2007). *Enhancing learning through the scholarship of teaching and learning.* San Francisco: Jossey-Bass.

National Network of Libraries of Medicine. (2011). *Health literacy.* Retrieved February 3, 2012, from http://nnlm.gov/outreach/consumer/hlthlit.html

Schon, D. A. (1987). *Educating the reflective practitioner.* San Francisco: Jossey-Bass.

Public welfare: Protection of human subjects, 45 CFR § 46 (2005).

U.S. Department of Education (2011). *Funding your education: The guide to federal student aid, 2012–13.* Retrieved February 3, 2012, from http://studentaid.ed.gov/students/attachments/siteresources/12–13_Guide.pdf

World Health Organization. (2010). *Framework for action on interprofessional education and collaborative practice.* Geneva: Author. Retrieved from http://whqlibdoc.who.int/hq/2010/WHO_HRH_HPN_10.3_eng.pdf

Concept Papers

A Descriptive Review of Occupational Therapy Education

Introduction

In an August 2002 Commission on Education (COE) meeting, COE members decided to design and write a *Guide to Occupational Therapy Education*. With the advent and passing of Resolution J—which became Resolution 670-99 at the 1999 Representative Assembly meeting of the American Occupational Therapy Association (Accreditation Council for Occupational Therapy Education [ACOTE], 1999b)—and new degree structures within the profession (i.e., professional/clinical doctorate), a guide to occupational therapy education is warranted. This guide, retitled *A Descriptive Review of Occupational Therapy Education*, is intended for practitioners, academicians, and potential occupational therapy program applicants to augment their understanding of occupational therapy education.

Organization of Review

The review is organized into eight sections. The first, the introductory section, describes the process of the development of the Descriptive Review. The second section distinguishes between professional and graduate education. This information provides the background and foundational groundwork for the Review. The next section includes the underpinning information that describes the levels of education in the United States as used by most colleges and universities. It is the common language used in all degree majors and programs and should be the guide for occupational therapy education language so that degrees in occupational therapy can be recognized and understood by fields other than occupational therapy.

The fourth section delineates the levels of education in occupational therapy in the United States from the technical level of education to the doctoral level, using the previous foundational information as the basis of the descriptions. The Review then lists suggested factors that should be considered when choosing an occupational therapy program.

The Review was written to describe the present state of occupational therapy education within the American educational system and is limited to this perspective only. It is purposefully written in a factual format and does not intend to promote one occupational therapy degree over any other, nor is it intended to resolve the multiple issues regarding the various degree levels or entry-level competencies. Those issues need to be addressed by a broad-based consensus group or other professional bodies.

Professional and Graduate Education

The terms *professional education* and *graduate education* are often used synonymously. Educational institutions have the prerogative to house degree programs in any appropriate organizational structure. For example, some master's-degree programs award the degree under the auspices of the graduate school, whereas others offer the degree from a professional school. However, a distinction between *graduate* and *professional* education is needed to understand the nature of the organizational context of occupational therapy educational programs within colleges and universities. Although there is a paucity of literature distinguishing the two types of education, Mayhew and Ford's (1974) *Reform in Graduate and Professional Education* was a welcomed resource to higher educational planners. Mayhew and Ford eloquently articulated the purposes and problems of both graduate and professional education.

Professional Education

Professional education is a term used to describe educational programs in which students are enrolled to study service delivery of a particular profession (e.g., dentistry, medicine, nursing, pharmacy, veterinary science). Studying a profession is different from studying a discipline (e.g., physics, theology, mathematics, biology, sociology) (Mayhew & Ford, 1971). A discipline has its own "unique epistemology" that serves as its foundation for autonomy (Knowles, 1977, p. 2209). Professional programs are highly influenced by the professions they serve. The professional standards are at a minimally acceptable level, and governance from the institution often requires higher and different standards (e.g., requirement of thesis, capstone project, electives, additional coursework, interdisciplinary classes).

The purpose of professional education is to admit and educate a sufficient number of students who meet minimum theoretical knowledge and practice skill competencies to practice a profession (Mayhew & Ford, 1974). "Professional education should be directed toward significant objectives, including professional competence, understanding of society, ethical behavior, and scholarly concern" (Mayhew & Ford, 1974, p. 3).

Graduate Education

Graduate education comprises the master's (e.g., MA, MS) degree and doctor of philosophy (PhD) degree (Carmichael, 1961). The graduate school is the organizational authority within colleges and universities that houses graduate educational programs. Traditionally, graduate education focused on advanced study and scholarship within a discipline; however, more recently, some graduate programs in professional fields have emerged (e.g., master's degree in nursing, PhD in rehabilitation).

Historically, graduate education was intended for four purposes (Mayhew & Ford, 1974). The first purpose of graduate education was character formation—to produce broadly learned graduates. The second purpose, preparation of college teachers, was traditionally the primary purpose of PhD programs. The paradox of this intent was that traditional PhD graduate education focused primarily on producing independent researchers and rarely addressed preparation for college teaching. A third purpose of graduate education was "to prepare people for research and scholarship in a specialized field" (Mayhew & Ford, 1974, p. 94). The fourth purpose of graduate education was to have graduates enter the work force and apply their research competencies in professional fields.

Levels of Education in the United States

One of the hallmarks of higher education in the United States is the diversity of institutions, degrees, and programs available. Levels of education are represented by the academic degree conferred to graduates. A degree is a credential or title "conferred by a college or university as official recognition for the completion of a program of studies" (Shafritz, Koeppe, & Soper, 1988, p. 145). Academic degree levels include associate, baccalaureate, master's, and doctoral.

Associate Degree

According to the National Center for Education Statistics, an *associate degree* is "an award that requires the completion of at least 2 but less than 4 full-time equivalent academic years of college-level work in an academic or occupationally specified field of study, and which meets institutional standards for otherwise satisfying the requirements for this degree level" (U.S. Department of Education [USDE], 2002, p. A-63).

Baccalaureate

A *baccalaureate degree* is an award requiring completion of 4 to 5 full-time equivalent academic years of college-level work in an academic or occupationally specific field of study, and which satisfies institutional standards of the requirement of the degree level (USDE, 2002, p. A-63). Two common baccalaureate degrees are the bachelor of arts (BA or AB, for the Latin *atrium baccalareus*) for programs in the humanities and the bachelor of science (BS) for programs in the sciences. Some institutions offer baccalaureate degrees in specialized areas, for example, bachelor of music (BMus) or bachelor of education (BEd) (Unger, 1996).

Master's

A *master's degree* typically requires approximately 36 credits of postbaccalaureate education in a subject field. Three master's degrees are commonly awarded. One type includes both the master of arts (MA) and the master of science (MS). MA and MS degrees are "awarded in liberal arts and sciences for advanced scholarship in a subject field or discipline and demonstrated ability to perform scholarly research" (USDE, 2002, p. 298). A second type of master's degree is conferred for completion of a professional entry-level program; for example, an MEd in education, an MBA in business administration, or an MFA in fine arts. In occupational therapy, the MOT, or master of occupational therapy, degree is awarded by some institutions. The third type of master's degree includes the award in professional fields for study beyond the first-professional (entry-level) degree, such as the master of laws (LLM) and the master of science (MS) in various medical professions. Occupational therapy has typically referred to this level of degree as a post-professional master's degree.

Various classifications of master's degrees exist, including *academic, professional,* and *experiential* (Glazer, 1988). Curricular requirements for master's degrees vary from institution to institution and from state to state. The diversity in master's degree curricula makes comparison of degree programs, fields, and credentials difficult (Glazer, 1988). For example, some master's-degree programs require a thesis, whereas others do not. The master's degree must be approached "as a class of degrees rather than as a generic model, and as a credential sought increasingly for its own merits rather than in relation to the bachelor's or doctoral degree" (Glazer, 1988, p. 1).

Historically, the purpose of a master's degree was to produce graduates with beginning research or inquiry skills. Not all professions offer a degree at the doctoral level, and thus the master's degree may be the *terminal degree* (highest degree conferred) for some professions.

During the 1980s, master's-degree programs were challenged by more convenient educational alternatives that were shorter in duration and less expensive (e.g., certificate programs). Such certificate alternatives typically did not result in the conferral of a graduate degree. To compete with certificate programs, some master's-degree programs were oriented toward practice rather than research. Currently, approximately 85% of all master's-degree programs in the United States are considered to be practice-oriented or professional degrees (LaPidus, 2000). These programs are specialized in their focus, applied in terms of their content, and decentralized in that they are frequently not housed under the auspices of a graduate school (LaPidus, 2000).

Doctorate: Professional and Research

A *doctoral degree* is the highest degree conferred by an institution of higher education. Most doctoral degrees require the equivalent of 3 years of full-time postbaccalaureate study (Kapel, Gifford, & Kapel, 1991). Commonly, universities require a minimum of 72 hours of postbaccalaureate study plus a residence requirement. "Doctorate entitles bearers to be addressed as 'Doctor' and to append their names with the appropriate letters of their degrees—that is, PhD (doctor of philosophy) or MD (doctor of medicine)" (Unger, 1996, p. 305). There are two types of doctoral degrees: the *research doctorate* and the *professional doctorate* (Shafritz et al., 1988; Unger, 1996). The professional doctorate is also referred to as a *clinical doctorate* in many health professions (Pierce & Peyton, 1999).

The *research doctorate* (also called the *academic doctorate*), or PhD, was originally awarded for the study of philosophy in the mid- to late 19th century. However, the degree was extended to include many disciplines of the humanities and sciences, with each PhD simply modified to indicate the field of study; for example, PhD in engineering, PhD in history, or PhD in chemistry. The purpose of the PhD degree is to develop graduates who are independent researchers and are knowledgeable in a specific area of study. Requirements for the PhD degree usually include a course of didactic study, followed by written or oral comprehensive examinations (upon passing, one applies for candidacy), and the completion of a dissertation in some area of new knowledge as deemed appropriate by a committee of senior faculty after an oral defense of the research (Shafritz et al., 1988).

The *doctor of science* (ScD) is an alternative doctoral degree similar to the PhD. Its curriculum is focused on the study of an applied science, such as audiology, occupational therapy, and so forth. ScD degree programs commonly include didactic coursework focused on the study of an applied science, an advanced clinical practicum, and a supervised clinical research project (Kidd, Cox, & Matthies, 2003). Other alternative doctoral degrees include the doctor of education (EdD) and the doctor of public health (DPH).

The professional doctorate reflects academic attainment and seldom requires a master's degree or dissertation (Unger, 1996). Unlike the PhD's focus on developing independent researchers, "sophisticated practice competencies" (Pierce & Peyton, 1999, p. 64) are emphasized in the professional doctorate degree. A person with a professional doctorate, such as an MD or doctor of jurisprudence (JD), must pass state or national qualifying examinations to obtain a license to practice (Unger, 1996). In the health sciences, the term *clinical doctorate* is synonymous with the term *professional doctorate* and the program of study typically requires "mentored advanced clinical experiences for autonomous practice competencies" (Edens & Labadie, 1987; Faut-Callahan, 1992; Hummer, Hunt, & Figuers, 1994; Pierce & Peyton, 1999; Watson, 1988).

Postdoctoral Education

With the growing complexity of knowledge and the need for scholars trained to high, creative levels, postdoctoral education has become increasingly popular to meet work demands in universities, industries, and government (Carmichael, 1961). However, postdoctoral education is widely misunderstood because there is little uniformity.

The adjective *postdoctoral* is frequently used to describe the variety of postdoctoral educational experiences. For example, terms such as *postdoctoral fellow, postdoctoral research associate,* and *postdoctoral trainee* are typically used. Despite the lack of uniformity among terms, postdoctoral is used to denote a *research* appointment after a doctoral degree has been awarded within a discipline or profession (Knowles, 1977).

Residencies

Although residencies are not common practice in occupational therapy, they are a form of postdoctoral education. "The purpose of postprofessional residency education is to advance the resident's preparation as a provider of patient care services in a defined (specialized) area of clinical practice" (DiFabio, 1999, p. 81). Residency training activities are designed to promote the integration of practice, research, and scholarly inquiry (Medeiros, 1998). Professions such as medicine, pharmacy (American Society of Health-System Pharmacists, 2001; Miller & Clarke, 2002), and physical therapy (DiFabio, 1999; Farrell, 1996; Medeiros, 2000) offer postdoctoral specialty residencies to qualified practitioners.

Levels of Education in Occupational Therapy Within the United States

Technical Level

OTA

Occupational therapy assistant (OTA) programs are classified as technical and obtain accreditation from the Accreditation Council for Occupational Therapy Education (ACOTE®). OTA programs are commonly offered at community colleges, private junior colleges, and some 4-year colleges and universities. All OTA programs must adhere to the *Standards for an Accredited Educational Program for the Occupational Therapy Assistant.* As articulated in the Preamble of the Standards, an entry-level OTA must

- Have acquired an educational foundation in the liberal arts and sciences, including a focus on issues related to diversity;

- Be educated as a generalist, with a broad exposure to the delivery models and systems utilized in settings where occupational therapy is currently practiced and where it is emerging as a service;

- Have achieved entry-level competence through a combination of academic andfieldwork education;

- Be prepared to work under the supervision of and in cooperation with the occupational therapist;

- Be prepared to articulate and apply occupational therapy principles, intervention approaches and rationales, and expected outcomes as these relate to occupation;

- Be prepared to be a lifelong learner and keep current with best practice;

- Uphold the ethical standards, values, and attitudes of the occupational therapy profession (ACOTE, 1999b, p. 583).

After completing the OTA didactic and fieldwork requirements, the OTA graduate is eligible to sit for the national certification examination for OTAs. On successful completion, the certified occupational therapy assistant (COTA) may apply for the appropriate state credential and, under specified supervision, render occupational therapy services at the technical level of practice.

Professional Level

Master's: Entry-Level and Postprofessional

As of January 2007, the master's degree is the lowest degree level at which one can enter the profession as an occupational therapist. In occupational therapy education, there are entry-level (or sometimes referred to as the *first professional degree*) and postprofessional master's-degree programs. Distinguishing between entry-level and postprofessional master's-degree programs is not typical in other professions and disciplines (Rogers, 1980a, 1980b). Entry-level master's-degree programs are the entrance into the profession of occupational therapy and are accredited by ACOTE. Some entry-level programs may require students to earn a baccalaureate degree in a related field before entering the master's-degree program in occupational therapy. Other entry-level programs may require extensive prerequisite coursework but not mandate a baccalaureate degree. For example, the course of study may be a 5-year program leading to a master's degree; or, in other programs, the study comprises two semesters beyond an undergraduate degree in a major such as occupational science. Coursework that may be considered remedial or prerequisite is not generally included in the total credits required for the master's degree. On successful completion of the academic and fieldwork requirements, the graduate is eligible to take the national certification examination, then apply for state licensure and provide occupational therapy services at the professional level.

Postprofessional master's-degree programs are available to individuals who have a professional degree in occupational therapy (e.g., baccalaureate, entry-level master's, or an entry-level doctorate degree). Such postprofessional degrees are typical of master's-degree programs in other disciplines with a range of 30 to 36 credits. Postprofessional programs are developed to enhance occupational therapy skills in a specific area (e.g., pediatrics, assistive technology, gerontology). Other master's-degree programs may provide a general program with a curricular emphasis (e.g., leadership, research).

Doctorate: Professional and Research

Currently, doctoral-level occupational therapy offerings include the professional (or clinical) and research doctorates. Some programs offer the PhD degree in occupational therapy. Other doctoral-degree programs related to occupational therapy exist, such as the PhD degree in rehabilitation sciences or occupational science or the ScD. Although many of these programs focus on the application of occupational therapy, it is beyond the scope of this document to describe the variations of doctoral programs closely aligned with occupational therapy.

The professional or clinical doctorate degree in occupational therapy confers the degree of *doctor of occupational therapy* (OTD) or *doctor of occupational therapy* (DrOT) degree to graduates. Two pathways exist for pursuing the clinical doctorate degree. The first is available to postprofessional students, that is, students who have an entry-level degree in occupational therapy. The second pathway leading to the clinical doctorate degree is an entry-level program. Entry-level clinical doctorate degree programs are available for individuals who do not have an entry-level degree in occupational therapy but who have completed specified prerequisite coursework and, as of 2010, a baccalaureate degree.

Although the clinical-doctorate-degree programs vary in philosophy and curriculum, typically the post-professional clinical-doctorate programs are shorter in duration than the entry-level clinical-doctorate programs. The rationale for the difference in program length is that postprofessional clinical-doctorate students have previously completed an entry-level occupational therapy degree.

Several occupational therapy programs offer the PhD degree in occupational therapy. These doctoral programs focus on preparing graduates who are independent researchers and who will develop original knowledge pertinent to occupational therapy.

Accreditation

There are two types of accreditation: institutional (or regional) accreditation and program (or specialized) accreditation (Kaplin & Lee, 1995). Accreditation of occupational therapy programs is completed by ACOTE, which is part of a larger accreditation context (Kramer & Graves, 2005).

Institutional Accreditation

Regional or national accrediting bodies do not accredit programs but rather accredit institutions. "Institutional accreditation applies to the entire institution and all its programs, departments, and schools" (Kaplin & Lee, 1995, p. 873). There are 6 regional agencies that accredit institutions located in distinct geographical areas. Accreditation standards from regional or national accrediting bodies influence ACOTE in that their standards must be aligned with requirements from the USDE and the Council for Higher Education Accreditation (CHEA) (Kramer & Graves, 2005). In postprofessional OT programs, there is no specialized accrediting body. However, institutional accrediting bodies can require a focus visit of a particular program. A focus visit does not result in the accrediting of a specific program.

Program or Specialized Accreditation

Program or specialized accreditation "applies to a particular school, department or program within the institution" and "may also apply to an entire institution if it is a free-standing, specialized institution … whose curriculum is all in the same program area" (Kaplin & Lee, 1995, p. 873). The USDE and the CHEA afford ACOTE "the distinction of being reflected as a national recognized accrediting agency that is seen as a reliable authority about the quality of education offered by the occupational therapy and occupational therapy assistant programs it accredits" (Kramer & Graves, 2005, p. 1). Currently, ACOTE accredits OTA and entry-level or first professional-degree programs in occupational therapy. Such accreditation endeavors are considered specialized, because the accrediting body, ACOTE, reviews OT and OTA programs to ensure quality and that educational standards are met. The educational standards are developed through ACOTE with input from stakeholders.

Suggested Considerations When Choosing an Occupational Therapy Educational Program

When choosing an occupational therapy educational program, important factors must be considered (see Table 1).

A variety of resources can help one to obtain information about specific education programs. Institutional Web sites can be helpful in acquiring information about the program's curriculum and faculty. Brochures, catalogs, and bulletin descriptions often present the program's mission, philosophy, curriculum, or policies. These materials can be requested from the admissions office of each institution. Contacting faculty within the program is frequently useful to answer specific questions. Prospective students may request contact with a current student or alumni to gain a consumer's perspective of the program.

Table 1. Considerations for Occupational Therapy Entry-Level and Postprofessional Education

- Location of program
- Tuition
- Length of program
- Availability of student scholarships
- Full- or part-time programs
- On-campus or distance-formatted programs
- Admission requirements
  - Interview
  - Entrance exams (e.g., Miller's Analogy, Graduate Record Exam)
  - Letters of recommendation, essays
  - Prerequisite classes or degree
  - Observation hours in occupational therapy
- Type of program
  - Degree awarded (e.g., AA, MS, MA, MOT, PhD, ScD, OTD)
  - Thesis requirement
  - Dissertation requirement
  - Curriculum (e.g., courses offered, course descriptions printed in catalog)
  - Program mission and philosophical grounding
  - Specialization (e.g., gerontology, pediatrics, entrepreneurialism)
  - Experiential components
    - Fieldwork, internships, rotations, etc.
    - Length of clinical preparation
    - Opportunities for postdegree experiences (e.g., residencies/fellowships)
- Institutional variables
  - Carnegie classification
  - Library resources
  - Information technology/computer support
  - Stability of program
  - Graduate or professional school
  - Ratings and rankings of programs
- Graduate/alumni accomplishments
  - Graduation rate
  - Employment rates, sites
  - Employer satisfaction with graduates
  - Consumer satisfaction with graduate performance
- Faculty
  - Faculty credentials (e.g., doctorally prepared, specialty certified)
  - Faculty-to-student ratios
  - Faculty accessibility
  - Faculty projects (e.g., grants, publications)
  - Faculty clinical practice

In addition, it is important to answer the following questions:
- What are my future career goals?
- Does the degree offered contribute to accomplishing my short-term and long-term goals?
- If considering an online program, do I have the necessary skills to be successful (e.g., motivation, self-initiative, technical skills)?

References and Resources

Accreditation Council for Occupational Therapy Education. (1999a, August). *ACOTE Motion* and *Resolution J* [Minutes at the meeting of the Accreditation Council for Occupational Therapy Education]. Bethesda, MD: Author.

Accreditation Council for Occupational Therapy Education. (1999b). Standards for an accredited educational program for the occupational therapy assistant. *American Journal of Occupational Therapy, 53,* 583–589.

American Occupational Therapy Association. (2001). *ACOTE sets timeline for post baccalaureate degree programs.* Retrieved June 19, 2001, from http://www.aota.org/nonmembers/area13/links/LINK16.asp

American Society of Health-System Pharmacists. (2001). *The residency learning system (RLS) model* (2nd ed.). Bethesda, MD: Author.

Carmichael, O. C. (1961). *Graduate education: A critique and a program.* New York: Harper & Brothers.

DiFabio, R. P. (1999). Clinical expertise and the DPT: A need for residency training. *Journal of Orthopaedic and Sports Physical Therapy, 29,* 80–82.

Edens, G. E., & Labadie, G. C. (1987). Opinions about the professional doctorate in nursing. *Nursing Outlook, 35,* 136–140.

Farrell, J. P. (1996). In search of clinical excellence. *Journal of Orthopaedic and Sports Physical Therapy, 24,* 115–121.

Faut-Callahan, M. (1992). Graduate education for nurse anesthetists: Master's versus a clinical doctorate. *Journal of the American Association of Nurse Anesthetists, 60,* 98–103.

Glazer, J. S. (1988). *The master's degree* (Report No. EDO-HE-88-3). Washington, DC: Office of Educational Research and Improvement. (ERIC Document Reproduction Service No. ED301140)

Hummer, L. A., Hunt, K. S., & Figuers, C. C. (1994). Predominant thought regarding entry-level doctor of physical therapy programs. *Journal of Physical Therapy Education, 8,* 60–66.

Kapel, D. E., Gifford, C. S., & Kapel, M. B. (1991). *American educators' encyclopedia* (rev. ed.). Westport, CT: Greenwood.

Kaplin, W. A., & Lee, B. A. (1995). *The law of higher education* (3rd ed.). San Francisco: Jossey-Bass.

Kidd, G. D., Cox, C. C., & Matthies, M. L. (2003). Boston University doctor of science degree program: Clinical doctorate in audiology. *American Journal of Audiology, 12,* 3–6.

Knowles, A. S. (1977). Postdoctoral education. In *The international encyclopedia of higher education* (Vol. 5, pp. 1923–1928). San Francisco: Jossey-Bass.

Kramer, P., & Graves, S. (2005, March). Accreditation 101: Understanding the broad world of accreditation. *Education Special Interest Section Quarterly, 15,* 1–2.

LaPidus, J. B. (2000). Postbaccalaureate and graduate education: A dynamic balance. In K. Kohl & J. LaPidus (Eds.), *Postbaccalaureate futures* (pp. 3–9). Phoenix, AZ: Oryx.

Mayhew, L. B., & Ford, P. J. (1971). *Changing the curriculum.* San Francisco: Jossey-Bass.

Mayhew, L. B., & Ford, P. J. (1974). *Reform in graduate and professional education.* San Francisco: Jossey-Bass.

Medeiros, J. M. (1998). Post professional clinical residency programs. *Journal of Manual and Manipulative Therapy, 6,* 10.

Medeiros, J. M. (2000). Educational standards for residency education. *Journal of Manual and Manipulative Therapy, 8,* 50.

Miller, S., & Clarke, A. (2002). Impact of postdoctoral specialty residencies in drug information on graduates' career paths. *American Journal of Health-System Pharmacy, 59,* 961–963.

Pierce, D., & Peyton, C. (1999). A historical cross-disciplinary perspective on the professional doctorate in occupational therapy. *American Journal of Occupational Therapy, 53,* 64–71.

Rogers, J. C. (1980a). Design of the master's degree in occupational therapy, part 1. A logical approach. *American Journal of Occupational Therapy, 34,* 113–118.

Rogers, J. C. (1980b). Design of the master's degree in occupational therapy, part 2. An empirical approach. *American Journal of Occupational Therapy, 34,* 176–184.

Shafritz, J. M., Koeppe, R. P., & Soper, E. W. (1988). *American educators' encyclopedia.* Westport, CT: Greenwood Press.

Unger, H. G. (1996). *Encyclopedia of American education.* New York: Facts on File.

U.S. Department of Education. (2002). *Classification of instructional programs: 2000 edition.* Washington, DC: Office of Educational Research and Improvement.

Watson, J. (1988). *The professional doctorate as an entry level into practice. Perspectives in nursing—1987–1989.* New York: National League for Nursing.

Authors

Brenda M. Coppard, PhD, OTR/L
Creighton University, Omaha, NE
Member, AOTA Commission on Education, 2002–2007
Anne Dickerson, PhD, OTR/L, FAOTA
East Carolina University, Greenville, NC
Member, AOTA Commission on Education, 2000–2006

for

The Commission on Education
Linda Fazio, PhD, OTR/L, FAOTA, *Chairperson*
Brenda M. Coppard, PhD, OTR/L, *Postprofessional Academic Educator*
Donna Costa, MS, OTR/L, *Academic Fieldwork Educator*
Linda Musselman, PhD, OTR, FAOTA, *Professional Program Director*
David Haynes, MBA, OTR/L, *OTA Program Director*
Kelly Fischer, OTR/L, *Fieldwork Educator*
Terrianne Jones, MA, OTR/L, *OTA Academic Educator*
Marc Freedman, *ASD Liaison*
Shirley Marino, COTA, AP, *OTA Educator*
Jaime Muñoz, PhD, OTR/L, FAOTA, *Professional Academic Educator*
René Padilla, PhD, OTR/L, FAOTA, *Chair-Elect*
Jyothi Gupta, PhD, OTR/L, *EDSIS Liaison*

Adopted by the Representative Assembly 2007C11

The Role of Occupational Therapy in Disaster Preparedness, Response, and Recovery: A Concept Paper

Purpose

The focus of occupational therapy is to support people's health and participation in life through engagement in occupations (American Occupational Therapy Association [AOTA], 2008). Natural and human-created disasters are increasing in frequency throughout the world (Rodriguez, Vos, Below, & Guha-Sapir, 2009) and have a significant negative impact, both short- and long-term, on the health and occupational engagement of individuals, families, and communities. The purpose of this concept paper is to provide occupational therapy practitioners[1] with a basic understanding of disasters so those occupational therapy practitioners can support people's health and participation in life across the spectrum of disaster preparedness, response, and recovery. Beyond reading this concept paper, time for additional training and reflecting on one's own preparedness and motivation is needed prior to engaging in this important work.

Overview

When a societal crisis occurs, individuals, families, communities, institutions, and society as a whole become "disabled"—that is, limited in their ability to perform normal daily activities; restricted by environmental barriers; prohibited from participating in usual life roles; threatened by personal and financial losses; and subjected to a variety of psychological reactions, including fear, helplessness, and loss of confidence (Scaffa, 2003). Along with other people who experience a natural or technological (human-made) disaster, occupational therapists and occupational therapy assistants are victims and survivors of these experiences. However, occupational therapy practitioners also have the opportunity to be part of the solution for helping people prepare for, respond to, and recover from the disaster. They can use their understanding of occupations, occupational disruption, and activity analysis to increase individual and community readiness for and response to the disaster; to minimize or prevent maladaptation or further injury; and, ultimately, to promote health and recovery through an occupation-based approach.

Occupational therapy scholars have proposed several ways in which occupation can mediate the effects of stressful situations and promote health (McColl, 2002). Occupation can contribute to a person's sense of mastery and reinforce identity. It can restore habits and normalcy and can re-establish routines and meaningful roles. Many occupations that focus on taking care of self and others are health-promoting and are essential in responding to and recovering from trauma. Finally, occupation is a means through which people support themselves and others and through which they connect to their larger communities and social networks.

In this paper, disasters are defined, and the five stages of a disaster are presented. Next, assumptions that inform occupational therapy practitioners' participation in disaster relief are identified, followed by a discussion of occupational therapy's potential contributions before and during times of disaster. The role

---

[1]When the term *occupational therapy practitioner* is used in this document, it refers to both occupational therapists and occupational therapy assistants (AOTA, 2006a). *Occupational therapists* are responsible for all aspects of occupational therapy service delivery and are accountable for the safety and effectiveness of the occupational therapy service delivery process. *Occupational therapy assistants* deliver occupational therapy services under the supervision of and in partnership with an occupational therapist (AOTA, 2009).

occupational therapy practitioners can play in the stages of disaster work—disaster preparedness, disaster response, and disaster recovery—is outlined and provides an overview of how to initiate involvement in any of these stages. Finally, the relationship of disaster preparedness and relief to the *Occupational Therapy Code of Ethics and Ethics Standards (2010)* (AOTA, 2010a) is provided, followed by a call for involvement in disaster work and research.

Definitions and Background

In 1961, Charles E. Fritz, a pioneer in disaster research, defined *disasters* as

> Actual or threatened accidental or uncontrollable events that are concentrated in time and space, in which a society or a relatively self-sufficient subdivision of a society undergoes severe danger, and incurs such losses to its members and physical appurtenances that the social structure is disrupted and the fulfillment of all or some of the essential functions of the society, or its subdivision, is prevented. (p. 655)

This definition describes not only the physical damage and personal injuries that are typically sustained during a disaster but also the potential widespread social and economic disruption of daily-life routines.

Typically, disasters are classified into two categories: (1) natural and (2) technological (or human-made). Natural disasters include earthquakes, fires or wildfires, floods, heat waves, hurricanes, landslides and debris flow, thunderstorms, tornadoes, tsunamis, volcanoes, and winter storms/extreme cold. Technological disasters include biological threats, chemical emergencies/threats, computer attacks/viruses, dam failure, explosions, hazardous material leaks (e.g., oil spills), mass transportation accidents, mining accidents, nuclear blasts, nuclear power plant emergencies, prolonged or widespread power failures, radiological dispersion device activations, and any other terrorist activities (Federal Emergency Management Agency [FEMA], 2010; Fischer, 1998; Schneid & Collins, 2001).

Disasters progress through five stages, each requiring different behavioral and organizational responses:

- In the first stage, the *pre-impact period*, a warning of impending disaster may allow for preparation. For example, the National Weather Service may issue a hurricane warning, which prompts individuals, families, and institutions to put disaster response plans in effect while time permits. In some cases, though, there is no warning, and the pre-impact stage is short or nonexistent, such as when a mass shooting at an academic institution or a massive oil spill occurs unexpectedly.

- The second stage, the *impact period*, is generally the shortest in duration but the most dangerous in the life cycle of a disaster. In this stage the disaster is experienced in full force. Research has shown that altruism and an outpouring of concern for the victims of natural disasters is the norm, and people tend to share food, equipment, and supplies and assist one another in recovery efforts. Perceptions that antisocial behavior and widespread panic occur immediately following a disaster have not been substantiated by the literature (Drabek & McEntire, 2003; Fischer, 2002; Tierney, Bevc, & Kuligowski, 2006).

- In the third stage, the *immediate post-impact period*, search-and-rescue and evacuation efforts are initiated, the media generate increasing coverage of the event, and emergency organizations begin to respond.

- During the fourth stage, the *recovery period*, clearance of debris is completed, essential services such as electricity and water are restored, preliminary reconstruction plans are initiated, and daily life routines begin to normalize.

- The fifth and final stage, the *reconstruction period*, may last from several months to several years depending on the scope and the severity of the disaster. Reconstruction involves the rebuilding not only of structures but also of individual lifestyles and a sense of community.

According to Fischer (1998), the mental health effects of disasters often last longer than the physical manifestations.

Assumptions

This paper is based on the following nine assumptions gathered from the literature:

1. Natural disasters have been increasing in frequency throughout the world since 1998 (Rodriguez et al., 2009) and deprive persons of their right to participate in life-sustaining and meaningful occupations.

2. When disaster strikes, already-difficult circumstances are exacerbated for marginalized populations, such as persons with disabilities, elderly individuals, people with chronic illnesses, children, the poor population, and indigenous groups. These groups are especially vulnerable and disproportionately affected by disasters (Smith & Notaro, 2009).

3. Disaster situations generate significant personal loss and environmental changes that can adversely affect adaptive occupational performance of individuals and communities across all areas of occupation (Rosenfeld, 1982, 1989; Tuchner, Meiner, Parush, & Hartman-Maier, 2010).

4. Disasters can generate significant traumatic stress (Diamond & Precin, 2003; Tuchner et al., 2010; Young, Ford, Ruzek, Friedman, & Gusman, 1998), and survivors' usual coping strategies may prove inadequate for disaster situations (Rosenfeld, 1982; Tuchner et al., 2010; Young et al., 1998).

5. Engagement in occupation can moderate the effects of disaster (McColl, 2002; Tuchner et al., 2010).

6. Occupational therapy practitioners can contribute to interdisciplinary efforts of disaster preparedness through their use of activity analysis, skills at grading and adaptation of tasks, knowledge of contexts, and an understanding of the occupational needs of individuals and families.

7. In disaster situations, the focus of occupational therapy is to facilitate engagement in occupations in order to enhance adaptive responses to the disaster and to resume valued life habits, routines, roles, and rituals (AOTA, 2008).

8. Occupational therapy practitioners can assist individuals, families (Tuchner et al., 2010), and communities in coping with disaster situations and in returning to optimal occupational performance (Rosenfeld, 1982, 1989).

9. Occupational therapists and occupational therapy assistants can identify disruptions in occupational performance patterns and help clients develop new, effective patterns of performance by facilitating the process of occupational adaptation (Rosenfeld, 1982).

Occupational Therapy Contributions in Times of Disaster

Occupational therapy practitioners can and should be involved in disaster preparedness, response, and recovery. In working with individuals, families, and communities affected by disasters, occupational therapy practitioners bring a set of core practice skills grounded on the importance of occupational engagement. Working together with the client, occupational therapy practitioners can plan and implement interventions that enable people to reestablish balance and engagement in as many areas of occupation (e.g., activities of daily living [ADLs], instrumental activities of daily living, rest and sleep, education, work, play, leisure, social participation) as possible by

- Evaluating people's occupational balance, occupational performance (functional abilities), and performance patterns;

- Configuring contexts (i.e., cultural, personal, temporal, virtual,) and environments (i.e., social, physical) to maximize occupational engagement and social participation; and

- Analyzing occupations and activities to determine the underlying requisites for effective performance.

In addition, occupational therapy practitioners have mental health knowledge and skills (in common with other professionals) that are useful in disaster management and response. Possession of this knowledge and skill facilitates inclusion of occupational therapy practitioners on mental health intervention teams in times of disaster.

Occupational Therapy Contributions in Disaster Preparedness

Disaster preparedness involves actions taken before a disaster that enable a community to respond effectively. This requires planning at the community, organizational, and household levels. Planned interventions designed to address system-level concerns, as well as direct service interventions for the individual, are necessary to ensure safety and facilitate normalization. Organizations and businesses should develop emergency response plans, train employees in how to handle emergency situations, acquire needed supplies and equipment, and conduct response drills and exercises (Tierney, Lindell, & Perry, 2001). Individuals must know what these plans entail so that they can proactively remain safe or seek help, when needed, in a timely and efficient way.

When interfacing with disaster response teams, it is important to know the hierarchical structure of agencies and organizations involved in planning, responding, and facilitating recovery from disasters. The National Disaster Medical System is a section within the FEMA in the U.S. Department of Homeland Security. It is responsible for managing and coordinating the federal medical response to major emergencies and federally declared disasters. Its focus is to ensure medical response to a disaster area in the form of providing teams, supplies, and equipment; moving injured people from disaster sites to unaffected areas; and identifying the types of medical care available at participating hospitals in unaffected areas.

All states are divided into local regions with Disaster Medical Assistance Teams (DMATs). These teams develop and implement plans to meet physical and mental health needs during disasters in their areas. State, county, and local agencies, businesses, and community organizations, as well as individuals, may assist these teams in disaster planning, response, and recovery. Participating in "table-top" and other mock disaster drills at the local, state, and national levels as a member of a team provides needed training. Becoming affiliated with local and national organizations, such as the American Red Cross, community emergency response teams (CERTs), mental health crisis services, critical incident stress management (CISM) teams, and employee assistance programs prior to a disaster increases the credibility of the occupational therapy practitioner and facilitates involvement when a disaster occurs.

Occupational therapy practitioners should select the level of involvement and role that best matches community need as well as their personal availability, skills, and knowledge. Practitioners can apply their expertise in several settings, including health care facilities, schools, businesses, and shelters. Those who work in health care facilities should participate in discussions of existing policies and procedures, as well as the role of occupational therapy in the promotion of the safety of clients during a fire or severe weather conditions, including consideration of what to do when these conditions continue for an extended period. For example, when a predicted hurricane arrives, plans are already in place for securing facilities, moving those with special needs, and providing food and shelter and necessary medications for the short term. But if the storm is fierce and has caused extensive destruction, then staff need to be able to design and adapt spaces, modify expectations, create new physical and social environments, and provide support services for those under their care for an unknown period of time.

Schools often are the most likely place that children will be when a disaster occurs. School disaster planning is essential and typically consists of identifying school crisis teams, delineating the roles of staff during an emergency, and establishing processes for reuniting children with their parents. Occupational therapy practitioners who work in academic settings (e.g., K–12 schools, universities) can assist in school planning regarding the requirements of students with special needs. For example, occupational therapists can assess the medical and mental health resources that are available in the school environment and assist in the development of individualized emergency care plans for students with disabilities (Asher & Pollak, 2009; American Academy of Pediatrics, Council on School Health, 2008). According to Asher and Pollak (2009), occupational therapists are uniquely qualified to identify the elements of an emergency care plan, including "how the student is transported, moved, and positioned;

any personal equipment that may need to accompany the student; where to exit the building; or when to stay in the building" (p. CE3). In addition, occupational therapy practitioners can offer their expertise in planning for disasters by recommending the use of compact, easily stored supplies for age-appropriate activities during disasters such as a prolonged "lock down," flu or disease outbreak, or blizzard.

Occupational therapy practitioners can help DMATs and employers design plans to evacuate workers with disabilities effectively in the event of an emergency and can train staff and volunteers to work in shelters for people with special needs prior to disasters. Occupational therapy practitioners planning system-level interventions can ensure that shelters and other emergency sites are organized in ways that minimize environmental barriers. For example, they can ensure that people with mobility limitations will be located near restrooms to facilitate independence in self-care. Such planning also decreases the number of environmental modifications or kinds of adaptive equipment that will be required to address self-care needs and privacy concerns. Occupational therapists have the expertise needed to plan, organize, and direct programs in shelters and to train and supervise volunteers. In addition, practitioners can work with individuals or groups of individuals with disabilities on their own emergency preparedness plans (Diamond & Precin, 2003).

Knowledge of available resources and understanding of local plans for responding to such disasters are critical to effective rapid humanitarian responses. Sensitivity to occupational performance needs and facilitating choice in occupational engagement is a unique marker of the services provided by occupational therapy practitioners (Stone, 2006) and dissimilar to any that are likely to be provided by other members of the response team. It also is essential that practitioners have in place appropriate plans for their family's care during the extended period when they may need to remain on duty at their institution to help prevent conflicting demands on their energies and emotions.

Occupational Therapy Contributions in Disaster Response

Emergency response involves actions taken just prior to, during, and shortly after disaster impact to address the immediate needs of victims and to reduce damage, destruction, and disruption. Emergency response activities include detection of threats, dissemination of warnings, and evacuation of vulnerable populations. In addition, they include search for and rescue of victims, provision of emergency medical care, and furnishing of food and shelter for displaced persons (Tierney et al., 2001). The daily concerns of older adults after Hurricane Katrina included "securing basic resources, facing communication difficulties, and finding transportation" (Henderson, Roberto, & Kano, 2010, p. 48). All disaster-related interventions should recognize and be delivered within the hierarchy of needs framework, typically survival, safety and security, and food and shelter needs are primary, followed by health, both physical and mental (National Institute of Mental Health [NIMH], 2002).

During times of disaster or emergency, all professionals are called on to provide their expertise voluntarily in the service of others. Occupational therapy practitioners are qualified to provide disaster response services to people with special needs. FEMA defines *special-needs populations* as people in the community with physical, mental, or medical care needs who may require assistance before, during, or after a disaster or an emergency, after exhausting their usual resources and support network. During a disaster, people with special needs may be moved to regular shelters or shelters for people with special needs, or they may *shelter-in-place* (i.e., remain in their personal homes or other residences, such as assisted living facilities, foster and group homes, and long-term care facilities). People with mobility or sensory disabilities often are moved to a temporary emergency location not specifically designed to accommodate their needs. Occupational therapy practitioners can—within their skill level and arena of practice—modify and adapt these environments to promote safety and more independent function. Occupational therapy services may include supervising staff and volunteers at special-needs shelters, making home visits or telephone calls to those sheltering-in-place, and facilitating support groups designed to reduce anxiety and stress.

Occupational therapy practitioners also may provide support for displaced, confused adults and children until their caregivers can be identified and located. Occupational therapists can identify children who are having difficulty coping and address their mental health concerns, as well as provide guidance for their caregivers.

Occupational therapy practitioners can provide a variety of services to individuals and families who have evacuated their homes and workplaces and are living in emergency shelters or who are sheltering-in-place. People who are displaced from their homes and workplaces to emergency shelters face a variety of challenges. People of various cultures and ethnic backgrounds with different beliefs and habits often are forced to live in one large room with no privacy. Children are bored, a general sense of uneasiness pervades, and stress levels increase. Using a client-centered approach, occupational therapy practitioners can evaluate the needs of people in the shelter and provide appropriate services. Interventions might include providing structure in daily routines, identifying and emphasizing people's strengths, encouraging creative expression of feelings, coordinating age-appropriate play for children, and providing opportunities for stress management (Newton, 2000).

In addition, occupational therapy practitioners with appropriate knowledge and skills who are part of a disaster response team can provide short-term, supportive mental health services to victims, families, first responders, and volunteers (AOTA, 2010c). This is referred to as *psychological first aid* (NIMH, 2008; Watson & Shalev, 2005) or *mental health first aid* and is provided only to those who seek the service. Mental health first aid can be defined as "help provided to a person developing a mental health problem or in a mental health crisis. The first aid is given until appropriate professional treatment is received or until the crisis resolves" (Kitchener & Jorm, 2007, p. 2). The goals of mental health first aid are to

* Prevent injury or death when a person is a danger to themselves or others,

* Protect survivors from further harm,

* Reduce distress,

* Prevent the mental health problem from developing into a more serious condition,

* Promote the recovery of positive mental health,

* Reduce physiological arousal,

* Provide comfort to the person coping with a mental health crisis,

* Facilitate reunion with loved ones, and

* Guide the person toward appropriate professional help (Kitchener & Jorm, 2007; NIMH, 2002).

The mental health first aid process generally consists of several components:

* Assessing risk of suicide or harm,

* Listening in an active empathic manner,

* Providing reassurance and information/education,

* Facilitating self-help strategies and access to community resources,

* Reducing secondary stressors, and

* Encouraging the person to seek appropriate professional help when needed (Kitchener & Jorm, 2007; Shalev, Tuval-Mashiach, & Hadar, 2004).

First responders, including firefighters, police, and emergency medical personnel, also may benefit from occupational therapy. These individuals work long hours under difficult circumstances and often are away from home. Occupational therapists can observe first responders and volunteers for signs of distress and can provide respite, psychological first aid, or other appropriate interventions (Newton, 2000).

Occupational therapy is based on the premise that engagement in occupations facilitates adaptation. Occupation can help disaster survivors reestablish their sense of control. Focused, constructive activity, such as helping others, moves people beyond shock and denial. This strategy is especially effective for survivors who are being disruptive. Engaging survivors as active participants in their ongoing survival and adjustment to change can help them regain their sense of mastery and overcome any sense of guilt from a perceived failure to prepare for the disaster or to protect their family. By engaging in play, vigorous physical activity, or valued leisure occupations, survivors can get a brief respite from recurring thoughts, worries, and concerns about the future.

Occupational Therapy Contributions in Disaster Recovery

Post-disaster recovery involves repair and rebuilding of property, reestablishment of public utilities, and restoration of disrupted social and economic activities, and routines. For example, the restoration of the school community provides age-appropriate occupational engagement for students (Hobfoll et al., 2007). According to the Council on School Health of the American Academy of Pediatrics (2008), "Although returning to the classroom does not ensure that children are ready to address learning tasks, evidence points to the restorative power of the educational routine in guiding children through emotional crises" (p. 898). Post-disaster recovery also includes efforts to reduce acute stress, foster resilience, re-establish roles and routines, and enhance the psychosocial well-being and the quality of life of the community members affected (Tierney et al., 2001).

Following disasters, many survivors experience acute stress reactions (see Table 1). Hobfoll et al. (2007) identified five essential elements to trauma intervention including: (1) promotion of sense of safety, (2) promotion of calming, (3) promotion of sense of self-efficacy and collective efficacy, (4) promotion of connectedness, and (5) promotion of hope. A sense of safety can be instilled by providing the facts of

Table 1. Common Acute Stress Reactions to Disaster

Emotional Effects	Cognitive Effects
Shock	Impaired concentration
Anger	Impaired decision-making ability
Despair	Memory impairment
Emotional numbing	Disbelief
Terror	Confusion
Guilt	Distortion
Grief or sadness	Decreased self-esteem
Irritability	Decreased self-efficacy
Helplessness	Self-blame
Loss of derived pleasure from regular activities	Intrusive thoughts and memories
Dissociation (e.g., perceptual experience seems "dreamlike," "tunnel vision," "spacey," or "on automatic pilot")	Worry
Mood swings	

Physical Effects	Interpersonal Effects
Fatigue	Alienation
Insomnia	Social withdrawal
Sleep disturbance	Increased conflict within relationships
Hyperarousal	Vocational impairment
Somatic complaints	School impairment
Impaired immune response	
Headaches	
Gastrointestinal problems	
Decreased appetite	
Decreased libido	
Startle response	

Note. From *Disaster Mental Health Services: A Guidebook for Clinicians and Administrators,* by B. H. Young, J. D. Ford, J. I. Ruzek, M. J. Friedman, & F. D. Gusman, 1998, Menlo Park, CA: National Center for Post-Traumatic Stress Disorder, Department of Veterans Affairs. Available at www.ncptsd.org/publications/disaster/.

the current situation without the hyperbole of some media reports. Calming is required for the occupational performance of restorative sleep, which is commonly adversely affected. Occupational therapists can promote a sense of self-efficacy as they help clients to problem-solve and successfully address disaster-related issues. It is imperative to facilitate connectedness to ensure social participation necessary for well-being. Finally, hope can be instilled by providing a realistic but noncatastrophic view of the future (Hobfoll et al., 2007).

Fostering resilience as well as psychological and social recovery are major goals in this stage of disaster. Strategies to facilitate resilience and psychological and social recovery include providing education on acute stress responses and coping skills training, fostering natural social supports, encouraging social interactions, facilitating spiritual support, and offering group and family interventions (AOTA, 2010b, 2010c; NIMH, 2002).

The profession of occupational therapy has long recognized the importance of roles, habits, and routines to occupational engagement (American Occupational Therapy Foundation [AOTF], 2010). Disasters can seriously disrupt role engagement and the habits and routines that sustain them. Roles help give people an identity and a sense of self, as well as identify the responsibilities associated with that identity (Deeny & McFetridge, 2005; Kielhofner, Forsyth, & Barrett, 2003). After a disaster, roles such as student, worker, leisure participant, or others may be lost. In the case of displacement from a person's home and community, some roles, like those of family member or friend, must be maintained from a distance, or worse, relinquished. Other roles may need to be expanded, such as homeowner, as insurance issues will require significant time and attention. Often, changes in context require the adoption of new roles, such as volunteer, renter, or home remodeler. Occupational therapy practitioners are adept at helping clients successfully negotiate periods of transition and can help clients adapt to role changes dictated by the disaster.

Occupation and activity can help clients cope with traumatic stress and meet survival needs. Occupational engagement reduces the intensity of stressful events and helps reestablish a sense of mastery in a situation in which a person feels a loss of control. The military has long used occupational therapy to help soldiers overcome occupational dysfunction due to the stress of war (Ellsworth, Laedtke, & McPhee, 1993; Laedtke, 1996), to support their role identity, and to restore their confidence in their ability to function (Gerardi, 1996, 1999; Gerardi & Newton, 2004). Participation in occupation facilitates restoration of adaptive habits and routines, supports a person's sense of identity, and helps establish a spiritual connection in the disaster situation (McColl, 2002). As part of the intervention team, occupational therapy practitioners can help clients develop coping skills to deal with the aftereffects of their experience. Additionally, through engagement in occupation, disaster survivors can restructure their habits and routines to cope more effectively with stress and anxiety, to enhance their sense of mastery over their environment, and to participate in their valued life roles.

Some survivors may experience lasting psychological effects from the traumatic stress of their experience. These posttraumatic stress symptoms may be severe enough to manifest themselves as depression or an anxiety disorder such as posttraumatic stress disorder (PTSD). Characteristic of PTSD is persistent re-experiencing of the event (e.g., in nightmares and flashbacks), avoidance of reminders of the trauma and numbing of emotions (e.g., difficulty recalling aspects of the trauma and detachment from others), and heightened physiological arousal (e.g., insomnia, irritability, exaggerated startle response), all lasting more than one month (American Psychiatric Association, 1994). In addition—and of primary concern to the occupational therapy practitioner—a person with PTSD may experience significant occupational dysfunction. Providing occupational therapy in a group format offers a supportive environment and can enhance function and provide a renewed sense of self-efficacy (Ziv & Roitman, 2008).

For persons diagnosed with PTSD, occupation can be used to recover and enhance skills required in daily life roles. Such interventions may focus on ADLs to enhance independent living; on coping skills (e.g., relaxation, biofeedback) to deal with stress, anxiety, and physiological arousal; and on socialization skills to decrease emotional and social withdrawal and to increase socialization (Davis & Kutter, 1998; Froelich, 1992; Rosenfeld, 1982, 1989; Short-Degraff & Engelman, 1992). Expressive media can be used to help clients re-experience their trauma in a safe supportive environment. This enables them to explore and discover how they have been affected by the event and to practice skills to deal more effectively with their physiological and emotional responses (Davis, 1999; Froelich, 1992; Morgan & Johnson, 1995; Short-Degraff & Engelman, 1992).

Contributions of Occupational Therapy Organizations in Times of Disaster

The AOTF, AOTA, and the World Federation of Occupational Therapists (WFOT) have been involved in disaster work. In 2002, following the terrorist attacks of 9/11, the AOTF established the Task Force on Occupation in Societal Crises. This group, made up of civilian and military personnel and occupational therapists from Canada and the United States, worked in collaboration with AOTA's Commission on Practice to write the first version of this concept paper (AOTA, 2006b).

AOTA has been responsive after hurricanes Katrina, Rita, and Ike, as well as other disasters. In large-scale disasters, where citizens of affected communities are simply struggling to survive, it is imperative that entities outside the immediate disaster zone provide assistance to ensure safe living arrangements, mental health support, job opportunities, and continued curriculum or equal educational opportunities. Local and regional, trained and networked occupational therapy practitioners are best prepared to help and to serve as conduits of information regarding needs to professional associations at the state, national, and international levels. However, before disasters occur, professional associations can provide guidance through official documents and other training materials. For example, in response to the 2004 Indian Ocean Tsunami, WFOT produced a Disaster Preparedness and Response information package and is supporting the development of a textbook on the same topic (WFOT, n.d.). AOTA also has produced disaster-related materials; links to these resources and those of the WFOT appear in Table 2. While professional associations have a role in educating members and society about the potential role of occupational therapy, ultimately it is individual occupational therapy practitioners who need to take the initiative to be trained and ready to serve if disaster occurs in their institution, community, or region (Stone, 2006).

Occupational Justice, Ethics, and Research in Disaster Preparedness, Response, and Recovery

The term *occupational justice* conveys the profession's commitment to populations and individuals in need as well as the strong belief that access to occupation is a right and a necessity for health and quality of life (AOTA, 2008; Townsend & Wilcock, 2004). Disaster survivors often are vulnerable and in need of the services of occupational therapy practitioners. Stone (2006) reports that the best method to provide recovery services is in the community (when possible) by local, pre-trained providers who are part of an established network.

To be able to assist in an ethical manner, occupational therapy practitioners must

• Be keenly aware of their motivations to engage in this type of work,

• Have an individual/family disaster plan in place,

• Seek out training and secure a position from an authorized agency,

• Be competent in the tasks and services they provide,

• Not expect special privileges, and

• Not unduly take advantage of the experience or capitalize on others' misfortune.

Communities affected by disaster can provide tremendous opportunities for research (Morris, 2008). However, special care must be taken to ensure research is done in an ethical and compassionate way. A group of social scientists met after Hurricane Katrina and established eight criteria to guide research on the disaster (Gill et al., 2007). While all eight criteria are relevant to occupational therapy research, the

Table 2. Disaster Resources

Title	Link	Description
American Academy of Pediatrics, "Children and Disasters: Disaster Preparedness to Meet Children's Needs"	www.aap.org/disasters	Web site on disaster preparedness to meet the needs of children
American Occupational Therapy Association	http://www.aota.org/Practitioners/Resources/Collections/Preparedness-Library/Emergency-Resources-.aspx	Emergency preparedness and response resources compiled for occupational therapy practitioners
American Red Cross, *Disaster Preparedness for Persons With Disabilities*	http://www.redcross.org/www-files/Documents/pdf/Preparedness/Fast%20Facts/Disaster_Preparedness_for_PwD-English.pdf	Booklet
American Red Cross, *Disaster Preparedness for Seniors by Seniors*	http://www.redcross.org/www-files/Documents/pdf/Preparedness/Fast%20Facts/Disaster_Preparedness_for_Srs-English.revised_7-09.pdf	Booklet
Center for an Accessible Society, "Disaster Mitigation for Persons With Disabilities"	www.accessiblesociety.org/topics/independentliving/disasterprep.htm	Web site of resources
Federal Emergency Management Agency	www.fema.gov	Web site
Federal Emergency Management Agency, *A Citizen Guide to Disaster Preparedness*	http://webharvest.gov/peth04/20041017185751/http://www.pueblo.gsa.gov/cic_text/family/disaster-guide/disasterguide.htm	Booklet
Federal Emergency Management Agency, National Preparedness Directorate, Emergency Management Institute	http://training.fema.gov/	Web site of nationwide training program of resident and nonresident courses to enhance U.S. emergency management practices
Inclusive Preparedness Center, "Emergency Preparedness for People With Disabilities and Other Vulnerable Populations"	http://www.inclusivepreparedness.org/	Web site focused on ensuring that all people are included in emergency planning, response, and recovery from natural and technological disasters
International Critical Incident Stress Foundation	www.icisf.org/	Web site of nonprofit, open-membership foundation dedicated to prevention and mitigation of disabling stress through provision of education, training, and support services for all emergency medical service professions; continuing education and training in emergency mental health services; and consultation in establishment of crisis and disaster response programs for varied organizations and communities worldwide
National Voluntary Organizations Active in Disaster	http://www.nvoad.org	A coalition of nonprofit organizations sharing knowledge and resources regarding disaster preparation, response, and recovery to help disaster survivors and their communities
Substance Abuse and Mental Health Services Administration, "Disaster Kit"	http://mentalhealth.samhsa.gov/disasterrelief/default.aspx	Publications on mental health and disaster
Substance Abuse and Mental Health Services Administration, *Training Manual for Mental Health and Human Service Workers in Major Disasters*	http://mentalhealth.samhsa.gov/publications/allpubs/ADM90-538/Default.asp	Manual

(continued)

Table 2. Disaster Resources *(cont.)*

Title	Link	Description
U.S. Department of Education, *Practical Information on Crisis Planning: A Guide for Schools and Communities*	www.ed.gov/admins/lead/safety/emergency plan/crisisplanning.pdf	Book
U.S. Department of Health and Human Services, "National Disaster Medical System"	http://ndms.dhhs.gov	Web site
World Federation of Occupational Therapists, *Disaster Preparedness and Response Information Package*	https://www.wfot.org/wfotshop/shop exd.asp?id=71	Educational CD-ROM available for purchase or free to those working in disaster relief and to countries without the financial resources to purchase
World Federation of Occupational Therapists, *WFOT Disaster Preparedness and Response Questionnaire*	http://www.wfot.org/singleNews.asp? id=163&name=WFOT%20Disaster%20 Preparedness%20and%20Response% 20-%20Questionnaire	Survey to gather information regarding disaster preparedness and relief activities around the world

following four resonate most strongly with the *Occupational Therapy Code of Ethics and Ethics Standards* (AOTA, 2010a) and occupational justice:

- "Reducing vulnerability of populations to disaster, promoting the sustainability of human and ecological systems, and enhancing the resiliency of communities" (p. 790).

- "Facilitating recovery of individuals and communities" (p. 791).

- "Enhancing stakeholder participation, collaboration, and empowerment" (p. 792).

- "Developing new knowledge of understudied disaster-related issues" (p. 792).

Conclusion

Occupational therapy practitioners can have a significant role in disaster preparedness, response, and recovery. For example, in preparation for disasters, occupational therapy practitioners can

- Participate in facility-level and community-wide planning efforts,

- Design special-needs shelters and train staff and volunteers, and

- Assist businesses and employers in developing plans for evacuating employees with disabilities.

Occupational therapy has much to offer individuals, families, organizations, institutions, and communities affected by disaster. The profession's holistic approach and its focus on occupational engagement and adaptation constitute its unique contribution to disaster management. During the disaster response, occupational therapy practitioners can

- Provide supportive mental health services to victims and their families;

- Provide supportive mental health services to first responders, such as police, firefighters, and military personnel;

- Manage special-needs shelters;

- Provide supportive services by telephone or visits to those sheltering-in-place;

- Provide occupational interventions in shelters; and

- Facilitate psychological and educational support groups to decrease anxiety and stress.

Throughout the disaster recovery phase, occupational therapy practitioners can provide occupation-based and mental health services for persons with acute stress reactions and PTSD. Interventions must be designed to be meaningful and purposeful to those engaged in them, and they must support the individual, family, community, or agency in responding to the unique characteristics of the disaster.

Occupational therapy practitioners can use their professional expertise and the power of occupational engagement to restore control, order, and quality of life and to normalize lives in crisis when individuals, families, institutions, and communities are disrupted by natural or technological disasters. However, to be effective in this arena, occupational therapy practitioners must

- Define and establish their role in disaster preparedness, response, and recovery (McDaniel, 1960);

- Be aware of existing hospital, institutional, work site, and community disaster plans;

- Be knowledgeable about how national, state, and local governments and private agencies involved in disaster management are organized and how to gain entry into these systems;

- Monitor the literature for evidence-based work on the efficacy of various approaches such as psychological/mental health first aid and other approaches;

- Develop skills and train for their role in disaster response and recovery; and

- Be personally and professionally prepared to respond effectively to disaster situations (see Table 2 for resources).

A quote from author C. S. Lewis written for another time remains relevant today as occupational therapy practitioners think about their response to disaster, both as private individuals and as professionals. When disaster comes, let it

> find us doing sensible and human things—praying, working, teaching, reading, listening to music, bathing the children, playing tennis, chatting to our friends over a pint and a game of darts . . . . (Lewis, 1986, pp. 73–74)

References

American Academy of Pediatrics, Council on School Health. (2008). Disaster planning for schools. *Pediatrics, 122*(4), 895–901.

American Occupational Therapy Association. (2006a). Policy 1.44: Categories of occupational therapy personnel. In *Policy manual* (2009 ed.). Bethesda, MD: Author.

American Occupational Therapy Association. (2006b). The role of occupational therapy in disaster preparedness, response, and recovery. *American Journal of Occupational Therapy, 60*(6), 642–649.

American Occupational Therapy Association. (2008). Occupational therapy practice framework: Domain and process (2nd ed.). *American Journal of Occupational Therapy, 62*, 625–683.

American Occupational Therapy Association. (2009). Guidelines for supervision, roles, and responsibilities during the delivery of occupational therapy services. *American Journal of Occupational Therapy, 63*, 796–803.

American Occupational Therapy Association. (2010a). Occupational therapy code of ethics and ethics standards (2010). *American Journal of Occupational Therapy, 64*(Suppl.), S17–S26.

American Occupational Therapy Association. (2010b). Occupational therapy services in the promotion of psychological and social aspects of mental health. *American Journal of Occupational Therapy, 64*(Suppl.), S78–S91.

American Occupational Therapy Association. (2010c). Specialized knowledge and skills in mental health promotion, prevention, and intervention in occupational therapy practice. *American Journal of Occupational Therapy, 64*(Suppl.), S30–S43.

American Occupational Therapy Foundation. (2010, January). The making of New Year's resolutions and a key concept of occupational therapy. *Research Resources: A Monthly Newsletter of the AOTF Institute for the Study of Occupation and Health.* Available online at http://www.aotf.org/Portals/0/documents/News/Research-Resources/January%2012%202010%20Research%20Resources.pdf

American Psychiatric Association. (1994). *Diagnostic and statistical manual of mental disorders* (4th ed., text rev.). Washington, DC: Author.

Asher, A., & Pollak, J. R. (2009). Planning emergency evacuations for students with unique needs: Role of occupational therapy. *OT Practice, 14*(21), CE1–CE7.

Davis, J. (1999). Effects of trauma on children: Occupational therapy to support recovery. *Occupational Therapy International, 6,* 126–142.

Davis, J., & Kutter, C. J. (1998). Independent living skills and posttraumatic stress disorder in women who are homeless: Implications for future practice. *American Journal of Occupational Therapy, 52,* 39–44.

Deeny, P., & McFetridge, B. (2005). The impact of disaster on culture, self, and identity: Increased awareness by health care professionals is needed. *Nursing Clinics of North America, 40*(3), 431–440.

Diamond, H., & Precin, P. (2003). Disabled and experiencing disaster: Personal and professional accounts. *Occupational Therapy in Mental Health, 19*(3/4), 27–42.

Drabek, T. E., & McEntire, D. A. (2003). Emergent phenomena and the sociology of disaster: Lessons, trends, and opportunities. *Disaster Prevention and Management, 12*(2), 97–112.

Ellsworth, P. D., Laedtke, M. E., & McPhee, S. D. (1993). Utilization of occupational therapy in combat stress control during the Persian Gulf War. *Military Medicine, 158,* 381–385.

Federal Emergency Management Agency. (2010). *Are you ready? An in-depth guide to citizen preparedness.* Retrieved March 18, 2010, from http://www.fema.gov/areyouready/

Fischer, H. W. (1998). *Response to disaster: Fact versus fiction and its perpetuation: The sociology of disaster* (2nd ed.). Lanham, MD: University Press of America.

Fischer, H. W. (2002). Terrorism and 11 September 2001: Does the "behavioral response to disaster" model fit? *Disaster Prevention and Management, 11*(2), 123–127.

Fritz, C. E. (1961). Disasters. In R. K. Merton & R. A. Nisbet (Eds.), *Contemporary social problems* (pp. 651–694). New York: Harcourt.

Froelich, J. (1992). Occupational therapy interventions with survivors of sexual abuse. *Occupational Therapy in Health Care, 8*(2/3), 1–25.

Gerardi, S. M. (1996). The management of battle-fatigued soldiers: An occupational therapy model. *Military Medicine, 161,* 483–488.

Gerardi, S. M. (1999). Part I. Work hardening for warriors: Occupational therapy for combat stress casualties. *Work, 13,* 185–195.

Gerardi, S. M., & Newton, S. M. (2004, July–September). The role of the occupational therapist in CSC (combat stress control) operations. *U.S. Army Medical Department Journal,* pp. 20–27.

Gill, D. A., Clarke, L., Cohen, M. J., Ritchie, L. A., Ladd, A. E., Meinhold, S., et al. (2007). Post-Katrina guiding principles of disaster social science research. *Sociological Spectrum, 27,* 789–792.

Henderson, T. L., Roberto, K. A., & Kamo, K. A. (2010). Older adults' responses to Hurricane Katrina: Daily hassles and coping strategies. *Journal of Applied Gerontology, 29*(1), 48–69.

Hobfoll, S. E., Watson, P., Bell, C. C., Bryant, R. A., Brymer, M. J., Friedman, M. J., et al. (2007). Five essential elements of immediate and mid-term mass trauma intervention: Empirical evidence. *Psychiatry, 70*(4), 283–315.

Kielhofner, G., Forsyth, K., & Barrett, L. (2003). The Model of Human Occupation. In E. B. Crepeau, E. S. Cohn, & B. A. Boyt Schell (Eds.), *Willard and Spackman's occupational therapy* (pp. 212–219). Philadelphia: Lippincott Williams & Wilkins.

Kitchener, B., & Jorm, A. (2007). *Mental health first aid manual.* Melbourne: University of Melbourne, ORYGEN Research Centre. Available online at http://www.burdekinmentalhealthfoundation.org/Mental%20Health%20First%20Aid%20Manual.pdf

Laedtke, M. E. (1996). Occupational therapy and the treatment of combat stress. In J. A. Martin, L. R. Sparacinco, & G. Belenky (Eds.), *The Gulf War and mental health: A comprehensive guide* (pp. 145–152). Westport, CT: Praeger.

Lewis, C. S. (1986). *Present concerns: A compelling collection of timely journalistic essays.* London: C. S. Lewis PTE.

McColl, M. A. (2002). Occupation in stressful times. *American Journal of Occupational Therapy, 56,* 350–353.

McDaniel, M. L. (1960). The role of the occupational therapist in natural disaster situations. *American Journal of Occupational Therapy, 14,* 195–198.

Morgan, C. A., & Johnson, D. R. (1995). Use of a drawing task in the treatment of nightmares in combat-related post-traumatic stress disorder. *Art Therapy, 12,* 244–247.

Morris, A. S. (2008). Making it through a traumatic life experience: Applications for teaching, research, and personal adjustment. *Training and Education in Professional Psychology, 2*(2), 89–95.

National Institute of Mental Health. (2002). *Mental health and mass violence: Evidence-based early intervention for victims/survivors of mass violence* (NIH Pub. 02-5138). Washington, DC: U.S. Government Printing Office.

National Institute of Mental Health. (2008). *Post-traumatic stress disorder (PTSD)* (NIH Pub. 08-6388). Washington, DC: U.S. Government Printing Office.

Newton, S. (2000, November). *Matching occupational therapy skills to new opportunities: Working on a natural disaster.* Poster session presented at the annual meeting of the Occupational Therapy Association of California.

Rodriguez, J., Vos, F., Below, R., & Guha-Sapir, D. (2009). *Annual disaster statistical review 2008.* Brussels, Belgium: Centre for Research on the Epidemiology of Disasters.

Rosenfeld, M. S. (1982). A model for activity intervention in disaster-stricken communities. *American Journal of Occupational Therapy, 36,* 229–235.

Rosenfeld, M. S. (1989). Occupational disruption and adaptation: A study of house fire victims. *American Journal of Occupational Therapy, 43,* 89–96.

Scaffa, M. (2003, Spring). Competence, mastery, and independence: Our cultural heritage. *American Occupational Therapy Foundation Connection, 10*(1), 6–7.

Schneid, T. D., & Collins, L. (2001). *Disaster management and preparedness.* Boca Raton, FL: Lewis.

Shalev, A.Y., Tuval-Mashiach, R., & Hadar, H. (2004). Posttraumatic stress disorder as a result of mass trauma. *Journal of Clinical Psychiatry, 65*(Suppl. 1), 4–10.

Short-Degraff, M. A., & Engelman, T. (1992). Activities in the treatment of combat-related post-traumatic stress disorder. *Occupational Therapy in Health Care, 8*(2/3), 27–47.

Smith, D. L., & Notaro, S. J. (2009). Personal emergency preparedness for people with disabilities from the 2006–2007 Behavioral Risk Factor Surveillance System. *Disability and Health Journal, 2*(2), 86–94.

Stone, G. V. M. (2006). Occupational therapy in times of disaster. *American Journal of Occupational Therapy, 60*(1), 7–8.

Tierney, K., Bevc, C., & Kuligowski, E. (2006). Metaphor matter: Disaster myths, media frames, and their consequences in Hurricane Katrina. *Annals of the American Academy of Political and Social Science, 604*(1), 57–81.

Tierney, K. J., Lindell, M. K., & Perry, R. W. (Eds.). (2001). *Facing the unexpected: Disaster preparedness and response in the United States.* Washington, DC: Joseph Henry Press & National Academy of Sciences.

Townsend, E., & Wilcock, A. (2004). Occupational justice and client-centered practice: A dialogue in progress. *Canadian Journal of Occupational Therapy, 71*(2), 75–87.

Tuchner, M., Meiner, Z., Parush, S., & Hartman-Maier, A. (2010). Relationships between sequela of injury, participation, and quality of life in survivors of terrorists' attacks. *OTJR: Occupation, Participation and Health, 20*(1), 29–38.

Watson, P. J., & Shalev, A. Y. (2005). Assessment and treatment of adult acute responses to traumatic stress following mass traumatic events. *CNS Spectrums, 10*(2), 123–131.

World Federation of Occupational Therapists. (n.d.). *WFOT Disaster Preparedness and Response Questionnaire.* Retrieved April 6, 2010, from http://www.wfot.org/singleNews.asp?id=163&name=WFOT%20Disaster%20Preparedness%20and%20Response%20-%20Questionnaire

Young, B. H., Ford J. D., Ruzek, J. I., Friedman, M. J., & Gusman, F. D. (1998). *Disaster mental health services: A guidebook for clinicians and administrators.* Menlo Park, CA, & White River Junction, VT: Department of Veterans Affairs, National Center for Post-Traumatic Stress Disorder. Available online at www.ncptsd.org//publications/disaster/

Ziv, N., & Roitman, D. M. (2008). Addressing the needs of elderly clients whose lives have been compounded by traumatic histories. *Occupational Therapy in Health Care, 22*(2/3), 85–93.

Authors

Marjorie E. Scaffa, PhD, OTR/L, FAOTA
S. Maggie Reitz, PhD, OTR/L, FAOTA
Theresa Marie Smith, PhD, OTR/L, CLVT

for

The Commission on Practice
Janet V. DeLany, DEd, OTR/L, FAOTA, *Chairperson*

Adopted by the Representative Assembly Coordinating Council (RACC) for the Representative Assembly. Revised by the Commission on Practice 2011.

This revision replaces the 2005 document *The Role of Occupational Therapy in Disaster Preparedness, Response, and Recovery: A Concept Paper* (previously published and copyrighted in 2006 by the American Occupational Therapy Association in the *American Journal of Occupational Therapy, 60,* 642–649).

Scholarship in Occupational Therapy

In this document, we present the position of the American Occupational Therapy Association (AOTA) on the importance of scholarship to the growth, development, and vitality of the profession, and we describe the range of scholarly activities that will advance the profession. In addition, this document serves to inform both internal and external audiences concerning the expectations for—and the role of—scholarship in occupational therapy practices.

It is important to distinguish between scholarly practice and scholarship. *Scholarly practice* involves using the knowledge base of the profession or discipline in one's practice. As occupational therapy practitioners we, call this scholarly practice *evidence-based practice.* When engaged in scholarly teaching, educators draw on the "knowledge base on teaching and learning" (McKinney, 2007, p. 9) and their discipline or professional knowledge bases. Occupational therapy practitioners engaged in scholarly practice or scholarly teaching are reflective practitioners who assess and discuss their actions in light of the current knowledge base (McKinney, 2007; Schön, 1983). In contrast, *scholarship* or *research* is "a systematic investigation... designed to develop or to contribute to generalizable knowledge" (U.S. Department of Health and Human Services, 2005). Scholarship is made public, subject to review, and part of the discipline or professional knowledge base (Glassick, Huber, & Maeroff, 1997). It allows others to build on it and further advance the field.

Occupational therapy practitioners view scholarship as a vitally important contribution to the profession, the academy, and ultimately to society. Hence, practitioners see that engaging in scholarship is a professional responsibility. Every occupational therapy practitioner should contribute independently or collaboratively to building the evidence base for occupational therapy practice and occupational therapy education (Accreditation Council for Occupational Therapy Education, 2008; AOTA, 2007).

Occupational therapy practitioners are committed to engagement in scholarship that honors societal ethical standards and adheres to the standards of rigor accepted by the scientific community. Occupational therapy scholars value empiricism as the means by which knowledge must emerge, recognizing that through a variety of experimental and naturalistic means one may achieve knowledge and understanding (DePoy & Gitlin, 2005; Kielhofner, 2006). Moreover, they recognize that knowledge is not established in isolation but through interdisciplinary collaboration and intellectual discourse (Yerxa, 1987). As providers of therapeutic and educational services, occupational therapy practitioners are committed to continually developing foundational and theoretical knowledge that underlies practice; understanding the process and outcomes of service; and finally, establishing evidence of efficacious therapy and educational outcomes (Kielhofner, 2006).

The profession recognizes the necessity of a broad range of scholarly endeavors that will serve to describe and interpret the scope of the profession, establish new knowledge, interpret and appropriately apply this knowledge to practice, and engage learners in their development and understanding of the profession. Therefore, we acknowledge the relevance and legitimacy of the variety of scholarly approaches as described by Boyer (1990): the Scholarship of Discovery, the Scholarship of Integration, the Scholarship of Application, and the Scholarship of Teaching. This range of scholarship is particularly relevant considering the diversity in the field of occupational therapy represented by stakeholders with varying educational backgrounds. The four types of scholarship are discussed in the order Boyer (1990) presented them in *Scholarship Reconsidered: Priorities for the Professoriate*. He did not identify a hierarchy among the four types of scholarship and none is intended in this document.

Scholarship of Discovery

According to Boyer (1990), the *Scholarship of Discovery* is the engagement in activity that leads to the development of "knowledge for its own sake" (p. 17). The Scholarship of Discovery encompasses original research that contributes to expanding the knowledge base of a discipline. It is the type of research that the academic community most easily recognizes and accepts, and as such, is often the expected vehicle for intellectual discourse within the academy. Traditionally, faculty members who are trained to be independent researchers in research universities conduct discovery scholarship. Such scholars are, according to Golde (2006), stewards of the discipline responsible for "*generating* new knowledge and defending knowledge claims against challenges and criticism; of *conserving* the most important ideas and findings that are a legacy of past and current work; and of *transforming* knowledge that has been generated and conserved by teaching well to a variety of audiences, including those outside formal classrooms."

Clearly, there is a need for scholarship in occupational therapy that expands overall understanding of the engagement in and meaning of human occupation and its role in attaining and maintaining health. Clark (2006) noted that the profession needed a critical mass of the scholarship of discovery to continue to build the theoretical and knowledge base for occupational therapy, to foster intellectual vitality, and to maintain and strengthen the central tenets of the discipline.

Scholarship of Integration

The *Scholarship of Integration* is concerned with making creative connections both within and across disciplines to integrate, synthesize, interpret, and create new perspectives and theories. This form of scholarship is the most similar to the Scholarship of Discovery, but the difference lies in the nature of the research questions. In this form of inquiry, the scholars' aim is to find the meaning of research findings and interpret the findings in ways that synthesize isolated facts from within and outside of the discipline and integrate them to provide a richer and more thorough understanding of the issues. In light of the complex nature of contemporary issues confronting the individual and society, the profession needs the scholarship of integration, which lies in the intersections of disciplinary boundaries, to generate new knowledge for occupational therapy to better understand and meet societal needs.

Scholarship of Application

Through the Scholarship of Application, practitioners apply the knowledge generated by Scholarship of Discovery or Integration to address real problems at all levels of society. In occupational therapy, an example would be the application of theoretical knowledge to practice interventions or to teaching in the classroom. Another example may be using knowledge about the value of occupations as a health determinant to address health disparities of populations. Some authors, in focusing their efforts on application, have coined the term *Scholarship of Practice* (Braveman, Helfrich, & Fisher, 2001; Kielhofner, 2005), which focuses on program development and occupational therapy intervention. Another dimension of the Scholarship of Application is the *Scholarship of Engagement* (1990), which focuses on an interactive, participatory scholarship with persons and organizations (Barker, 2004; Boyer, 1996). In this form of scholarship, multiple stakeholders, including community members, produce knowledge. Regardless of differing terms, these activities fit best under Boyer's (1990) scholarship of application.

Scholarship of Teaching and Learning

Boyer (1990) identified a fourth area of scholarship, the *Scholarship of Teaching.* Over time it has been expanded to the *Scholarship of Teaching and Learning,* recognizing the interrelatedness of teaching and learning. The Scholarship of Teaching and Learning implies a "research agenda," and "involves the systematic study of teaching and/or learning and the public sharing and review of such work through presentations, publications, and performances" (McKinney, 2007, p. 10). Contributions must meet the rigorous standards of all forms of scholarship, be public, and be open to critical review.

Scholarship and Practice Roles

Scholarship must be generated, evaluated, and used to inform the many practice roles of occupational therapy. All occupational therapists and occupational therapy assistants, regardless of their individual practice roles, have the professional responsibility to not only use that evidence to inform their professional decision making but also to generate new evidence through independent or collaborative research, or both. For example, research through the Scholarships of Discovery and of Integration will contribute to the improved understanding of the constructs, processes, and theories (e.g., occupation and its therapeutic use) that provide the foundation for meeting society's complex occupational needs. At other times, through the Scholarship of Application, practitioners will establish evidence concerning the effectiveness of a specific intervention or the reliability, validity, and utility of an assessment tool and appropriately use the intervention or assessment on the basis of the strength of that evidence. Finally, they may develop and use evidence derived from the Scholarship of Teaching and Learning in client education to support participation in meaningful occupations. Practitioners challenge occupational therapy educators—including academic educators, academic fieldwork educators, and fieldwork educators—to find better ways to prepare diverse students to be competent professionals who advance the profession. Through the Scholarship of Teaching and Learning and the Scholarship of Application, they can empirically determine and apply better instructional methodologies to prepare students to meet the demands of a rapidly changing and increasingly complex health care environment, where consumers expect evidence-based practice and continuous professional development of all practitioners. Finally, administrators can contribute to, and benefit from, evidence produced through the Scholarship of Application when determining how best to meet the needs of clients in a cost-effective manner or how to better mentor or supervise others. Additional examples and benchmarks of scholarship are provided in Appendix A.

References

Accreditation Council for Occupational Therapy Education. (2008). *Accreditation Council for Occupational Therapy Education standards and interpretive guidelines.* Retrieved November 14, 2008, from http://www.aota.org/Educate/Accredit/StandardsReview/guide/42369.aspx

American Occupational Therapy Association. (2007). *AOTA's Centennial Vision.* Retrieved November 14, 2008, from http://www.aota.org/News/Centennial.aspx

Barker, D. (2004). The scholarship of engagement: A taxonomy of five emerging practices. *Journal of Higher Education Outreach and Engagement, 9,* 123–137.

Boyer, E. L. (1990). *Scholarship reconsidered: Priorities of the professoriate.* San Francisco: Jossey-Bass.

Boyer, E. L. (1996). The scholarship of engagement. *Journal of Public Service and Outreach, 1,* 11–20.

Braveman, B. H., Helfrich, C. A., & Fisher, G. S. (2001). Developing and maintaining community partnerships within "A Scholarship of Practice." *Occupational Therapy in Health Care, 15,* 109–125.

Clark, F. (2006). One person's thoughts on the future of occupational science. *Journal of Occupational Science, 13*(3), 167–179.

DePoy, E., & Gitlin, L. N. (2005). *Introduction to research: Understanding and applying multiple strategies* (3rd ed.). St. Louis, MO: Elsevier/Mosby.

Glassick, C. E., Huber, M. T., & Maeroff, G. I. (1997). *Scholarship assessed: Evaluation of the professoriate.* San Francisco: Jossey-Bass.

Golde, C. (2006). *Preparing stewards of the discipline.* The Carnegie Foundation for the advancement of teaching. Retrieved September, 2008 from http://www.carnegiefoundation.org/perspectives/sub.asp?key= 245&subkey=1811

Kielhofner, G. (2005). A scholarship of practice: Creating discourse between theory, research, and practice. *Occupational Therapy in Health Care, 19,* 7–16.

Kielhofner, G. (2006). *Research in occupational therapy: Methods of inquiry for enhancing practice.* Philadelphia: F. A. Davis.

McKinney, K. (2007). *Enhancing learning through the scholarship of teaching and learning.* San Francisco: Jossey-Bass.

Schön, D. A. (1983). *The reflective practitioner.* New York: Basic Books.

U.S. Department of Health Human Services. (2005). Part 46—Protection of human subjects. Code of Federal Regulations Title 45—Public Welfare. Available online at http://www.hhs.gov/ohrp/documents/ OHRPRegulation.pdf

Yerxa, E. (1987). Research: The key to the development of occupational therapy as an academic discipline. *American Journal of Occupational Therapy, 41,* 415–419.

The Commission on Education:
René Padilla, PhD, OTR/L, FAOTA, *Chairperson*
Andrea Bilics, PhD, OTR/L
Judith C. Blum, MS, OTR/L
Paula C. Bohr, PhD, OTR/L, FAOTA
Jennifer C. Coyne, COTA/L
Jyothi Gupta, PhD, OTR/L
Linda Musselman, PhD, OTR, FAOTA
Linda Orr, MPA, OTR/L
Abbey Sipp (ASD)
Patricia Stutz-Tanenbaum, MS, OTR
Neil Harvison, PhD, OTR/L, *Staff Liaison*

Adopted by the Representative Assembly 2009FebCS114

This document replaces the document *Scholarship and Occupational Therapy* 2003M42T.

Appendix A.
Characteristics of Scholarship in Occupational Therapy

Type of Scholarship	Examples	Demonstration of Scholarship	Documentation
Scholarship of Discovery Contributes to the development or creation of new knowledge	• Primary empirical research • Historical research • Theory development • Methodological studies • Philosophical inquiry	• Peer-reviewed publications of research, theory, or philosophical essays • Peer-reviewed/invited professional presentations of research, theory, or philosophical essays • Grant awards in support of research or scholarship • Positive peer evaluations of the body of work	• Bibliographic citation of the accomplishments • Positive external evaluation of the body of work
Scholarship of Integration Contributes to the critical analysis and review of knowledge within disciplines or the creative synthesis of insights contained in different disciplines or fields of study	• Inquiry that advances knowledge across a range of theories, practice areas, techniques, or methodologies • Includes works that interface among occupational therapy and a variety of disciplines, including but not limited to occupational science	• Peer-reviewed publications of research, policy analysis, case studies, integrative reviews of the literature, and others • Copyrights, licenses, patents, or products • Published books • Positive peer evaluations of contributions to integrative scholarship • Reports of interdisciplinary programs or services • Interdisciplinary grant awards • Peer-reviewed/invited professional presentations • Policy papers designed to influence organizations or governments • Service on editorial board or as peer reviewer	• Bibliographic citation of the accomplishments • Positive external evaluation of the body of work • Documentation of role in editorial/review processes

(continued)

Appendix A.
Characteristics of Scholarship in Occupational Therapy *(cont.)*

Type of Scholarship	Examples	Demonstration of Scholarship	Documentation
Scholarship of Application, Practice, or Engagement Applies findings generated through the Scholarship of Integration or discovery to solve real problems in the professions, industry, government, and community	• Development of clinical knowledge • Application of technical or research skills to address problems • Participatory action research involving collaboration with community groups • Efficacy of treatment approach • Developing valid outcome measures	• Peer-reviewed publications of research, policy analysis, case studies, integrative reviews of the literature, and others • Activities related to the faculty member's area of expertise (e.g., consultation, technical assistance, policy analysis, program evaluation, development of practice patterns) • Peer-reviewed/invited professional presentations related to practice • Consultation reports • Reports compiling and analyzing patient or health services outcomes • Products, patents, license copyrights • Peer reviews of practice • Grant awards in support of practice • Reports of meta-analyses related to practice problems • Reports of clinical demonstration projects • Policy papers related to practice	• Formal documentation of a record of the activity and positive formal evaluation by users of the work • Bibliographic citation of the accomplishments • Positive external evaluation of the body of work • Documentation of role in multi-authored products

Appendix A.
Characteristics of Scholarship in Occupational Therapy *(cont.)*

Type of Scholarship	Examples	Demonstration of Scholarship	Documentation
Scholarship of Teaching and Learning Contributes to the development of critically reflective knowledge about teaching and learning	• Application of knowledge of the discipline or specialty applied in teaching–learning in the academic and/or fieldwork setting • Development of innovative teaching and evaluation methods • Program development and learning outcome evaluation of academic and/or fieldwork education • Professional role modeling	• Peer-reviewed publications of research related to teaching methodology or learning outcomes, case studies related to teaching–learning, learning theory development, and development or testing of educational models or theories • Educational effectiveness studies such as those found in comprehensive programs reports • Successful applications of technology to teaching and learning • Positive peer evaluations of innovations in teaching • Published textbooks or other learning aids • Grant awards in support of teaching and learning • Peer-reviewed/invited professional presentations related to teaching and learning	• Bibliographic citation of the accomplishments • Positive external evaluation of the body of work

Note. Adapted from http://www.clt.uts.edu.au/Scholarship/A.Model.html, http://aacn.nche.edu/Publications/positions/scholar.htm, http://www.apta.org/AM/Template.cfm?Section=CAPTE3&Template=/CM/ContentDisplay.cfm&ContentID=23140

Ethics

Enforcement Procedures for the *Occupational Therapy Code of Ethics and Ethics Standards*

1. Introduction

The principal purposes of the *Occupational Therapy Code of Ethics and Ethics Standards* (hereinafter referred to as the *Code and Ethics Standards*) are to help protect the public and to reinforce its confidence in the occupational therapy profession rather than to resolve private business, legal, or other disputes for which there are other more appropriate forums for resolution. The *Code and Ethics Standards* also is an aspirational document to guide occupational therapists, occupational therapy assistants, and occupational therapy students toward appropriate professional conduct in all aspects of their diverse roles. It applies to any conduct that may affect the performance of occupational therapy as well as to behavior that an individual may do in another capacity that reflects negatively on the reputation of occupational therapy.

The *Enforcement Procedures for the Occupational Therapy Code of Ethics and Ethics Standards* (formerly the *Enforcement Procedures for the Occupational Therapy Code of Ethics*) have undergone a series of revisions by the American Occupational Therapy Association's (AOTA's) Ethics Commission (hereinafter referred to as the *EC*) since their initial adoption. The most recent update was in 2009. This public document articulates the procedures that are followed by the EC as it carries out its duties to enforce the *Code and Ethics Standards*. A major goal of these *Enforcement Procedures* is to ensure objectivity and fundamental fairness to all individuals who may be parties in an ethics complaint.

The *Enforcement Procedures* are used to help ensure compliance with the *Code and Ethics Standards*, which represent the values and principles that members of the profession have identified as important. Acceptance of AOTA membership commits individuals to adherence to the *Code and Ethics Standards* and cooperation with its *Enforcement Procedures*. These are established and maintained by the EC: The EC and AOTA's Ethics Office make the *Enforcement Procedures* public and available to members of the profession, state regulatory boards, consumers, and others for their use.

The EC urges particular attention to the following issues:

1.1. **Professional Responsibility, Other Processes**—All occupational therapy personnel have an obligation to maintain the *Code and Ethics Standards* of their profession and to promote and support these Standards among their colleagues. Each AOTA member must be alert to practices that undermine these Standards and is obligated to take action that is appropriate in the circumstances. At the same time, members must carefully weigh their judgments as to potentially unethical practice to ensure that they are based on objective evaluation and not on personal bias or prejudice, inadequate information, or simply differences of professional viewpoint. It is recognized that individual occupational therapy personnel may not have the authority or ability to address or correct all situations of concern. Whenever feasible and appropriate, members should first pursue other corrective steps within the relevant institution or setting and discuss ethical concerns directly with the potential Respondent before resorting to AOTA's ethics complaint process.

1.2. **Jurisdiction**—The *Code and Ethics Standards* apply to persons who are or were AOTA members at the time of the conduct in question. Later nonrenewal or relinquishment of membership does not affect

Association jurisdiction. The *Enforcement Procedures* that shall be utilized in any complaint shall be those in effect at the time the complaint is initiated.

1.3. **Disciplinary Actions/Sanctions (Pursuing a Complaint)**—If the EC determines that unethical conduct has occurred, it may impose sanctions, including reprimand, censure, probation (with terms), suspension, or permanent revocation of AOTA membership. In all cases, except those involving only reprimand, the Association will report the conclusions and sanctions in its official publications and also will communicate to any appropriate persons or entities. The potential sanctions are defined as follows:

    1.3.1. **Reprimand**—A formal expression of disapproval of conduct communicated privately by letter from the EC Chairperson that is nondisclosable and noncommunicative to other bodies (e.g., state regulatory boards [SRBs], National Board for Certification in Occupational Therapy,® [NBCOT®]).

    1.3.2. **Censure**—A formal expression of disapproval that is public.

    1.3.3. **Probation of Membership Subject to Terms**—Failure to meet terms will subject an AOTA member to any of the disciplinary actions or sanctions.

    1.3.4. **Suspension**—Removal of AOTA membership for a specified period of time.

    1.3.5. **Revocation**—Permanent denial of AOTA membership.

        1.3.5.1. If an individual is on either the Roster of Fellows (ROF) or the Roster of Honor (ROH), the EC Chairperson (via the EC Staff Liaison) shall notify the Recognitions Committee Chairperson (and AOTA Executive Director) of their membership revocation. That individual shall have their name removed from either the ROF or the ROH and no longer has the right to use the designated credential of FAOTA or ROH.

1.4. **Educative Letters**—If the EC determines that the alleged conduct may or may not be a true breach of the *Code and Ethics Standards* but in any event does not warrant any of the sanctions set forth in Section 1.3.or is not completely in keeping with the aspirational nature of the *Code and Ethics Standards* or within the prevailing standards of practice or good professionalism, the EC may send a letter to educate the Respondent about relevant standards of practice and/or appropriate professional behavior. In addition, a different educative letter, if appropriate, may be sent to the Complainant.

1.5. **Advisory Opinions**—The EC may issue general advisory opinions on ethical issues to inform and educate the AOTA membership. These opinions shall be publicized to the membership and are available in the *Reference Guide to the Occupational Therapy Code of Ethics and Ethics Standards* as well as in other locations.

1.6. **Rules of Evidence**—The EC proceedings shall be conducted in accordance with fundamental fairness. However, formal rules of evidence that are used in legal proceedings do not apply to these *Enforcement Procedures*. The Disciplinary Council (see Section 5) and the Appeal Panel (see Section 6) can consider any evidence that they deem appropriate and pertinent.

1.7. **Confidentiality and Disclosure**—The EC develops and adheres to strict rules of confidentiality in every aspect of its work. This requires that participants in the process refrain from any communication relating to the existence and subject matter of the complaint other than with those directly involved in the enforcement process. Maintaining confidentiality throughout the investigation and enforcement process of a formal ethics complaint is essential in order to ensure fairness to all parties involved. These rules of confidentiality pertain not only to the EC but also apply to others involved in the complaint process. Beginning with the EC Staff Liaison and support staff, strict rules of confidentiality are followed. These same rules of confidentiality apply to Complainants, Respondents and their attorneys, and witnesses involved with the EC's investigatory process. Due diligence must be exercised by everyone involved in the investigation to avoid compromising the confidential nature of the process. Any AOTA member who breaches these rules of confidentiality may become subject to an ethics complaint/investigatory process himself or herself. Non–AOTA members may lodge an ethics complaint against an Association member, and these individuals are still expected to adhere to the Association's confidentiality rules. The Association reserves the right to take appropriate action against non–AOTA members who violate confidentiality rules, including notification of their appropriate licensure boards.

    1.7.1. Disclosure—When the EC investigates a complaint, it may request information from a variety of sources. The process of obtaining additional information is carefully executed in order to maintain confidentiality. The EC may request information from a variety of sources, including state licensing agencies, academic councils, courts, employers, and other persons and entities. It is within the EC's purview to determine what disclosures are appropriate for particular parties in order to effectively implement its investigatory obligations. Public sanctions by the EC, Disciplinary Council, or Appeal Panel will be publicized as provided in these *Enforcement Procedures*. Normally, the EC does not disclose information or documentation reviewed in the course of an investigation unless the EC determines that disclosure is necessary to obtain additional, relevant evidence or to administer the ethics process or is legally required.

Individuals who file a complaint (i.e., *Complainant*) and those who are the subject of one (i.e., *Respondent*) must not disclose to anyone outside of those involved in the complaint process their role in an ethics complaint. Disclosing this information in and of itself may jeopardize the ethics process and violate the rules of fundamental fairness by which all parties are protected. Disclosure of information related to any case under investigation by the EC is prohibited and, if done, will lead to repercussions as outlined in these *Enforcement Procedures* (see Section 2.2.3.).

2. Complaints

2.1. Interested Party Complaints

    2.1.1. Complaints stating an alleged violation of the *Code and Ethics Standards* may originate from any individual, group, or entity within or outside AOTA. All complaints must be in writing, signed by the Complainant(s), and submitted to the EC Chairperson at the address of the AOTA Headquarters. Complainants must complete the Formal Statement of Complaint Form at the end of this document. All complaints shall identify the person against whom the complaint is directed (the Respondent), the ethical principles that the Complainant believes have been violated, and the key facts and date(s) of the alleged ethical violations. If lawfully available, supporting documentation should be attached.

    2.1.2. Within 90 days of receipt of a complaint, the EC shall make a preliminary assessment of the complaint and decide whether it presents sufficient questions as to a potential ethics violation that an investigation is warranted in accordance with Section 3. Commencing an investigation does not imply a conclusion that an ethical violation has in fact occurred or any judgment as to the ultimate sanction, if any, that may be appropriate. In the event the EC determines at the completion of an investigation that the complaint does rise to the level of an ethical violation, the EC may initiate a charge as set forth in Section 4 below. In the event the EC determines that the complaint does not rise to the level of an ethical violation, the EC may direct the parties to utilize *Roberts Rules* and/or other conflict resolution resources via an educative letter. This applies to all complaints including those involving AOTA elected/volunteer leadership related to their official roles.

2.2. Complaints Initiated by the EC

2.2.1. The EC itself may initiate a complaint (a *sua sponte complaint*) when it receives information from a governmental body, certification or similar body, public media, or other source indicating that a person subject to its jurisdiction may have committed acts that violate the *Code and Ethics Standards*. The Association will ordinarily act promptly after learning of the basis of a sua sponte complaint, but there is no specified time limit.

If the EC passes a motion to initiate a sua sponte complaint, the AOTA Staff Liaison to the EC will complete the Formal Statement of Complaint Form (at the end of this document) and will describe the nature of the factual allegations that led to the complaint and the manner in which the EC learned of the matter. The Complaint Form will be signed by the EC Chairperson on behalf of the EC. The form will be filed with the case material in the Association's Ethics Office.

2.2.2. De Jure Complaints—Where the source of a sua sponte complaint is the findings and conclusions of another official body, the EC classifies such sua sponte complaints as *de jure*. The procedure in such cases is addressed in Section 4.2.

2.2.3. The EC shall have the jurisdiction to investigate, charge, or sanction any matter or person for violations based on information learned in the course of investigating a complaint under Section 2.2.2.

2.3. Continuation of Complaint Process—If an AOTA member relinquishes membership, fails to renew membership, or fails to cooperate with the ethics investigation, the EC shall nevertheless continue to process the complaint, noting in its report the circumstances of the Respondent's action. Such actions shall not deprive the EC of jurisdiction. All correspondence related to the EC complaint process is in writing and sent by certified mail, return receipt requested. In the event that any written correspondence does not have delivery confirmation, the AOTA Ethics Office will make an attempt to search for an alternate address or make a second attempt to send to the original address. If Respondent does not claim correspondence after two attempts to deliver, delivery cannot be confirmed, or correspondence is returned to the Association as undeliverable, the EC shall consider that it has made good-faith effort and shall proceed with the ethics enforcement process.

3. EC Review and Investigations

3.1. Initial Action—The purpose of the preliminary review is to decide whether or not the information submitted with the complaint warrants opening the case. If in its preliminary review of the complaint the EC determines that an investigation is not warranted, the Complainant will be so notified.

3.2. Dismissal of Complaints—The EC may at any time dismiss a complaint for any of the following reasons:

3.2.1. Lack of Jurisdiction—The EC determines that it has no jurisdiction over the Respondent (e.g., a complaint against a person who is or was not an AOTA member at the time of the alleged incident or who has never been a member).

3.2.2. Absolute Time Limit/Not Timely Filed—The EC determines that the violation of the *Code and Ethics Standards* is alleged to have occurred more than 7 years prior to the filing of the complaint.

3.2.3. Subject to Jurisdiction of Another Authority—The EC determines that the complaint is based on matters that are within the authority of and are more properly dealt with by another governmental or nongovernmental body, such as an SRB, NBCOT, an Association component other than the EC, an employer, or a court (e.g., accusing a superior of sexual harassment at work, accusing someone of anticompetitive practices subject to the antitrust laws).

3.2.4. No Ethics Violation—The EC finds that the complaint, even if proven, does not state a basis for action under the *Code and Ethics Standards* (e.g., simply accusing someone of being unpleasant or rude on an occasion).

3.2.5. Insufficient Evidence—The EC determines that there clearly would not be sufficient factual evidence to support a finding of an ethics violation.

3.2.6. Corrected Violation—The EC determines that any violation it might find already has been or is being corrected and that this is an adequate result in the given case.

3.2.7. Other Good Cause.

3.3. Investigator (Avoidance of Conflict of Interest)—The investigator chosen shall not have a conflict of interest (i.e., shall never have had a substantial professional, personal, financial, business, or volunteer relationship with either the Complainant or the Respondent). In the event that the EC Staff Liaison has such a conflict, the EC Chairperson shall appoint an alternate investigator who has no conflict of interest.

3.4. Investigation—If an investigation is deemed warranted, the EC Chairperson shall do the following within thirty (30) days: Appoint the EC Staff Liaison at the AOTA Headquarters to investigate the complaint and notify the Respondent (by certified, return-receipt mail) that a complaint has been received and an investigation is being conducted. A copy of the complaint and supporting documentation shall be enclosed with this notification. The Complainant also will receive notification by certified, return-receipt mail that the complaint is being investigated.

3.4.1. Ordinarily, the Investigator will send questions formulated by the EC to be answered by the Complainant and/or the Respondent.

3.4.2. The Complainant shall be given thirty (30) days from receipt of the questions to respond in writing to the investigator.

3.4.3. The Respondent shall be given thirty (30) days from receipt of the questions to respond in writing to the Investigator.

3.4.4. The EC ordinarily will notify the Complainant of any substantive new evidence adverse to the Complainant's initial complaint that is discovered in the course of the ethics investigation and allow the Complainant to respond to such adverse evidence. In such cases, the Complainant will be given a copy of such evidence and will have fourteen (14) days in which to submit a written response. If the new evidence clearly shows that there has been no ethics violation, the EC may terminate the proceeding. In addition, if the investigation includes questions for both the Respondent and the Complainant, the evidence submitted by each party in response to the investigatory questions shall be provided to the Respondent and available to the Complainant on request. The EC may request reasonable payment for copying expenses depending on the volume of material to be sent.

3.4.5. The Investigator, in consultation with the EC, may obtain evidence directly from third parties without permission from the Complainant or Respondent.

3.5. Investigation Timeline—The investigation will be completed within ninety (90) days after receipt of notification by the Respondent or his or her designee that an investigation is being conducted, unless the EC determines that special circumstances warrant additional time for the investigation. All timelines noted here can be extended for good cause at the discretion of the EC, including the EC's schedule and additional requests of the Respondent. The Respondent and the Complainant shall be notified in writing if a delay occurs or if the investigational process requires more time.

3.6. Case Files—The investigative files shall include the complaint and any documentation on which the EC relied in initiating the investigation.

3.7. Cooperation by Member—Every AOTA member has a duty to cooperate reasonably with enforcement processes for the *Code and Ethics Standards*. Failure of the Respondent to participate and/or cooperate with the investigative process of the EC shall not prevent continuation of the ethics process, and this behavior itself may constitute a violation of the *Code and Ethics Standards*.

3.8. Referral of Complaint—The EC may at any time refer a matter to NBCOT, the SRB, or other recognized authorities for appropriate action. Despite such referral to an appropriate authority, the EC shall retain jurisdiction. EC action may be stayed for a reasonable period pending notification of a decision by that authority, at the discretion of the EC (and such delays will extend the time periods under these *Procedures*). A stay in conducting an investigation shall not constitute a waiver by the EC of jurisdiction over the matters. The EC shall provide written notice by mail (requiring signature and proof of date of receipt) to the Respondent and the Complainant of any such stay of action.

4. EC Review and Decision

4.1. Regular Complaint Process

4.1.1. Charges—The EC shall review the relevant materials resulting from the investigation and shall render a decision on whether a charge by the EC is warranted within 90 days of receipt. The EC may, in the conduct of its review, take whatever further investigatory actions it deems necessary. If the EC determines that an ethics complaint warrants a charge, the EC shall proceed with a disciplinary proceeding by promptly sending a notice of the charge(s) to the Respondent and Complainant by mail with signature and proof of date received. The notice of the charge(s) shall describe the alleged conduct that, if proven in accordance with these *Enforcement Procedures,* would constitute a violation of the *Code and Ethics Standards*. The notice of charge(s) shall describe the conduct in sufficient detail to inform the Respondent of the nature of the unethical behavior that is alleged. The EC may indicate in the notice its preliminary view (absent contrary facts or mitigating circumstances) as to what sanction would be warranted if the violation is proven in accordance with these *Enforcement Procedures*.

4.1.2. Respondent's Response—Within 30 days of notification of the EC's decision to charge, and proposed sanction, if any, the Respondent shall

    4.1.2.1. Advise the EC Chairperson in writing that he or she accepts the EC's charge of an ethics violation and the proposed sanction and waives any right to a Disciplinary Council hearing, or

    4.1.2.2. Advise the EC Chairperson in writing that he or she accepts the EC's charge of an ethics violation but believes the sanction is not justified or should be reduced with a rationale to support a reduced sanction.

    4.1.2.3. Advise the EC Chairperson in writing that he or she contests the EC's charge and the proposed sanction and requests a hearing before the Disciplinary Council.

Failure of the Respondent to take one of these actions within the time specified will be deemed to constitute acceptance of the charge and proposed sanction. If the Respondent requests a Disciplinary Council hearing, it will be scheduled. If the Respondent does not request a Disciplinary Council hearing but accepts the decision, the EC will notify all relevant parties and implement the sanction.

4.2. De Jure Complaint Process

4.2.1. The EC Staff Liaison will present to the EC any findings from external sources (as described above) that come to his or her attention and that may warrant sua sponte complaints pertaining to individuals who are or were AOTA members at the time of the alleged incident.

4.2.2. Because *de jure complaints* are based on the findings of fact or conclusions of another official body, the EC will decide whether or not to act based on such findings or conclusions and will not ordinarily initiate another investigation, absent clear and convincing evidence that such findings and conclusions were erroneous or not supported by substantial evidence. Based on the information presented by the EC Staff Liaison, the EC will determine whether the findings of the public body also are sufficient to demonstrate an egregious violation of the *Code and Ethics Standards* and therefore warrant an ethics charge.

4.2.3. If the EC decides that a formal charge is warranted, the EC Chairperson will notify the Respondent in writing of the formal charge and the proposed education and/or disciplinary action. In response to the de jure sua sponte charge by the EC, the Respondent may

> **4.2.3.1.** Accept the decision of the EC (as to both the ethics violation and the sanction) based solely on the findings of fact and conclusions of the EC or the public body, or

> **4.2.3.2.** Accept the charge that the Respondent committed unethical conduct but within thirty (30) days submit to the EC a statement setting forth the reasons why any sanction should not be imposed or reasons why the sanction should be mitigated or reduced.

> **4.2.3.3.** Within thirty (30) days, present information showing the findings of fact of the official body relied on by the EC to initiate the charge are clearly erroneous and request reconsideration by the EC. The EC may have the option of opening an investigation or modifying the sanction in the event they find clear and convincing evidence that the findings and the conclusions of the other body are erroneous.

4.2.4. In cases of de jure complaints, a Disciplinary Council hearing can later be requested (pursuant to Section 5 below) only if the Respondent has first exercised Options 4.2.3.2 or 4.2.3.3.

4.2.5. Respondents in an ethics case may utilize Options 4.2.3.2 or 4.2.3.3 (reconsideration) once in responding to the EC. Following one review of the additional information submitted by the Respondent, if the EC reaffirms its original sanction, the Respondent has the option of accepting the violation and proposed sanction or requesting a Disciplinary Council hearing. Repeated requests for reconsideration will not be accepted by the EC.

5. The Disciplinary Council

5.1. **Purpose**—The purpose of the Disciplinary Council (hereinafter to be known as *the Council*) hearing is to provide the Respondent an opportunity to present evidence and witnesses to answer and refute the charge and/or the proposed sanction and to permit the EC Chairperson or designee to present evidence and witnesses in support of his or her charge. The Council shall consider the matters alleged in the complaint; the matters raised in defense as well as other relevant facts, ethical principles, and federal or state law, if applicable. The Council may question the parties concerned and determine ethical issues arising from the factual matters in the case even if those specific ethical issues were not raised by the Complainant. The Council also may choose to apply Principles or other language from the AOTA *Code and Ethics Standards* not originally identified by the EC. The Council may affirm the decision of the EC or reverse or modify it if it finds that the decision was clearly erroneous or a material departure from its written procedure.

5.2. Parties—The parties to a Council Hearing are the Respondent and the EC Chairperson.

5.3. Criteria and Process for Selection of Council Chairperson

    5.3.1. Criteria

        5.3.1.1. Must have experience in analyzing/reviewing cases.

        5.3.1.2. May be selected from the pool of candidates for the Council or a former EC member who has been off the EC for at least three (3) years.

        5.3.1.3. The EC Chairperson shall not serve as the Council Chairperson.

    5.3.2. Process

        5.3.2.1. The Representative Assembly (RA) Speaker (in consultation with EC Staff Liaison) will select the Council Chairperson.

        5.3.2.2. If the RA Speaker needs to be recused from this duty, the RA Vice Speaker will select the Council Chairperson.

5.4. Criteria and Process for Selection of Council Members

    5.4.1. Criteria

        5.4.1.1. AOTA Administrative SOP guidelines in Policy 2.6 shall be considered in the selection of qualified potential candidates for the Council, which shall be composed of qualified individuals and AOTA members drawn from a pool of candidates who meet the criteria outlined below. In the interest of financial prudence and efficiency, every effort will be made to assemble Council members who meet the criteria below but also who are within geographic proximity to the AOTA Headquarters.

        5.4.1.2. Members ideally will have some knowledge or experience in the areas of activity that are at issue in the case. They also will have experience in disciplinary hearings and/or general knowledge about ethics as demonstrated by education, presentations, and/or publications.

        5.4.1.3. No conflict of interest may exist with either the Complainant or the Respondent (refer to Association Policy 1.22—Conflict of Interest for guidance).

        5.4.1.4. No individual may serve on the Council who is currently a member of the EC or the AOTA Board of Directors.

        5.4.1.5. No individual may serve on the Council who has previously been the subject of an ethics complaint that resulted in a specific EC disciplinary action.

        5.4.1.6. The public member on the Council shall have knowledge of the profession and ethical issues.

        5.4.1.7. The public member shall not be an occupational therapy practitioner, educator, or researcher.

    5.4.2. Process

        5.4.2.1. Potential candidates for the Council pool will be recruited through public postings in AOTA publications and via the electronic forums. Association leadership will be encouraged to recruit qualified candidates. Potential members of the Council shall be interviewed to ascertain the following:

a. Willingness to serve on the Council and availability for a period of three (3) years and

b. Qualifications per criteria outlined in Section 5.3.1.

5.4.2.2. The AOTA President and EC Staff Liaison will maintain a pool of no less than six (6) and no more than twelve (12) qualified individuals.

5.4.2.3. The President, with input from the EC Staff Liaison, will select from the pool the members of each Council within thirty (30) days of notification by a Respondent that a Council is being requested.

5.4.2.4. Each Council shall be composed of three (3) AOTA members in good standing and a public member.

5.4.2.5. The EC Staff Liaison will remove anyone with a potential conflict of interest in a particular case from the potential Council pool.

5.5. Notification of Parties (EC Chairperson, Complainant, Respondent, Council Members)

5.5.1. The EC Staff Liaison shall schedule a hearing date in coordination with the Council Chairperson.

5.5.2. The Council (via the EC Staff Liaison) shall notify all parties at least forty-five (45) days prior to the hearing of the date, time, and place.

5.5.3. Case material will be sent to all parties and the Council members by national delivery service or mail with signature required and proof of date received with return receipt.

5.6. Hearing Witnesses, Materials, and Evidence

5.6.1. Within thirty (30) days of notification of the hearing, the Respondent shall submit to the Council a written response to the charges, including a detailed statement as to the reasons that he or she is appealing the decision and a list of potential witnesses (if any) with a statement indicating the subject matter they will be addressing.

5.6.2. The Complainant before the Council also will submit a list of potential witnesses (if any) to the Council with a statement indicating the subject matter they will be addressing. Only under limited circumstances may the Council consider additional material evidence from the Respondent or the Complainant not presented or available prior to the issuance of their proposed sanction. Such new or additional evidence may be considered by the Council if the Council is satisfied that the Respondent or the Complainant has demonstrated the new evidence was previously unavailable and provided it is submitted to all parties in writing no later than fifteen (15) days prior to the hearing.

5.6.3. The Council Chairperson may permit testimony by conference call (at no expense to the participant), limit participation of witnesses in order to curtail repetitive testimony, or prescribe other reasonable arrangements or limitations. The Respondent may elect to appear (at Respondent's own expense) and present testimony. If alternative technology options are available for the hearing, the Respondent, Council members, and EC Chairperson shall be so informed when the hearing arrangements are sent.

5.7. Counsel—The Respondent may be represented by legal counsel at his or her own expense. AOTA's Legal Counsel shall advise and represent the Association at the hearing. AOTA's Legal Counsel also may advise the Council regarding procedural matters to ensure fairness to all parties. All parties and the AOTA Legal Counsel (at the request of the EC or the Council) shall have the opportunity to question witnesses.

5.8. Hearing

5.8.1. The Council hearing shall be recorded by a professional transcription service or telephone recording transcribed for Council members and shall be limited to two (2) hours.

5.8.2. The Council Chairperson will conduct the hearing and does not vote except in the case of a tie.

5.8.3. Each person present shall be identified for the record, and the Council Chairperson will describe the procedures for the Council hearing. An oral affirmation of truthfulness will be requested from each participant who gives factual testimony in the Council hearing.

5.8.4. The Council Chairperson shall allow for questions.

5.8.5. The EC Chairperson shall present the ethics charge, a summary of the evidence resulting from the investigation, and the EC proposed disciplinary action against the Respondent.

5.8.6. The Respondent may present a defense to the charges(s) after the EC presents its case.

5.8.7. Each party and/or his or her legal representative shall have the opportunity to call witnesses to present testimony and to question any witnesses including the EC Chairperson or his or her designee. The Council Chairperson shall be entitled to provide reasonable limits on the extent of any witnesses' testimony or any questioning.

5.8.8. The Council Chairperson may recess the hearing at any time.

5.8.9. The Council Chairperson shall call for final statements from each party before concluding the hearing.

5.8.10. Decisions of the Council will be by majority vote.

5.9. Disciplinary Council Decision

5.9.1. An official copy of the transcript shall be sent to each Council member, the EC Chairperson, the AOTA Legal Counsel, the EC Staff Liaison, and the Respondent and his or her counsel as soon as it is available from the transcription company.

5.9.2. The Council Chairperson shall work with the EC Staff Liaison and the AOTA Legal Counsel in preparing the text of the final decision.

5.9.3. The Council shall issue a decision in writing to the AOTA Executive Director within thirty (30) days of receiving the written transcription of the hearing (unless special circumstances warrant additional time). The Council decision shall be based on the record and evidence presented and may affirm, modify, or reverse the decision of the EC, including increasing or decreasing the level of sanction or determining that no disciplinary action is warranted.

5.10. Action, Notification, and Timeline Adjustments

5.10.1. A copy of the Council's official decision and appeal process (Section 6) is sent to the Respondent, the EC Chairperson, and other appropriate parties within fifteen (15) business days via mail (with signature and proof of date received) after notification of the AOTA Executive Director.

5.10.2. The time limits specified in the *Enforcement Procedures for the Occupational Therapy Code and Ethics Standards* may be extended by mutual consent of the Respondent, Complainant, and Council Chairperson for good cause by the Chairperson.

5.10.3. Other features of the preceding *Enforcement Procedures* may be adjusted in particular cases in light of extraordinary circumstances, consistent with fundamental fairness.

5.11. Appeal—Within thirty (30) days after notification of the Council's decision, a Respondent upon whom a sanction was imposed may appeal the decision as provided in Section 6. Within thirty (30) days after notification of the Council's decision, the EC also may appeal the decision as provided in Section 6. If no appeal is filed within that time, the AOTA Executive Director or EC Staff Liaison shall publish the decision in accordance with these procedures and make any other notifications deemed necessary.

6. Appeal Process

6.1. Appeals—Either the EC or the Respondent may appeal. Appeals shall be written, signed by the appealing party, and sent by certified mail to the AOTA Executive Director in care of the AOTA Ethics Office. The grounds for the appeal shall be fully explained in this document. When an appeal is requested, the other party will be notified.

6.2. Grounds for Appeal—Appeals shall generally address only the issues, procedures, or sanctions that are part of the record before the Council. However, in the interest of fairness, the Appeal Panel may consider newly available evidence relating to the original charge only under extraordinary circumstances.

6.3. Composition and Leadership of Appeal Panel—The AOTA Vice-President, Secretary, and Treasurer shall constitute the Appeal Panel. In the event of vacancies in these positions or the existence of a conflict of interest, the Vice President shall appoint replacements drawn from among the other AOTA Board of Directors members. If the entire Board has a conflict of interest (e.g., the Complainant or Respondent is or was recently a member of the Board), the Board Appeal process shall be followed. The President shall not serve on the Appeal Panel. No individual may serve on the Council who has previously been the subject of an ethics complaint that resulted in a specific EC disciplinary action.

The Appeal Panel Chairperson will be selected by its members from among themselves.

6.4. Appeal Process—The AOTA Executive Director shall forward any letter of appeal to the Appeal Panel within fifteen (15) business days of receipt. Within thirty (30) days after the Appeal Panel receives the appeal, the Panel shall determine whether a hearing is warranted. If the Panel decides that a hearing is warranted, timely notice for such hearing shall be given to the parties. Participants at the hearing shall be limited to the Respondent and legal counsel (if so desired), the EC Chairperson, the Council Chairperson, the AOTA Legal Counsel, or others approved in advance by the Appeal Panel as necessary to the proceedings.

6.5. Decision

6.5.1. The Appeal Panel shall have the power to (a) affirm the decision; or (b) modify the decision; or (c) reverse or remand to the EC, but only if there were procedural errors materially prejudicial to the outcome of the proceeding or if the Council decision was against the clear weight of the evidence.

6.5.2. Within thirty (30) days after receipt of the appeal if no hearing was granted, or within thirty (30) days after receipt of the transcript if a hearing was held, the Appeal Panel shall notify the AOTA Executive Director of its decision. The AOTA Executive Director shall promptly notify the Respondent, the original Complainant, appropriate Association bodies, and any other parties deemed appropriate (e.g., SRB, NBCOT). For Association purposes, the decision of the Appeal Panel shall be final.

7. Notifications

All notifications referred to in these *Enforcement Procedures* shall be in writing and shall be delivered by national delivery service or mail with signature and proof of date of receipt required.

8. Records and Reports

At the completion of the enforcement process, the written records and reports that state the initial basis for the complaint, material evidence, and the disposition of the complaint shall be retained in the AOTA Ethics Office for a period of five (5) years.

9. Publication

Final decisions will be publicized only after any Appeal Panel process has been completed.

10. Modification

AOTA reserves the right to (a) modify the time periods, procedures, or application of these *Enforcement Procedures* for good cause consistent with fundamental fairness in a given case and (b) modify its *Code and Ethics Standards* and/or these *Enforcement Procedures,* with such modifications to be applied only prospectively.

Adopted by the Representative Assembly 2009CONov146 as Attachment A of the Standard Operating Procedures (SOP) of the Ethics Commission.

Reviewed by BPPC 1/04, 1/05, 9/06, 1/07, 9/09

Adopted by RA 4/96, 5/04, 5/05, 11/06, 4/07, 11/09

Revised by SEC 4/98, 4/00, 1/02, 1/04, 12/04, 9/06

Revised by EC 12/06, 2/07, 8/09

Note. The Commission on Standards and Ethics (SEC) changed to Ethics Commission (EC) in September 2005 as per Association Bylaws.

Copyright © 2010, by the American Occupational Therapy Association. Previously published in the *American Journal of Occupational Therapy, 64*(Suppl.), S4–S16. http://dx.doi.org/10.5014/ajot.2010.64S4

AMERICAN OCCUPATIONAL THERAPY ASSOCIATION
ETHICS COMMISSION

Formal Complaint of Alleged Violation of the
Occupational Therapy Code of Ethics and Ethics Standards

If an investigation is deemed necessary, a copy of this form will be provided to the individual against whom the complaint is filed.

Date _____

Complainant: (Information regarding individual filing the complaint)

_____   _____
NAME   SIGNATURE

_____   _____
ADDRESS   TELEPHONE

_____   _____
                                              E-MAIL ADDRESS

Respondent: (Information regarding individual against whom the complaint is directed)

_____   _____
NAME   SIGNATURE

_____   _____
ADDRESS   TELEPHONE

_____   _____
                                              E-MAIL ADDRESS

1. **Summarize** in an written attachment the **facts and circumstances, including dates and events,** which support a violation of the *Code of Ethics and Ethics Standards* and this complaint. Include steps if any, that have been taken to resolve this complaint before filing.

2. **Please sign and date all documents you have written and are submitting.** *Do not include confidential documents such as patient or employment records.*

3. **If you have filed a complaint about this same matter with any other agency (e.g., NBCOT; SRB; academic institution; any federal, state, or local official), indicate to whom it was submitted, the approximate date(s) and resolution if known.**

I certify that the statements/information within this complaint are correct and truthful to the best of my knowledge and are submitted in good faith, not for resolution of private business, legal, or other disputes for which other appropriate forums exist.

_____
Signature

Send completed form, with accompanying documentation, **IN AN ENVELOPE MARKED** *CONFIDENTIAL* **to:**

Ethics Commission
American Occupational Therapy Association, Inc.
Attn: Staff Liaison to the EC/Ethics Office
4720 Montgomery Lane, PO Box 31220
Bethesda, MD 20824-1220

Office Use Only:

Membership Verified? ❑ Yes ❑ No

By: _____

Occupational Therapy Code of Ethics and Ethics Standards (2010)

Preamble

The American Occupational Therapy Association (AOTA) *Occupational Therapy Code of Ethics and Ethics Standards (2010)* ("Code and Ethics Standards") is a public statement of principles used to promote and maintain high standards of conduct within the profession. Members of AOTA are committed to promoting inclusion, diversity, independence, and safety for all recipients in various stages of life, health, and illness and to empower all beneficiaries of occupational therapy. This commitment extends beyond service recipients to include professional colleagues, students, educators, businesses, and the community.

Fundamental to the mission of the occupational therapy profession is the therapeutic use of everyday life activities (occupations) with individuals or groups for the purpose of participation in roles and situations in home, school, workplace, community, and other settings. "Occupational therapy addresses the physical, cognitive, psychosocial, sensory, and other aspects of performance in a variety of contexts to support engagement in everyday life activities that affect health, well-being, and quality of life" (AOTA, 2004, p. 694). Occupational therapy personnel have an ethical responsibility primarily to recipients of service and secondarily to society.

The *Occupational Therapy Code of Ethics and Ethics Standards (2010)* was tailored to address the most prevalent ethical concerns of the profession in education, research, and practice. The concerns of stakeholders including the public, consumers, students, colleagues, employers, research participants, researchers, educators, and practitioners were addressed in the creation of this document. A review of issues raised in ethics cases, member questions related to ethics, and content of other professional codes of ethics were utilized to ensure that the revised document is applicable to occupational therapists, occupational therapy assistants, and students in all roles.

The historical foundation of this Code and Ethics Standards is based on ethical reasoning surrounding practice and professional issues, as well as on empathic reflection regarding these interactions with others (see e.g., AOTA, 2005, 2006). This reflection resulted in the establishment of principles that guide ethical action, which goes beyond rote following of rules or application of principles. Rather, *ethical action* it is a manifestation of moral character and mindful reflection. It is a commitment to benefit others, to virtuous practice of artistry and science, to genuinely good behaviors, and to noble acts of courage.

While much has changed over the course of the profession's history, more has remained the same. The profession of occupational therapy remains grounded in seven core concepts, as identified in the *Core Values and Attitudes of Occupational Therapy Practice* (AOTA, 1993): *altruism, equality, freedom, justice, dignity, truth,* and *prudence.* *Altruism* is the individual's ability to place the needs of others before their own. *Equality* refers to the desire to promote fairness in interactions with others. The concept of *freedom* and personal choice is paramount in a profession in which the desires of the client must guide our interventions. Occupational therapy practitioners, educators, and researchers relate in a fair and impartial manner to individuals with whom they interact and respect and adhere to the applicable laws and standards regarding their area of practice, be it direct care, education, or research *(justice)*. Inherent in the practice of occupational therapy is the promotion and preservation of the individuality and *dignity* of the client, by assisting him or her to engage in occupations that are meaningful to him or her regardless of level of disability. In all situations, occupational therapists, occupational therapy assistants, and students must provide accurate information, both in oral and written form *(truth)*. Occupational therapy personnel use their clinical and ethical reasoning skills, sound judgment, and reflection to make decisions to direct them in their area(s) of practice *(prudence)*. These seven core values provide a foundation by which occupational therapy personnel guide their interactions with others, be they students, clients, colleagues, research participants, or communities. These values also define the ethical principles to which the profession is committed and which the public can expect.

The *Occupational Therapy Code of Ethics and Ethics Standards (2010)* is a guide to professional conduct when ethical issues arise. Ethical decision making is a process that includes awareness of how the outcome will impact occupational therapy clients in all spheres. Applications of Code and Ethics Standards Principles are considered situation-specific, and where a conflict exists, occupational therapy personnel will pursue responsible efforts for resolution. These Principles apply to occupational therapy personnel engaged in any professional role, including elected and volunteer leadership positions.

The specific purposes of the *Occupational Therapy Code of Ethics and Ethics Standards (2010)* are to

1. Identify and describe the principles supported by the occupational therapy profession.

2. Educate the general public and members regarding established principles to which occupational therapy personnel are accountable.

3. Socialize occupational therapy personnel to expected standards of conduct.

4. Assist occupational therapy personnel in recognition and resolution of ethical dilemmas.

The *Occupational Therapy Code of Ethics and Ethics Standards (2010)* define the set of principles that apply to occupational therapy personnel at all levels:

DEFINITIONS

- **Recipient of service:** Individuals or groups receiving occupational therapy.

- **Student:** A person who is enrolled in an accredited occupational therapy education program.

- **Research participant:** A prospective participant or one who has agreed to participate in an approved research project.

- **Employee:** A person who is hired by a business (facility or organization) to provide occupational therapy services.

- **Colleague:** A person who provides services in the same or different business (facility or organization) to which a professional relationship exists or may exist.

- **Public:** The community of people at large.

BENEFICENCE

Principle 1. Occupational therapy personnel shall demonstrate a concern for the well-being and safety of the recipients of their services.

Beneficence includes all forms of action intended to benefit other persons. The term *beneficence* connotes acts of mercy, kindness, and charity (Beauchamp & Childress, 2009). Forms of beneficence typically include altruism, love, and humanity. Beneficence requires taking action by helping others, in other words, by promoting good, by preventing harm, and by removing harm. Examples of beneficence include protecting and defending the rights of others, preventing harm from occurring to others, removing conditions that will cause harm to others, helping persons with disabilities, and rescuing persons in danger (Beauchamp & Childress, 2009).

Occupational therapy personnel shall

A. Respond to requests for occupational therapy services (e.g., a referral) in a timely manner as determined by law, regulation, or policy.

B. Provide appropriate evaluation and a plan of intervention for all recipients of occupational therapy services specific to their needs.

C. Reevaluate and reassess recipients of service in a timely manner to determine if goals are being achieved and whether intervention plans should be revised.

D. Avoid the inappropriate use of outdated or obsolete tests/assessments or data obtained from such tests in making intervention decisions or recommendations.

E. Provide occupational therapy services that are within each practitioner's level of competence and scope of practice (e.g., qualifications, experience, the law).

F. Use, to the extent possible, evaluation, planning, intervention techniques, and therapeutic equipment that are evidence-based and within the recognized scope of occupational therapy practice.

G. Take responsible steps (e.g., continuing education, research, supervision, training) and use careful judgment to ensure their own competence and weigh potential for client harm when generally recognized standards do not exist in emerging technology or areas of practice.

H. Terminate occupational therapy services in collaboration with the service recipient or responsible party when the needs and goals of the recipient have been met or when services no longer produce a measurable change or outcome.

I. Refer to other health care specialists solely on the basis of the needs of the client.

J. Provide occupational therapy education, continuing education, instruction, and training that are within the instructor's subject area of expertise and level of competence.

K. Provide students and employees with information about the Code and Ethics Standards, opportunities to discuss ethical conflicts, and procedures for reporting unresolved ethical conflicts.

L. Ensure that occupational therapy research is conducted in accordance with currently accepted ethical guidelines and standards for the protection of research participants and the dissemination of results.

M. Report to appropriate authorities any acts in practice, education, and research that appear unethical or illegal.

N. Take responsibility for promoting and practicing occupational therapy on the basis of current knowledge and research and for further developing the profession's body of knowledge.

NONMALEFICENCE

Principle 2. Occupational therapy personnel shall intentionally refrain from actions that cause harm.

Nonmaleficence imparts an obligation to refrain from harming others (Beauchamp & Childress, 2009). The principle of nonmaleficence is grounded in the practitioner's responsibility to refrain from causing harm, inflicting injury, or wronging others. While beneficence requires action to incur benefit, nonmaleficence requires non-action to avoid harm (Beauchamp & Childress, 2009). Nonmaleficence also includes an obligation to not impose risks of harm even if the potential risk is without malicious or harmful intent. This principle often is examined under the context of *due care*. If the standard of due care outweighs the benefit of treatment, then refraining from treatment provision would be ethically indicated (Beauchamp & Childress, 2009).

Occupational therapy personnel shall

A. Avoid inflicting harm or injury to recipients of occupational therapy services, students, research participants, or employees.

B. Make every effort to ensure continuity of services or options for transition to appropriate services to avoid abandoning the service recipient if the current provider is unavailable due to medical or other absence or loss of employment.

C. Avoid relationships that exploit the recipient of services, students, research participants, or employees physically, emotionally, psychologically, financially, socially, or in any other manner that conflicts or interferes with professional judgment and objectivity.

D. Avoid engaging in any sexual relationship or activity, whether consensual or nonconsensual, with any recipient of service, including family or significant other, student, research participant, or employee, while a relationship exists as an occupational therapy practitioner, educator, researcher, supervisor, or employer.

E. Recognize and take appropriate action to remedy personal problems and limitations that might cause harm to recipients of service, colleagues, students, research participants, or others.

F. Avoid any undue influences, such as alcohol or drugs, that may compromise the provision of occupational therapy services, education, or research.

G. Avoid situations in which a practitioner, educator, researcher, or employer is unable to maintain clear professional boundaries or objectivity to ensure the safety and well-being of recipients of service, students, research participants, and employees.

H. Maintain awareness of and adherence to the Code and Ethics Standards when participating in volunteer roles.

I. Avoid compromising client rights or well-being based on arbitrary administrative directives by exercising professional judgment and critical analysis.

J. Avoid exploiting any relationship established as an occupational therapist or occupational therapy assistant to further one's own physical, emotional, financial, political, or business interests at the expense of the best interests of recipients of services, students, research participants, employees, or colleagues.

K. Avoid participating in bartering for services because of the potential for exploitation and conflict of interest unless there are clearly no contraindications or bartering is a culturally appropriate custom.

L. Determine the proportion of risk to benefit for participants in research prior to implementing a study.

AUTONOMY, CONFIDENTIALITY

Principle 3. Occupational therapy personnel shall respect the right of the individual to self-determination.

The principle of autonomy and confidentiality expresses the concept that practitioners have a duty to treat the client according to the client's desires, within the bounds of accepted standards of care and to protect the client's confidential information. Often *autonomy* is referred to as the *self-determination* principle. However, respect for autonomy goes beyond acknowledging an individual as a mere agent and also acknowledges a "person's right to hold views, to make choices, and to take actions based on personal values and beliefs" (Beauchamp & Childress, 2009, p. 103). Autonomy has become a prominent principle in health care ethics; the right to make a determination regarding care decisions that directly impact the life of the service recipient should reside with that individual. The principle of autonomy and confidentiality also applies to students in an educational program, to participants in research studies, and to the public who seek information about occupational therapy services.

Occupational therapy personnel shall

A. Establish a collaborative relationship with recipients of service, including families, significant others, and caregivers in setting goals and priorities throughout the intervention process. This includes full disclosure of the benefits, risks, and potential outcomes of any intervention; the personnel who will be providing the intervention(s); and/or any reasonable alternatives to the proposed intervention.

B. Obtain consent before administering any occupational therapy service, including evaluation, and ensure that recipients of service (or their legal representatives) are kept informed of the progress in meeting goals specified in the plan of intervention/care. If the service recipient cannot give consent, the practitioner must be sure that consent has been obtained from the person who is legally responsible for that recipient.

C. Respect the recipient of service's right to refuse occupational therapy services temporarily or permanently without negative consequences.

D. Provide students with access to accurate information regarding educational requirements and academic policies and procedures relative to the occupational therapy program/educational institution.

E. Obtain informed consent from participants involved in research activities, and ensure that they understand the benefits, risks, and potential outcomes as a result of their participation as research subjects.

F. Respect research participant's right to withdraw from a research study without consequences.

G. Ensure that confidentiality and the right to privacy are respected and maintained regarding all information obtained about recipients of service, students, research participants, colleagues, or employees. The only exceptions are when a practitioner or staff member believes that an individual is in serious foreseeable or imminent harm. Laws and regulations may require disclosure to appropriate authorities without consent.

H. Maintain the confidentiality of all verbal, written, electronic, augmentative, and non-verbal communications, including compliance with HIPAA regulations.

I. Take appropriate steps to facilitate meaningful communication and comprehension in cases in which the recipient of service, student, or research participant has limited ability to communicate (e.g., aphasia or differences in language, literacy, culture).

J. Make every effort to facilitate open and collaborative dialogue with clients and/or responsible parties to facilitate comprehension of services and their potential risks/benefits.

SOCIAL JUSTICE

Principle 4. Occupational therapy personnel shall provide services in a fair and equitable manner.

Social justice, also called *distributive justice*, refers to the fair, equitable, and appropriate distribution of resources. The principle of social justice refers broadly to the distribution of all rights and responsibilities in society (Beauchamp & Childress, 2009). In general, the principle of social justice supports the concept of achieving justice in every aspect of society rather than merely the administration of law. The general idea is that individuals and groups should receive fair treatment and an impartial share of the benefits of society. Occupational therapy personnel have a vested interest in addressing unjust inequities that limit opportunities for participation in society (Braveman & Bass-Haugen, 2009). While opinions differ regarding the most ethical approach to addressing distribution of health care resources and reduction of health disparities, the issue of social justice continues to focus on limiting the impact of social inequality on health outcomes.

Occupational therapy personnel shall

A. Uphold the profession's altruistic responsibilities to help ensure the common good.

B. Take responsibility for educating the public and society about the value of occupational therapy services in promoting health and wellness and reducing the impact of disease and disability.

C. Make every effort to promote activities that benefit the health status of the community.

D. Advocate for just and fair treatment for all patients, clients, employees, and colleagues, and encourage employers and colleagues to abide by the highest standards of social justice and the ethical standards set forth by the occupational therapy profession.

E. Make efforts to advocate for recipients of occupational therapy services to obtain needed services through available means.

F. Provide services that reflect an understanding of how occupational therapy service delivery can be affected by factors such as economic status, age, ethnicity, race, geography, disability, marital status, sexual orientation, gender, gender identity, religion, culture, and political affiliation.

G. Consider offering *pro bono* ("for the good") or reduced-fee occupational therapy services for selected individuals when consistent with guidelines of the employer, third-party payer, and/or government agency.

PROCEDURAL JUSTICE

Principle 5. Occupational therapy personnel shall comply with institutional rules, local, state, federal, and international laws and AOTA documents applicable to the profession of occupational therapy.

Procedural justice is concerned with making and implementing decisions according to fair processes that ensure "fair treatment" (Maiese, 2004). Rules must be impartially followed and consistently applied to generate an unbiased decision. The principle of procedural justice is based on the concept that procedures and processes are organized in a fair manner and that policies, regulations, and laws are followed. While *the law* and *ethics* are not synonymous terms, occupational therapy personnel have an ethical responsibility to uphold current reimbursement regulations and state/territorial laws governing the profession. In addition, occupational therapy personnel are ethically bound to be aware of organizational policies and practice guidelines set forth by regulatory agencies established to protect recipients of service, research participants, and the public.

Occupational therapy personnel shall

A. Be familiar with and apply the Code and Ethics Standards to the work setting, and share them with employers, other employees, colleagues, students, and researchers.

B. Be familiar with and seek to understand and abide by institutional rules, and when those rules conflict with ethical practice, take steps to resolve the conflict.

C. Be familiar with revisions in those laws and AOTA policies that apply to the profession of occupational therapy and inform employers, employees, colleagues, students, and researchers of those changes.

D. Be familiar with established policies and procedures for handling concerns about the Code and Ethics Standards, including familiarity with national, state, local, district, and territorial procedures for handling ethics complaints as well as policies and procedures created by AOTA and certification, licensing, and regulatory agencies.

E. Hold appropriate national, state, or other requisite credentials for the occupational therapy services they provide.

F. Take responsibility for maintaining high standards and continuing competence in practice, education, and research by participating in professional development and educational activities to improve and update knowledge and skills.

G. Ensure that all duties assumed by or assigned to other occupational therapy personnel match credentials, qualifications, experience, and scope of practice.

H. Provide appropriate supervision to individuals for whom they have supervisory responsibility in accordance with AOTA official documents and local, state, and federal or national laws, rules, regulations, policies, procedures, standards, and guidelines.

I. Obtain all necessary approvals prior to initiating research activities.

J. Report all gifts and remuneration from individuals, agencies, or companies in accordance with employer policies as well as state and federal guidelines.

K. Use funds for intended purposes, and avoid misappropriation of funds.

L. Take reasonable steps to ensure that employers are aware of occupational therapy's ethical obligations as set forth in this Code and Ethics Standards and of the implications of those obligations for occupational therapy practice, education, and research.

M. Actively work with employers to prevent discrimination and unfair labor practices, and advocate for employees with disabilities to ensure the provision of reasonable accommodations.

N. Actively participate with employers in the formulation of policies and procedures to ensure legal, regulatory, and ethical compliance.

O. Collect fees legally. Fees shall be fair, reasonable, and commensurate with services delivered. Fee schedules must be available and equitable regardless of actual payer reimbursements/contracts.

P. Maintain the ethical principles and standards of the profession when participating in a business arrangement as owner, stockholder, partner, or employee, and refrain from working for or doing business with organizations that engage in illegal or unethical business practices (e.g., fraudulent billing, providing occupational therapy services beyond the scope of occupational therapy practice).

VERACITY

Principle 6. Occupational therapy personnel shall provide comprehensive, accurate, and objective information when representing the profession.

Veracity is based on the virtues of truthfulness, candor, and honesty. The principle of *veracity* in health care refers to comprehensive, accurate, and objective transmission of information and includes fostering the client's understanding of such information (Beauchamp & Childress, 2009). Veracity is based on respect owed to others. In communicating with others, occupational therapy personnel implicitly promise to speak truthfully and not deceive the listener. By entering into a relationship in care or research, the recipient of service or research participant enters into a contract that includes a right to truthful information (Beauchamp & Childress, 2009). In addition, transmission of information is incomplete without also ensuring that the recipient or participant understands the information provided. Concepts of veracity must be carefully balanced with other potentially competing ethical principles, cultural beliefs, and organizational policies. Veracity ultimately is valued as a means to establish trust and strengthen professional relationships. Therefore, adherence to the Principle also requires thoughtful analysis of how full disclosure of information may impact outcomes.

Occupational therapy personnel shall

A. Represent the credentials, qualifications, education, experience, training, roles, duties, competence, views, contributions, and findings accurately in all forms of communication about recipients of service, students, employees, research participants, and colleagues.

B. Refrain from using or participating in the use of any form of communication that contains false, fraudulent, deceptive, misleading, or unfair statements or claims.

C. Record and report in an accurate and timely manner, and in accordance with applicable regulations, all information related to professional activities.

D. Ensure that documentation for reimbursement purposes is done in accordance with applicable laws, guidelines, and regulations.

E. Accept responsibility for any action that reduces the public's trust in occupational therapy.

F. Ensure that all marketing and advertising are truthful, accurate, and carefully presented to avoid misleading recipients of service, students, research participants, or the public.

G. Describe the type and duration of occupational therapy services accurately in professional contracts, including the duties and responsibilities of all involved parties.

H. Be honest, fair, accurate, respectful, and timely in gathering and reporting fact-based information regarding employee job performance and student performance.

I. Give credit and recognition when using the work of others in written, oral, or electronic media.

J. Not plagiarize the work of others.

FIDELITY

Principle 7. Occupational therapy personnel shall treat colleagues and other professionals with respect, fairness, discretion, and integrity.

The principle of fidelity comes from the Latin root *fidelis* meaning loyal. Fidelity refers to being faithful, which includes obligations of loyalty and the keeping of promises and commitments (Veatch & Flack, 1997). In the health professions, fidelity refers to maintaining good-faith relationships between various service providers and recipients. While respecting fidelity requires occupational therapy personnel to meet the client's reasonable expectations (Purtillo, 2005), Principle 7 specifically addresses fidelity as it relates to maintaining collegial and organizational relationships. Professional relationships are greatly influenced by the complexity of the environment in which occupational therapy personnel work. Practitioners, educators, and researchers alike must consistently balance their duties to service recipients, students, research participants, and other professionals as well as to organizations that may influence decision making and professional practice.

Occupational therapy personnel shall

A. Respect the traditions, practices, competencies, and responsibilities of their own and other professions, as well as those of the institutions and agencies that constitute the working environment.

B. Preserve, respect, and safeguard private information about employees, colleagues, and students unless otherwise mandated by national, state, or local laws or permission to disclose is given by the individual.

C. Take adequate measures to discourage, prevent, expose, and correct any breaches of the Code and Ethics Standards, and report any breaches of the former to the appropriate authorities.

D. Attempt to resolve perceived institutional violations of the Code and Ethics Standards by utilizing internal resources first.

E. Avoid conflicts of interest or conflicts of commitment in employment, volunteer roles, or research.

F. Avoid using one's position (employee or volunteer) or knowledge gained from that position in such a manner that gives rise to real or perceived conflict of interest among the person, the employer, other Association members, and/or other organizations.

G. Use conflict resolution and/or alternative dispute resolution resources to resolve organizational and interpersonal conflicts.

H. Be diligent stewards of human, financial, and material resources of their employers, and refrain from exploiting these resources for personal gain.

References

American Occupational Therapy Association. (1993). Core values and attitudes of occupational therapy practice. *American Journal of Occupational Therapy, 47,* 1085–1086.

American Occupational Therapy Association. (2004). Policy 5.3.1: Definition of occupational therapy practice for state regulation. *American Journal of Occupational Therapy, 58,* 694–695.

American Occupational Therapy Association. (2005). Occupational therapy code of ethics (2005). *American Journal of Occupational Therapy, 59,* 639–642.

American Occupational Therapy Association. (2006). Guidelines to the occupational therapy code of ethics. *American Journal of Occupational Therapy, 60,* 652–658.

Beauchamp, T. L., & Childress, J. F. (2009). *Principles of biomedical ethics* (6th ed.). New York: Oxford University Press.

Braveman, B., & Bass-Haugen, J. D. (2009). Social justice and health disparities: An evolving discourse in occupational therapy research and intervention. *American Journal of Occupational Therapy, 63,* 7–12.

Maiese, M. (2004). *Procedural justice.* Retrieved July 29, 2009, from http://www.beyondintractability.org/essay/procedural_justice/

Purtillo, R. (2005). *Ethical dimensions in the health professions* (4th ed.). Philadelphia: Elsevier/Saunders.

Veatch, R. M., & Flack, H. E. (1997). *Case studies in allied health ethics.* Upper Saddle River, NJ: Prentice-Hall.

Authors

Ethics Commission (EC):

Kathlyn Reed, PhD, OTR, FAOTA, MLIS, *Chairperson*
Barbara Hemphill, DMin, OTR, FAOTA, FMOTA, *Chair-Elect*
Ann Moodey Ashe, MHS, OTR/L
Lea C. Brandt, OTD, MA, OTR/L
Joanne Estes, MS, OTR/L
Loretta Jean Foster, MS, COTA/L
Donna F. Homenko, RDH, PhD
Craig R. Jackson, JD, MSW
Deborah Yarett Slater, MS, OT/L, FAOTA, *AOTA Staff Liaison*

Adopted by the Representative Assembly 2010CApr17.

Note. This document replaces the following rescinded Ethics documents 2010CApril18: the *Occupational Therapy Code of Ethics (2005)* (*American Journal of Occupational Therapy, 59,* 639–642); the *Guidelines to the Occupational Therapy Code of Ethics* (*American Journal of Occupational Therapy, 60,* 652–658); and the *Core Values and Attitudes of Occupational Therapy Practice* (*American Journal of Occupational Therapy, 47,* 1085–1086).

Guidelines

Guidelines for Documentation of Occupational Therapy

Documentation of occupational therapy services is necessary whenever professional services are provided to a client. Occupational therapists and occupational therapy assistants[1] determine the appropriate type of documentation structure and then record the services provided within their scope of practice. This document, based on the *Occupational Therapy Practice Framework: Domain and Process* (2nd ed.; American Occupational Therapy Association [AOTA], 2008), describes the components and purpose of professional documentation used in occupational therapy.

AOTA's (2010) *Standards of Practice for Occupational Therapy* states that an occupational therapy practitioner[2] documents the occupational therapy services and "abides by the time frames, format, and standards established by the practice settings, government agencies, external accreditation programs, payers, and AOTA documents" (p. S108). These requirements apply to both electronic and written forms of documentation. Documentation should reflect the nature of services provided and the clinical reasoning of the occupational therapy practitioner, and it should provide enough information to ensure that services are delivered in a safe and effective manner. Documentation should describe the depth and breadth of services provided to meet the complexity of individual client[3] needs. The client's diagnosis or prognosis should not be used as the sole rationale for occupational therapy services.

The purpose of documentation is to

- Communicate information about the client from the occupational therapy perspective;

- Articulate the rationale for provision of occupational therapy services and the relationship of those services to client outcomes, reflecting the occupational therapy practitioner's clinical reasoning and professional judgment; and

- Create a chronological record of client status, occupational therapy services provided to the client, client response to occupational therapy intervention, and client outcomes.

Types of Documentation

Table 1 outlines common types of documentation reports. Reports may be named differently or combined and reorganized to meet the specific needs of the setting. Occupational therapy documentation should always record the practitioner's activity in the areas of screening, evaluation, intervention, and outcomes (AOTA, 2008) in accordance with payer, facility, and state and federal guidelines.

---

[1]*Occupational therapists* are responsible for all aspects of occupational therapy service delivery and are accountable for the safety and effectiveness of the occupational therapy service delivery process. *Occupational therapy assistants* deliver occupational therapy services under the supervision of and in partnership with an occupational therapist (AOTA, 2009).

[2]When the term *occupational therapy practitioner* is used in this document, it refers to both occupational therapists and occupational therapy assistants (AOTA, 2006).

[3]In this document, *client* may refer to an individual, organization, or population.

Table 1. Common Types of Occupational Therapy Documentation Reports

Process Areas	Type of Report
I. Screening	A. Screening Report
II. Evaluation	A. Evaluation Report
	B. Reevaluation Report
III. Intervention	A. Intervention Plan
	B. Contact Report Note or Communiqué
	C. Progress Report/Note
	D. Transition Plan
IV. Outcomes	A. Discharge/Discontinuation Report

Content of Reports

I. Screening

    A. Documents referral source, reason for occupational therapy screening, and need for occupational therapy evaluation and service.

        1. Phone referrals should be documented in accordance with payer, facility, and state and federal guidelines and include

            a. Names of individuals spoken with,

            b. Purpose of screening,

            c. Date of request,

            d. Number of contact for referral source, and

            e. Description of client's prior level of occupational performance.

    B. Consists of an initial brief assessment to determine client's need for an occupational therapy evaluation or for referral to another service if not appropriate for occupational therapy services.

    C. Suggested content:

        1. *Client information*—Name/agency; date of birth; gender; health status; and applicable medical/educational/developmental diagnoses, precautions, and contraindications

        2. *Referral information*—Date and source of referral, services requested, reason for referral, funding source, and anticipated length of service

        3. *Brief occupational profile*—Client's reason for seeking occupational therapy services, current areas of occupation that are successful and problematic, contexts and environments that support and hinder occupations, medical/educational/work history, occupational history (e.g., patterns of living, interest, values), client's priorities, and targeted goals

        4. *Assessments used and results*—Types of assessments used and results (e.g., interviews, record reviews, observations)

        5. *Recommendation*—Professional judgments regarding appropriateness of need for complete occupational therapy evaluation.

II. Evaluation

A. Evaluation Report

1. Documents referral source and data gathered through the evaluation process in accordance with payer, facility, state, and/or federal guidelines. Includes

   a. Analysis of occupational performance and identification of factors that support and hinder performance and participation and

   b. Identification of specific areas of occupation and occupational performance to be addressed, interventions, and expected outcomes.

2. Suggested content:

   a. *Client information*—Name; date of birth; gender; health status; medical history; and applicable medical/educational/developmental diagnoses, precautions, and contraindications

   b. *Referral information*—Date and source of referral, services requested, reason for referral, funding source, and anticipated length of service

   c. *Occupational profile*—Client's reason for seeking occupational therapy services, current areas of occupation that are successful and problematic, contexts and environments that support or hinder occupations, medical/educational/work history, occupational history (e.g., patterns of living, interest, values), client's priorities, and targeted outcomes

   d. *Assessments used and results*—Types of assessments used and results (e.g., interviews, record reviews, observations, standardized and/or nonstandardized assessments)

   e. *Analysis of occupational performance*—Description of and judgment about performance skills, performance patterns, contexts and environments, activity demands, outcomes from standardized measures and/or nonstandardized assessments,[4] and client factors that will be targeted for intervention and outcomes expected

   f. *Summary and analysis*—Interpretation and summary of data as related to occupational profile and referring concern

   g. *Recommendation*—Judgment regarding appropriateness of occupational therapy services or other services.

   Note. The intervention plan, including intervention goals addressing anticipated outcomes, objectives, and frequency of therapy, is described in the "Intervention Plan" section that follows.

B. Reevaluation Report

1. Documents the results of the reevaluation process. Frequency of reevaluation depends on the needs of the setting, the progress of the client, and client changes.

2. Suggested content:

   a. *Client information*—Name; date of birth; gender; and applicable medical/educational/developmental diagnoses, precautions, and contraindications

   b. *Occupational profile*—Updates on current areas of occupation that are successful and problematic, contexts and environments that support or hinder occupations, summary of any new

---

[4]*Nonstandardized assessment tools* are considered a valid form of information gathering that allows for flexibility and individualization when measuring outcomes related to the status of an individual or group through an intrapersonal comparison. Although not uniform in administration or scoring or possessing full and complete psychometric data, nonstandardized assessment tools possess strong internal validity and represent an evidence-based approach to occupational therapy practice (Hinojosa, Kramer, & Christ, 2010). Nonstandardized tools should be selected on the basis of the best available evidence and the clinical reasoning of the practitioner.

medical/educational/work information, and updates or changes to client's priorities and targeted outcomes

c. *Reevaluation results*—Focus of reevaluation, specific types of outcome measures from standardized and/or nonstandardized assessments used, and client's performance and subjective responses

d. *Analysis of occupational performance*—Description of and judgment about performance skills, performance patterns, contexts and environments, activity demands, outcomes from standardized measures and/or nonstandardized assessments, and client factors that will be targeted for intervention and outcomes expected

e. *Summary and analysis*—Interpretation and summary of data as related to referring concern and comparison of results with previous evaluation results

f. *Recommendations*—Changes to occupational therapy services, revision or continuation of interventions, goals and objectives, frequency of occupational therapy services, and recommendation for referral to other professionals or agencies as applicable.

III. Intervention

A. Intervention Plan

1. Documents the goals, intervention approaches, and types of interventions to be used to achieve the client's identified targeted outcomes and is based on results of evaluation or reevaluation processes. Includes recommendations or referrals to other professionals and agencies in adherence with each payer source documentation requirements (e.g., pain levels, time spent on each modality).

2. Suggested content:

a. *Client information*—Name, date of birth, gender, precautions, and contraindications

b. *Intervention goals*—Measurable and meaningful occupation-based long-term and short-term objective goals directly related to the client's ability and need to engage in desired occupations

c. *Intervention approaches and types of interventions to be used*—Intervention approaches that include create/promote, establish/restore, maintain, modify, and/or prevent; types of interventions that include consultation, education process, advocacy, and/or the therapeutic use of occupations or activities

d. *Service delivery mechanisms*—Service provider, service location, and frequency and duration of services

e. *Plan for discharge*—Discontinuation criteria, discharge setting (e.g., skilled nursing facility, home, community, classroom) and follow-up care

f. *Outcome measures*—Tools that assess occupational performance, adaptation, role competence, improved health and wellness, improved quality of life, self-advocacy, and occupational justice. Standardized and/or nonstandardized assessments used at evaluation should be readministered periodically to monitor measurable progress and report functional outcomes as required by client's payer source and/or facility requirements.

g. *Professionals responsible and date of plan*—Names and positions of persons overseeing plan, date plan was developed, and date when plan was modified or reviewed.

B. Service Contacts

1. Documents contacts between the client and the occupational therapy practitioner. Records the types of interventions used and client's response, which can include telephone contacts, interventions, and meetings with others.

    2. Suggested content:

        a. *Client information*—Name; date of birth; gender; and diagnosis, precautions, and contraindications

        b. *Therapy log*—Date, type of contact, names/positions of persons involved, summary or significant information communicated during contacts, client attendance and participation in intervention, reason service is missed, types of interventions used, client's response, environmental or task modification, assistive or adaptive devices used or fabricated, statement of any training education or consultation provided, and the client's present level of performance. Documentation of services provided should reflect the complexity of the client and the professional clinical reasoning and expertise of an occupational therapy practitioner required to provide an effective outcome in occupational performance. The client's diagnosis or prognosis should not be the sole rationale for the skilled interventions provided. Measures used to assess outcomes should be repeated in accordance with payer and facility requirements and documented to demonstrate measurable functional progress of the client.

        c. *Intervention/procedure coding* (i.e., CPT™),[5] if applicable.

C. Progress Report/Note

    1. Summarizes intervention process and documents client's progress toward achievement of goals. Includes new data collected; modifications of treatment plan; and statement of need for continuation, discontinuation, or referral.

    2. Suggested content:

        a. *Client information*—Name; date of birth; gender; and diagnosis, precautions, and contraindications

        b. *Summary of services provided*—Brief statement of frequency of services and length of time services have been provided; techniques and strategies used; measurable progress or lack thereof using age-appropriate current functional standardized and/or nonstandardized outcome measures; environmental or task modifications provided; adaptive equipment or orthotics provided; medical, educational, or other pertinent client updates; client's response to occupational therapy services; and programs or training provided to the client or caregivers

        c. *Current client performance*—Client's progress toward the goals and client's performance in areas of occupations

        d. *Plan or recommendations*—Recommendations and rationale as well as client's input to changes or continuation of plan.

D. Transition Plan

    1. Documents the formal transition plan and is written when client is transitioning from one service setting to another within a service delivery system.

    2. Suggested content:

        a. *Client information*—Name; date of birth; gender; and diagnosis, precautions, and contraindications

        b. *Client's current status*—Client's current performance in occupations

        c. *Transition plan*—Name of current service setting and name of setting to which client will transition, reason for transition, time frame in which transition will occur, and outline of activities to be carried out during the transition plan

---

[5]*CPT* is a trademark of the American Medical Association (AMA). *CPT* five-digit codes, nomenclature, and other data are copyright © 2011 by the AMA. All rights reserved.

    d. *Recommendations*—Recommendations and rationale for occupational therapy services, modifications or accommodations needed, and assistive technology and environmental modifications needed.

IV. Outcomes

    A. Discharge Report—Summary of Occupational Therapy Services and Outcomes

      1. Summarizes the changes in client's ability to engage in occupations between the initial evaluation and discontinuation of services and makes recommendations as applicable.

      2. Suggested content with examples include

        a. *Client information*—name/agency, date of birth, gender, diagnosis, precautions, and contraindications

        b. *Summary of intervention process*—date of initial and final service; frequency, number of sessions, summary of interventions used; summary of progress toward goals; and occupational therapy outcomes—initial client status and ending status regarding engagement in occupations, client's assessment of efficacy of occupational therapy services

        c. *Recommendations*—recommendations pertaining to the client's future needs; specific follow-up plans, if applicable; and referrals to other professionals and agencies, if applicable.

Each occupational therapy client has a client record maintained as a permanent file. The record is maintained in a professional and legal fashion (i.e., organized, legible, concise, clear, accurate, complete, current, grammatically correct, and objective; see Box 1 for more information).

Box 1. Fundamentals of Documentation

- Client's full name and case number (if applicable) on each page of documentation
- Date
- Identification of type of documentation (e.g., evaluation report, progress report/note)
- Occupational therapy practitioner's signature with a minimum of first name or initial, last name, and professional designation
- When applicable, signature of the recorder directly after the documentation entry. If additional information is needed, a signed addendum must be added to the record.
- Cosignature of an occupational therapist or occupational therapy assistant on student documentation, as required by payer policy, governing laws and regulations, and/or employer
- Compliance with all laws, regulations, payer, and employer requirements
- Acceptable terminology defined within the boundaries of setting
- Abbreviations usage as acceptable within the boundaries of setting
- All errors noted and signed
- Adherence to professional standards of technology, when used to document occupational therapy services with electronic claims or records.
- Disposal of records (electronic and traditionally written) within law or agency requirements
- Compliance with confidentiality standards
- Compliance with agency or legal requirements of storage of records
- Documentation should reflect professional clinical reasoning and expertise of an occupational therapy practitioner and the nature of occupational therapy services delivered in a safe and effective manner. The client's diagnosis or prognosis should not be the sole rationale for occupational therapy services.

References

American Medical Association. (2010). *Current procedural terminology.* Chicago: Author.

American Occupational Therapy Association. (2006). Policy 1.41. Categories of occupational therapy personnel. In *Policy manual* (2011 ed.). Bethesda, MD: Author.

American Occupational Therapy Association. (2008). Occupational therapy practice framework: Domain and process (2nd ed.). *American Journal of Occupational Therapy, 62,* 625–683. http://dx.doi.org/10.5014/ajot.62.6.625

American Occupational Therapy Association. (2009). Guidelines for supervision, roles, and responsibilities during the delivery of occupational therapy services. *American Journal of Occupational Therapy, 63,* 797–803. http://dx.doi.org/10.5014/ajot.63.6.797

American Occupational Therapy Association. (2010). Standards of practice for occupational therapy. *American Journal of Occupational Therapy, 64*(Suppl.), S106–S111. http://dx.doi.org/10.5014/ajot.2010.64S106

Hinojosa, J., Kramer, P., & Crist, P. (2010). *Evaluation: Obtaining and interpreting data* (3rd ed.). Bethesda, MD: AOTA Press.

Authors

Gloria Frolek Clark, MS, OTR/L, FAOTA
Mary Jane Youngstrom, MS, OTR/L, FAOTA

for

The Commission on Practice
Sara Jane Brayman, PhD, OTR/L, FAOTA, *Chairperson*

Adopted by the Representative Assembly 2003M16

Edited by the Commission on Practice 2007

Edited by the Commission on Practice 2012
Debbie Amini, EdD, OTR/L, CHT, *Chairperson*

Adopted by the Representative Assembly Coordinating Council (RACC) for the Representative Assembly, 2012

Note. This revision replaces the 2007 document previously published and copyrighted 2008, by the American Occupational Therapy Association in the *American Journal of Occupational Therapy, 62,* 684–690.

To be published and copyrighted in 2013 by the American Occupational Therapy Association in the *American Journal of Occupational Therapy, 67*(Suppl.).

Guidelines for Supervision, Roles, and Responsibilities During the Delivery of Occupational Therapy Services

This document contains four sections that direct the delivery of occupational therapy services. These sections are General Supervision, Supervision of Occupational Therapists and Occupational Therapy Assistants, Roles and Responsibilities of Occupational Therapists and Occupational Therapy Assistants During the Delivery of Occupational Therapy Services, and Supervision of Occupational Therapy Aides.

General Supervision

These guidelines provide a definition of supervision and outline parameters regarding effective supervision as it relates to the delivery of occupational therapy services. These supervision guidelines are to assist in the appropriate and effective provision of occupational therapy services. The guidelines themselves cannot be interpreted to constitute a standard of supervision in any particular locality. Occupational therapists, occupational therapy assistants, and occupational therapy aides are expected to meet applicable state and federal regulations, adhere to relevant workplace policies and the *Occupational Therapy Code of Ethics* (AOTA, 2005) and participate in ongoing professional development activities to maintain continuing competency.

In these guidelines, *supervision* is viewed as a cooperative process in which two or more people participate in a joint effort to establish, maintain, and or elevate a level of competence and performance. Supervision is based on mutual understanding between the supervisor and the supervisee about each other's competence, experience, education, and credentials. It fosters growth and development, promotes effective utilization of resources, encourages creativity and innovation, and provides education and support to achieve a goal (AOTA, 2004). Within the scope of occupational therapy practice, supervision is a process aimed at ensuring the safe and effective delivery of occupational therapy services and fostering professional competence and development.

Supervision of Occupational Therapists and Occupational Therapy Assistants

Occupational Therapists

Based on their education and training, occupational therapists, after initial certification, are autonomous practitioners who are able to deliver occupational therapy services independently. Occupational therapists are responsible for all aspects of occupational therapy service delivery and are accountable for the safety and effectiveness of the occupational therapy service delivery process. Occupational therapists are encouraged to seek supervision and mentoring to develop best practice approaches and promote professional growth.

Occupational Therapy Assistants

Based on their education and training, occupational therapy assistants must receive supervision from an occupational therapist to deliver occupational therapy services. Occupational therapy assistants deliver occupational therapy services under the supervision of and in partnership with occupational therapists. Occupational therapists and occupational therapy assistants are responsible for collaboratively developing a plan for supervision.

General Principles

1. Supervision involves guidance and oversight related to the delivery of occupational therapy services and the facilitation of professional growth and competence. It is the responsibility of occupational therapists and occupational therapy assistants to seek the appropriate quality and frequency of supervision to ensure safe and effective occupational therapy service delivery.

2. To ensure safe and effective occupational therapy services, it is the responsibility of occupational therapists and occupational therapy assistants to recognize when supervision is needed and to seek supervision that supports current and advancing levels of competence.

3. The specific frequency, methods, and content of supervision may vary by practice setting and are dependent on the

   a. Complexity of client needs,

   b. Number and diversity of clients,

   c. Skills of the occupational therapist and the occupational therapy assistant,

   d. Type of practice setting,

   e. Requirements of the practice setting, and

   f. Other regulatory requirements.

4. Supervision that is more frequent than the minimum level required by the practice setting or regulatory agencies may be necessary when

   a. The needs of the client and the occupational therapy process are complex and changing,

   b. The practice setting provides occupational therapy services to a large number of clients with diverse needs, or

   c. The occupational therapist and occupational therapy assistant determine that additional supervision is necessary to ensure safe and effective delivery of occupational therapy services.

5. A variety of types and methods of supervision should be used. Methods may include direct, face-to-face contact and indirect contact. Examples of methods or types of supervision that involve direct face-to-face contact include observation, modeling, co-treatment, discussions, teaching, and instruction. Examples of methods or types of supervision that involve indirect contact include phone conversations, written correspondence, and electronic exchanges.

6. Occupational therapists and occupational therapy assistants must abide by agency and state requirements regarding the documentation of a supervision plan and supervision contacts. Documentation may include the

   a. Frequency of supervisory contact,

   b. Method(s) or type(s) of supervision,

   c. Content areas addressed,

   d. Evidence to support areas and levels of competency, and

   e. Names and credentials of the persons participating in the supervisory process.

7. Supervision related to professional growth, such as leadership and advocacy development, may differ from that needed to provide occupational therapy services. The person providing this supervision, as

well as the frequency, method, and content of supervision, should be responsive to the supervisee's advancing levels of professional growth.

Supervision Outside the Delivery of Occupational Therapy Services

The education and expertise of occupational therapists and occupational therapy assistants prepare them for employment in arenas other than those related to the delivery of occupational therapy. In these other arenas, supervision may be provided by non–occupational therapy professionals.

1. The guidelines of the setting, regulatory agencies, and funding agencies direct the supervision requirements.

2. The occupational therapist and occupational therapy assistant should obtain and use credentials or job titles commensurate with their roles in these other employment arenas.

3. The following are used to determine whether the services provided are related to the delivery of occupational therapy:

   a. State practice acts;

   b. Regulatory agency standards and rules;

   c. Domain of occupational therapy practice; and

   d. Written and verbal agreement among the occupational therapist, the occupational therapy assistant, the client, and the agency or payer about the services provided.

Roles and Responsibilities of Occupational Therapists and Occupational Therapy Assistants During the Delivery of Occupational Therapy Services

General Statement

The focus of occupational therapy is to support the client's "health and participation in life through engagement in occupation" (AOTA, 2008, p. 626). Occupational therapy addresses the needs and goals of the client related to engaging in areas of occupation and considers the performance skills, performance patterns, context and environment, activity demands, and client factors that may influence performance in various areas of occupation.

1. The occupational therapist is responsible for all aspects of occupational therapy service delivery and is accountable for the safety and effectiveness of the occupational therapy service delivery process. The occupational therapy service delivery process involves evaluation, intervention planning, intervention implementation, intervention review, and outcome evaluation.

2. The occupational therapist must be directly involved in the delivery of services during the initial evaluation and regularly throughout the course of intervention and outcome evaluation.

3. The occupational therapy assistant delivers occupational therapy services under the supervision of and in partnership with the occupational therapist.

4. It is the responsibility of the occupational therapist to determine when to delegate responsibilities to an occupational therapy assistant. It is the responsibility of the occupational therapy assistant who performs the delegated responsibilities to demonstrate service competency.

5. The occupational therapist and the occupational therapy assistant demonstrate and document service competency for clinical reasoning and judgment during the service delivery process as well as for the performance of specific techniques, assessments, and intervention methods used.

6. When delegating aspects of occupational therapy services, the occupational therapist considers the following factors:

   a. Complexity of the client's condition and needs;

   b. Knowledge, skill, and competence of the occupational therapy practitioner;

   c. Nature and complexity of the intervention; and

   d. Needs and requirements of the practice setting.

Roles and Responsibilities

Regardless of the setting in which occupational therapy services are delivered, occupational therapists and occupational therapy assistants assume the following generic responsibilities during evaluation, intervention, and outcomes evaluation.

Evaluation

1. The occupational therapist directs the evaluation process.

2. The occupational therapist is responsible for directing all aspects of the initial contact during the occupational therapy evaluation, including

   a. Determining the need for service,

   b. Defining the problems within the domain of occupational therapy that need to be addressed,

   c. Determining the client's goals and priorities,

   d. Establishing intervention priorities,

   e. Determining specific further assessment needs, and

   f. Determining specific assessment tasks that can be delegated to the occupational therapy assistant.

3. The occupational therapist initiates and directs the evaluation, interprets the data, and develops the intervention plan.

4. The occupational therapy assistant contributes to the evaluation process by implementing delegated assessments and by providing verbal and written reports of observations and client capacities to the occupational therapist.

5. The occupational therapist interprets the information provided by the occupational therapy assistant and integrates that information into the evaluation and decision-making process.

Intervention Planning

1. The occupational therapist has overall responsibility for the development of the occupational therapy intervention plan.

2. The occupational therapist and the occupational therapy assistant collaborate with the client to develop the plan.

3. The occupational therapy assistant is responsible for being knowledgeable about evaluation results and for providing input into the intervention plan, based on client needs and priorities.

Intervention Implementation

1. The occupational therapist has overall responsibility for implementing the intervention.

2. When delegating aspects of the occupational therapy intervention to the occupational therapy assistant, the occupational therapist is responsible for providing appropriate supervision.

3. The occupational therapy assistant is responsible for being knowledgeable about the client's occupational therapy goals.

4. The occupational therapy assistant selects, implements, and makes modifications to therapeutic activities and interventions that are consistent with demonstrated competency levels, client goals, and the requirements of the practice setting.

Intervention Review

1. The occupational therapist is responsible for determining the need for continuing, modifying, or discontinuing occupational therapy services.

2. The occupational therapy assistant contributes to this process by exchanging information with and providing documentation to the occupational therapist about the client's responses to and communications during intervention.

Outcome Evaluation

1. The occupational therapist is responsible for selecting, measuring, and interpreting outcomes that are related to the client's ability to engage in occupations.

2. The occupational therapy assistant is responsible for being knowledgeable about the client's targeted occupational therapy outcomes and for providing information and documentation related to outcome achievement.

3. The occupational therapy assistant may implement outcome measurements and provide needed client discharge resources.

Supervision of Occupational Therapy Aides[1]

An *aide*, as used in occupational therapy practice, is an individual who provides supportive services to the occupational therapist and the occupational therapy assistant. Aides do not provide skilled occupational therapy services. An aide is trained by an occupational therapist or an occupational therapy assistant to perform specifically delegated tasks. The occupational therapist is responsible for the overall use and actions of the aide. An aide first must demonstrate competency to be able to perform the assigned, delegated client and non-client tasks.

1. The occupational therapist must oversee the development, documentation, and implementation of a plan to supervise and routinely assess the ability of the occupational therapy aide to carry out non-client- and client-related tasks. The occupational therapy assistant may contribute to the development and documentation of this plan.

2. The occupational therapy assistant can supervise the aide.

3. Non-client-related tasks include clerical and maintenance activities and preparation of the work area or equipment.

4. Client-related tasks are routine tasks during which the aide may interact with the client. The following factors must be present when an occupational therapist or occupational therapy assistant delegates a selected client-related task to the aide:

---

[1]Depending on the setting in which service is provided; aides may be referred to by various names. Examples include, but are not limited to, *rehabilitation aides, restorative aides, extenders, paraprofessionals,* and *rehab techs* (AOTA, 2004).

    a. The outcome anticipated for the delegated task is predictable.

    b. The situation of the client and the environment is stable and will not require that judgment, interpretations, or adaptations be made by the aide.

    c. The client has demonstrated some previous performance ability in executing the task.

    d. The task routine and process have been clearly established.

5. When performing delegated client-related tasks, the supervisor must ensure that the aide

    a. Is trained and able to demonstrate competency in carrying out the selected task and using equipment, if appropriate;

    b. Has been instructed on how to specifically carry out the delegated task with the specific client; and

    c. Knows the precautions, signs, and symptoms for the particular client that would indicate the need to seek assistance from the occupational therapist or occupational therapy assistant.

6. The supervision of the aide needs to be documented. Documentation includes information about frequency and methods of supervision used the content of supervision and the names and credentials of all persons participating in the supervisory process.

Summary

These guidelines about supervision, roles, and responsibilities are to assist in the appropriate utilization of occupational therapists, occupational therapy assistants, and occupational therapy aides and in the appropriate and effective provision of occupational therapy services. It is expected that occupational therapy services are delivered in accordance with applicable state and federal regulations, relevant workplace policies, the *Occupational Therapy Code of Ethics* (AOTA, 2005), and continuing competency and professional development guidelines.

References

American Occupational Therapy Association. (2004). Guidelines for supervision, roles, and responsibilities during the delivery of occupational therapy services. *American Journal of Occupational Therapy, 58,* 663–667.

American Occupational Therapy Association. (2005). Occupational therapy code of ethics (2005). *American Journal of Occupational Therapy, 59,* 639–642.

American Occupational Therapy Association. (2008). Occupational therapy practice framework: Domain and process (2nd ed.). *American Journal of Occupational Therapy, 62,* 625–683.

Additional Reading

American Occupational Therapy Association. (2005). Standards of practice for occupational therapy. *American Journal of Occupational Therapy, 59,* 663–665.

Authors
Sara Jane Brayman, PhD, OTR/L, FAOTA, *Chairperson, 2002–2005*
Gloria Frolek Clark, MS, OTR/L, FAOTA
Janet V. DeLany, DEd, OTR/L
Eileen R. Garza, PhD, OTR, ATP
Mary V. Radomski, MA, OTR/L, FAOTA
Ruth Ramsey, MS, OTR/L
Carol Siebert, MS, OTR/L

Kristi Voelkerding, BS, COTA/L

Patricia D. LaVesser, PhD, OTR/L, *SIS Liaison*

Lenna Aird, *ASD Liaison*

Deborah Lieberman, MHSA, OTR/L, FAOTA, *AOTA Headquarters Liaison*

for

The Commission on Practice

Sara Jane Brayman, PhD, OTR/L, FAOTA, *Chairperson*

Adopted by the Representative Assembly 2004C24

Edited by the Commission on Practice 2009

This replaces the 2004 document *Guidelines for Supervision, Roles, and Responsibilities During the Delivery of Occupational Therapy Services* (previously published and copyrighted in 2004 in the *American Journal of Occupational Therapy, 58,* 663–667).

Guidelines for Re-Entry Into the Field of Occupational Therapy

Purpose of the Guidelines

These guidelines are designed to assist occupational therapists and occupational therapy assistants who have left the field of occupational therapy for an extended period of time and have chosen to return to the profession and deliver occupational therapy services. The guidelines represent minimum recommendations only and are designed to support practitioners in meeting their ethical obligations to "take responsibility for maintaining high standards and continuing competence in practice, education and research" (American Occupational Therapy Association [AOTA], 2010a, 2010b).

It is expected that practitioners will identify and meet requirements outlined in applicable state and federal regulations, relevant workplace policies, the *Occupational Therapy Code of Ethics and Ethics Standards (2010)* (AOTA, 2010a), and continuing competence and professional development guidelines prior to re-entering the field.

Clarification of Terms

Re-Entry—For the purpose of this document, re-entering occupational therapists and occupational therapy assistants are individuals who

- Have practiced in the field for a minimum of 1 year (individuals who have practiced for less than 1 year are considered entry-level); and

- Have not engaged in the practice of occupational therapy (may include direct intervention, supervision, teaching, consultation, administration, case or care management, community programming, or research) for a minimum of 18 months; and

- Wish to return to the profession in the capacity of delivering occupational therapy services to clients.

Formal Learning—Refers to any learning that has established goals and objectives that are measureable. This may include activities such as

- Attending workshops, seminars, lectures, and professional conferences

- Auditing or participating in formal academic coursework

- Participating in external self-study series (e.g., AOTA Self-Paced Clinical Course)

- Participating in independent distance learning (asynchronous) continuing education (CE) (e.g., CE articles, video, audio, or online courses) with established goals and objectives that are measurable

- Participating in interactive distance learning (synchronous) CE with established goals and objectives that are measurable.

Supervised Service Delivery—For this document, refers to provision of occupational therapy services under the supervision of a qualified occupational therapist. *Supervision* is "a cooperative process in which two or more people participate in a joint effort to establish, maintain, and or elevate a level of competence and performance…. Within the scope of occupational therapy practice, supervision is a process aimed at ensuring the safe and effective delivery of occupational therapy services and fostering professional competence and development" (AOTA, 2009, p. 797).

Specific Guidelines for Re-Entry

1. Engage in a formalized process of self-assessment (e.g., self-assessment tools, such as using AOTA's [2003] *Professional Development Tool*), and complete a professional development plan that addresses the *Standards for Continuing Competence* (AOTA, 2010b).

2. Attend a minimum of 10 hours of formal learning related to occupational therapy service delivery for each year out of practice, at least 20 of which must have occurred within the past 24 months of re-entry.

3. Attain relevant updates to core knowledge of the profession of occupational therapy and the responsibilities of occupational therapy practitioners that are consistent with material found in AOTA official documents such as the *Occupational Therapy Practice Framework* (AOTA, 2008), *Occupational Therapy Code of Ethics and Ethics Standards (2010)* (AOTA, 2010a), *Standards for Continuing Competence* (AOTA, 2010b), *Standards of Practice* (AOTA, 2010c), and *Guidelines for Supervision, Roles, and Responsibilities during the Delivery of Occupational Therapy Services* (AOTA, 2009).

4. *For practitioners who have been out of practice more than 3 years:* Within the parameters present in a practitioner's workplace setting and applicable state regulations, complete a minimum of 30 hours of documented supervised practice in occupational therapy within the 12 months prior to anticipated reentry or within 30 days of employment as a practitioner delivering occupational therapy services.

    a. The re-entering practitioner, in conjunction with the supervising occupational therapy practitioners, should establish specific goals and objectives for the 30 hours. Goals, objectives, and related assessment of performance may be developed or adapted from a variety of sources, including competency and performance review resources existing within the setting, as well as AOTA resources such as the *Fieldwork Performance Evaluation for the Occupational Therapy Student©* forms (AOTA, 2002a, 2002b).

    b. The supervised practice experience should focus on the area of practice to which the practitioner intends to return.

    c. Supervised practice should occur with a practitioner at the same or greater professional level.

    d. Supervision should be direct face-to-face contact, which may include observation, modeling, co-treatment, discussions, teaching, and instruction (AOTA, 2009), and may be augmented by indirect methods such as telephone and e-mail communications.

Ongoing Continuing Competence

Once practitioners have successfully returned to the delivery of occupational therapy services, they are encouraged to engage in activities that support them in their ongoing continuing competence, such as

*   Seeking mentoring, consultation, or supervision—especially during the first year of return to practice.

*   Engaging in relevant AOTA Special Interest Section forums to build a professional network and facilitate opportunities for practice guidance.

- Exploring relevant AOTA Board and Specialty Certifications, and use the identified competencies and criteria as a blueprint for ongoing professional development.

- Joining and becoming active in both AOTA and state occupational therapy association to stay informed of practice trends and increase opportunities for networking.

References and Resources

American Occupational Therapy Association. (2002a). *Fieldwork performance evaluation for the occupational therapy assistant student*. Bethesda, MD: AOTA Press.

American Occupational Therapy Association. (2002b). *Fieldwork performance evaluation for the occupational therapy student*. Bethesda, MD: AOTA Press.

American Occupational Therapy Association. (2003). *Professional development tool*. Retrieved January 12, 2010, from http://www.aota.org/pdt

American Occupational Therapy Association. (2008). Occupational therapy practice framework: Domain and process (2nd ed.). *American Journal of Occupational Therapy, 62*, 625–683. http://dx.doi.org/10.5014/ajot.62.6.625

American Occupational Therapy Association. (2009). Guidelines for supervision, roles, and responsibilities during the delivery of occupational therapy services. *American Journal of Occupational Therapy, 63*, 797–803. http://dx.doi.org/10.5014/ajot.63.6.797

American Occupational Therapy Association. (2010a). Occupational therapy code of ethics and ethics standards (2010). *American Journal of Occupational Therapy, 64*(Suppl.), S17–S26. http://dx.doi.org/10.5014/ajot.2010.64S17

American Occupational Therapy Association. (2010b). Standards for continuing competence. *American Journal of Occupational Therapy, 64*(Suppl.), S103–S105. http://dx.doi.org/10.5014/ajot.2010.64S103

American Occupational Therapy Association. (2010c). Standards of practice for occupational therapy. *American Journal of Occupational Therapy, 64*(Suppl.), S106–S111. http://dx.doi.org/10.5014/ajot.2010.64S106

Authors

Jan Davis, MS, OTR/L, *Chair*
Gloria Frolek Clark, MS, OTR/L, BCP, FAOTA
Mary Kay Currie, OT, BCPR
Nancy Richman, OTR, FAOTA
Pamela Roberts, PhD, OTR/L, SCFES, CPHQ, FAOTA
Barbara A. Schell, PhD, OT, FAOTA
Winifred Schultz-Krohn, PhD, OTR/L, BCP, FAOTA
Carol Siebert, MS, OTR/L, FAOTA
Maria Elena E. Louch, OT, *AOTA Staff Liaison*

for

The Commission on Continuing Competence and Professional Development
Barbara A. Schell, PhD, OT, FAOTA, *Chairperson*

Adopted by the Representative Assembly 2010CApr11

OCCUPATIONAL THERAPY PRACTICE
FRAMEWORK:
Domain & Process
2nd Edition

Contents

INTRODUCTION

The *Occupational Therapy Practice Framework: Domain and Process, 2nd Edition* (*Framework–II*) is an official document of the American Occupational Therapy Association (AOTA). Intended for internal and external audiences, it presents a summary of interrelated constructs that define and guide **occupational therapy**[1] practice. The *Framework* was developed to articulate occupational therapy's contribution to promoting the **health** and **participation** of people, organizations, and populations through **engagement** in **occupation.** It is not a taxonomy, theory, or model of occupational therapy and therefore must be used in conjunction with the knowledge and evidence relevant to occupation and occupational therapy. The revisions included in this second edition are intended to refine the document and include language and concepts relevant to current and emerging occupational therapy practice.

Implicit within this summary are the profession's core beliefs in the positive relationship between occupation and health and its view of people as occupational beings. "All people need to be able or enabled to engage in the occupations of their need and choice, to grow through what they do, and to experience **independence** or **interdependence,** equality, participation, security, health, and well-being" (Wilcock & Townsend, 2008, p. 198). With this aim, occupational therapy is provided to **clients,** the entity that receives occupational therapy services. Clients may be categorized as

- **Persons,** including families, caregivers, teachers, employers, and relevant others;
- **Organizations,** such as businesses, industries, or agencies; and
- **Populations** within a community, such as refugees, veterans who are homeless, and people with chronic health disabling conditions (Moyers & Dale, 2007).

The *Framework* is divided into two major sections: (1) the ***domain,*** which outlines the profession's purview and the areas in which its mem-

---

[1]Many of the terms that appear in **bold** are defined in the glossary.

"The *Framework* was developed to articulate occupational therapy's contribution to promoting the health and participation of people, organizations, and populations through engagement in occupation."

bers have an established body of knowledge and expertise (see Figure 1), and (2) the dynamic occupation and client-centered *process* used in the delivery of occupational therapy services (see Figure 2). The domain and process of occupational therapy direct occupational therapy practitioners[2] to focus on performance of occupations that results from the dynamic intersection of the client, the context and environment, and the client's occupations (Christiansen & Baum, 1997; Christiansen, Baum, & Bass-Hagen, 2005; Law, Baum, & Dunn, 2005). Although the domain and process are described separately, in actuality, they are inextricably linked in a transactional relationship (see Figure 3).

Numerous resource materials, including an appendix, a glossary, references, and a bibliography, are supplied at the end of the document. Although the *Framework* includes a glossary of defined terms, it does not contain an exhaustive or uniform list of terms used in the profession nor all

of the definitions of these terms discussed in the literature.

Domain of Occupational Therapy
Overview

This edition of the *Framework* begins with a description of the occupational therapy profession's domain. The overarching statement—**supporting health and participation in life through engagement in occupation**—describes the domain in its fullest sense. Within this diverse profession, the defining contribution of occupational therapy is the application of core values, knowledge, and skills to assist clients (people, organizations, and populations) to engage in everyday activities or occupations that they want and need to do in a manner that supports health and participation. Figure 4 identifies the aspects of the domain and illustrates the dynamic interrelatedness among them. All aspects of the domain are of equal value, and together they interact to influence the client's engagement in occupations, participation, and health.

Occupational therapists are educated to evaluate aspects of the occupational therapy domain and their **transactional** relationships. Occupational therapists and occupational therapy assistants are educated about the aspects of the occupational therapy domain and apply this knowledge to the intervention process as they work to support the health and participation of their clients. Occupational therapists are responsible for all aspects of occupational therapy service delivery and are accountable for the safety and effectiveness of that service delivery process. Occupational therapy assistants deliver occupational therapy service under the supervision of and in collaboration with an occupational therapist (AOTA, 2004b).

---

[2]When the term *occupational therapy practitioner* is used in this document, it refers to occupational therapists and occupational therapy assistants (AOTA, 2006).

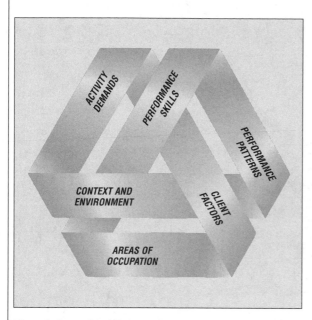

Figure 1. Occupational Therapy's Domain.
Supporting health and participation in life through engagement in occupation.

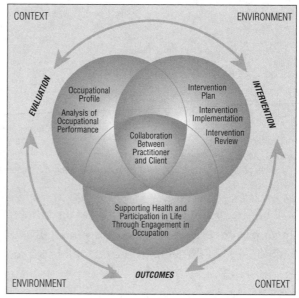

Figure 2. Occupational Therapy's Process.
Collaboration between the practitioner and the client is central to the interactive nature of service delivery.

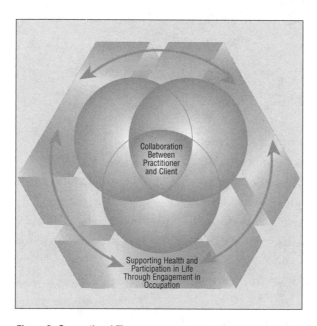

Figure 3. Occupational Therapy.
The domain and process are inextricably linked.

Note: Mobius in figures 1 and 3 originally designed by Mark Dow. Used with permission.

AREAS OF OCCUPATION	CLIENT FACTORS	PERFORMANCE SKILLS	PERFORMANCE PATTERNS	CONTEXT AND ENVIRONMENT	ACTIVITY DEMANDS
Activities of Daily Living (ADL)* Instrumental Activities of Daily Living (IADL) Rest and Sleep Education Work Play Leisure Social Participation *Also referred to as *basic activities of daily living (BADL)* or *personal activities of daily living (PADL).*	Values, Beliefs, and Spirituality Body Functions Body Structures	Sensory Perceptual Skills Motor and Praxis Skills Emotional Regulation Skills Cognitive Skills Communication and Social Skills	Habits Routines Roles Rituals	Cultural Personal Physical Social Temporal Virtual	Objects Used and Their Properties Space Demands Social Demands Sequencing and Timing Required Actions Required Body Functions Required Body Structures

Figure 4. Aspects of Occupational Therapy's Domain.
All aspects of the domain transact to support engagement, participation, and health. This figure does not imply a hierarchy.

The discussion that follows provides a brief explanation of each aspect identified in Figure 4. Tables included throughout provide full lists and definitions of terms.

Supporting Health and Participation in Life Through Engagement in Occupation

The profession of occupational therapy uses the term *occupation* to capture the breadth and meaning of "everyday **activity.**" Occupational therapy is founded on an understanding that engaging in occupations structures everyday life and contributes to health and well-being. Occupational therapy practitioners believe that occupations are multidimensional and complex. Engagement in occupation as the focus of occupational therapy intervention involves addressing both subjective (emotional and psychological) and objective (physically observable) aspects of performance. Occupational therapy practitioners understand engagement from this dual and holistic perspective and address all aspects of performance when providing interventions.

Occupational science, a discipline devoted to the study of occupation, informs occupational therapy practice by expanding the understanding of occupation (Zemke & Clark, 1996). Occupations are central to a client's (person, organization, or pop-

> "All aspects of the domain are of equal value, and together they interact to influence the client's engagement in occupations, participation, and health."

ulation) identity and sense of competence and have particular meaning and value to the client. They influence how clients spend time making decisions. Several definitions of occupation can be found in the literature that adds to an understanding of this core concept. *Occupation* has been defined as

- "Goal-directed pursuits that typically extend over time, have meaning to the performance, and involve multiple tasks" (Christiansen et al., 2005, p. 548).
- "Daily activities that reflect cultural values, provide structure to living, and meaning to

individuals; these activities meet human needs for self-care, enjoyment, and participation in society" (Crepeau, Cohn, & Schell, 2003, p. 1031).

- "Activities that people engage in throughout their daily lives to fulfill their time and give life meaning. Occupations involve mental abilities and skills and may or may not have an observable physical dimension" (Hinojosa & Kramer, 1997, p. 865).
- "[A]ctivities…of everyday life, named, organized, and given value and meaning by individuals and a culture. Occupation is everything people do to occupy themselves, including looking after themselves…enjoying life…and contributing to the social and economic fabric of their communities" (Law, Polatajko, Baptiste, & Townsend, 1997, p. 32).
- "A dynamic relationship among an occupational form, a person with a unique developmental structure, subjective meanings and purpose, and the resulting occupational performance" (Nelson & Jepson-Thomas, 2003, p. 90).
- "[C]hunks of daily activity that can be named in the lexicon of the culture" (Zemke & Clark, 1996, p. vii).

Sometimes occupational therapy practitioners use the terms *occupation* and *activity* interchangeably to describe participation in daily life pursuits. Some scholars have proposed that the two terms are different (Christiansen & Townsend, 2004; Hinojosa & Kramer, 1997; Pierce, 2001; Reed, 2005). In the *Framework,* the term occupation encompasses activity.

Occupational engagement occurs individually or with others. A client may be considered independent when the client performs or directs the actions necessary to participate regardless of the amount or kind of assistance desired or required. In contrast with narrower definitions of indepen-

dence, occupational therapy practitioners consider a client as independent whether the client solely performs the activities, performs the activities in an adapted or modified environment, makes use of various devices or alternative strategies, or oversees activity completion by others (AOTA, 2002a). For example, people with a spinal cord injury can direct a personal care assistant to assist them with their activities of daily living (ADLs), demonstrating independence in this essential aspect of their lives.

Occupations often are shared. Those that implicitly involve two or more individuals may be termed *co-occupations* (Zemke & Clark, 1996). Care giving is a co-occupation that involves active participation on the part of the caregiver and the recipient of care. For example, the co-occupations required during mothering, such as the socially interactive routines of eating, feeding, and comforting, may involve the parent, a partner, the child, and significant others (Olsen, 2004). The activities intrinsic to this social interaction are reciprocal, interactive, and nested "co-occupations" (Dunlea, 1996; Esdaile & Olson, 2004). Clients also may perform several occupations simultaneously, enfolding them into one another such as when a caregiver concurrently helps with homework, pays the bills, and makes dinner. Consideration of co-occupation supports an integrated view of the client's engagement in relationship to significant others within context.

Occupational therapy practitioners recognize that health is supported and maintained when clients are able to engage in occupations and activities that allow desired or needed participation in home, school, workplace, and community life. Thus, occupational therapy practitioners are concerned not only with occupations but also the complexity of factors that empower and make possible clients' engagement and participation in positive health-promoting occupations (Wilcock &

Townsend, 2008). In 2003, Townsend applied the concept of **social justice** to occupational therapy's focus and coined the term ***occupational justice*** to describe the profession's concern with ethical, moral, and civic factors that can support or hinder health-promoting engagement in occupations and participation in home and community life. *Occupational justice* ensures that clients are afforded the opportunity for full participation in those occupations in which they choose to engage (Christiansen & Townsend, 2004, p. 278). Occupational therapy practitioners interested in occupational justice recognize and work to support social policies, actions, and laws that allow people to engage in occupations that provide purpose and meaning in their lives.

Occupational therapy's focus on engaging in occupations and occupational justice complements the World Health Organization's (WHO) perspective of health. WHO, in its effort to broaden the understanding of the effects of disease and disability on health, has recognized that health can be affected by the inability to carry out activities and participate in life situations caused by environmental barriers, as well as by problems that exist with body structures and body functions (WHO, 2001). As members of a global community, occupational therapy practitioners advocate for the well-being of all persons, groups, and populations with a commitment to inclusion and nondiscrimination (AOTA, 2004c).

Areas of Occupation

When occupational therapy practitioners work with clients, they consider the many types of occupations in which clients might engage. The broad range of activities or occupations are sorted into categories called "**areas of occupation**"—*activities of daily living, instrumental activities of daily living, rest and sleep, education, work, play, leisure, and social participation* (see Table 1).

Individual differences in the way in which clients view their occupations reflect the complexity and multidimensionality of each occupation. The client's perspective of how an occupation is categorized varies depending on that client's needs and interests. For example, one person may perceive doing laundry as work, while another may consider it an instrumental activity of daily living (IADL). One population may engage in a quiz game and view their participation as play, while another population may engage in the same quiz game and view it as an educational occupation.

The way in which clients prioritize engagement in areas of occupation may vary at different times. For example, a community psychiatric rehabilitation organization may prioritize member voter registration during a presidential campaign and celebration preparations during holiday periods. The extent and nature of the engagement is as important as the engagement itself; for example, excessive work without sufficient regard to other aspects of life such as sleep or relationships places clients at risk for health problems (Hakansson, Dahlin-Ivanoff, & Sonn, 2006).

Client Factors

Client factors are specific abilities, characteristics, or beliefs that reside within the client and may affect performance in areas of occupation. Because occupational therapy practitioners view clients holistically, they consider client factors that involve the values, beliefs, and spirituality; body functions; and body structures. These underlying client factors are affected by the presence or absence of illness, disease, deprivation, and disability. They affect and are affected by performance skills, performance patterns, activity demands, and contextual and environmental factors.

Despite their importance, the presence or absence of specific body functions and body

TABLE 1. AREAS OF OCCUPATION
Various kinds of life activities in which people, populations, or organizations engage, including ADL, IADL, rest and sleep, education, work, play, leisure, and social participation.

■ ACTIVITIES OF DAILY LIVING (ADLs)

Activities that are oriented toward taking care of one's own body (adapted from Rogers & Holm, 1994, pp. 181–202). ADL also is referred to as *basic activities of daily living (BADLs)* and *personal activities of daily living (PADLs)*. These activities are "fundamental to living in a social world; they enable basic survival and well-being" (Christiansen & Hammecker, 2001, p. 156).

- **Bathing, showering**—Obtaining and using supplies; soaping, rinsing, and drying body parts; maintaining bathing position; and transferring to and from bathing positions.
- **Bowel and bladder management**—Includes completing intentional control of bowel movements and urinary bladder and, if necessary, using equipment or agents for bladder control (Uniform Data System for Medical Rehabilitation, 1996, pp. III–20, III–24).
- **Dressing**—Selecting clothing and accessories appropriate to time of day, weather, and occasion; obtaining clothing from storage area; dressing and undressing in a sequential fashion; fastening and adjusting clothing and shoes; and applying and removing personal devices, prostheses, or orthoses.
- **Eating**—"The ability to keep and manipulate food or fluid in the mouth and swallow it; *eating* and *swallowing* are often used interchangeably" (AOTA, 2007b).
- **Feeding**—"The process of setting up, arranging, and bringing food [or fluid] from the plate or cup to the mouth; sometimes called *self-feeding*" (AOTA, 2007b).
- **Functional mobility**—Moving from one position or place to another (during performance of everyday activities), such as in-bed mobility, wheelchair mobility, and transfers (e.g., wheelchair, bed, car, tub, toilet, tub/shower, chair, floor). Includes functional ambulation and transporting objects.
- **Personal device care**—Using, cleaning, and maintaining personal care items, such as hearing aids, contact lenses, glasses, orthotics, prosthetics, adaptive equipment, and contraceptive and sexual devices.
- **Personal hygiene and grooming**—Obtaining and using supplies; removing body hair (e.g., use of razors, tweezers, lotions); applying and removing cosmetics; washing, drying, combing, styling, brushing, and trimming hair; caring for nails (hands and feet); caring for skin, ears, eyes, and nose; applying deodorant; cleaning mouth; brushing and flossing teeth; or removing, cleaning, and reinserting dental orthotics and prosthetics.
- **Sexual activity**—Engaging in activities that result in sexual satisfaction.
- **Toilet hygiene**—Obtaining and using supplies; clothing management; maintaining toileting position; transferring to and from toileting position; cleaning body; and caring for menstrual and continence needs (including catheters, colostomies, and suppository management).

■ INSTRUMENTAL ACTIVITIES OF DAILY LIVING (IADLs)

Activities to support daily life within the home and community that often require more complex interactions than self-care used in ADL.

- **Care of others (including selecting and supervising caregivers)**—Arranging, supervising, or providing the care for others.
- **Care of pets**—Arranging, supervising, or providing the care for pets and service animals.
- **Child rearing**—Providing the care and supervision to support the developmental needs of a child.
- **Communication management**—Sending, receiving, and interpreting information using a variety of systems and equipment, including writing tools, telephones, typewriters, audiovisual recorders, computers, communication boards, call lights, emergency systems, Braille writers, telecommunication devices for the deaf, augmentative communication systems, and personal digital assistants.
- **Community mobility**—Moving around in the community and using public or private transportation, such as driving, walking, bicycling, or accessing and riding in buses, taxi cabs, or other transportation systems.
- **Financial management**—Using fiscal resources, including alternate methods of financial transaction and planning and using finances with long-term and short-term goals.
- **Health management and maintenance**—Developing, managing, and maintaining routines for health and wellness promotion, such as physical fitness, nutrition, decreasing health risk behaviors, and medication routines.
- **Home establishment and management**—Obtaining and maintaining personal and household possessions and environment (e.g., home, yard, garden, appliances, vehicles), including maintaining and repairing personal possessions (clothing and household items) and knowing how to seek help or whom to contact.
- **Meal preparation and cleanup**—Planning, preparing, and serving well-balanced, nutritional meals and cleaning up food and utensils after meals.
- **Religious observance**—Participating in *religion,* "an organized system of beliefs, practices, rituals, and symbols designed to facilitate closeness to the sacred or transcendent" (Moreira-Almeida & Koenig, 2006, p. 844).
- **Safety and emergency maintenance**—Knowing and performing preventive procedures to maintain a safe environment as well as recognizing sudden, unexpected hazardous situations and initiating emergency action to reduce the threat to health and safety.
- **Shopping**—Preparing shopping lists (grocery and other); selecting, purchasing, and transporting items; selecting method of payment; and completing money transactions.

(Continued)

TABLE 1. AREAS OF OCCUPATION

(Continued)

■ REST AND SLEEP

Includes activities related to obtaining restorative rest and sleep that supports healthy active engagement in other areas of occupation.

- **Rest**—Quiet and effortless actions that interrupt physical and mental activity resulting in a relaxed state (Nurit & Michel, 2003, p. 227). Includes identifying the need to relax; reducing involvement in taxing physical, mental, or social activities; and engaging in relaxation or other endeavors that restore energy, calm, and renewed interest in engagement.

- **Sleep**—A series of activities resulting in going to sleep, staying asleep, and ensuring health and safety through participation in sleep involving engagement with the physical and social environments.

- **Sleep preparation**—(1) Engaging in routines that prepare the self for a comfortable rest, such as grooming and undressing, reading or listening to music to fall asleep, saying goodnight to others, and meditation or prayers; determining the time of day and length of time desired for sleeping or the time needed to wake; and establishing sleep patterns that support growth and health (patterns are often personally and culturally determined).

  (2) Preparing the physical environment for periods of unconsciousness, such as making the bed or space on which to sleep; ensuring warmth/coolness and protection; setting an alarm clock; securing the home, such as locking doors or closing windows or curtains; and turning off electronics or lights.

- **Sleep participation**—Taking care of personal need for sleep such as cessation of activities to ensure onset of sleep, napping, dreaming, sustaining a sleep state without disruption, and nighttime care of toileting needs or hydration. Negotiating the needs and requirements of others within the social environment. Interacting with those sharing the sleeping space such as children or partners, providing nighttime care giving such as breastfeeding, and monitoring the com-

fort and safety of others such as the family while sleeping.

■ EDUCATION

Includes activities needed for learning and participating in the environment.

- **Formal educational participation**—Including the categories of academic (e.g., math, reading, working on a degree), nonacademic (e.g., recess, lunchroom, hallway), extracurricular (e.g., sports, band, cheerleading, dances), and vocational (prevocational and vocational) participation.

- **Informal personal educational needs or interests exploration (beyond formal education)**—Identifying topics and methods for obtaining topic-related information or skills.

- **Informal personal education participation**—Participating in classes, programs, and activities that provide instruction/training in identified areas of interest.

■ WORK

Includes activities needed for engaging in remunerative employment or volunteer activities (Mosey, 1996, p. 341).

- **Employment interests and pursuits**—Identifying and selecting work opportunities based on assets, limitations, likes, and dislikes relative to work (adapted from Mosey, 1996, p. 342).

- **Employment seeking and acquisition**—Identifying and recruiting for job opportunities; completing, submitting, and reviewing appropriate application materials; preparing for interviews; participating in interviews and following up afterward; discussing job benefits; and finalizing negotiations.

- **Job performance**—Job performance including work skills and patterns; time management; relationships with co-workers, managers, and customers; creation, production, and distribution of products and services; initiation, sustainment, and completion of work; and compliance with work norms and procedures.

- **Retirement preparation and adjustment**—Determining aptitudes, developing interests and skills, and selecting appropriate avocational pursuits.

- **Volunteer exploration**—Determining community causes, organizations, or opportunities for unpaid "work" in relationship to personal skills, interests, location, and time available.

- **Volunteer participation**—Performing unpaid "work" activities for the benefit of identified selected causes, organizations, or facilities.

■ PLAY

"Any spontaneous or organized activity that provides enjoyment, entertainment, amusement, or diversion" (Parham & Fazio, 1997, p. 252).

- **Play exploration**—Identifying appropriate play activities, which can include exploration play, practice play, pretend play, games with rules, constructive play, and symbolic play (adapted from Bergen,1988, pp. 64–65).

- **Play participation**—Participating in play; maintaining a balance of play with other areas of occupation; and obtaining, using, and maintaining toys, equipment, and supplies appropriately.

■ LEISURE

"A nonobligatory activity that is intrinsically motivated and engaged in during discretionary time, that is, time not committed to obligatory occupations such as work, self-care, or sleep" (Parham & Fazio, 1997, p. 250).

- **Leisure exploration**—Identifying interests, skills, opportunities, and appropriate leisure activities.

- **Leisure participation**—Planning and participating in appropriate leisure activities; maintaining a balance of leisure activities with other areas of occupation; and obtaining, using, and maintaining equipment and supplies as appropriate.

TABLE 1. AREAS OF OCCUPATION
(Continued)

■ **SOCIAL PARTICIPATION**

"Organized patterns of behavior that are characteristic and expected of an individual or a given position within a social system" (Mosey, 1996, p. 340).

• **Community**—Engaging in activities that result in successful interaction at the community level (i.e., neighborhood, organizations, work, school).

• **Family**—Engaging in "[activities that result in] successful interaction in specific

required and/or desired familial roles" (Mosey, 1996, p. 340).

• **Peer, friend**—Engaging in activities at different levels of intimacy, including engaging in desired sexual activity.

Note. Some of the terms used in this table are from, or adapted from, the rescinded *Uniform Terminology for Occupational Therapy—Third Edition* (AOTA, 1994, pp. 1047–1054).

---

structures do not necessarily ensure a client's success or difficulty with daily life occupations. Factors that influence performance such as supports in the physical or social environment may allow a client to manifest skills in a given area even when body functions or structure are absent or deficient. It is in the process of observing a client engaging in occupations and activities that the occupational therapy practitioner is able to determine the transaction between client factors and performance.

Client factors are substantively different at the person, organization, and population levels. Following are descriptions of client factors for each level.

Person

• **Values, beliefs, and spirituality** influence a client's motivation to engage in occupations and give his or her life meaning. *Values* are principles, standards, or qualities considered worthwhile by the client who holds them. *Beliefs* are cognitive content held as true (Moyers & Dale, 2007, p. 28). *Spirituality* is "the personal quest for understanding answers to ultimate questions about life, about meaning and about relationship with the sacred or transcendent, which may (or may not) lead to or arise from the development of religious rituals and the formation of community" (Moreira-Almeida & Koenig, 2006, p. 844).

• *Body functions* refer to the "physiological function of body systems (including psychological functions)" (WHO, 2001, p. 10). Examples include sensory, mental (affective, cognitive, perceptual), cardiovascular, respiratory, and endocrine functions (see Table 2 for complete list).

• *Body structures* are the "anatomical parts of the body such as organs, limbs, and their components" (WHO, 2001, p. 10). Body structures and body functions are interrelated (e.g., the heart and blood vessels are body structures that support cardiovascular function; see Table 2).

The categorization of body function and body structure client factors outlined in Table 2 is based on the *International Classification of Functioning, Disability, and Health* proposed by the WHO (2001). The classification was selected because it has received wide exposure and presents a language that is understood by external audiences.

Organization

• *Values and beliefs* include the vision statement, code of ethics, value statements, and esprit de corps.

• *Functions* include planning, organizing, coordinating, and operationalizing the mission, products or services, and productivity.

• *Structures* include departments and departmental relationships, leadership and management, performance measures, and job titles.

Population

- *Values and beliefs* can be viewed as including emotional, purposive, and traditional perspectives (Foucault, 1973).
- *Functions* include economic, political, social, and cultural capital (Weber, 1978).
- *Structure* may include constituents such as those with similar genetics, sexual orientation, and health-related conditions (Baum, Bass-Haugen, & Christiansen, 2005, p. 381).

Activity Demands

Activity demands refer to the specific features of an activity that influence the type and amount of effort required to perform the activity. Occupational therapy practitioners analyze activities to understand what is required of the client and determine the relationship of the activity's requirements to engagement in occupation. Activity demands include the specific objects and their properties used in the activity, the physical space requirements of the activity,

TABLE 2. CLIENT FACTORS

Client factors include (1) values, beliefs, and spirituality; (2) body functions; and (3) body structures that reside within the client and may affect performance in areas of occupation.

▓ VALUES, BELIEFS, AND SPIRITUALITY

Category and Definition	Examples
Values: Principles, standards, or qualities considered worthwhile or desirable by the client who holds them.	**Person** 1. Honesty with self and with others 2. Personal religious convictions 3. Commitment to family. **Organization** 1. Obligation to serve the community 2. Fairness. **Population** 1. Freedom of speech 2. Equal opportunities for all 3. Tolerance toward others.
Beliefs: Cognitive content held as true.	**Person** 1. He or she is powerless to influence others 2. Hard work pays off. **Organization** 1. Profits are more important than people 2. Achieving the mission of providing service can effect positive change in the world. **Population** 1. People can influence government by voting 2. Accessibility is a right, not a privilege.
Spirituality: The "personal quest for understanding answers to ultimate questions about life, about meaning, and the sacred" (Moyers & Dale, 2007, p. 28).	**Person** 1. Daily search for purpose and meaning in one's life 2. Guiding actions from a sense of value beyond the personal acquisition of wealth or fame. **Organization and Population** (see "Person" examples related to individuals within an organization and population).

TABLE 2. CLIENT FACTORS

(Continued)

■ **BODY FUNCTIONS:** "[T]he physiological functions of body systems (including psychological functions)" (WHO, 2001, p. 10). The "Body Functions" section of the table below is organized according to the classifications of the *International Classification of Functioning, Disability, and Health (ICF)* classifications. For fuller descriptions and definitions, refer to WHO (2001).

Categories	Body Functions Commonly Considered by Occupational Therapy Practitioners *(Not intended to be all-inclusive list)*
Mental functions (affective, cognitive, perceptual)	
• **Specific mental functions**	**Specific mental functions**
○ Higher-level cognitive	Judgment, concept formation, metacognition, cognitive flexibility, insight, attention, awareness
○ Attention	Sustained, selective, and divided attention
○ Memory	Short-term, long-term, and working memory
○ Perception	Discrimination of sensations (e.g., auditory, tactile, visual, olfactory, gustatory, vestibular–proprioception), including multi-sensory processing, sensory memory, spatial, and temporal relationships (Calvert, Spence, & Stein, 2004)
○ Thought	Recognition, categorization, generalization, awareness of reality, logical/coherent thought, and appropriate thought content
○ Mental functions of sequencing complex movement	Execution of learned movement patterns
○ Emotional	Coping and behavioral regulation (Schell, Cohn, & Crepeau, 2008)
○ Experience of self and time	Body image, self-concept, self-esteem
• **Global mental functions**	**Global mental functions**
○ Consciousness	Level of arousal, level of consciousness
○ Orientation	Orientation to person, place, time, self, and others
○ Temperament and personality	Emotional stability
○ Energy and drive	Motivation, impulse control, and appetite
○ Sleep (physiological process)	
Sensory functions and pain	**Sensory functions and pain**
• Seeing and related functions, including visual acuity, visual stability, visual field functions	Detection/registration, modulation, and integration of sensations from the body and environment
	Visual awareness of environment at various distances
• Hearing functions	Tolerance of ambient sounds; awareness of location and distance of sounds such as an approaching car
• Vestibular functions	Sensation of securely moving against gravity
• Taste functions	Association of taste
• Smell functions	Association of smell
• Proprioceptive functions	Awareness of body position and space
• Touch functions	Comfort with the feeling of being touched by others or touching various textures such as food
• Pain (e.g., diffuse, dull, sharp, phantom)	Localizing pain
• Temperature and pressure	Thermal awareness

(continued)

217

TABLE 2. CLIENT FACTORS

(Continued)

■ **BODY FUNCTIONS:** *(Continued)*

Categories	Body Functions Commonly Considered by Occupational Therapy Practitioners *(Not intended to be all-inclusive list)*
Neuromusculoskeletal and movement-related functions	**Neuromusculoskeletal and movement-related functions**
• Functions of joints and bones	
○ Joint mobility	Joint range of motion
○ Joint stability	Postural alignment (this refers to the physiological stability of the joint related to its structural integrity as compared to the motor skill of aligning the body while moving in relation to task objects)
○ Muscle power	Strength
○ Muscle tone	Degree of muscle tone (e.g., flaccidity, spasticity, fluctuating)
○ Muscle endurance	Endurance
○ Motor reflexes	Stretch, asymmetrical tonic neck, symmetrical tonic neck
○ Involuntary movement reactions	Righting and supporting
○ Control of voluntary movement	Eye–hand/foot coordination, bilateral integration, crossing the midline, fine- and gross-motor control, and oculomotor (e.g., saccades, pursuits, accommodation, binocularity)
○ Gait patterns	Walking patterns and impairments such as asymmetric gait, stiff gait. (*Note:* Gait patterns are considered in relation to how they affect ability to engage in occupations in daily life activities.)
Cardiovascular, hematological, immunological, and respiratory system function	**Cardiovascular, hematological, immunological, and respiratory system function**
• Cardiovascular system function	Blood pressure functions (hypertension, hypotension, postural hypotension), and heart rate
• Hematological and immunological system function	
• Respiratory system function	(*Note:* Occupational therapy practitioners have knowledge of these body functions and understand broadly the interaction that occurs between these functions to support health and participation in life through engagement in occupation. Some therapists may specialize in evaluating and intervening with a specific function as it is related to supporting performance and engagement in occupations and activities targeted for intervention.)
• Additional functions and sensations of the cardiovascular and respiratory systems	Rate, rhythm, and depth of respiration
	Physical endurance, aerobic capacity, stamina, and fatigability
Voice and speech functions	(*Note:* Occupational therapy practitioners have knowledge of these body functions and understand broadly the interaction that occurs between these functions to support health and participation in life through engagement in occupation. Some therapists may specialize in evaluating and intervening with a specific function, such as incontinence and pelvic floor disorders, as it is related to supporting performance and engagement in occupations and activities targeted for intervention.)
• Voice functions	
• Fluency and rhythm	
• Alternative vocalization functions	
Digestive, metabolic, and endocrine system function	
• Digestive system function	
• Metabolic system and endocrine system function	
Genitourinary and reproductive functions	
• Urinary functions	
• Genital and reproductive functions	

TABLE 2. CLIENT FACTORS

(Continued)

■ **BODY FUNCTIONS:** *(Continued)*

Categories	Body Functions Commonly Considered by Occupational Therapy Practitioners *(Not intended to be all-inclusive list)*
Skin and related-structure functions • Skin functions • Hair and nail functions	**Skin and related-structure functions** Protective functions of the skin—presence or absence of wounds, cuts, or abrasions Repair function of the skin—wound healing (*Note:* Occupational therapy practitioners have knowledge of these body functions and understand broadly the interaction that occurs between these functions to support health and participation in life through engagement in occupation. Some therapists may specialize in evaluating and intervening with a specific function as it is related to supporting performance and engagement in occupations and activities targeted for intervention.)

■ **BODY STRUCTURES:** *Body structures* are "anatomical parts of the body, such as organs, limbs, and their components [that support body function]" (WHO, 2001, p. 10). The "Body Structures" section of the table below is organized according to the *ICF* classifications. For fuller descriptions and definitions, refer to WHO (2001).

Categories	Examples are not delineated in the "Body Structure" section of this table.
Structure of the nervous system **Eyes, ear, and related structures** **Structures involved in voice and speech** **Structures of the cardiovascular, immunological, and respiratory systems** **Structures related to the digestive, metabolic, and endocrine systems** **Structure related to the genitourinary and reproductive systems** **Structures related to movement** **Skin and related structures**	(*Note:* Occupational therapy practitioners have knowledge of body structures and understand broadly the interaction that occurs between these structures to support health and participation in life through engagement in occupation. Some therapists may specialize in evaluating and intervening with a specific structure as it is related to supporting performance and engagement in occupations and activities targeted for intervention.)

Note. Some data adapted from the *ICF* (WHO, 2001).

TABLE 3. ACTIVITY DEMANDS

The aspects of an activity, which include the objects and their properties, space, social demands, sequencing or timing, required actions and skills, and required underlying body functions and body structure needed to carry out the activity.

Activity Demand Aspects	Definition	Examples
Objects and their properties	Tools, materials, and equipment used in the process of carrying out the activity	• Tools (e.g., scissors, dishes, shoes, volleyball) • Materials (e.g., paints, milk, lipstick) • Equipment (e.g., workbench, stove, basketball hoop) • Inherent properties (e.g., heavy, rough, sharp, colorful, loud, bitter tasting)
Space demands (relates to physical context)	Physical environmental requirements of the activity (e.g., size, arrangement, surface, lighting, temperature, noise, humidity, ventilation)	• Large, open space outdoors required for a baseball game • Bathroom door and stall width to accommodate wheelchair • Noise, lighting, and temperature controls for a library
Social demands (relates to social environment and cultural contexts)	Social environment and cultural contexts that may be required by the activity	• Rules of game • Expectations of other participants in activity (e.g., sharing supplies, using language appropriate for the meeting)

Sequence and timing	Process used to carry out the activity (e.g., specific steps, sequence, timing requirements)	• *Steps to make tea:* Gather cup and tea bag, heat water, pour water into cup, and so forth.
		  ○ *Sequence:* Heat water before placing tea bag in water.
		  ○ *Timing:* Leave tea bag to steep for 2 minutes.
		• *Steps to conduct a meeting:* Establish goals for meeting, arrange time and location for meeting, prepare meeting agenda, call meeting to order.
		  ○ *Sequence:* Have people introduce themselves before beginning discussion of topic.
		  ○ *Timing:* Allot sufficient time for discussion of topic and determination of action items.

Required actions and performance skills	The usual skills that would be required by any performer to carry out the activity. Sensory, perceptual, motor, praxis, emotional, cognitive, communication, and social performance skills should each be considered. The performance skills demanded by an activity will be correlated with the demands of the other activity aspects (e.g., objects, space)	• Feeling the heat of the stove • Gripping handlebar • Choosing the ceremonial clothes • Determining how to move limbs to control the car • Adjusting the tone of voice • Answering a question
Required body functions	"[P]hysiological functions of body systems (including psychological functions)" (WHO, 2001, p. 10) that are required to support the actions used to perform the activity	• Mobility of joints • Level of consciousness
Required body structures	"Anatomical parts of the body such as organs, limbs, and their components [that support body function]" (WHO, 2001, p. 10) that are required to perform the activity	• Number of hands • Number of eyes

the social demands, sequence and timing, the required actions or skills needed to perform the activity, and the required body functions and structures used during the performance of the activity (see Table 3 for definitions and examples.)

Activity demands are specific to each activity. A change in one feature of an activity may change the extent of the demand in another feature. For example, an increase in the number of the steps or sequence of steps in an activity increases the demand on attention skills.

Performance Skills

Various approaches have been used to describe and categorize *performance skills*. The occupational therapy literature from research and practice offers multiple perspectives on the complexity and types of skills used during performance.

According to Fisher (2006), *performance skills* are observable, concrete, goal-directed actions clients use to engage in daily life occupations. Fisher further defines these skills as small, measurable units in a chain of actions that are observed as a person performs meaningful tasks. They are learned and developed over time and are situated in specific contexts and environments. Fisher categorized performance skills as follows: Motor Skills, Process Skills, and Communication/Interaction Skills. Rogers and Holm (2008) have proposed that during task-specific performance skills, various body functions and structures coalesce into unique combinations and emerge to affect performance in real life.

Given that **performance skills** are described and categorized in multiple ways, within the *Occupational Therapy Practice Framework* they are defined as the abilities clients demonstrate in the actions they perform. The categories of a person's performance skills are interrelated and include

- **Motor and praxis skills**
- **Sensory–perceptual skills**
- **Emotional regulation skills**
- **Cognitive skills**
- **Communication and social skills.**

Numerous body functions and structures underlie and enable performance (Rogers & Holm, 2008). Whereas body functions such as mental (affective, cognitive, perceptual), sensory, neuromuscular, and movement-related body functions (WHO, 2001) reflect the capacities that reside within the body, performance skills are the clients' demonstrated abilities. For example, praxis skills can be observed through client actions such as imitating, sequencing, and constructing; cognitive skills can be observed as the client demonstrates organization, time management, and safety; and emotional regulation skills can be observed through the behaviors the client displays to express emotion appropriately. Numerous body functions underlie each performance skill.

Multiple factors, such as the context in which the occupation is performed, the specific demands of the activity being attempted, and the client's body functions and structures, affect the client's ability to acquire or demonstrate performance skills. Performance skills are closely linked and are used in combination with one another to allow the client to perform an occupation. A change in one performance skill can affect other performance skills. In practice and in some literature, performance skills often are labeled in various combinations such as perceptual–motor skills and social–emotional skills. Table 4 provides definitions and selected examples under each category.

Occupational therapy practitioners observe and analyze performance skills in order to understand the transactions among underlying factors that support or hinder engagement in occupations and occupational performance. For example, when observing a person writing a check, the occupational therapy practitioner observes the

TABLE 4. PERFORMANCE SKILLS

Performance skills are the abilities clients demonstrate in the actions they perform.

Skill	Definition	Examples
Motor and praxis skills	*Motor:* Actions or behaviors a client uses to move and physically interact with tasks, objects, contexts, and environments (adapted from Fisher, 2006). Includes planning, sequencing, and executing new and novel movements. *Praxis:* Skilled purposeful movements (Heilman & Rothi, 1993). Ability to carry out sequential motor acts as part of an overall plan rather than individual acts (Liepmann, 1920). Ability to carry out learned motor activity, including following through on a verbal command, visual–spatial construction, ocular and oral–motor skills, imitation of a person or an object, and sequencing actions (Ayres, 1985; Filley, 2001). Organization of temporal sequences of actions within the spatial context, which form meaningful occupations (Blanche & Parham, 2002).	• *Bending* and *reaching* for a toy or tool in a storage bin • *Pacing* tempo of movements to clean the room • *Coordinating* body movements to complete a job task • *Maintaining balance* while walking on an uneven surface or while showering • *Anticipating or adjusting posture and body position* in response to environmental circumstances, such as obstacles • *Manipulating* keys or lock to open the door
Sensory–perceptual skills	Actions or behaviors a client uses to locate, identify, and respond to sensations and to select, interpret, associate, organize, and remember sensory events based on discriminating experiences through a variety of sensations that include visual, auditory, proprioceptive, tactile, olfactory, gustatory, and vestibular.	• *Positioning the body* in the exact location for a safe jump • *Hearing and locating* the voice of your child in a crowd • *Visually* determining the correct size of a storage container for leftover soup • *Locating* keys by touch from many objects in a pocket or purse (i.e., *stereognosis*) • *Timing the appropriate moment* to cross the street safely by determining one's own position and speed relative to the speed of traffic • *Discerning* distinct flavors within foods or beverages
Emotional regulation skills	Actions or behaviors a client uses to identify, manage, and express feelings while engaging in activities or interacting with others	• *Responding* to the feelings of others by acknowledgment or showing support • *Persisting* in a task despite frustrations • *Controlling* anger toward others and reducing aggressive acts • *Recovering* from a hurt or disappointment without lashing out at others • *Displaying* the emotions that are appropriate for the situation • *Utilizing* relaxation strategies to cope with stressful events
Cognitive skills	Actions or behaviors a client uses to plan and manage the performance of an activity	• *Judging* the importance or appropriateness of clothes for the circumstance • *Selecting* tools and supplies needed to clean the bathroom • *Sequencing* tasks needed for a school project • *Organizing* activities within the time required to meet a deadline • *Prioritizing* steps and *identifying* solutions to access transportation • *Creating* different activities with friends that are fun, novel, and enjoyable • *Multitasking*—doing more than one thing at a time, necessary for tasks such as work, driving, and household management

TABLE 4. PERFORMANCE SKILLS

(Continued)

Skill	Definition	Examples
Communication and social skills	Actions or behaviors a person uses to communicate and interact with others in an interactive environment (Fisher, 2006)	• *Looking* where someone else is pointing or gazing • *Gesturing* to emphasize intentions • *Maintaining* acceptable physical space during conversation • *Initiating and answering* questions with relevant information • *Taking turns* during an interchange with another person verbally and physically • *Acknowledging* another person's perspective during an interchange

motor skills of gripping and manipulating objects and the cognitive skills of initiating and sequencing the steps of the activity. The observed skills are supported by underlying body functions related to movement and cognition and by the environmental context of the bank. Proficient occupational performance observed in playing a game of tennis or playing the piano requires multiple sets of performance skills.

Further resources informing occupational therapy practice related to performance skills include Fisher (2006); Bloom, Krathwohl, and Masia (1984); Harrow (1972); and Chapparo and Ranka (1997). Detailed information about the way that skills are used in occupational therapy practice also may be found in the literature on specific theories such as sensory integration theory (Ayres, 1972, 2005) and motor learning and motor control theory (Shumway-Cook & Wollacott, 2007).

Performance Patterns

Performance patterns refer to **habits, routines, roles,** and **rituals** used in the process of engaging in occupations or activities. *Habits* refer to specific, automatic behaviors that can be useful, dominating, or impoverished (Clark, 2000; Neistadt & Crepeau, 1998), whereas *routines* are established sequences of occupations or activities that provide a structure for daily life. Routines also can be

health promoting or damaging (Fiese et al., 2002; Segal, 2004). *Roles* are sets of behaviors expected by society, shaped by culture, and may be further conceptualized and defined by the client. Roles can provide guidance in selecting occupations or can lead to stereotyping and restricted engagement patterns. Jackson (1998a, 1998b) cautioned that describing people by their roles can be limiting and can promote segmented rather than

> "...only occupational therapy practitioners focus this process toward the end-goal of supporting health and participation in life through engagement in occupations."

enfolded occupations. When considering roles within occupational therapy, occupational therapy practitioners are concerned with the way clients construct their occupations to fulfill their perceived roles and identity and reinforce their

"Occupational therapy practitioners apply theory, evidence, knowledge, and skills regarding the therapeutic use of occupations to positively affect the client's health, well-being, and life satisfaction."

values and beliefs. *Rituals* are symbolic actions with spiritual, cultural, or social meaning that contribute to the client's identity and reinforce the client's values and beliefs (Fiese et al., 2002; Segal, 2004). Habits, routines, roles, and rituals can support or hinder occupational performance.

People, organizations, and populations demonstrate performance patterns in daily life. They develop over time and are influenced by all other aspects of the domain. When practitioners consider the client's patterns of performance, they are better able to understand the frequency and manner in which performance skills and occupations are integrated into the client's life. While a client may have the ability or capacity for skilled performance, if he or she does not embed those skills in a productive set of engagement patterns, health and participation may be negatively affected. For example, a client who has the skills and resources to engage in appropriate grooming, bathing, and meal preparation but does not embed them into a consistent

routine, may struggle with poor nutrition and social isolation. Tables 5a, 5b, and 5c provide examples of performance patterns for persons, organizations, and populations.

Context and Environment

A client's engagement in occupation takes place within a social and physical environment situated within context. In the literature, the terms *environment* and *context* often are used interchangeably. In the *Framework,* both terms are used to reflect the importance of considering the wide variety of interrelated conditions both internal and external to the client that influence performance.

The term **environment** refers to the external physical and social environments that surround the client and in which the client's daily life occupations occur. **Physical environment** refers to the natural and built nonhuman environment and the objects in them. The **social environment** is constructed by the presence, relationships, and expectations of persons, groups, and organizations with whom the client has contact.

The term *context* refers to a variety of interrelated conditions that are within and surrounding the client. These interrelated contexts often are less tangible than physical and social environments but nonetheless exert a strong influence on performance. Contexts, as described in the *Framework,* are **cultural, personal, temporal,** and **virtual.** *Cultural context* includes customs, beliefs, activity patterns, behavior standards, and expectations accepted by the society of which the client is a member. *Personal context* refers to demographic features of the individual such as age, gender, socioeconomic status, and educational level that are not part of a health condition (WHO, 2001). *Temporal context* includes stages of life, time of day or year, duration, rhythm of activity, or history. *Virtual context* refers to interactions in simulated, real-time, or near-time situ-

TABLE 5A. PERFORMANCE PATTERNS—PERSON

Patterns of behavior related to an individual's or significant other's daily life activities that are habitual or routine.

	Examples
HABITS—"Automatic behavior that is integrated into more complex patterns that enable people to function on a day-to-day basis" (Neistadt & Crepeau, 1998, p. 869). Habits can be useful, dominating, or impoverished and either support or interfere with performance in areas of occupation.	– Automatically puts car keys in the same place. – Spontaneously looks both ways before crossing the street – Repeatedly rocks back and forth when asked to initiate a task – Repeatedly activates and deactivates the alarm system before entering the home – Maintains the exact distance between all hangers when hanging clothes in a closet
ROUTINES—Patterns of behavior that are observable, regular, repetitive, and that provide structure for daily life. They can be satisfying, promoting, or damaging. Routines require momentary time commitment and are embedded in cultural and ecological contexts (Fiese et al., 2002; Segal, 2004).	– Follows the morning sequence to complete toileting, bathing, hygiene, and dressing – Follows the sequence of steps involved in meal preparation
RITUALS—Symbolic actions with spiritual, cultural, or social meaning, contributing to the client's identity and reinforcing values and beliefs. Rituals have a strong affective component and represent a collection of events (Fiese et al., 2002; Segal, 2004).	– Uses the inherited antique hairbrush and brushes her hair with 100 strokes nightly as her mother had done – Prepares the holiday meals with favorite or traditional *accoutrements*, using designated dishware – Kisses a sacred book before opening the pages to read
ROLES—A set of behaviors expected by society, shaped by culture, and may be further conceptualized and defined by the client.	– Mother of an adolescent with developmental disabilities – Student with learning disability studying computer technology – Corporate executive returning to work after experiencing a stroke

Note. Information for "Habits" section of this table adapted from Dunn (2000b).

TABLE 5B. PERFORMANCE PATTERNS—ORGANIZATION

Patterns of behavior related to the daily functioning of an organization.

	Examples
ROUTINES—Patterns of behavior that are observable, regular, repetitive, and that provide structure for daily life. They can be satisfying, promoting, or damaging. Routines require momentary time commitment and are embedded in cultural and ecological contexts (Fiese et al., 2002; Segal, 2004).	– Holds regularly scheduled meetings for staff, directors, executive boards – Follows documentation practices for annual reports, timecards, and strategic plans – Turns in documentation on a scheduled basis – Follows the chain of command – Follows safety and security routines (e.g., signing in/out, using pass codes) – Maintains dress codes (e.g., casual Fridays) – Socializes during breaks, lunch, at the water cooler – Follows beginning or ending routines (e.g., opening/closing the facility) – Offers activities to meet performance expectations or standards

(Continued)

TABLE 5B. PERFORMANCE PATTERNS—ORGANIZATION

(Continued)

	Examples
RITUALS—Symbolic actions that have meaning, contributing to the organization's identity and reinforcing values and beliefs (adapted from Fiese et al., 2002; Segal, 2004).	– Holds holiday parties, company picnics – Conducts induction, recognition, and retirement ceremonies – Organizes annual retreats or conferences – Maintains fundraising activities for organization to support local charities
ROLES—A set of behaviors by the organization expected by society, shaped by culture, and may be further conceptualized and defined by the client.	– Nonprofit organization provides housing for persons living with mental illness – Humanitarian organization distributes food and clothing donations to refugees – University educates and provides service to the surrounding community

Note. In this document, habits are addressed only in Table 5A (Person).

TABLE 5C. PERFORMANCE PATTERNS—POPULATION

Patterns of behavior related to a population.

	Examples
ROUTINES—Patterns of behavior that are observable, regular, repetitive, and that provide structure for daily life. They can be satisfying, promoting, or damaging. Routines require momentary time commitment and are embedded in cultural and ecological contexts (Fiese et al., 2002; Segal, 2004).	– Follows health practices, such as scheduled immunizations for children and yearly health screenings for adults – Follows business practices, such as provision of services for the disadvantaged populations (e.g., loans to underrepresented groups) – Follows legislative procedures, such as those associated with IDEA and Medicare – Follows social customs for greeting
RITUALS—Rituals are shared social actions with traditional, emotional, purposive, and technological meaning, contributing to values and beliefs within the population.	– Holds cultural celebrations – Has parades or demonstrations – Shows national affiliations/allegiances – Follows religious, spiritual, and cultural practices, such as touching the mezuzah or using holy water when leaving/entering, praying to Mecca
ROLES	– SEE DESCRIPTION OF THESE AREAS FOR INDIVIDUALS WITHIN THE POPULATION

Note. In this document, habits are addressed only in Table 5A (Person).

TABLE 6. CONTEXTS AND ENVIRONMENTS

Context and *environment* (including cultural, personal, temporal, virtual, physical, and social) refers to a variety of interrelated conditions within and surrounding the client that influence performance.

The term *context* refers to a variety of interrelated conditions that are within and surrounding the client. Contexts include cultural, personal, temporal, and virtual. The term *environment* refers to the external physical and social environments that surround the client and in which the client's daily life occupations occur.

Context and Environment	Definition	Examples
Cultural	Customs, beliefs, activity patterns, behavior standards, and expectations accepted by the society of which the client is a member. Includes ethnicity and values as well as political aspects, such as laws that affect access to resources and affirm personal rights. Also includes opportunities for education, employment, and economic support.	*Person:* Shaking hands when being introduced *Organization:* Employees marking the end of the work week with casual dress on Friday *Population:* Celebrating Independence Day
Personal	"[F]eatures of the individual that are not part of a health condition or health status" (WHO, 2001, p. 17). Personal context includes age, gender, socioeconomic status, and educational status. Can also include organizational levels (e.g., volunteers and employees) and population levels (e.g., members of society).	*Person:* Twenty-five-year-old unemployed man with a high school diploma *Organization:* Volunteers working in a homeless shelter *Population:* Teenage women who are pregnant or new mothers
Temporal	"Location of occupational performance in time" (Neistadt & Crepeau, 1998, p. 292). The experience of time as shaped by engagement in occupations. The temporal aspects of occupation "which contribute to the patterns of daily occupations" are "the rhythm…tempo…synchronization…duration…and sequence" (Larson & Zemke, 2004, p. 82; Zemke, 2004, p. 610). Includes stages of life, time of day or year, duration, rhythm of activity, or history.	*Person:* A person retired from work for 10 years *Organization:* Annual fundraising campaign *Population:* Engaging in siestas or high teas
Virtual	Environment in which communication occurs by means of airways or computers and an absence of physical contact. Includes simulated or real-time or near-time existence of an environment via chat rooms, email, video-conferencing, radio transmissions.	*Person:* Text message to a friend *Organization:* Video conference, telephone conference call, instant message, interactive white boards among all the members *Population:* Virtual community of gamers
Physical	Natural and built nonhuman environment and the objects in them: • Natural environment includes geographic terrain, sensory qualities of environment, plants and animals • Built environment and objects includes buildings, furniture, tools or devices.	*Person:* Individual's house, apartment *Organization:* Office building, factory *Population:* Transportation system
Social	Is constructed by presence, relationships, and expectations of persons, organizations, populations. • Availability and expectations of significant individuals, such as spouse, friends, and caregivers • Relationships with individuals, groups, or organizations • Relationships with systems (e.g., political, legal, economic, institutional) that are influential in establishing norms, role expectations, and social routines.	*Person:* Friends, colleagues *Organization:* Advisory board *Population:* City government

---

EVALUATION

Occupational profile—The initial step in the evaluation process that provides an understanding of the client's occupational history and experiences, patterns of daily living, interests, values, and needs. The client's problems and concerns about performing occupations and daily life activities are identified, and the client's priorities are determined.

Analysis of occupational performance—The step in the evaluation process during which the client's assets, problems, or potential problems are more specifically identified. Actual performance is often observed in context to identify what supports performance and what hinders performance. Performance skills, performance patterns, context or contexts, activity demands, and client factors are all considered, but only selected aspects may be specifically assessed. Targeted outcomes are identified.

INTERVENTION

Intervention plan—A plan that will guide actions taken and that is developed in collaboration with the client. It is based on selected theories, frames of reference, and evidence. Outcomes to be targeted are confirmed.

Intervention implementation—Ongoing actions taken to influence and support improved client performance. Interventions are directed at identified outcomes. Client's response is monitored and documented.

Intervention review—A review of the implementation plan and process as well as its progress toward targeted outcomes.

OUTCOMES (Supporting Health and Participation in Life Through Engagement in Occupation)

Outcomes—Determination of success in reaching desired targeted outcomes. Outcome assessment information is used to plan future actions with the client and to evaluate the service program (i.e., program evaluation).

Figure 5. Process of Service Delivery.
The process of service delivery is applied within the profession's domain to support the client's health and participation.

ations absent of physical contact. Some contexts are external to the client (e.g., virtual), some are internal to the client (e.g., personal), and some may have both external features and internalized beliefs and values (e.g., cultural).

Clients' engagement in occupations evolves within their social and physical environments and reflects their interdependence with these environments. Cultural contexts often influence how occupations are chosen, prioritized, and organized. Contexts and environments affect a client's accessibility to occupations and influence the quality of performance and satisfaction with performance. A client who has difficulty performing effectively in one environment or context may be successful when the environment or context is changed. The context within which the engagement in occupations occurs is unique for each client. Contexts and environments are interrelated both with each other and all other aspects of the domain (see Table 6 for a description of the different kinds of contexts and environments).

Process of Occupational Therapy

Overview

This second section of the *Occupational Therapy Practice Framework* describes the process that outlines the way in which occupational therapy practitioners operationalize their expertise to provide services to clients (see Figure 5). This process includes evaluation, intervention, and outcome monitoring; occurs within the purview of the domain; and involves collaboration among the occupational therapist, occupational therapy assistant, and the client. Occupational therapy practitioners are required to maintain appropriate credentials and abide by ethical standards, existing laws, and regulatory requirements for each step of the occupational therapy process.

Many professions use the process of evaluating, intervening, and targeting intervention **outcomes.** However, only occupational therapy practitioners focus this process toward the end-goal of supporting health and participation in life through engagement in occupations. Occupational therapy practitioners also use occupations as a method of intervention implementation by engaging clients throughout the process in occupations that are therapeutically selected. The profession's use of occupation as both means and end is a unique application of the process (Trombly, 1995).

Although for the purpose of organization the *Framework* describes the process in a linear manner, in reality, the process does not occur in a sequenced, step-by-step fashion (see Table 7). Instead, it is fluid and dynamic, allowing occupational therapy practitioners to operate with an ongoing focus on outcomes while continually reflecting on and changing an overall plan to accommodate new developments and insights along the way.

Occupational therapy involves facilitating interactions among the client, the environments or contexts, and the activities or occupations in order to help the client reach the desired outcomes that support health and participation in life. Occupational therapy practitioners apply theory, evidence, knowledge, and skills regarding the therapeutic use of occupations to positively affect the client's health, well-being, and life satisfaction.

The broader definition of *client* included in this document is indicative of the profession's increasing involvement in providing services not only to a person but also to organizations and populations. Regardless of whether the client is a person, organization, or population, the client's wants, needs, occupational risks, and problems are evaluated, and information is gathered, synthesized, and framed from an occupational perspective. This perspective is based on the theories, knowledge, and skills generated and used by the profession and informed by available evidence. Client concerns are viewed relative to problems or risks in occupational performance.

Occupational therapy practitioners develop a collaborative relationship with clients in order to understand their experiences and desires for intervention, as noted in Figure 2. The collaborative approach, which is used throughout the process, honors the contributions of the client and the occupational therapy practitioner. Clients bring knowledge about their life experiences and their **hopes** and dreams for the future. They identify and share their needs and priorities. Occupational therapy practitioners bring their knowledge about how engagement in occupation affects health and performance. This information is coupled with the practitioner's **clinical reasoning** and theoretical perspectives to critically observe, analyze, describe, and interpret human performance. Occupational therapy practitioners also apply knowledge and skills to reduce the effects of disease, disability, and deprivation and to promote health and well-being. Together, practitioners and clients identify and prioritize the focus of the intervention plan. This collaboration may include family, significant others, community members, and stakeholders who affect or are affected by the client's engagement in occupation, health, and participation.

Rarely is an individual the exclusive focus of the intervention. For example, the needs of an at-risk infant may be the initial impetus for intervention, but the concerns and priorities of the parent, the extended family, and funding agencies also are considered. Similarly, services addressing independent-living skills for adults coping with serious and persistent mental illness may involve the needs and expectations of state and local services agencies as well as business groups.

Throughout the process, the occupational therapy practitioner is engaged continually in clinical reasoning about the client's engagement in occupation. Clinical reasoning enables the occupational therapy practitioner to (1) identify

229

TABLE 7. OPERATIONALIZING THE OCCUPATIONAL THERAPY PROCESS

Evaluation		Intervention			Outcomes
					Supporting Health and Participation in Life through Engagement in Occupation
Occupational Profile ⟷	*Analysis of Occupational Performance*	*Intervention Plan*	*Intervention Implementation*	*Intervention Review*	

Identify
• Who is the client?
• Why is the client seeking services?
• What occupations and activities are successful or are causing problems?
• What contexts and environments support or inhibit desired outcomes?
• What is the client's occupational history?
• What are the client's priorities and targeted outcomes?
	• Synthesize information from the occupational profile.
	• Observe client's performance in desired occupation/activity.
	• Note the effectiveness of performance skills and patterns and select assessments to identify factors (context or contexts, activity demands, client factors) that may be influencing performance skills and patterns.
	• Interpret assessment data to identify facilitators and barriers to performance.
	• Develop and refine hypotheses about client's occupational performance strengths and weaknesses.
	• Collaborate with client to create goals that address targeted outcomes.
	• Delineate areas for intervention based on best practice and evidence.
		• Develop plan that includes
		  –Objective and measurable goals with time frame,
		  –Occupational therapy intervention approach based on theory and evidence, and
		  –Mechanisms for service delivery.
		• Consider discharge needs and plan.
		• Select outcome measures.
		• Make recommendation or referral to others as needed.
			• Determine types of occupational therapy interventions to be used and carry them out.
			• Monitor client's response according to ongoing assessment and reassessment.
				• Reevaluate plan relative to achieving targeted outcomes.
				• Modify plan as needed.
				• Determine need for continuation, discontinuation, or referral.
					• Focus on outcomes as they relate to supporting health and participation in life through engagement in occupation.
					• Select outcome measures.
					• Measure and use outcomes.

⟵———— Continue to renegotiate intervention plans and targeted outcomes. ————⟶

⟵———— Ongoing interaction among evaluation, intervention, and outcomes occurs throughout the process. ————⟶

the multiple demands, skills, and potential meanings of the activity and (2) gain a deeper understanding of the interrelationships between aspects of the domain that affect performance and those that will support client-centered interventions and outcomes.

Evaluation

The **evaluation** process begins with an evaluation conducted by the occupational therapist and is focused on finding out what the client wants and needs to do, determining what the client can do and has done, and identifying those factors that act as supports or barriers to health and participation. Evaluation often occurs both formally and informally during all interactions with the client. The type and focus of the evaluation differs depending on the practice setting.

The evaluation consists of the **occupational profile** and **analysis of occupational performance.** The *occupational profile* includes information about the client and the client's needs, problems, and concerns about performance in areas of occupation. The *analysis of occupational performance* focuses on collecting and interpreting information using **assessment** tools designed to observe, measure, and inquire about factors that support or hinder occupational performance. Although the ways occupational therapists collect client information are described separately and sequentially in the *Framework,* the exact manner is influenced by the client needs and the practice setting. Information related to the occupational profile is gathered throughout the occupational therapy process.

The occupational therapist's knowledge and skills, as well as theoretical principles and available evidence, guide his or her clinical reasoning for the selection and application of various theories and frames of reference throughout the evaluation process. Concurrently, the occupational therapist's

knowledge and skills in these areas influence the information that is collected during the evaluation. Knowledge and evidence about occupational performance problems and diagnostic conditions are used to guide information gathering and synthesis of information for interpretation and intervention planning. The occupational therapist's skilled interpretation of assessment results relative to the whole evaluation leads to a clear delineation of the strengths and limitations affecting the client's occupational performance. The occupational therapy assistant contributes to the evaluation process based on established competencies and under the supervision of an occupational therapist.

Occupational Profile

An *occupational profile* is defined as a summary of information that describes the client's occupational history and experiences, patterns of daily living, **interests,** values, and needs. Because the profile is designed to gain an understanding of the client's perspective and background, its format varies depending on whether the client is a person, organization, or population. Using a **client-centered approach,** the occupational therapy practitioner gathers information to understand what is currently important and meaningful to the client. The profile includes inquiry related to what the client wants and needs to do in the present or future as well as past experiences and interests that may assist in identifying strengths and limitations. Refinement of the information collected during the occupational profile subsequently refines the intervention plan and identified outcomes.

During the process of collecting this information, the client's priorities and desired outcomes that will lead to engagement in occupation for improved health are identified. Clients identify occupations that give meaning to their lives and select the **goals** and priorities important to them. Valuing and respecting the client's collaboration in the therapeutic process helps foster client involvement and more efficiently guide interventions.

The process and timing of completing the occupational profile varies depending on the circumstances. Occupational therapy practitioners may gather information formally and informally in one session or over a longer period while working with the client. Obtaining information through both formal interview and casual conversation helps establish a therapeutic relationship with the client. Ideally, the information obtained during the development of the occupational profile leads to a more client-centered approach in the evaluation, intervention planning, and intervention implementation stages.

Specifically, the information collected answers the following questions:

- Who is the client (person, including family, caregivers, and significant others; population; or organization)?
- Why is the client seeking services, and what are the client's current concerns relative to engaging in occupations and in daily life activities?
- What areas of occupation are successful, and what areas are causing problems or risks (see Table 1)?
- What contexts and environments support or inhibit participation and engagement in desired occupations?
- What is the client's occupational history (i.e., life experiences, values, interests, previous patterns of engagement in occupations and in daily life activities, the meanings associated with them)?
- What are the client's priorities and desired outcomes?

Once the profile data are collected and documented, the occupational therapist reviews the information; identifies the client's strengths, limitations, and needs; and develops a working hypothe-

sis regarding possible reasons for identified problems and concerns. The occupational therapy assistant contributes to this process. The information from the occupational therapy profile often guides the selection of outcome measures. If an organization or population is the identified client, the strengths and needs are those that affect the collective entity rather than the individual.

Analysis of Occupational Performance

Occupational performance is the accomplishment of the selected occupation resulting from the dynamic transaction among the client, the context and environment, and the activity. Evaluation of occupational performance involves one or more of the following:

- Synthesizing information from the occupational profile to focus on specific areas of occupation and contexts that need to be addressed;
- Observing the client's performance during activities relevant to desired occupations, noting effectiveness of the performance skills and performance patterns;
- Selecting and using specific assessments to measure performance skills and performance patterns, as appropriate;
- Selecting assessments, as needed, to identify and measure more specifically contexts or environments, activity demands, and client factors influencing performance skills and performance patterns;
- Interpreting the assessment data to identify what supports performance and what hinders performance;
- Developing and refining hypotheses about the client's occupational performance strengths and limitations;
- Creating goals in collaboration with the client that address the desired outcomes;
- Determining procedures to measure the outcomes of intervention; and

• Delineating a potential intervention approach or approaches based on best practices and available evidence.

Multiple methods often are used during the evaluation process to assess the client, the context, the occupation or activity, and the occupational performance. Methods may include an interview with the client and significant others, observation of performance and context, record review, and direct assessment of specific aspects of performance. Formal and informal, structured and unstructured, and standardized criterion or norm-referenced assessment tools can be used. Standardized assessments are preferred, when appropriate, to provide objective data about the various aspects of the domain influencing engagement and performance. "Obtaining reliable and valid information [through the use of standard assessments] provides a high level of support that can justify the need for occupational therapy services" (Gutman, Mortera, Hinojosa, & Kramer, 2007, p. 121).

Activity analysis is an important process used by occupational therapy practitioners to understand the demands that a specific desired activity places on a client. "Activity analysis addresses the typical demands of an activity, the range of skills involved in its performance, and the various cultural meanings that might be ascribed to it" (Crepeau, 2003, p. 192). When activity analysis is completed and the demands of a specific activity that the client wants and needs to do are understood, the client's specific skills and abilities are then compared with the selected activity's demands.

> Occupation-based activity analysis places the person [client] in the foreground. It takes into account the particular person's [client's] interests, goals, abilities, and contexts, as well as the demands of the activity itself. These considerations shape the practitioner's efforts to help the...person [client] reach his/her goals through carefully designed evaluation and intervention. (Crepeau, 2003, p. 193)

Examining the environments and contexts in which occupational performance can or does occur provides insights into overarching, underlying, and embedded influences on engagement. The external environments and context (e.g., physical and social environment, virtual context) provide resources that support or inhibit the client's performance (e.g., doorway widths as part of the physical environment that allow for wheelchair passage, presence or absence of a caregiver as part of the social environment, access to a computer to communicate with others as part of the virtual context). Different environments (e.g., community, institution, home) provide different supports and resources for service delivery (e.g., assessment of an infant or toddler in the hospital without the primary caregivers present yields different results than while at home with a parent).

The client's personal context affects service delivery by influencing personal beliefs, perceptions, and expectations. The cultural context exists within small groups of related individuals, such as a nuclear family, and within larger groups of people, such as populations of a country or ethnic group. The expectations, beliefs, and customs of various cultures can affect a client's **identity** and activity choices and need to be considered when determining how and when services may be delivered. Note that in Figure 2, context and environment are depicted as surrounding and underlying the process.

Analyzing occupational performance requires an understanding of the complex and dynamic interaction among performance skills, performance patterns, contexts and environments, activity demands, and client factors. Occupational therapy practitioners attend to each aspect and gauge the influence of each aspect on the others—individually and collectively. By understanding how these aspects dynamically influence each other, occupational therapists can better evaluate how they contribute to the client's performance-related concerns, and how they

"Supporting health
and participation
in life through
engagement in
occupation is the
broad, overarching
outcome of the
occupational therapy
intervention process."

potentially contribute to interventions that support occupational performance. When working with an organization or population, occupational therapy practitioners consider the collective occupational performance abilities of the respective members.

Intervention

The **intervention** process consists of the skilled actions taken by occupational therapy practitioners in collaboration with the client to facilitate engagement in occupation related to health and participation. Occupational therapy practitioners use the information about the client gathered during the evaluation and from theoretical principles to direct occupation-centered interventions. Intervention is provided then to assist the client in reaching a state of physical, mental, and social well-being; to identify and realize aspirations; to satisfy needs; and to change or cope with the environment. A variety of types of occupational therapy interventions are discussed in Table 8.

Intervention is intended to be health-promoting. *Health promotion* is "the process of enabling people to increase control over, and to improve, their health" (WHO, 1986). Wilcock (2006) states

[F]ollowing an occupation-focused health promotion approach to well-being embraces a belief that the potential range of what people can do, be, and strive to become is the primary concern and that health is a by-product. A varied and full occupational lifestyle will coincidentally maintain and improve health and well-being if it enables people to be creative and adventurous physically, mentally, and socially. (p. 315)

Interventions vary depending on the client—person, organization, or population—and the context of service delivery (Moyers & Dale, 2007). The actual term used for clients receiving occupational therapy varies among practice settings and delivery models. For example, when working in a hospital, the person might be referred to as a *patient,* and in a school, the client might be a *student, teacher, parent,* or *administrator.* When providing services to an organization, the client may be called the *consumer.* When serving a population, the client may be specific entities, such as disability groups, veterans who are homeless, or refugees.

The term *person* includes others who also may help or be served indirectly, such as caregiver, teacher, parent, employer, or spouse. When addressing the person or a small group of persons who support or care for the client in need of services (e.g., caregiver, teacher, partner, employer, spouse), the practitioners address the interaction among client factors, performance skills, performance patterns, contexts and environments, and activity demands that influence occupational performance within those occupations the person needs and wants to do. The intervention focus is on modifying the environment/contexts and activity demands or patterns, promoting health, establishing or restoring and maintaining occupational performance, and preventing further disability and occupational performance problems.

Interventions provided to *organizations* are designed to affect the organization to more efficiently and effectively meet the needs of the clients or

TABLE 8. TYPES OF OCCUPATIONAL THERAPY INTERVENTIONS

THERAPEUTIC USE OF SELF—An occupational therapy practitioner's planned use of his or her personality, insights, perceptions, and judgments as part of the therapeutic process (adapted from Punwar & Peloquin, 2000, p. 285).

THERAPEUTIC USE OF OCCUPATIONS AND ACTIVITIES[a]—Occupations and activities selected for specific clients that meet therapeutic goals. To use occupations/activities therapeutically, context or contexts, activity demands, and client factors all should be considered in relation to the client's therapeutic goals. Use of assistive technologies, application of universal-design principles, and environmental modifications support the ability of clients to engage in their occupations.

Occupation-based intervention	*Purpose:* Client engages in client-directed occupations that match identified goals. *Examples:* • Completes morning dressing and hygiene using adaptive devices • Purchases groceries and prepares a meal • Utilizes the transportation system • Applies for a job • .Plays on playground and community recreation equipment • Participates in a community festival • Establishes a pattern of self-care and relaxation activities in preparation for sleep
Purposeful activity	*Purpose:* Client engages in specifically selected activities that allow the client to develop skills that enhance occupational engagement. *Examples:* • Practices how to select clothing and manipulate clothing fasteners • Practices safe ways to get in and out of a bathtub • Practices how to prepare a food list and rehearses how to use cooking appliances • Practices how to use a map and transportation schedule • Rehearses how to write answers on an application form • .Practices how to get on and off playground and recreation equipment • Role plays when to greet people and initiates conversation • Practices how to use adaptive switches to operate home environmental control system
Preparatory methods	*Purpose:* Practitioner selects directed methods and techniques that prepare the client for occupational performance. Used in preparation for or concurrently with purposeful and occupation-based activities. *Examples:* • Provides sensory enrichment to promote alertness • Administers physical agent modalities to prepare muscles for movement • Provides instruction in visual imagery and rhythmic breathing to promote rest and relaxation • Issues orthotics/splints to provide support and facilitate movement • Suggests a home-based conditioning regimen using Pilates and yoga • Provides hand-strengthening exercises using therapy putty and theraband • Provides instruction in assertiveness to prepare for self-advocacy

(Continued)

TABLE 8. TYPES OF OCCUPATIONAL THERAPY INTERVENTIONS

(Continued)

CONSULTATION PROCESS—A type of intervention in which occupational therapy practitioners use their knowledge and expertise to collaborate with the client. The collaborative process involves identifying the problem, creating possible solutions, trying solutions, and altering them as necessary for greater effectiveness. When providing consultation, the practitioner is not directly responsible for the outcome of the intervention (Dunn, 2000a, p. 113).

Person	• Advises a family about architectural options • Advises family how to create pre-sleep nighttime routines for their children
Organization	• Recommends work pattern modifications and ergonomically designed workstations for a company • Recommends disaster evacuation strategies for a residential community related to accessibility and reduced environmental barriers
Population	• Advises senior citizens on older driver initiatives

EDUCATION PROCESS—An intervention process that involves imparting knowledge and information about occupation, health, and participation and that does not result in the actual performance of the occupation/activity.

Person	• Instructs a classroom teacher on sensory regulation strategies
Organization	• Teaches staff at a homeless shelter how to structure daily living, play, and leisure activities for shelter members
Population	• Instructs town officials about the value of and strategies for making walking and biking paths accessible for all community members

ADVOCACY—Efforts directed toward promoting occupational justice and empowering clients to seek and obtain resources to fully participate in their daily life occupations.

Person	• Collaborates with a person to procure reasonable accommodations at worksite
Organization	• Serves on policy board of an organization to procure supportive housing accommodations for persons with disabilities
Population	• Collaborates with adults with serious mental illness to raise public awareness of the impact of this stigma • Collaborates with and educates federal funding sources for the disabled population to include cancer patients prior to their full remission

[a]Information adapted from Pedretti and Early (2001).

consumers and stakeholders. Practitioners address features of the organization or agency such as its mission, values, organizational culture and structure, policies and procedures, and built and natural environments. Practitioners evaluate how each of these features either supports or inhibits the overall performance of individuals within the organization. For example, to enable the staff at a skilled-nursing facility to provide better services, an occupational therapy practitioner may recommend the walls in each hallway be painted a different color, enabling residents to more easily locate their rooms.

Interventions provided to *populations* are directed to all the members of the group collectively rather than individualized to specific people within the group. Practitioners direct their interventions toward current or potential health problems and disabling conditions within the population and community. Their goal is to enhance the health of all people within the population by addressing services and supports within the community that can be implemented to improve the population's performance. The intervention focus often is on health promotion activities, self-management educational services, and environmental modification. For instance, the occupational therapy practitioner may design developmentally based day care programs run by college student volunteers for homeless shelters catering to families in a large metropolitan area. Practitioners may work with a wide variety of populations experiencing difficulty in accessing and engaging in health occupations due to conditions such as poverty, homelessness, and discrimination.

The intervention process is divided into three steps: (1) intervention plan, (2) intervention implementation, and (3) intervention review. During the intervention process, information from the evaluation is integrated with theory, practice models, frames of reference, and evidence. This information guides the clinical reasoning of the occupa-

tional therapist and the occupational therapy assistant in the development, implementation, and review of the intervention plan.

Intervention Plan

The intervention plan directs the actions of the occupational therapist and occupational therapy assistant. It describes the selected occupational therapy approaches and types of interventions for reaching the client's identified outcomes. The intervention plan is developed collaboratively with the client and is based on the client's goals and priorities. Depending on whether the client is a person, organization, or population, others such as family members, significant others, board members, service providers, and community groups also may collaborate in the development of the plan.

The design of the intervention plan is directed by the

- Client's goals, values, beliefs, and occupational needs;
- Client's health and well-being;
- Client's performance skills and performance patterns;
- Collective influence of the context, environment, activity demands, and client factors on the client;
- Context of service delivery in which the intervention is provided (e.g., caregiver expectations, organization's purpose, payer's requirements, applicable regulations); and
- Best available evidence.

The selection and design of the intervention plan and goals are directed toward addressing the client's current and potential problems related to engagement in occupations or activities.

Intervention planning includes the following steps:

1. *Developing the plan.* The occupational therapist develops the plan with the client, and the

occupational therapy assistant contributes to the plan's development. The plan includes

- Objective and measurable goals with a time-frame
- Occupational therapy **intervention approach** or approaches (see Table 9)
  –Create or promote
  –Establish or restore
  –Maintain
  –Modify
  –Prevent.
- Mechanisms for service delivery
  –People providing the intervention
  –Types of interventions
  –Frequency and duration of service.

2. *Considering potential discharge needs and plans*
3. *Selecting outcome measures*
4. *Making recommendation or referral to others as needed.*

Intervention Implementation

Intervention implementation is the process of putting the plan into action. It involves the skilled process of altering factors in the client, activity, and context and environment for the purpose of effecting positive change in the client's desired engagement in occupation, health, and participation.

Interventions may focus on a single aspect of the domain, such as a specific performance pattern, or several aspects of the domain, such as performance patterns, performance skills, and context. Given that the factors are interrelated and influence one another in a continuous, dynamic process, occupational therapy practitioners expect that the client's ability to adapt, change, and develop in one area will affect other areas. Because of this dynamic interrelationship, assessment and intervention planning continue throughout the implementation process. Intervention implementation includes the following steps:

1. Determining and carrying out the type of occupational therapy intervention or interventions to be used (see Table 8)
   - Therapeutic use of self
   - Therapeutic use of occupations or activities
     – **Occupation-based interventions**
     – **Purposeful activity**
     – **Preparatory methods.**
   - **Consultation process**
   - **Education process**
   - **Advocacy.**
2. Monitoring the client's response to interventions based on ongoing assessment and reassessment of the client's progress toward goals.

Intervention Review

Intervention review is the continuous process of reevaluating and reviewing the intervention plan, the effectiveness of its delivery, and the progress toward outcomes. As during intervention planning, this process includes collaboration with the client based on his or her goals. Depending on whether the client is a person, organization, or population, various stakeholders, such as family members, significant others, board members, other service providers, and community groups, also may collaborate in the intervention review. **Re-evaluation** and review may lead to change in the intervention plan.

The intervention review includes the following steps:

1. Re-evaluating the plan and how it is implemented relative to achieving outcomes
2. Modifying the plan as needed
3. Determining the need for continuation or discontinuation of occupational therapy services and for referral to other services.

The intervention review may include program evaluations that critique the way that occupational therapy services are provided. This may include a review of client satisfaction and the client's perception of the benefits of receiving occupational ther-

TABLE 9. OCCUPATIONAL THERAPY INTERVENTION APPROACHES

Specific strategies selected to direct the process of intervention that are based on the client's desired outcome, evaluation data, and evidence.

Approach	Focus of Intervention	Examples
Create, promote (health promotion)[a]—An intervention approach that does not assume a disability is present or that any factors would interfere with performance. This approach is designed to provide enriched contextual and activity experiences that will enhance performance for all persons in the natural contexts of life (adapted from Dunn, McClain, Brown, & Youngstrom, 1998, p. 534).	**Performance skills**	• Create a parenting class to help first-time parents engage their children in developmentally appropriate play
	Performance patterns	• Promote effective handling of stress by creating time use routines with healthy clients
	Context or contexts or physical environments	• Promote a diversity of sensory play experiences by recommending a variety of equipment for playgrounds and other play areas
	Activity demands	• Serve food family style in the congregate dining area to increase the opportunities for socialization
	Client factors (body functions, body structures)	• Promote increased endurance by recommending year-round daily outdoor recess for all school children • Design a dance program for senior citizens that will enhance strength and flexibility
Establish, restore (remediation, restoration)[a]—An intervention approach designed to change client variables to establish a skill or ability that has not yet developed or to restore a skill or ability that has been impaired (adapted from Dunn et al., 1998, p. 533).	**Performance skills**	• Provide adjustable desk chairs to improve client sitting posture • Work with senior community centers to offer driving educational programs targeted at improving driving skills for persons ages 65 or older
	Performance patterns	• Collaborate with clients to help them establish morning routines needed to arrive at school or work on time • Provide classes in fatigue management for cancer patients and their families • Collaborate with clients to help them establish healthy sleep–wake patterns • Develop walking programs at the local mall for employees and community members
	Client factors (body functions, body structures)	• Support daily physical education classes for entire population of children in a school aimed at improving physical strength and endurance • Collaborate with schools and businesses to establish universal-design models in their buildings, classrooms, and so forth • Gradually increase time required to complete a computer game to increase client's attention span

(Continued)

TABLE 9. OCCUPATIONAL THERAPY INTERVENTION APPROACHES

(Continued)

Approach	Focus of Intervention	Examples
Maintain—An intervention approach designed to provide the supports that will allow clients to preserve the performance capabilities they have regained, that continue to meet their occupational needs, or both. The assumption is that, without continued maintenance intervention, performance would decrease, occupational needs would not be met, or both, thereby affecting health and quality of life.	**Performance skills**	• Maintain the ability of the client to organize tools by providing a tool outline painted on a pegboard • Develop a refresher safety program for industrial organizations to remind workers of need to continue to use safety skills on the job • Provide a program for community-dwelling older adults to maintain motor and praxis skills
	Performance patterns	• Enable client to maintain appropriate medication schedule by providing a timer to aid with memory • Establish occupational performance patterns to maintain a healthy lifestyle after significant weight loss
	Context or contexts or physical environments	• Maintain safe and independent access for persons with low vision by recommending increased hallway lighting • During a natural disaster, work with facilities identified as "shelters" to provide play and leisure activities for displaced people to allow a constructive outlet and semblance of normalcy • Incorporate principles of universal design in homes to allow people to age in place
	Activity demands	• Maintain independent gardening for persons with arthritic hands by recommending tools with modified grips, long-handled tools, seating alternatives, raised gardens, and so forth
	Client factors **(body functions, body structures)**	• Provide multisensory activities in which nursing-home residents may participate to maintain alertness • Provide hand-based thumb splint for client use during periods of stressful or prolonged intensive activity to maintain pain-free joints
Modify (compensation, adaptation)[a]—An intervention approach directed at "finding ways to revise the current context or activity demands to support performance in the natural setting, [including] compensatory techniques, [such as]...enhancing some features to provide cues or reducing other features to reduce distractibility" (Dunn et al., 1998, p. 533).	**Performance patterns**	• Provide a visual schedule to help a student follow routines and transition easily between activities at home and school • Simplify task sequence to help a person with cognitive issues complete a morning self-care routine
	Context or contexts or physical environments	• Assist a family in determining requirements for building a ramp at home for a family member who is returning home after physical rehabilitation • Consult with builders in designing homes that will allow families the ability to provide living space for aging parents (e.g., bedroom and full bath on the main floor of a multilevel dwelling) • Modify the number of people in a room to decrease client's distractibility

TABLE 9. OCCUPATIONAL THERAPY INTERVENTION APPROACHES

(Continued)

Approach	Focus of Intervention	Examples
	Activity demands	• Adapt writing surface used in classroom by fourth grader by adding adjustable incline board • Assist a patient with a terminal illness and his or her family in modifying tasks to maintain engagement • Consult with school teams on placement of switches to increase students' access to computers, augmentative communication devices, environmental devices, and so forth • Provide a seat at the assembly station to allow a client with decreased standing tolerance to be able to continue to perform
Prevent (disability prevention)[a]—An intervention approach designed to address clients with or without a disability who are at risk for occupational performance problems. This approach is designed to prevent the occurrence or evolution of barriers to performance in context. Interventions may be directed at client, context, or activity variables (adapted from Dunn et al., 1998, p. 534).	**Performance skills**	• Prevent poor posture when sitting for prolonged periods by providing a chair with proper back support
	Performance patterns	• Aid in the prevention of illicit chemical substance use by introducing self-initiated routine strategies that support drug-free behavior
	Context or contexts or physical environments	• Prevent social isolation of employees by promoting participation in after-work group activities • Reduce risk of falls by modifying the environment and removing known hazards in the home (e.g., throw rugs)
	Activity demands	• Prevent back injury by providing instruction in proper lifting techniques
	Client factors (body functions, body structures)	• Prevent repetitive stress injury by suggesting that clients wear a wrist support splint when typing • Consultation with hotel chain to provide an ergonomics educational program designed to prevent back injuries in housekeepers

[a]Parallel language used in Moyers and Dale (2007, p. 34).

apy services (adapted from Maciejewski, Kawiecki, & Rockwood, 1997). Examples may include (1) a letter of thanks from the family of a child with spinal bifida (person); (2) a request for additional occupational therapy services at a homeless shelter for their clients (organizations); and (3) procurement of funds to implement support groups for caregivers of people with Alzheimer's disease throughout the United States (populations).

Outcomes

Supporting health and participation in life through engagement in occupation is the broad, overarching outcome of the occupational therapy intervention process. This outcome statement acknowledges the profession's belief that active engagement in occupation promotes, facilitates, and maintains health and participation. *Outcomes* are defined as important dimensions of health, attributed to interventions, and include the ability to function, health perceptions, and satisfaction with care (adapted from Request for Planning Ideas, 2001). Outcomes are the end-result of the occupational therapy process and describe what occupational therapy intervention can achieve with clients.

The three interrelated concepts included in the profession's overarching outcome are defined as

1. *Health*—"[A] positive concept emphasizing social and personal resources, as well as physical capacities" (WHO, 1986).
2. *Participation*—That is, "involvement in a life situation" (WHO, 2001, p. 10). Participation naturally occurs when clients are actively involved in carrying out occupations or daily life activities they find purposeful and meaningful in desired contexts. More specific outcomes of occupational therapy intervention (see Table 10) are multidimensional and support the end-result of participation.
3. *Engagement in occupation*—The commitment made to performance in occupations as the result of choice, motivation, and meaning and includes objective and subjective aspects of carrying out activities meaningful and purposeful to the individual person, organization, or population. Occupational therapy intervention focuses on creating or facilitating opportunities to engage in these occupations.

To determine the client's success in achieving health and participation in life through engagement in occupation, occupational therapy practitioners assess observable outcomes. This assessment takes into consideration the hypothesized relationships among various aspects of occupational performance. For example, a client's improved ability to embed performance skills into a routine (performance pattern) and improved strength or range of motion (body functions) enables engagement in managing a home (IADL).

Implicit in any outcome assessment used by occupational therapy practitioners are the client's beliefs systems and underlying assumptions regarding their desired occupational performance. The assessment tools and the variables measured often become the operational definition for the outcome. Therefore, occupational therapy practitioners select outcome assessments pertinent to the needs and desires of clients, congruent with the practitioner's theoretical model of practice, based on knowledge of the psychometric properties of standardized measures or the rationale and protocols of non-standardized measures and the available evidence. In addition, the client's perception of success in engaging in desired occupations is vital to any outcomes assessment. As a point of comparison and in collaboration with the client, the occupational therapist may revisit the occupational profile to assess change.

The benefits of occupational therapy are multifaceted and may occur in all aspects of the domain of concern. Supporting health and participation in life through engagement in occupation is the broad outcome of intervention. Clients' improved performance of occupations, perceived happiness, self-efficacy, and hopefulness about their life and abilities are valuable outcomes. For example, parents whose children received occupational therapy valued understanding their child's' behaviors in new ways and had greater perceived efficacy about their parenting (Cohn, 2001; Cohn, Miller, & Tickle-Degnan, 2000). Interventions designed for caregivers who provide care for people with dementia improve the quality of life for both the care recipient and the caregiver. Caregivers who received intervention reported fewer declines in the occupational performance of care recipients and less need for help and enhanced mastery and skill, self-efficacy, and well-being for themselves (Gitlin & Corcoran, 2005; Gitlin, Corcoran, Winter, Boyce, & Hauck, 2001; Gitlin et al., 2003).

Outcomes for people may include subjective impressions related to goals such as an improved outlook, confidence, hope, playfulness, self-efficacy, sustainability of valued occupations, resilience, or perceived well-being. Outcomes also may include measurable increments of progress in factors related to occupational performance such as skin integrity, amount of sleep, endurance, desire, initiation, balance, visual–motor skills, and at the participation level, activity participation and community re-integration. Outcomes for organizations may include increased workplace morale, productivity, reduced injuries, and improved worker satisfaction. Outcomes for populations may include health promotion, social justice, and access to services. The definitions and connotations of outcomes are specific to clients, groups, and organizations as well as to payers and regulators. Specific outcomes as well as documentation of those outcomes vary by practice setting and are influenced by the particular stakeholders in each setting.

The focus on outcomes is interwoven throughout the process of occupational therapy. The occupational therapist and client collaborate during the evaluation to identify the client's initial desired outcomes related to engagement in valued occupations or daily life activities. During intervention implementation and re-evaluation, the client and therapist and, when appropriate, the occupational therapy assistant, may modify desired outcomes to accommodate changing needs, contexts, and performance abilities. As further analysis of occupational performance and the development of the intervention plan occur, the occupational therapist and client may redefine the desired outcomes.

Implementation of the outcomes process includes the following steps:

1. Selecting types of outcomes and measures, including but not limited to **occupational performance, adaptation, health and wellness, participation, prevention, self-advocacy, quality of life, and occupational justice** (see Table 10).
   - Selecting outcome measures early in the intervention process (see "Evaluation" above)
   - Selecting outcome measures that are valid, reliable, and appropriately sensitive to change in the client's occupational performance and are consistent with the outcomes
   - Selecting outcome measures or instruments for a particular client that are congruent with client goals
   - Selecting outcome measures that are based on their actual or purported ability to predict future outcomes.

2. Using outcomes to measure progress and adjust goals and interventions
   - Comparing progress toward goal achievement to outcomes throughout the intervention process
   - Assessing outcome use and results to make decisions about the future direction of intervention (e.g., continue intervention, modify intervention, discontinue intervention, provide follow-up, refer to other services).

TABLE 10. TYPES OF OUTCOMES

The examples listed specify how the broad outcome of engagement in occupation may be operationalized. The examples are not intended to be all-inclusive.

Outcome	Description
Occupational performance	The act of doing and accomplishing a selected activity or occupation that results from the dynamic transaction among the client, the context, and the activity. Improving or enabling skills and patterns in occupational performance leads to engagement in occupations or activities (adapted in part from Law et al., 1996, p. 16).
	• *Improvement*—Used when a performance limitation is present. These outcomes document increased occupational performance for the person, organization, or population. Outcome examples may include (1) the ability of a child with autism to play interactively with a peer (person); (2) the ability of an older adult to return to the home from a skilled-nursing facility (person); (3) decreased incidence of back strain in nursing personnel as a result of an in-service education program in body mechanics for carrying out job duties that require bending, lifting, and so forth (organizations); and (d) construction of accessible playground facilities for all children in local city parks (populations).
	• *Enhancement*—Used when a performance limitation is not currently present. These outcomes document the development of performance skills and performance patterns that augment existing performance or prevent potential problems from developing in life occupations. Outcome examples may include (1) increased confidence and competence of teenage mothers to parent their children as a result of structured social groups and child development classes (person); (2) increased membership of the local senior citizen center as a result of diverse social wellness and exercise programs (organization); (3) increased ability by school staff to address and manage school-age youth violence as a result of conflict resolution training to address "bullying" (organizations); and (4) increased opportunities for seniors to participate in community activities due to ride share programs (populations).
Adaptation	A change in response approach that the client makes when encountering an occupational challenge. "This change is implemented when the [client's] customary response approaches are found inadequate for producing some degree of mastery over the challenge" (adapted from Schultz & Schkade, 1997, p. 474). Examples of adaptation outcomes include (1) clients modifying their behaviors to earn privileges at an adolescent treatment facility (person); (2) a company redesigning the daily schedule to allow for an even workflow and to decrease times of high stress (organizations); and (3) a community making available accessible public transportation and erecting public and "reserved" benches for older adults to socialize and rest (populations).
Health and wellness	Health is a resource for everyday life, not the objective of living. For individuals, it is a state of physical, mental, and social well-being, as well as a positive concept emphasizing social and personal resources and physical capacities (WHO, 1986). Health of organizations and populations includes these individual aspects but also includes social responsibility of members to society as a whole. *Wellness* is "[a]n active process through which individuals [organizations or populations] become aware of and make choices toward a more successful existence" (Hettler, 1984, p. 1170). Wellness is more than a lack of disease symptoms; it is a state of mental and physical balance and fitness (adapted from *Taber's Cyclopedic Medical Dictionary,* 1997, p. 2110). Outcome examples may include (1) participation in community outings by a client with schizophrenia in a group home (person); (2) implementation of a company-wide program to identify problems and solutions for balance among work, leisure, and family life (organizations); and (3) decreased incidence of childhood obesity (populations).
Participation	Engagement in desired occupations in ways that are personally satisfying and congruent with expectations within the culture.

TABLE 10. TYPES OF OUTCOMES

(Continued)

Outcome	Description
Prevention	"[H]ealth promotion is equally and essentially concerned with creating the conditions necessary for health at individual, structural, social, and environmental levels through an understanding of the determinants of health: peace, shelter, education, food, income, a stable ecosystem, sustainable resources, social justice, and equity" (Kronenberg, Algado, & Pollard, 2005, p. 441). Occupational therapy promotes a healthy lifestyle at the individual, group, organizational, community (societal), and governmental or policy level (adapted from Brownson & Scaffa, 2001). Outcome examples may include (1) appropriate seating and play area for a child with orthopedic impairments (person); (2) implementation of a program of leisure and educational activities for a drop-in center for adults with severe mental illness (organizations); and (3) access to occupational therapy services in underserved areas regardless cultural or ethnic backgrounds (populations).
Quality of life	The dynamic appraisal of the client's life satisfaction (perceptions of progress toward one's goals), hope (the real or perceived belief that one can move toward a goal through selected pathways), self-concept (the composite of beliefs and feelings about oneself), health and functioning (including health status, self-care capabilities, and socioeconomic factors, e.g., vocation, education, income; adapted from Radomski, 1995; Zhan, 1992). Outcomes may include (1) full and active participation of a deaf child from a hearing family during a recreational activity (person); (2) residents being able to prepare for outings and travel independently as a result of independent-living skills training for care providers of a group (organization); and (3) formation of a lobby to support opportunities for social networking, advocacy activities, and sharing scientific information for stroke survivors and their families (population).
Role competence	The ability to effectively meet the demands of roles in which the client engages.
Self-advocacy	Actively promoting or supporting oneself or others (individuals, organizations, or populations); requires an understanding of strengths and needs, identification of goals, knowledge of legal rights and responsibilities, and communicating these aspects to others (adapted from Dawson, 2007). Outcomes may include (1) a student with a learning disability requesting and receiving reasonable accommodations such as textbooks on tape (person); (2) a grassroots employee committee requesting and procuring ergonomically designed keyboards for their computers at work (organization); and (3) people with disabilities advocating for universal design with all public and private construction (population).
Occupational justice	Access to and participation in the full range of meaningful and enriching occupations afforded to others. Includes opportunities for social inclusion and the resources to participate in occupations to satisfy personal, health, and societal needs (adapted from Townsend & Wilcock, 2004). Outcomes may include (1) people with intellectual disabilities serving on an advisory board to establish programs offered by a community recreation center (person); (2) workers who have enough of break time to have lunch with their young children at day care centers (organization); (3) people with persistent mental illness welcomed by community recreation center due to anti-stigma campaign (organization); and (4) alternative adapted housing options for older adult to "age in place" (populations).

Historical and Future Perspectives on the *Occupational Therapy Practice Framework*

The *Occupational Therapy Practice Framework* emerged out of the examination of documents related to *Uniform Terminology*. The first document was the *Occupational Therapy Product Output Reporting System and Uniform Terminology for Reporting Occupational Therapy Services* (AOTA, 1979). This original text created consistent terminology that could be used in official documents, practice, and education. The second edition of *Uniform Terminology for Occupational Therapy* (AOTA, 1989) was adopted by the AOTA Representative Assembly (RA) and published in 1989. The document focused on delineating and defining only the occupational performance areas and occupational performance components that are addressed in occupational therapy direct services. The last revision, *Uniform Terminology for Occupational Therapy—Third Edition* (UT–III; AOTA, 1994), was adopted by the RA in 1994 and was "expanded to reflect current practice and to incorporate contextual aspects of performance" (p. 1047). Each revision reflected changes in current practice and provided consistent terminology that could be used by the profession. Originally a document that responded to a federal requirement to develop a uniform reporting system, the text gradually shifted to describing and outlining the domain of concern of occupational therapy.

In the fall of 1998, the AOTA Commission on Practice (COP) embarked on the journey that culminated in the *Occupational Therapy Practice Framework: Domain and Process* (*Framework; AOTA, 2002b). During that time, AOTA published *The Guide to Occupational Therapy Practice* (Moyers, 1999), which outlined many of the contemporary shifts of the day, and the COP carefully reviewed this document. In light of those changes and the feedback received during the review process of *UT–III,* the COP decided that practice needs had changed and that it was time to develop a different kind of document.

Because the *Framework* is an official AOTA document, it is reviewed on a 5-year cycle. During the review period, the COP collected feedback from membership, scholars, authors, and practitioners to determine the needed changes. Revisions ensued to maintain the integrity of the *Framework* and change only what was necessary. The revisions reflect the contributions of the current COP, refinement of the writing of the document, and emerging concepts and changes in occupational therapy. The rationale for specific changes is listed in Table 11.

The *Framework* is an evolving document and will undergo another review in 5 years, which again will examine the usefulness of the document and need for further refinements and change. The next iteration likely will change as the result of the profession's progress toward AOTA's 2017 *Centennial Vision* of "occupational therapy [as] a powerful, widely recognized, science-driven, and evidence-based profession with a globally connected and diverse workforce meeting society's occupational needs" (AOTA, 2007a).

Although the *Framework* represents the latest in the profession's evolution, it builds on a set of values that the profession of occupational therapy has held since its founding in 1917. This founding vision had at its center a profound belief in the value of therapeutic occupations as a way to remediate illness and maintain health (Slagle, 1924). It emphasized the importance of establishing a therapeutic relationship with each client and designing a treatment plan based on knowledge about the individual's environment, values, goals, and desires (Meyer, 1922). And it advocated for a scientific practice based on systematic observation

TABLE 11. SUMMARY OF SIGNIFICANT *FRAMEWORK* REVISIONS

Domain Area	Change	Intended Benefit	Rationale
Title	Supporting Health and Participation in Life Through Engagement in Occupation	Increase clarity of intent	Changing from the original title of Figure 1, Engagement in Occupation to Support Participation in Context or Contexts, emphasizes that the vehicle for occupational therapy to health and participation is engagement in occupation. Deleted "in context" to shorten the title, because it is discussed in the text and implied by the definition of occupation.
Spirituality	Move from Context to Client Factor	Reflect the way in which occupational therapy practitioners view and analyze meaning, values, and beliefs of a broad range of clients	More commonly, individuals consider spirituality residing within the client rather than as part of a context. Moreira-Almeida and Koenig (2006) discussed spirituality, religion, and personal beliefs as components of quality of life. Their definitions are included in the text.
Performance Skills	Broaden categories with more generic language	Provide language inclusive of a broad range of assessments and interventions as well as commonly used terms in the literature related to skills	Based on her work with the Assessment of Motor and Process Skills (AMPS), Fisher (2006) provides the most distinct categories and definitions of skill functions. An attempt is made in this revision to address critiques of the 2002 *Framework* that Fisher's categories are limited. To broaden skill categories to more generic and inclusive language, the COP considered at length the differences among *body functions, abilities, capacities, skills, levels of skills,* and *components of occupations.* In most articles, authors use terms related to skills interchangeably with *abilities* and *capacities,* confusing the issue. To add to the difficulty in providing readers with a list of performance skills, the proposed categories are not completely distinct from one another. Without creating an artificial distinction between categories, it is necessary to tolerate the overlap in these skill areas. For example, according to Filley (2001), "skill learning and acquisition of praxis may well be identical phenomena" (p. 89). Perception often is discussed in cognitive literature; social cognition implies a specific skill set, as do social–emotional skills; and sensory–motor skills are often considered together.
Rest and Sleep	Move from ADL to Area of Occupation	Highlight the importance of rest and sleep, especially as they relate to supporting or hindering engagement in other areas of occupation	Rest and sleep are two of the four main categories of occupation discussed by Adolf Meyer (1922). Unlike any other area of occupation, all people rest as a result of engaging in occupations and engage in sleep for multiple hours per day throughout their life span. Within the occupation of rest and sleep are activities such as preparing the self and environment for sleep, interactions with others who share the sleeping space, reading or listening to music to fall asleep, napping, dreaming, nighttime care of toileting needs, nighttime caregiving duties, and ensuring safety. Sleep significantly affects all other areas of occupation. Jonsson (2007) suggested that providing sleep prominence in the framework as an area of occupation will promote the consideration of lifestyle choices as an important aspect of participation and health.
Context	Change to context and environment	Allow use of broader language consistent with external audiences and existing occupational therapy theories	The terms *context* and *environment* are not the same but often are used interchangeably. In the general literature, environment is used more frequently. Occupational therapy theories often use environment rather than context. This change allows for a cross-walk between the two terms. In the narrative, context is used to include environment.

(Continued)

247

TABLE 11. SUMMARY OF SIGNIFICANT *FRAMEWORK* REVISIONS

(Continued)

Domain Area	Change	Intended Benefit	Rationale
Occupational justice	Include narrative about the importance of social justice specific to occupational therapy	Highlight the importance of occupational therapy values in the global community	The discussion of concepts of occupational justice encourages practitioners to examine the multiple contributors to engagement and social participation. Townsend and Wilcock (2004) are leaders in our understanding of this important concept. Gupta and Walloch (2006) provide a nice summary of this work.

Process Area	Change	Intended Benefit	Rationale
Client	Include person, organization, population	Broaden the scope of occupational therapy services and provides language consistent with advocacy and policy-making groups.	Consistent with *The Guide to Occupational Therapy Practice* (Moyers & Dale, 2007). Language in occupational therapy literature often is focused on the individual or person. This change highlights the way in which occupational therapy contributes to groups of persons, populations, and organizations, often in nontraditional practice arenas.
Clinical Reasoning	Identify the way in which the practitioner's view of the client is informed via knowledge, skills, and evidence	Highlight the importance of the practitioner's problem-solving skills in the interaction with the client	Clinical reasoning was expanded in the document to emphasize its importance throughout the occupational therapy process. Intrinsic to any interaction between the practitioner and the client is the critical thinking implicit within clinical-reasoning skills that inform and guide the intervention.
Activity Analysis Activity Synthesis	Include discussion about analyzing activities in and of themselves and in relation to the client	Highlight the importance of this critical skill that informs intervention	Occupational therapy practitioners have a high level of skill in identifying the demands of an activity and then synthesizing this information by comparing it with the client's needs and abilities to identify specific occupational performance difficulties.
Self-Advocacy	Include self-advocacy as an outcome	Provide focus on empowerment as a key feature in health and participation	When working with individuals, populations, or organizations, occupational therapy provides intervention, which promotes self-advocacy as a means toward improved health and participation.
Evidence-based practice	Emphasize the role of research in informing practice	Articulate the value of a science-driven profession	Occupational therapy is a profession founded on basic and applied science informing practice.

TABLE 11. SUMMARY OF SIGNIFICANT *FRAMEWORK* REVISIONS

(Continued)

Terminology	Change	Intended Benefit	Rationale
Transactive and interactive	Include the idea that areas of the domain are transactive and the client is interactive	Create distinction between the relationships of concepts within the domain and interactions between clients and practitioners	*Transactive* is used to describe the dynamic way in which the areas of the occupational therapy domain intersect. *Interactive* is the way in which clients and occupational therapy practitioners engage together or with others. Occupational therapy is therefore the interaction between practitioners and clients within one or more areas of the domain to meet the overarching objective of engagement in occupation to support health and participation.
Activity/ occupation and purposeful activity	Use occupation to include activity in the narrative	To increase readability of the document	Recognizing the work of scholars in the field, the authors acknowledge the differences in activity and occupation. However, this document does not engage in this debate. In the *Framework,* occupation is used to include activity. Activity is used specific to tasks considered in isolation of the client. Purposeful activity is used to describe a type of intervention determined by the therapist to be "purposeful" for achieving the goals of intervention, not in judging whether or not a client's chosen activity is purposeful or not.

Outcomes	Change	Intended Benefit	Rationale
Outcomes	Added occupational justice and self-advocacy to Table 10: Types of Outcomes	To acknowledge occupational therapy's commitment to occupational justice and self-determination for all people	Recognizing that an important outcome of occupational therapy intervention may be enabling all individuals to be able to meet basic needs and to have equal opportunities and life chances to reach toward his or her potential through engagement in diverse and meaningful occupation.

and treatment (Dunton, 1934). Paraphrased using today's lexicon, the founders proposed a vision that was occupation-based, client-centered, contextual, and evidence-based—the vision articulated in the *Framework* today.

Acknowledgments

The Commission on Practice (COP) expresses sincere appreciation to all those who participated in the development of the *Occupational Therapy Practice Framework: Domain and Process, 2nd Edition.* This new edition represents the combined efforts of numerous esteemed colleagues providing a collective description of the architecture of occupational therapy within which the ecology of the profession occurs. In addition to those named below, the COP wishes to thank everyone who has contributed to the dialogue, feedback, and concepts presented in the document.

Sincere and heartfelt appreciation is extended to Wendy Schoen for all her support; to AOTA's past-president, Carolyn Baum, PhD, OTR/L, FAOTA, and current president Penelope A. Moyers Cleveland, EdD, OTR/L, BCMH, FAOTA, for their insights and direction; the Representative Assembly Coordinating Council (RACC) members, especially Brent Braveman, PhD, OTR/L, FAOTA, and Wendy Hildenbrand, MPH, OTR/L, FAOTA; to those providing significant content and reviews, including Ina Elfant Asher, MS, OTR/L; Kathleen Barker Schwartz, EdD, OTR/L, FAOTA; Mary Frances Baxter, PhD, OTR/L; Christine Beall, OTR/L; Stefanie

Bodison, MA, OTR/L; Sarah Burton, MS, OT/L; Denea S. Butts, OTD, OTR/L; Jane Case-Smith, EdD, OTR, BCP, FAOTA; Florence Clark, PhD, OTR/L, FAOTA; Gloria Frolek Clark, MS, OTR/L, FAOTA; Elizabeth Crepeau, PhD, OTR, FAOTA; Anne E. Dickerson, PhD, OTR/L, FAOTA; Winifred Dunn, PhD, OTR, FAOTA; Lisa Ann Fagan, MS, OTR/L; Anne G. Fisher, PhD, OTR, FAOTA; Naomi Gil, MSc, OT; Lou Ann Griswald, PhD, OTR, FAOTA; Sharon A. Gutman, PhD, OTR/L; Jim Hinojosa, PhD, OT, FAOTA; Hans Jonsson, PhD, OT(Reg); Paula Kramer, PhD, OTR/L, FAOTA; Patricia LaVesser, PhD, OTR/L; Donna Lucente-Surber, OTR/L; Stephen H. Luster, MS, OTR, CHT; Zoe Mailloux, MA, OTR/L, FAOTA; Jean McKinley-Vargas, MS, OTR/L; David Nelson, PhD, OTR/L, FAOTA; L. Diane Parham, PhD, OTR/L, FAOTA; Marta Pelczarski, OTR; Kathlyn L. Reed, PhD, OTR, FAOTA; Barbara Schell, PhD, OTR/L, FAOTA; Camille Skubik-Peplaski, MS, OTR/L, BCP; Virginia Carroll Stoffel, PhD, OT, BCMH, FAOTA; Marjorie Vogeley, OTR/L; and Naomi Weintraub, PhD, OTR.

Glossary

A

Activities of daily living (ADLs)

Activities oriented toward taking care of one's own body (adapted from Rogers & Holm, 1994, pp. 181–202). **ADL** also is referred to as *basic activities of daily living (BADL)* and *personal activities of daily living (PADL)*. These activities are "fundamental to living in a social world; they enable basic survival and well-being" (Christiansen & Hammecker, 2001, p. 156) (see Table 1 for definitions of terms).

Activity (Activities)

A class of human actions that are goal directed.

Activity analysis

"...addresses the typical demands of an activity, the range of skills involved in its performance, and the various cultural meanings that might be ascribed to it" (Crepeau, 2003, p. 192).

Activity demands

The aspects of an activity, which include the objects and their physical properties, space, social demands, sequencing or timing, required actions or skills, and required underlying body functions and body structures needed to carry out the activity (see Table 3).

Adaptation

The response approach the client makes encountering an occupational challenge. "This change is implemented when the individual's customary response approaches are found inadequate for producing some degree of mastery over the challenge" (Schultz & Schkade, 1997, p. 474).

Advocacy

The "pursuit of influencing outcomes—including public policy and resource allocation decisions within political, economic, and social systems and institutions—that directly affect people's lives" (Advocacy Institute, 2001, as cited in Goodman-Lavey & Dunbar, 2003, p. 422).

Analysis of occupational performance

Part of the evaluation process. Collecting information via assessment tools designed to observe, measure, and inquire about selected factors that support or hinder occupational performance.

Areas of occupations

Various kinds of life activities in which people engage, including the following categories: ADLs, IADLs, rest and sleep, education, work, play, leisure, and social participation (see Table 1).

Assessment

"Specific tools or instruments that are used during the evaluation process" (AOTA, 2005, p. 663).

B

Belief

Any cognitive content held as true by the client (Moyers & Dale, 2007).

Body functions

"The physiological functions of body systems (including psychological functions)" (WHO, 2001, p. 10) (see Table 2).

Body structures

"Anatomical parts of the body such as organs, limbs, and their components [that support body function]" (WHO, 2001, p. 10) (see Table 2).

C

Client

The entity that receives occupational therapy services. Clients may include (1) individuals and other persons relevant to the individual's life, including family, caregivers, teachers, employers, and others who also may help or be served indirectly; (2) organizations such as business, industries, or agencies; and (3) populations within a community (Moyers & Dale, 2007).

Client-centered approach

An orientation that honors the desires and priorities of clients in designing and implementing interventions (adapted from Dunn, 2000a, p. 4).

Client factors

Those factors residing within the client that may affect performance in areas of occupation. Client factors include values, beliefs, and spirituality; body functions; and body structures (see Table 2).

Clinical reasoning

"Complex multi-faceted cognitive process used by practitioners to plan, direct, perform, and reflect on intervention" (Crepeau et al., 2003, p. 1027).

Communication and social skills

Actions or behaviors a person uses to communicate and interact with others in an interactive environment (Fisher, 2006).

Cognitive skills

Actions or behaviors a client uses to plan and manage the performance of an activity.

Context

Refers to a variety of interrelated conditions within and surrounding the client that influence performance. Contexts include cultural, personal, temporal, and virtual (see Table 6).

Co-occupations

Activities that implicitly involve at least two people (Zemke & Clark, 1996).

Cultural (context)

"Customs, beliefs, activity patterns, behavior standards, and expectations accepted by the society of which the [client] is a member. Includes ethnicity and values as well as political aspects, such as laws that affect access to resources and affirm personal rights. Also includes opportunities for education, employment, and economic support" (AOTA, 1994, p. 1054).

D

Domain

A sphere of activity, concern, or function (*American Heritage Dictionary*, 2006).

E

Education

Includes learning activities needed when participating in an environment (see Table 1).

Emotional regulation skills

Actions or behaviors a client uses to identify, manage, and express feelings while engaging in activities or interacting with others.

Engagement

The act of sharing activities.

Environment

The external physical and social environment that surrounds the client and in which the client's daily life occupations occur (see Table 6).

Evaluation

"The process of obtaining and interpreting data necessary for intervention. This includes planning for and documenting the evaluation process and results" (AOTA, 2005, p. 663).

G

Goals

"The result or achievement toward which effort is directed; aim; end" (*Webster's Encyclopedic Unabridged Dictionary of the English Language*, 1994, p. 605).

H

Habits

"Automatic behavior that is integrated into more complex patterns that enable people to function on a day-to-day basis..." (Neistadt & Crepeau, 1998, p. 869). Habits can be useful, dominating, or impoverished and either support or interfere with performance in areas of occupation.

Health

Health is a resource for everyday life, not the objective of living. It is a state of complete physical, mental, and social well-being, as well as a positive concept emphasizing social and personal resources, as well as physical capacities (adapted from WHO, 1986).

Health promotion

"[T]he process of enabling people to increase control over, and to improve, their health. To reach a state of complete physical, mental, and social well-being, an individual or group must be able to identify and realize aspirations, to satisfy needs, and to change or cope with the environment" (WHO, 1986).

"[C]reating the conditions necessary for health at individual, structural, social, and environmental levels through an understanding of the determinants of health: peace, shelter, education, food, income, a stable ecosystem, sustainable resources, social justice, and equity" (Trentham & Cockburn, 2005, p. 441).

Hope

The real or perceived belief that one can move toward a goal through selected pathways (Lopez et al., 2004).

I

Identity

"A composite definition of the self and includes an interpersonal aspect...an aspect of possibility or potential (who we might become), and a values aspect (that suggests importance and provides a stable basis for choices and decisions).... Identity can be viewed as the superordinate view of ourselves that includes both self-esteem and self-concept but also importantly reflects and is influenced by the larger social world in which we find ourselves" (Christiansen, 1999, pp. 548–549).

Independence

"A self-directed state of being characterized by an individual's ability to participate in necessary and preferred occupations in a satisfying manner irrespective of the amount or kind of external assistance desired or required

- Self-determination is essential to achieving and maintaining independence;
- An individual's independence is unrelated to whether he or she performs the activities related to an occupation himself or herself, performs the activities in an adapted or modified environment, makes use of various devices or alternative strategies, or oversees activity completion by others;
- Independence is defined by the individual's culture and values, support systems, and ability to direct his or her life; and
- An individual's independence should not be based on preestablished criteria, perception of outside observers, or how independence is accomplished" (AOTA, 2002a, p. 660).

Instrumental activities of daily living (IADLs)

Activities to support daily life within the home and community that often require more complex interactions than self-care used in ADL (see Table 1).

Interdependence

The "reliance that people have on each other as a natural consequence of group living" (Christiansen & Townsend, 2004, p. 277). "Interdependence engenders a spirit of social inclusion, mutual aid, and a moral commitment and responsibility to recognize and support difference" (p. 146).

Interests

"What one finds enjoyable or satisfying to do" (Kielhofner, 2002, p. 25).

Intervention

The process and skilled actions taken by occupational therapy practitioners in collaboration with the client to facilitate engagement in occupation related to health and participation. The intervention process includes the plan, implementation, and review (see Table 7).

Intervention approaches

Specific strategies selected to direct the process of interventions that are based on the client's desired outcome, evaluation date, and evidence (see Table 9).

L

Leisure

"A nonobligatory activity that is intrinsically motivated and engaged in during discretionary time, that is, time not committed to obligatory occupations such as work, self-care, or sleep" (Parham & Fazio, 1997, p. 250).

M

Motor and praxis skills

Motor

Actions or behaviors a client uses to move and physically interact with tasks, objects, contexts, and environments (adapted from Fisher, 2006). Includes planning, sequencing, and executing novel movements.

Also see Praxis.

O

Occupation

"Goal-directed pursuits that typically extend over time have meaning to the performance, and involve multiple tasks" (Christiansen et al., 2005, p. 548).

"Daily activities that reflect cultural values, provide structure to living, and meaning to individuals; these activities meet human needs for self-care, enjoyment, and participation in society" (Crepeau et al., 2003, p. 1031).

"Activities that people engage in throughout their daily lives to fulfill their time and give life

meaning. Occupations involve mental abilities and skills and may or may not have an observable physical dimension" (Hinojosa & Kramer, 1997, p. 865).

"[A]ctivities…of everyday life, named, organized, and given value and meaning by individuals and a culture. Occupation is everything people do to occupy themselves, including looking after themselves…enjoying life…and contributing to the social and economic fabric of their communities" (Law et al., 1997, p. 32).

"A dynamic relationship among an occupational form, a person with a unique developmental structure, subjective meanings and purpose, and the resulting occupational performance" (Nelson & Jepson-Thomas, 2003, p. 90).

"[C]hunks of daily activity that can be named in the lexicon of the culture" (Zemke & Clark, 1996, p. vii).

Occupation-based intervention

A type of occupational therapy intervention—a client-centered intervention in which the occupational therapy practitioner and client collaboratively select and design activities that have specific relevance or meaning to the client and support the client's interests, need, health, and participation in daily life.

Occupational justice

"Justice related to opportunities and resources required for occupational participation sufficient to satisfy personal needs and full citizenship" (Christiansen & Townsend, 2004, p. 278). To experience meaning and enrichment in one's occupations; to participate in a range of occupations for health and social inclusion; to make choices and share decision-making power in daily life; and to receive equal privileges for diverse participation in occupations (Townsend & Wilcock, 2004).

Occupational performance

The act of doing and accomplishing a selected activity or occupation that results from the dynamic transaction among the client, the context, and the activity. Improving or enabling skills and patterns in occupational performance leads to engagement in occupations or activities (adapted in part from Law et al., 1996, p. 16).

Occupational profile
A summary of the client's occupational history, patterns of daily living, interests, values, and needs.

Occupational science
An interdisciplinary academic discipline in the social and behavioral sciences dedicated to the study of the form, the function, and the meaning of human occupations (Zemke & Clark, 1996).

Occupational therapy
The practice of occupational therapy means the therapeutic use of everyday life activities (occupations) with individuals or groups for the purpose of participation in roles and situations in home, school, workplace, community, and other settings. Occupational therapy services are provided for the purpose of promoting health and wellness and to those who have or are at risk for developing an illness, injury, disease, disorder, condition, impairment, disability, activity limitation, or participation restriction. Occupational therapy addresses the physical, cognitive, psychosocial, sensory, and other aspects of performance in a variety of contexts to support engagement in everyday life activities that affect health, well-being, and quality of life (AOTA, 2004a).

Organizations
Entities with a common purpose or enterprise such as businesses, industries, or agencies.

Outcomes
What occupational therapy actually achieves for the consumers of its services (adapted from Fuhrer, 1987). Change desired by the client that can focus on any area of the client's occupational performance (adapted from Kramer, McGonigel, & Kaufman, 1991).

P

Participation
"Involvement in a life situation" (WHO, 2001, p. 10).

Performance patterns
Patterns of behavior related to daily life activities that are habitual or routine. They can include habits, routines, rituals, and roles (see Table 5).

Performance skills
The abilities clients demonstrate in the actions they perform (see Table 4).

Persons
Individuals, including families, caregivers, teachers, employees, and relevant others.

Personal
"Features of the individual that are not part of a health condition or health status" (WHO, 2001, p. 17). Personal context includes age, gender, socioeconomic, and educational status. Can also include organizational levels (i.e., volunteers, employees) and population levels (i.e., members of a society).

Physical environment
The natural and built nonhuman environment and objects in them.

Play
"Any spontaneous or organized activity that provides enjoyment, entertainment, amusement, or diversion" (Parham & Fazio, 1997, p. 252) (see Table 1).

Populations
Large groups as a whole, such as refugees, homeless veterans, and people who need wheelchairs.

Praxis
Skilled purposeful movements (Heilman & Rothi, 1993). The ability to carry out sequential motor acts as part of an overall plan rather than individual acts (Liepmann, 1920). The ability to carry out learned

motor activity, including following through on a verbal command, visual spatial construction, ocular and oral–motor skills, imitation of a person or an object, and sequencing actions (Ayres, 1985; Filley, 2001). Organization of temporal sequences of actions within the spatial context; which form meaningful occupations (Blanche & Parham, 2002).
Also see Motor.

Preparatory methods

Methods and techniques that prepare the client for occupational performance. Used in preparation for or concurrently with purposeful and occupation-based activities.

Prevention

"[H]ealth promotion is equally and essentially concerned with creating the conditions necessary for health at individual, structural, social, and environmental levels through an understanding of the determinants of health: peace, shelter, education, food, income, a stable ecosystem, sustainable resources, social justice, and equity" (Kronenberg, Algado, & Pollard, 2005, p. 441).

Promoting a healthy lifestyle at the individual, group, organizational, community (societal), governmental/policy level (adapted from Brownson & Scaffa, 2001).

Process

A description of the way in which occupational therapy practitioners operationalize their expertise to provide services to clients. The process includes evaluation, intervention, and outcome monitoring; occurs within the purview of the domain; and involves collaboration among the occupational therapist, occupational therapy assistant, and the client.

Purposeful activity

A goal-directed behavior or activity within a therapeutically designed context that leads to an occu-

pation or occupations. Specifically selected activities that allow the client to develop skills that enhance occupational engagement.

Q

Quality of life

A client's dynamic appraisal of life satisfactions (perceptions of progress toward identified goals), self-concept (the composite of beliefs and feelings about themselves), health and functioning (including health status, self-care capabilities), and socioeconomic factors (e.g., vocation, education, income) (adapted from Radomski, 1995; Zhan, 1992).

R

Re-evaluation

A reassessment of the client's performance and goals to determine the type and amount of change.

Rest

Quiet and effortless actions that interrupt physical and mental activity, resulting in a relaxed state (Nurit & Michel, 2003, p. 227).

Ritual

Symbolic actions with spiritual, cultural, or social meaning, contributing to the client's identity and reinforcing the client's values and beliefs (Fiese et al., 2002; Segal, 2004). Rituals are highly symbolic, with a strong affective component and representative of a collection of events.

Roles

Roles are sets of behaviors expected by society, shaped by culture, and may be further conceptualized and defined by the client.

Routines

Patterns of behavior that are observable, regular, repetitive, and that provide structure for daily life. They can be satisfying, promoting, or damaging. Routines require momentary time commitment and are embedded in cultural and ecological contexts (Fiese et al., 2002; Segal, 2004).

S

Self-advocacy

Understanding your strengths and needs, identifying your personal goals, knowing your legal rights and responsibilities, and communicating these to others (Dawson, 2007).

Sensory–perceptual skills

Actions or behaviors a client uses to locate, identify, and respond to sensations and to select, interpret, associate, organize, and remember sensory events via sensations that include visual, auditory, proprioceptive, tactile, olfactory, gustatory, and vestibular sensations.

Sleep

"A natural periodic state of rest for the mind and body, in which the eyes usually close and consciousness is completely or partially lost, so that there is a decrease in bodily movement and responsiveness to external stimuli. During sleep the brain in humans and other mammals undergoes a characteristic cycle of brain-wave activity that includes intervals of dreaming" (*The Free Dictionary*, 2007) (see Table 1).

A series of activities resulting in going to sleep, staying asleep, and ensuring health and safety through participation in sleep involving engagement with the physical and social environments.

Social environment

Is constructed by the presence, relationships, and expectations of persons, organizations, and populations.

Social justice

"Ethical distribution and sharing of resources, rights, and responsibilities between people, recognizing their equal worth as citizens. [It recognizes] 'their equal right to be able to meet basic needs, the need to spread opportunities and life chances as widely as possible, and finally the requirement that we reduce and where possible eliminate unjustified inequalities'" (Commission on Social Justice, 1994, p. 1).

"The promotion of social and economic change to increase individual, community, and political awareness, resources, and opportunity for health and well-being" (Wilcock, 2006, p. 344).

Social participation

"Organized patterns of behavior that are characteristic and expected of an individual in a given position within a social system" (Mosey, 1996, p. 340) (see Table 1).

Spirituality

"[T]he personal quest for understanding answers to ultimate questions about life, about meaning, and about relationship with the sacred or transcendent, which may (or may not) lead to or arise from the development of religious rituals and the formation of community" (Moreira-Almeida & Koenig, 2006, p. 844).

T

Temporal

"Location of occupational performance in time" (Neistadt & Crepeau, 1998, p. 292). The experience of time as shaped by engagement in occupations. The temporal aspects of occupations "which contribute to the patterns of daily occupations" are "the rhythm...tempo...synchronization...duration...and sequence" (Larson & Zemke, 2004, p. 82; Zemke, 2004, p. 610). It includes stages of life, time of day, duration, rhythm of activity, or history.

Transactional

A process that involves two or more individuals or elements that reciprocally and continually influence and affect one another through the ongoing relationship (Dickie, Cutchin, & Humphry, 2006).

V

Values

Principles, standards, or qualities considered worthwhile or desirable by the client who holds them (Moyers & Dale, 2007).

Virtual

Environment in which communication occurs by means of airways or computers and an absence of physical contact. Includes simulated or real-time or near-time existence of an environment, such as chat rooms, email, video conferencing, and radio transmissions.

W

Wellness

"An active process through which individuals become aware of and make choices toward a more successful existence" (Hettler, 1984, p. 1117). Wellness is more than a lack of disease symptoms. It is a state of mental and physical balance and fitness (adapted from *Taber's Cyclopedic Medical Dictionary*, 1997, p. 2110).

Work

"Activities needed for engaging in remunerative employment or volunteer activities" (Mosey, 1996, p. 341) (see Table 1).

References

American Heritage Dictionary of the English Language (4th ed.). (2006). Boston: Houghton-Mifflin.

American Occupational Therapy Association. (1979). *Occupational therapy product output reporting system and uniform terminology for reporting occupational therapy services.* (Available from American Occupational Therapy Association, 4720 Montgomery Lane, PO Box 31220, Bethesda, MD 20824-1220)

American Occupational Therapy Association. (1989). *Uniform terminology for occupational therapy* (2nd ed.). (Available from American Occupational Therapy Association, 4720 Montgomery Lane, PO Box 31220, Bethesda, MD 20824-1220)

American Occupational Therapy Association. (1994). Uniform terminology for occupational therapy (3rd ed.). *American Journal of Occupational Therapy, 48,* 1047–1054.

American Occupational Therapy Association. (2002a). Broadening the construct of independence [Position Paper]. *American Journal of Occupational Therapy, 56,* 660.

American Occupational Therapy Association. (2002b). Occupational therapy practice framework: Domain and process. *American Journal of Occupational Therapy, 56,* 609–639.

American Occupational Therapy Association. (2004a). *Definition of occupational therapy practice for the AOTA Model Practice Act.* Bethesda, MD: Author. (Available from the State Affairs Group, 4720 Montgomery Lane, PO Box 31220, Bethesda, MD 20824–1220)

American Occupational Therapy Association. (2004b). Guidelines for supervision, roles, and responsibilities during the delivery of occupational therapy services. *American Journal of Occupational Therapy, 58,* 663–667.

American Occupational Therapy Association. (2004c). Occupational therapy's commitment to nondiscrimination and inclusion (edited 2004). *American Journal of Occupational Therapy, 58,* 666.

American Occupational Therapy Association. (2005). Standards of practice for occupational therapy. *American Journal of Occupational Therapy, 59,* 663–665.

American Occupational Therapy Association. (2006). Policy 1.44: Categories of occupational therapy personnel. In *Policy manual* (2007 ed., pp. 33–34). Bethesda, MD: Author.

American Occupational Therapy Association. (2007a). AOTA Centennial Vision and executive summary. *American Journal of Occupational Therapy, 61,* 613–614.

American Occupational Therapy Association. (2007b). Specialized knowledge and skills in feeding, eating, and swallowing for occupational therapy practice. *American Journal of Occupational Therapy, 61,* 686–700.

Ayres, A. J. (1972). *Sensory integration and learning disorders.* Los Angeles: Western Psychological Services.

Ayres, A. J. (1985). *Developmental dyspraxia and adult onset apraxia.* Torrance, CA: Sensory Integration International.

Ayres, A. J. (2005). *Sensory integration and the child.* Los Angeles: Western Psychological Services.

Baum, C. M., Bass-Haugen, J., & Christiansen, C. H. (2005). Person–environment–occupation–performance: A model for planning interventions for individuals and organizations. In C. H. Christiansen, C. M. Baum, & J. Bass-Haugen (Eds.), *Occupational therapy: Performance, participation, and well-being* (3rd ed., pp. 373–392). Thorofare, NJ: Slack.

Bergen, D. (Ed.). (1988). *Play as a medium for learning and development: A handbook of theory and practice.* Portsmouth, NH: Heinemann.

Blanche, E. I., & Parham, L. D. (2002). Praxis and organization of behavior in time and space. In S. Smith Roley, E. I. Blanche, & R. C. Schaaf (Eds.), *Understanding the nature of sensory integration with diverse populations* (pp. 183–200). San Antonio, TX: Therapy Skill Builders.

Bloom, B. S., Krathwohl, D. R., & Masia, B. B. (1984). *Taxonomy of educational objectives: The classification of educational goals.* New York: Longman.

Brownson, C. A., & Scaffa, M. E. (2001). Occupational therapy in the promotion of health and the prevention of disease and disability. *American Journal of Occupational Therapy, 55,* 656–660.

Calvert, G., Spence, C., & Stein, B. E. (Eds.). (2004). *The handbook of multisensory processes.* Cambridge, MA: MIT Press.

Chapparo, C., & Ranka, J. (1997). The perceive, recall, plan, perform (PRPP) system of task analysis. In C. Chapparo & J. Ranka (Eds.), *Occupational performance model* (Australian Monograph 1, pp. 189–197). Sydney: Occupational Performance Network.

Christiansen, C. H. (1999). Defining lives: Occupation as identity—An essay on competence, coherence, and the creation of meaning [1999 Eleanor Clarke Slagle Lecture]. *American Journal of Occupational Therapy, 53,* 547–558.

Christiansen, C. H., & Baum, M. C. (Eds.). (1997). *Occupational therapy: Enabling function and well-being.* Thorofare, NJ: Slack.

Christiansen, C., Baum, M. C., & Bass-Haugen, J. (Eds.). (2005). *Occupational therapy: Performance, participation, and well-being.* Thorofare, NJ: Slack.

Christiansen, C. H., & Hammecker, C. L. (2001). Self care. In B. R. Bonder & M. B. Wagner (Eds.), *Functional performance in older adults* (pp. 155–175). Philadelphia: F. A. Davis.

Christiansen, C. H., & Townsend, E. A. (Eds.). (2004). *Introduction to occupation: The art and science of living.* Upper Saddle River, NJ: Prentice Hall.

Clark, F. A. (2000). The concept of habit and routine: A preliminary theoretical synthesis. *Occupational Therapy Journal of Research, 20,* 123S–137S.

Cohn, E. S. (2001). Parent perspectives of occupational therapy using a sensory integration approach. *American Journal of Occupational Therapy, 55,* 285–294.

Cohn, E. S., Miller, L. J., & Tickle-Degnan, L. (2000). Parental hopes for therapy outcomes: Children with sensory modulation disorders. *American Journal of Occupational Therapy, 54,* 36–43.

Commission on Social Justice. (1994). *Social justice: Strategies for national renewal. The report of the Commission on Social Justice.* London: Vintage.

Crepeau, E. (2003). Analyzing occupation and activity: A way of thinking about occupational performance. In E. Crepeau, E. Cohn, & B. Schell (Eds.), *Willard and Spackman's occupational therapy* (10th ed., pp. 189–198). Philadelphia: Lippincott Williams & Wilkins.

Crepeau, E., Cohn, E., & Schell, B. (Eds.). (2003). *Willard and Spackman's occupational therapy.* Philadelphia: Lippincott Williams & Wilkins.

Dawson, J. (2007). *Self-advocacy: A valuable skill for your teenager.* Retrieved January 20, 2007, from www.schwablearning.org

Dickie, V., Cutchin, M. P., & Humphry, R. (2006). Occupation as transactional experience: A critique of individualism in occupational science. *Journal of Occupational Science, 13,* 83–93.

Dunlea, A. (1996). An opportunity for co-adaptation: The experience of mothers and their infants who are blind. In R. Zemke & F. Clark (Eds.), *Occupational science: The evolving discipline* (pp. 227–342). Philadelphia: F. A. Davis.

Dunn, W. (2000a). *Best practice in occupational therapy in community service with children and families.* Thorofare, NJ: Slack.

Dunn, W. (2000b, Fall). Habit: What's the brain got to do with it? *Occupational Therapy Journal of Research, 20*(Suppl. 1), 6S–20S.

Dunn, W., McClain, L. H., Brown, C., & Youngstrom, M. J. (1998). The ecology of human performance. In M. E. Neistadt & E. B. Crepeau (Eds.), *Willard and Spackman's occupational therapy* (9th ed., pp. 525–535). Philadelphia: Lippincott Williams & Wilkins.

Dunton, W. R. (1934). The need for and value of research in occupational therapy. *Occupational Therapy and Rehabilitation, 13,* 325–328.

Esdaile, S. A., & Olson J. A. (2004). *Mothering occupations: Challenge, agency, and participation.* Philadelphia: F. A. Davis.

Fiese, B. H., Tomcho, T. J., Douglas, M., Josephs, K., Poltrock, S., & Baker, T. (2002). A review of 50 years of research on naturally occurring family routines and rituals: Cause for celebration? *Journal of Family Psychology, 16,* 381–390.

Filley, C. M. (2001). *Neurobehavioral anatomy.* Boulder: University Press of Colorado.

Fisher, A. (2006). Overview of performance skills and client factors. In H. Pendleton & W. Schultz-Krohn (Eds.), *Pedretti's occupational therapy: Practice skills for physical dysfunction* (pp. 372–402). St. Louis: Mosby/Elsevier.

Foucault, M. (1973). *The birth of the clinic: An archaeology of medical perception.* New York: Pantheon Books.

Fuhrer, M. J. (Ed.). (1987). *Rehabilitation outcomes analysis and measurement.* Baltimore: Brookes.

Gitlin, L. N., & Corcoran, M. A. (2005). *Occupational therapy and dementia care: The Home Environmental Skill-Building Program for individuals and families.* Bethesda, MD: AOTA Press.

Gitlin, L. N., Corcoran, M. A., Winter, L., Boyce, A., & Hauck, W. W. (2001). A randomized controlled trail of a home environmental intervention to enhance self-efficacy and reduce upset in family caregivers of persons with dementia. *The Gerontologist, 41,* 15–30.

Gitlin, L. N., Winter, L., Corcoran, M., Dennis, M., Schinfeld, S., & Hauck, W. (2003). Effects of the Home Environmental Skill-Building Program on the caregiver–care recipient dyad: Six-month outcomes from the Philadelphia REACH initiative. *The Gerontologist, 43,* 532–546.

Goodman-Lavey, M., & Dunbar, S. (2003). Federal legislative advocacy. In G. McCormack, E. Jaffe, & M. Goodman-Lavey (Eds.), *The occupational therapy manager* (4th ed., pp. 421–438). Bethesda, MD: AOTA Press.

Gupta, J., & Walloch, C. (2006). Process of infusing social justice into the practice framework: A case study. *OT Practice, 11*(15), CE1–CE8.

Gutman, S. A., Mortera, M. H., Hinojosa, J., & Kramer, P. (2007). Revision of the occupational therapy practice framework. *American Journal of Occupational Therapy, 61,* 119–126.

Hakansson, C., Dahlin-Ivanoff, S., & Sonn, U. (2006). Achieving balance in everyday life. *Journal of Occupational Science, 13,* 74–82.

Harrow, A. J. (1972). *A taxonomy of the psychomotor domain: A guide for developing behavioral objectives.* New York: McKay.

Heilman, K. M., & Rothi, L. J. G. (1993). *Clinical neuropsychology* (3rd ed.). New York: Oxford University Press.

Hettler, W. (1984). Wellness—The lifetime goal of a university experience. In J. D. Matarazzo, S. M. Weiss, J. A. Herd, N. E. Miller, & S. M. Weiss (Eds.), *Behavioral health: A handbook of health enhancement and disease prevention* (p. 1117). New York: Wiley.

Hinojosa, J., & Kramer, P. (1997). Fundamental concepts of occupational therapy: Occupation, purposeful activity, and function [Statement]. *American Journal of Occupational Therapy, 51,* 864–866.

Jackson, J. (1998a). Contemporary criticisms of role theory. *Journal of Occupational Science, 5*(2), 49–55.

Jackson, J. (1998b). Is there a place for role theory in occupational science? *Journal of Occupational Science 5*(2), 56–65.

Jonsson, H. (2007). *Towards a new direction in the conceptualization and categorization of occupation* [Wilma West Lecture, Occupational Science Symposium]. Los Angeles: University of Southern California, Occupational Science and Occupational Therapy.

Kielhofner, G. (2002). Motives, patterns, and performance of occupation: Basic concepts. In G. Kielhofner (Ed.), *A model of human occupation: Theory and application* (3rd ed., pp. 13–27). Philadelphia: Lippincott Williams & Wilkins.

Kramer, S., McGonigel, M., & Kaufmann, R. (1991). Developing the IFSP: Outcomes, strategies, activities, and services. In M. McGonigel, R. Kaufmann, & B. Johnson (Eds.), *Guidelines and recommended practices for the individualized family service plan* (2nd ed., pp. 41–49). Bethesda, MD: Association for the Care of Children's Health.

Kronenberg, F., Algado, S. S., & Pollard, N. (2005). *Occupational therapy without borders: Learning from the spirit of survivors*. Philadelphia: Elsevier/Churchill Livingstone.

Larson, E., & Zemke, R. (2004). Shaping the temporal patterns of our lives: The social coordination of occupation. *Journal of Occupational Science, 10,* 80–89.

Law, M., Baum, M. C., & Dunn, W. (2005). *Measuring occupational performance: Supporting best practice in occupational therapy* (2nd ed.). Thorofare, NJ: Slack.

Law, M., Cooper, B., Strong, S., Stewart, D., Rigby, P., & Letts, L. (1996). Person–environment–occupation model: A transactive approach to occupational performance. *Canadian Journal of Occupational Therapy, 63,* 9–23.

Law, M., Polatajko, H., Baptiste, W., & Townsend, E. (1997). Core concepts of occupational therapy. In E. Townsend (Ed.), *Enabling occupation: An occupational therapy perspective* (pp. 29–56). Ottawa, ON: Canadian Association of Occupational Therapists.

Liepmann, H. (1920). Apraxie. *Ergebnisse der Gesamten Medizin, 1,* 516–543.

Lopez, S. J., Snyder, C. R., Magyar-Moe, J., Edwards, L. M., Pedrotti, J. T., Janowski, K., et al. (2004). Strategies for accentuating hope. In P. A. Linley & S. Joseph (Eds.), *Positive psychology in practice* (pp. 388–404). Hoboken, NJ: John Wiley & Sons.

Maciejewski, M., Kawiecki, J., & Rockwood, T. (1997). Satisfaction. In R. L. Kane (Ed.), *Understanding health care outcomes research* (pp. 67–89). Gaithersburg, MD: Aspen.

Meyer, A. (1922). The philosophy of occupational therapy. *Archives of Occupational Therapy, 1,* 1–10.

Moreira-Almeida, A., & Koenig, H. G. (2006). Retaining the meaning of the words religiousness and spirituality: A commentary on the WHOQOL SRPB group's "A cross-cultural study of spirituality, religion, and personal beliefs as components of quality of life" (62:6, 2005, pp. 1486–1497). *Social Science and Medicine, 63,* 843–845.

Mosey, A. C. (1996). *Applied scientific inquiry in the health professions: An epistemological orientation* (2nd ed.). Bethesda, MD: American Occupational Therapy Association.

Moyers, P. A. (1999). The guide to occupational therapy practice. *American Journal of Occupational Therapy, 53,* 247–322.

Moyers, P. A., & Dale, L. M. (2007). *The guide to occupational therapy practice* (2nd ed.). Bethesda, MD: AOTA Press.

Neistadt, M. E., & Crepeau, E. B. (Eds.). (1998). *Willard and Spackman's occupational therapy* (9th ed.). Philadelphia: Lippincott Williams & Wilkins.

Nelson, D., & Jepson-Thomas, J. (2003). Occupational form, occupational performance, and a conceptual framework for therapeutic occupation. In P. Kramer, J. Hinojosa, & C. Brasic Royeen (Eds.), *Perspectives in human occupation: Participation in life* (pp. 87–155). Philadelphia: Lippincott Williams & Wilkins.

Nurit, W., & Michel, A. B. (2003). Rest: A qualitative exploration of the phenomenon. *Occupational Therapy International, 10,* 227–238.

Olsen, J. A. (2004). Mothering co-occupations in caring for infants and young children. In S. A. Esdaile & J. A. Olson (Eds.), *Mothering occupations* (pp. 28–51). Philadelphia: F. A. Davis.

Parham, L. D., & Fazio, L. S. (Eds.). (1997). *Play in occupational therapy for children.* St. Louis, MO: Mosby.

Pedretti, L. W., & Early, M. B. (2001). Occupational performance and model of practice for physical dysfunction. In L. W. Pedretti & M. B. Early (Eds.), *Occupational therapy practice skills for physical dysfunction* (pp. 7–9). St. Louis, MO: Mosby.

Pierce, D. (2001). Untangling occupation and activity. *American Journal of Occupational Therapy, 55,* 138–146.

Punwar, A. J., & Peloquin, S. M. (2000). *Occupational therapy principles and practice* (3rd ed.). Philadelphia: Lippincott Williams & Wilkins.

Radomski, M. V. (1995). There is more to life than putting on your pants. *American Journal of Occupational Therapy, 49,* 487–490.

Reed, K. L. (2005). An annotated history of the concepts used in occupational therapy. In C. H. Christiansen, M. C. Baum, & J. Bass-Haugen (Eds.), *Occupational therapy: Performance, participation, and well-being* (3rd ed., pp. 567–626). Thorofare, NJ: Slack.

Request for Planning Ideas for the Development of the Children's Health Outcomes Initiative, 66 Fed. Reg. 11296 (2001).

Rogers, J. C., & Holm, M. B. (1994). Assessment of self-care. In B. R. Bonder & M. B. Wagner (Eds.), *Functional performance in older adults* (pp. 181–202). Philadelphia: F. A. Davis.

Rogers, J. C., & Holm, M. B. (2008). The occupational therapy process: Evaluation and intervention. In E. B. Crepeau, E. S. Cohn, & B. A. B. Schell (Eds.), *Willard and Spackman's occupational therapy* (11th ed., pp. 478–518). Baltimore: Lippincott Williams & Wilkins.

Schell, B. A. B., Cohn, E. S., & Crepeau, E. B. (2008). Overview of personal factors affecting performance. In E. B. Crepeau, E. S. Cohn, & B. A. B. Schell (Eds.), *Willard and Spackman's occupational therapy* (11th ed., pp. 650–657). Baltimore: Lippincott Williams & Wilkins.

Schultz, S., & Schkade, J. (1997). Adaptation. In C. Christiansen & M. C. Baum (Eds.), *Occupational therapy: Enabling function and well-being* (p. 474). Thorofare, NJ: Slack.

Segal, R. (2004). Family routines and rituals: A context for occupational therapy interventions. *American Journal of Occupational Therapy, 58,* 499–508.

Shumway-Cook, A., & Wollacott, M. H. (2007). *Motor control: Translating research into clinical practice* (3rd ed.). Philadelphia: Lippincott Williams & Wilkins.

Slagle, E. C. (1924). A year's development of occupational therapy in New York state hospitals. *Modern Hospital, 22*(1), 98–104.

Sleep. (2007). *The free dictionary.* Retrieved June 1, 2007, from http://freedictionary.org

Taber's cyclopedic medical dictionary. (1997). Philadelphia: F. A. Davis.

Townsend, E. A., & Wilcock, A. A. (2004). Occupational justice. In C. H. Christiansen & E. A. Townsend (Eds.), *Introduction to occupation: The art and science of living* (pp. 243–273). Upper Saddle River, NJ: Prentice Hall.

Trentham, B., & Cockburn, L. (2005). Participating in action research: Creating new knowledge and opportunities for occupational engagement. In F. Kronenberg, S. S. Algado, & N. Pollard (Eds.), *Occupational therapy without borders: Learning from the spirit of survivors* (pp. 440–453). Philadelphia: Elsevier/Churchill Livingstone.

Trombly, C. (1995). Occupation: Purposefulness and meaningfulness as therapeutic mechanism. *American Journal of Occupational Therapy, 49,* 960–972.

Uniform Data System for Medical Rehabilitation. (1996). *Guide for the uniform data set for medical rehabilitation (including the FIM instrument).* Buffalo, NY: Author.

Weber, M. (1978). *Economy and society: An outline of interpretive sociology* (G. Roth & C. Wittich, Eds.; E. Fischoff et al., Trans.). Berkeley: University of California Press.

Webster's encyclopedic unabridged dictionary of the English language. (1994). Avenel, NJ: Gramercy Books.

Wilcock, A. A. (2006). *An occupational perspective of health* (2nd ed.). Thorofare, NJ: Slack.

Wilcock, A. A., & Townsend, E. A. (2008). Occupational justice. In E. B. Crepeau, E. S. Cohn, & B. B. Schell (Eds.), *Willard and Spackman's occupational therapy* (11th ed., pp. 192–199). Baltimore: Lippincott Williams & Wilkins.

World Health Organization. (1986, November 21). *The Ottawa Charter for Health Promotion.* First International Conference on Health Promotion, Ottawa. Retrieved February 4, 2008, from http://www.who.int/healthpromotion/conferences/previous/ottawa/en/print.html

World Health Organization. (2001). *International classification of functioning, disability, and health (ICF).* Geneva: Author.

Zemke, R. (2004). Time, space, and the kaleidoscopes of occupation [Eleanor Clarke Slagle Lecture]. *American Journal of Occupational Therapy, 58,* 608–620.

Zemke R., & Clark, F. (1996). *Occupational science: An evolving discipline.* Philadelphia: F. A. Davis.

Zhan, L. (1992). Quality of life: Conceptual and measurement issues. *Journal of Advanced Nursing, 17,* 795–800.

Bibliography

Accreditation Council for Occupational Therapy Education. (2007a). Accreditation standards for a doctoral-degree-level educational program for the occupational therapist. *American Journal of Occupational Therapy, 61,* 641–651.

Accreditation Council for Occupational Therapy Education. (2007b). Accreditation standards for an educational program for the occupational therapy assistant. *American Journal of Occupational Therapy, 61,* 662–671.

Accreditation Council for Occupational Therapy Education. (2007c). Accreditation standards for a master's-degree-level educational program for the occupational therapist. *American Journal of Occupational Therapy, 61,* 652–661.

American Occupational Therapy Association. (1995). Occupation: A position paper. *American Journal of Occupational Therapy, 49,* 1015–1018.

Baum, M. C. (1999, November). *At the core of our profession: Occupation-based practice* [Overhead presentation]. Presented at the AOTA Practice Conference, Reno, Nevada.

Blanche, E. I. (1999). *Play and process: The experience of play in the life of the adult.* Ann Arbor: University of Michigan.

Blount, M. L., Blount, W., & Hinojosa, J (2004). Perspectives. In J. Hinojosa & M. L. Blount (Eds.), *The texture of life: Purposeful activities in occupational therapy* (2nd ed., pp. 17–38). Bethesda, MD: AOTA Press.

Borg, B., & Bruce, M. (1991). Assessing psychological performance factors. In C. H. Christiansen & C. M. Baum (Eds.), *Occupational therapy: Overcoming human performance deficits* (pp. 538–586). Thorofare, NJ: Slack.

Borst, M. J., & Nelson, D. L. (1993). Use of uniform terminology by occupational therapists. *American Journal of Occupational Therapy, 47,* 611–618.

Buckley, K. A., & Poole, S. E. (2004). Activity analysis. In J. Hinojosa & M. L. Blount (Eds.), *The texture of life: Purposeful activities in occupational ther-*

apy (2nd ed., pp. 69–114). Bethesda, MD: AOTA Press.

Canadian Association of Occupational Therapists. (1997). *Enabling occupation: An occupational therapy perspective.* Ottawa, ON: CAOT Publications ACE.

Christiansen, C. H. (1997). Acknowledging a spiritual dimension in occupational therapy practice. *American Journal of Occupational Therapy, 51,* 169–172.

Christiansen, C. H., & Matuska, K. M. (2004). The importance of everyday activities. In C. H. Christiansen & K. M. Matuska (Eds.), *Ways of living: Adaptive strategies for special needs* (3rd ed., pp. 1–20). Bethesda, MD: AOTA Press.

Clark, F. A., Parham, D., Carlson, M. C., Frank, G., Jackson, J., Pierce, D., et al. (1991). Occupational science: Academic innovation in the service of occupational therapy's future. *American Journal of Occupational Therapy, 45,* 300–310.

Clark, F. A., Wood, W., & Larson, E. (1998). Occupational science: Occupational therapy's legacy for the 21st century. In M. E. Neistadt & E. B. Crepeau (Eds.), *Willard and Spackman's occupational therapy* (9th ed., pp. 13–21). Philadelphia: Lippincott Williams & Wilkins.

Culler, K. H. (1993). Occupational therapy performance areas: Home and family management. In H. L. Hopkins & H. D. Smith (Eds.), *Willard and Spackman's occupational therapy* (8th ed., pp. 207–269). Philadelphia: Lippincott Williams & Wilkins.

Dunn, W., Brown, C., & McGuigan, A. (1994). The ecology of human performance: A framework for considering the effect of context. *American Journal of Occupational Therapy, 48,* 595–607.

Gardner, H. (1999). *Intelligence reframed: Multiple intelligences for the 21st century.* New York: Basic Books.

Hill, J. (1993). Occupational therapy performance areas. In H. L. Hopkins & H. D. Smith (Eds.), *Willard and Spackman's occupational therapy* (8th ed., pp. 191–268). Philadelphia: Lippincott.

Hinojosa, J., & Blount, M. L. (2004). Purposeful activities within the context of occupational therapy. In J. Hinojosa & M. L. Blount (Eds.), *The texture of life: Purposeful activities in occupational ther-*

apy (2nd ed., pp. 1–16). Bethesda, MD: AOTA Press.

Holm, M. B., Rogers, J. C., & Stone, R. G. (1998). Treatment of performance contexts. In M. E. Neistadt & E. B. Crepeau (Eds.), *Willard and Spackman's occupational therapy* (9th ed., pp. 471–517). Philadelphia: Lippincott Williams & Wilkins.

Horsburgh, M. (1997). Towards an inclusive spirituality: Wholeness, interdependence, and waiting. *Disability and Rehabilitation, 19,* 398–406.

Intagliata, S. (1993). Rehabilitation centers. In H. L. Hopkins & H. D. Smith (Eds.), *Willard and Spackman's occupational therapy* (8th ed., pp. 784–789). Philadelphia: Lippincott.

Kane, R. L. (1997). Approaching the outcomes question. In R. L. Kane (Ed.), *Understanding health care outcomes research* (pp. 1–15). Gaithersburg, MD: Aspen.

Kielhofner, G. (1992). *Conceptual foundations of occupational therapy.* Philadelphia: F. A. Davis.

Kielhofner, G. (2002). Habituation: Patterns of daily occupation. In G. Kielhofner (Ed.), *Model of human occupation: Theory and application* (3rd ed., pp. 63–80). Philadelphia: Lippincott Williams & Wilkins.

Law, M. (1991). The environment: A focus for occupational therapy. *Canadian Journal of Occupational Therapy, 58,* 171–179.

Law, M. (1993). Evaluating activities of daily living: Directions for the future. *American Journal of Occupational Therapy, 47,* 233–237.

Law, M. (1998). Assessment in client-centered occupational therapy. In M. Law (Ed.), *Client-centered occupational therapy* (pp. 89–106). Thorofare, NJ: Slack.

Lifson, L. E., & Simon, R. I. (Eds.). (1998). *The mental health practitioner and the law: A comprehensive handbook.* Cambridge, MA: Harvard University Press.

Llorens, L. (1993). Activity analysis: Agreement between participants and observers on perceived factors and occupation components. *Occupational Therapy Journal of Research, 13,* 198–211.

Ludwig, F. M. (1993). Anne Cronin Mosey. In R. J. Miller & K. F. Walker (Eds.), *Perspectives on theory for the practice of occupational therapy* (pp. 41–63). Gaithersburg, MD: Aspen.

Mosey, A. C. (1981). Legitimate tools of occupational therapy. In A. Mosey (Ed.), *Occupational therapy: Configuration of a profession* (pp. 89–118). New York: Raven.

Mosey, A. C. (1986). *Psychosocial components of occupational therapy.* New York: Raven.

Nelson, D. L. (1988). Occupation: Form and performance. *American Journal of Occupational Therapy, 42,* 633–641.

Pierce, D. (1999, September). Putting occupation to work in occupational therapy curricula. *Education Special Interest Section Quarterly, 9*(3), 1–4.

Pollock, N., & McColl, M. A. (1998). Assessments in client-centered occupational therapy. In M. Law (Ed.), *Client-centered occupational therapy* (pp. 89–105). Thorofare, NJ: Slack.

Reed, K., & Sanderson, S. (1999). *Concepts of occupational therapy* (4th ed.). Philadelphia: Lippincott Williams & Wilkins.

Schell, B. B. (1998). Clinical reasoning: The basis of practice. In M. E. Neistadt & E. B. Crepeau (Eds.), *Willard and Spackman's occupational therapy* (9th ed., pp. 90–100). Philadelphia: Lippincott Williams & Wilkins.

Scherer, M. J., & Cushman, L. A. (1997). A functional approach to psychological and psychosocial factors and their assessment in rehabilitation. In S. S. Dittmar & G. E. Gresham (Eds.), *Functional assessment and outcomes measurement for the rehabilitation health professional* (pp. 57–67). Gaithersburg, MD: Aspen.

Urbanowski, R., & Vargo, J. (1994). Spirituality, daily practice, and the occupational performance model. *Canadian Journal of Occupational Therapy, 61,* 88–94.

Watson, D. E., & Wilson, S. A. (2003). *Task analysis: An individual and population approach* (2nd ed.). Bethesda, MD: AOTA Press.

Yerxa, E. J. (1980). Occupational therapy's role in creating a future climate of caring. *American Journal of Occupational Therapy, 34,* 529–534.

Authors

THE COMMISSION ON PRACTICE:

Susanne Smith Roley, MS, OTR/L, FAOTA,
Chairperson, 2005–2008

Janet V. DeLany, DEd, OTR/L, FAOTA,
Chairperson-Elect, 2007–2008

Cynthia J. Barrows, MS, OTR/L

Susan Brownrigg, OTR/L

DeLana Honaker, PhD, OTR/L, BCP

Deanna Iris Sava, MS, OTR/L

Vibeke Talley, OTR/L

Kristi Voelkerding, BS, COTA/L, ATP

Deborah Ann Amini, MEd, OTR/L, CHT,
SIS Liaison

Emily Smith, MOT, *ASD Liaison*

Pamela Toto, MS, OTR/L, BCG, FAOTA,
Immediate-Past SIS Liaison

Sarah King, MOT, OTR, *Immediate-Past
ASD Liaison*

Deborah Lieberman, MHSA, OTR/L, FAOTA,
AOTA Headquarters Liaison

With contributions from

M. Carolyn Baum, PhD, OTR/L, FAOTA

Ellen S. Cohn, ScD, OTR/L, FAOTA

Penelope A. Moyers Cleveland, EdD, OTR/L,
BCMH, FAOTA

Mary Jane Youngstrom, MS, OTR, FAOTA

for

THE COMMISSION ON PRACTICE

Susanne Smith Roley MS, OTR/L, FAOTA,
Chairperson

Adopted by the Representative Assembly 2008C5.

This document replaces the 2002 *Occupational
Therapy Practice Framework: Domain and Process.*

Specialized Knowledge and Skills Papers

Specialized Knowledge and Skills in Adult Vestibular Rehabilitation for Occupational Therapy Practice

Introduction

People with impairments of the vestibular system often have subtle problems that have profound ramifications for their ability to engage in daily life tasks and activities at home and to participate in society outside the home. Vestibular impairment often restricts an individual's ability to participate in everyday occupations, affecting not only that individual but also significant others, including family members, friends, coworkers, and caregivers. Occupational therapy facilitates increased independence in daily life tasks and participation in work and social occupations. For these reasons, occupational therapy is an appropriate intervention for clients needing vestibular rehabilitation to decrease symptoms and increase independence in all aspects of their lives. Thus, vestibular rehabilitation is within the scope of practice for occupational therapists and occupational therapy assistants[1] who have specialized knowledge and skills in this area. This document provides an understanding of the essential knowledge and skills needed by practitioners working with individuals with vestibular impairments and will be of interest to payers, practitioners, or consumers who wish to know more about occupational therapy practice using vestibular rehabilitation techniques.

People with vestibular disorders may present with symptoms including vertigo, oscillopsia, nausea, disequilibrium, spatial disorientation, visual motion sensitivity, decreased dynamic visual acuity, decreased concentration, and decreased skill in dual task performance. Spatial orientation deficits and disequilibrium may be manifested as head and body tilt while sitting or standing, perception of tilt while sitting or standing, veering or drifting to the side while walking or steering a vehicle, or a sense of not knowing which way is up. These problems may result in fear of falling. These symptoms may affect occupational performance and can result in social withdrawal and depression. For example, visual motion sensitivity may cause disequilibrium, vertigo, nausea, and disorientation, leading to slower or more awkward performance of self-care skills, decreased participation in social activities, and decreased ability to perform home management tasks outside of the home, such as grocery shopping. Vertigo, disequilibrium, and other symptoms may interfere with job skills as they cause difficulty standing, reaching, walking, turning the head to scan the environment, or making social gestures with the head such as nodding.

Definition

The term *vestibular rehabilitation* refers to intervention to decrease symptoms and increase independence, safety, and participation in people with specific disorders of the peripheral vestibular apparatus, the central vestibular pathways, and age-related disequilibrium. Interventions include, but are not limited to, exercise and activity programs to reduce vertigo and oscillopsia, repositioning interventions for positional vertigo, exercises and activities to improve standing and walking balance during activities, and safety

---

[1]*Occupational therapists* are responsible for all aspects of occupational therapy service delivery and are accountable for the safety and effectiveness of the occupational therapy service delivery process. *Occupational therapy assistants* deliver occupational therapy services under the supervision of and in partnership with an occupational therapist (AOTA, 2004).

training at home and at work. A client receiving occupational therapy including vestibular rehabilitation techniques may also receive occupational therapy using other interventions. For example, a client with a head injury may also receive perceptual, motor, or life skills training.

Vestibular rehabilitation is used to treat the sequelae of specific medical conditions, and provides an alternative or adjunct to pharmacologic and surgical intervention by the physician. Clients who receive vestibular rehabilitation have specific medical conditions that can be demonstrated with objective diagnostic tests or otherwise medically determined. Most people who are referred for vestibular rehabilitation are adults. They have a wide variety of health conditions including, but not limited to, benign paroxysmal positional vertigo (BPPV); acute, chronic, and recurrent labyrinthitis; vestibular neuronitis; some autoimmune disorders; postconcussion vertigo; postoperative vertigo; Ménierè's disease; bilateral vestibular weakness or total vestibular loss due to ototoxicity; presbystasis or disequilibrium of aging; some cases of strokes, some cases of multiple sclerosis, some cases of Parkinson's disease, some Parkinsonian syndromes, and some cases of migraine.

Although the focus of this document is on adult vestibular rehabilitation, we note that the same or similar vestibular impairments may occur in children. The literature has few papers on the efficacy of vestibular rehabilitation in children. These disorders are difficult to diagnose because children may not be able to describe their symptoms and because, for technical reasons, young children cannot always be tested with standard objective diagnostic tests. Vestibular disorders that occur in childhood that may respond to vestibular rehabilitation include childhood paroxysmal vertigo, which may be related to migraine; BPPV; labyrinthitis; vestibular neuronitis; bilateral impairment due to ototoxicity; some autoimmune disorders; and congenital malformations of the inner ear. In pediatric vestibular rehabilitation, treatment activities must be age appropriate.

Knowledge and Skills for Entry-Level and Advanced Practitioners

Clients with vestibular disorders have a complex combination of physiological and psychological problems. The effects of vestibular impairments are subtle and pervasive. Many people with these problems are not able to describe the sensations they have or the motions that elicit vertigo or disequilibrium. Therefore, rehabilitation of most individuals with vestibular impairments requires skills beyond entry-level competence. The specialized nature of this intervention requires specific, advanced-level knowledge. Intervention may require specific techniques that focus directly on the vestibular impairment. Advanced skills build on earlier competencies in knowledge, performance, critical reasoning, interpersonal abilities, and ethical reasoning and additional competencies developed during independent study of the literature, continuing education coursework, and additional practice.

An in-depth understanding of the structure and function of the vestibular system, visual/vestibular/proprioceptive interactions, and the principles of motor control is essential when providing vestibular rehabilitation. Occupational therapy entry-level education provides a foundation in functional anatomy, neuroscience, and motor control that assists the practitioner in understanding the types of complex problems experienced by clients with vestibular impairments. Practitioners need further training, however, to address the subtle problems of clients with these disorders. Advanced-level skills are necessary for evaluation of the deficits and specific manipulations that alter vestibular function. This knowledge and these skills are not provided to occupational therapists at the entry level. Appendix 1 outlines the basic science knowledge necessary for advanced practice.

Occupational therapists use knowledge of vestibular system anatomy and physiology when determining underlying problems that affect occupational performance. An individual's central nervous system uses information about head movement to help control four classes of behavior: (a) postural reflexes for control of balance, (b) vestibulo-ocular reflexes to stabilize gaze so the individual can see clearly, (c) coding of spatial coordinates for object orientation and navigation, and (d) some autonomic responses to prepare for "fight-or-flight" behavior. Appendix 2 outlines the applied science knowledge necessary for advanced practice.

The occupational therapist must be highly skilled at evaluating the consequences of subtle vestibular deficits, such as balance disturbances due to head movements while sitting, standing, walking, reaching, and performing transfers between positions. Understanding the potential impact of vestibular impairment on participation in healthy occupations requires knowledge of the effect of vestibular impairment on the life of the person. See Appendices 3–8 for specific examples of how vestibular impairments impact performance in occupation (AOTA, 2002).

Refined skills in activity analysis are essential for evaluation of and intervention planning for these clients. The occupational therapist uses knowledge of body structure and function in conjunction with observation and activity analysis when evaluating subtle decrements in performance during typical daily activities. At the entry level, occupational therapists and occupational therapy assistants are familiar with the location of the vestibular labyrinth and know that the symptoms of vestibular disorders include vertigo, poor balance, and fear of falling. Their use of the occupational profile helps to determine which tasks elicit those symptoms. They are able to determine if clients would benefit from adaptive safety equipment; to recommend equipment appropriate for the home; and to educate clients about other safety concerns, such as appropriate clothing and shoes. They also are able to evaluate many activities of daily living directly to determine if training is needed and provide training when necessary. Appendix 9 outlines the essential evaluation skills for the advanced practitioner. Appendix 10 outlines specific information on intervention using vestibular rehabilitation methods.

Occupation therapy practitioners who do vestibular rehabilitation may seek reimbursement through Medicare and other third-party payers. Examples of possible *Current Procedural Technology (CPT)* codes include, but are not limited to, codes for neuromuscular reeducation of movement, balance, coordination, and/or posture for sitting and/or standing activities (97112); manual therapy (97140); and therapeutic activities to improve functional performance (97530) (American Medical Association, 2006).

The occupational therapist assumes the ultimate responsibility for the delivery of occupational therapy services, including evaluation of the person and development of the intervention plan. The advanced occupational therapist may delegate certain selected interventions to an entry-level occupational therapist or to an occupational therapy assistant who has demonstrated service competency in those interventions. All practitioners should know when and how to refer clients to other health professionals when needed, including but not limited to: specialty physicians, certified driving rehabilitation specialists, psychologists, physical therapists, audiologists, and social workers.

Brief Review of the Research Literature

Vestibular rehabilitation in occupational therapy practice is supported by the literature, although considerable research remains to be done. This section is not an exhaustive review of the research but gives an overview of the research on vestibular impairment and vestibular rehabilitation that is relevant to occupational therapy. Suggested readings not cited here are listed in the "Additional Reading" list.

In the first paper describing the use of exercises for vertigo, Cawthorne (1944) indicated that some patients with postconcussion vertigo are rendered "helpless and immobile," preceding later work by occupational therapists and their collaborators showing that patients with disorders that cause vertigo have significantly reduced independence in activities of daily living (Cohen, 1992; Cohen, Ewell, & Jenkins, 1995; Cohen & Jerabek, 1999; Cohen & Kimball, 2000; Cohen, Kimball, & Adams, 2000; Cohen, Wells, Kimball, & Owsley, 2003; Farber, 1989; Morris, 1991).

In Cooksey's first paper describing vestibular rehabilitation exercises (Cooksey, 1945), he mentioned the need for teamwork by rehabilitation staff, including occupational therapists. Cooksey specifically noted the role of occupational therapy in the early resumption of purposeful activity. In his 1946 paper, Cooksey indicated that purposeful activity should be incorporated into the daily exercise program for these patients. Structured, purposeful activity is an effective treatment modality for reducing vertigo, improving balance, and increasing independence in activities of daily living (Cohen, Kane-Wineland, Miller, & Hatfield, 1995; Cohen, Miller, Kane-Wineland, & Hatfield, 1995). Vertigo habituation exercises are also effective in decreasing symptoms, improving spatial orientation skills, and increasing independence and ability to perform purposeful activity that involves repetitive head movements (Cohen & Kimball, 2002, 2003, 2004b, 2004c). Thus, exercises and purposeful activities may be components of a successful rehabilitation program for many patients with vertigo. For a critical review of more recent studies on vertigo habituation treatments and other issues, see Cohen's 2006 review paper.

A series of studies has shown that patients with vestibular disorders also have high rates of anxiety and other psychosocial problems (Eagger, Luxon, Davies, Coelho, & Ron, 1992; Yardley & Hallam, 1996; Yardley, Luxon, & Haacke, 1994; Yardley & Putman, 1992). Many of these kinds of problems might be appropriate for intervention by occupational therapists, combining our understanding of physical and psychosocial disorders.

Patients with benign paroxysmal positional vertigo are best treated with passive maneuvers of the head that are thought to reposition otoconial particles that have become displaced from one compartment to another. Occupational therapists and their collaborators have been in the forefront of investigators showing that these repositioning maneuvers are effective treatments (Cohen & Jerabek, 1999; Cohen Kimball, 2004a, 2005; Macias, Lambert, Massingale, Ellensohn, & Fritz, 2000; Steenerson & Cronin, 1996; Steenerson, Cronin, & Marbach, 2005).

Appendixes

The following Appendixes outline the basic knowledge needed to understand and treat vestibular disorders, the effects of vestibular disorders on occupational performance, and the types of interventions occupational therapists use. The appendices are not exhaustive. Further knowledge of specific conditions may be needed in some circumstances, particularly when clients have more than one diagnosis or health condition. Also, by the nature of growth in clinical skills, the division between entry-level and advanced knowledge is somewhat fluid as the practitioner learns more and advances in clinical knowledge and skill. Furthermore, the knowledge base listed here is not absolute. Research in basic and applied science continues to expand the available knowledge base. Therefore, practitioners continue to read the literature, attend continuing education courses, and otherwise engage in activities to maintain and improve their knowledge and understanding of intervention in this area, to support their evidence-based practice.

Vestibular disorders decrease the ability to be independent in many activities of daily living. In general, tasks that require rapid or repeated head movements, tasks that require good postural control, especially while standing or walking, and tasks that require good spatial orientation may be affected. Clients who have fallen or who are at risk for falls may severely restrict their movements and may actually increase their risk of falling as a result. These people often cease participation in exercise programs for strengthening, cardiovascular conditioning, weight loss, or bone health. In a few rare instances, avoiding motions or positions that elicit vertigo may even mean delaying necessary surgical procedures due to potential discomfort during postoperative bed rest.

Clients with vestibular impairments often require more time to complete routine self-care skills. They may need to adapt the environment for safety or change the way in which they perform some tasks (e.g., to sit rather than stand or to hold an object for safety while standing). They may need to reduce the amount of extraneous stimulation in the environment during task performance since divided attention becomes

Appendix 1. Basic Science Knowledge for Vestibular Rehabilitation

Detailed knowledge of the structure of the ear and vestibular labyrinth, including semicircular canals, otoliths, and vestibular nerve

Detailed knowledge of the physiology of the vestibular labyrinth, including basic understanding of the inertial mechanisms of the semicircular canals and otoliths

Understanding of central vestibular projections, including vestibular nuclei, vestibulocerebellar projections, vestibulospinal projections, vestibulo-ocular projections, and vestibulocortical projections

Understanding of multisensory interactions, including visual, vestibular, haptic, and proprioceptive

Understanding of vestibulo-autonomic interactions

Manifestations of the vestibular influence on postural control (e.g., vestibulopostural responses)

Manifestations of vestibulooocular control (e.g., vestibuloocular reflex)

Understanding of other eye movements and oculomotor responses: saccades, smooth pursuit, optokinetic responses, fixation/suppression, and interaction of vestibulo-ocular reflex with other eye movements

Manifestations of vestibular influence on spatial orientation: vertical orientation and path integration

Manifestations of vestibulo-autonomic responses

Appendix 2. Applied Science Knowledge for Vestibular Rehabilitation

Familiarity with symptoms of vestibular disorders: vertigo and oscillopsia, balance deficits, path integration impairments, autonomic signs, cognitive problems, psychosocial problems, hearing loss, and auditory/perceptual illusions on rare occasions

Familiarity with principles of objective diagnostic tests: low-frequency sinusoidal tests of the vestibuloocular reflex, bithermal caloric tests, vestibular-evoked myogenic potentials, Dix-Hallpike and side-lying tests, and computerized dynamic posturography. Advanced practitioners should be familiar with the standard techniques for recording eye movements, including electrooculography/electronystagmography and infrared videooculography. Advanced practitioners should also be familiar with related oculomotor tests and auditory screening tests.

Familiarity with peripheral vestibular disorders: Labyrinthitis/vestibular neuronitis; acute, self-limiting, recurrent, and chronic benign paroxysmal positional vertigo, Ménierè's disease, perilymph fistula, acoustic neuroma, Tullio's phenomenon, ototoxicity, and other causes of bilateral vestibular impairment

Familiarity with central vestibular disorders: presbystasis, cerebellopontine angle tumor, Arnold Chiari malformation, medulloblastoma, migraine, multiple sclerosis, Parkinson's disease and the Parkinsonian syndromes, lateral medullary syndrome and other cerebrovascular accidents, traumatic brain injury, and vertebrobasilar insufficiency

Familiarity with systemic disorders: diabetes, autoimmune disorders, especially those causing connective tissue disorders

Understanding of relevant physician subspecialties: otology/neurotology and otoneurology

Understanding of cognitive strategies and problems in dual- and multitask performance

more difficult, so they may require reduced noise, less visual clutter, or fewer tasks requiring simultaneous attention. Therefore, they may become less efficient when performing tasks.

Many clients deliberately constrain their lives, becoming less active within and outside the home. So, they may abandon activities that they consider to be nonessential and reduce their participation in essential tasks. Many people stop driving or drive only within their neighborhoods and avoid highway driving. They may even change jobs to reduce travel or to avoid other job-related requirements that elicit vertigo or disequilibrium. Many people with vestibular disorders stop socializing or attending worship services because they are embarrassed by their ataxic gaits and do not want to give the appearance of intoxication. Some clients, who have vertigo when they bow during required prayers or who are unable to kneel while praying, may feel spiritually bereft. These problems can affect relationships with family, friends, and coworkers. Even the most understanding spouses may become upset when intimate sexual activity is interrupted by vertigo, quiet time together while taking a walk is made unpleasant due to repeated stumbling or drifting back and forth, and the affected individual may no longer be able to participate in shared sports or other exercise activities. See Appendixes 3–8 for further examples.

Specific evaluation and intervention skills are used in vestibular rehabilitation. The occupational therapy practitioner who works in this specialty must be familiar with the evaluation skills in Appendix 9 and the intervention skills in Appendix 10.

Appendix 3. Examples of Impact on Activities of Daily Living

Eating: Leaning across a table to pass something

Bathing: Bending to reach the legs, feet, perineal area, closing eyes to wash hair

Toileting: Bending to wipe, bending to pull garments up or down, maintaining balance while standing to urinate (males), twisting to reach toilet paper if behind toilet

Transferring: Sit-to-stand transfers from toilet, other seats

Grooming and hygiene: Bending the head forward to groom hair or brush teeth

Taking medication: Bending the head back to swallow medication

Sexual activity: Being in the superior position and weight shifting or moving the head rapidly; stability on water bed or other positioning furniture

Sleep: Head movements during sleep, changing sleeping positions, or maintaining the head in certain positions during sleep will elicit vertigo and cause waking, possibly nausea, and disequilibrium while groggy

Instrumental Activities of Daily Living

Meal preparation, cleaning, other home management skills: Bending down, looking into high or low cabinets or shelves, and tasks that require repetitive head movements may all elicit symptoms. Task performance may be compromised or the task may be abandoned altogether.

Gardening, yard work: Tasks may be performed less efficiently or abandoned; falls may occur on uneven ground.

Vehicle care: Car washing and changing oil and filters may be difficult or impossible.

Child, elder, and pet care: Tasks that involve picking up and carrying loads, bending rapidly, performing or assisting in transfers, diaper changing, cleaning up messes on floor

Community mobility: Driving will be more difficult, especially under conditions of reduced visibility, and may be abandoned or performed only for limited errands.

Shopping: Navigating stores, carrying packages, bending to pick up items, scanning shelves for items will be more difficult and may be abandoned.

Safety: Ascending/descending fire escapes and stairs, dim areas with only emergency lighting

Play, leisure, social participation, religious activities: Visual motion sensitivity, difficulty kneeling, navigating in crowds, vertigo elicited by repetitive head movements or bending the head down; activities and rituals may be severely restricted or abandoned.

Work, either paid employment or volunteer jobs: Symptoms elicited by a wide range of tasks will cause reduced efficiency and sometimes total inability to perform some jobs, depending on task demands.

Appendix 4. Examples of Performance Skills Affected by Vestibular Impairments

Posture: Standing balance is impaired in most people with vestibular impairments. People may tilt the head and/or body off the vertical. They may have difficulty attaining and maintaining upright standing. This skill is particularly difficult when visual cues are absent or decreased. Static head and trunk posture while seated are sometimes impaired; dynamic sitting balance may also be impaired.

Mobility: Mobility skills are manifested as veering toward one side while walking, ataxic gait, and falling or stumbling, particularly on uneven surfaces. Load compensation skills are impaired. Clients may need to use light touch to improve orientation and stability.

Coordination: Dual-task performance skill is decreased.

Energy: Routine tasks take more energy than usual, and endurance is decreased.

Appendix 5. Examples of Performance Patterns Affected by Vestibular Impairments

Habits: Skill components of habits may be disrupted, and performance efficiency may be reduced, increasing the cognitive load and increasing the difficulty of performing habitual skills that were previously easy to perform (e.g., basic activities of daily living may have to be performed with modifications).

Routines: Due to effects on performance skills, routines are less efficient and may need to be changed or abandoned altogether (e.g., hair washing may require supervision for safety and may take too long in the morning before work, so the client's morning and evening routines may be changed).

Roles: Some roles may be reduced or even abandoned, with consequent detrimental economic and psychosocial effects (e.g., clients with Ménierè's disease may have to leave their jobs).

Appendix 6. Examples of Context Affected by Vestibular Impairments

Physical: The physical environment may require modifications for safety (e.g., installing bathroom grab bars), or the home environment may require significant change (e.g., removing throw rugs, changing lighting patterns).

Social: Misunderstanding of symptoms and problems by family, friends, and significant others may lead to hard feelings, reduced participation in socialization, changes in preferred social environments. These problems may occur due to decreased self-confidence, fear of falling, and a history of falls.

Spiritual: Falls, vertigo, decreased concentration, and decreased ability in dual task performance, which all lead to decreased performance in vocational and vocational activities and decreased participation in the community, can cause decreased sense of self-worth, self-doubt, and decreased joy in life.

Virtual: Visual motion sensitivity may lead to avoidance of virtual environments.

Appendix 7. Examples of Activity Demands Affected by Vestibular Impairments

Timing: Tasks may take longer than before.

Space demands: Lighting, flooring, and support surfaces may have to be changed.

Social demands: Reduced social interaction per task may be required due to reduced tolerance for auditory and visual noise.

Required bodily functions: Reduced function of vestibulo-ocular reflex, vestibulospinal reflex, and reduced spatial orientation skills all affect functional performance.

Appendix 8. Examples of Client Factors Affected by Vestibular Impairments

Mental functions: Reduced attention skills, reduced ability for dual task performance

Sensory functions: Reduced vestibular function, sometimes reduced auditory function

Neuromuscular functions: Reduced postural control, reduced dynamic visual acuity, impaired gait

Vestibular labyrinth: In some instances, structural abnormalities in the physical labyrinth may be present, but these features cannot be observed; they may only be inferred.

Appendix 9. Occupational Therapy Evaluation Skills for Vestibular Rehabilitation

Detailed occupational and health histories relevant to symptoms

Objective clinical tests involving the vestibuloocular reflex head thrusts, Dix-Hallpike and sidelying maneuvers, and other tests of positional vertigo in lateral and anterior canals

Tests of path integration skill

Oculomotor tests: saccades, pursuit, optokinetic nystagmus, vergence, visual/vestibuloocular reflex interaction, evaluation of spontaneous nystagmus

Standardized and nonstandardized tests of standing and walking balance, including Clinical Test of Sensory Organization on Balance, Functional Reach, Berg Balance Scale, Get Up and Go/Timed Up and Go, Dynamic Gait Index, expert observation of other gait and balance skills including stair climbing, subtle gait deficits, and weight-shifting deficits

Qualitative self-evaluations of ADL independence: Activities-Specific Balance Confidence scale, Dizziness Handicap Inventory, and Vestibular Disorders Activities of Daily Living scale

Tests of dynamic visual acuity and oscillopsia

Measures to evaluate vertigo: head shaking, repetitive activities

Cognitive and psychosocial assessments: qualitative assessments and self-report on scales

Evaluation of independence in activities of daily living, including subtle changes and problems

Home, work, and driving safety

Appendix 10. Occupational Therapy Intervention Skills for Vestibular Rehabilitation

Repositioning treatments for benign paroxysmal positional vertigo, including canalith repositioning, liberatory maneuvers, log-rolling maneuvers, Brandt Daroff exercises, other repositioning exercises and activities

Vertigo habituation exercises and activity programs

Gaze stabilization exercises and activities, including eye–head coordination tasks

Balance therapy: exercises and activities for "static" standing, weight shifting, and balance control; exercises and activities for "dynamic" balance control during translation through space, leading to independence in dual task performance and safety during obstacle avoidance tasks

Home and work safety, including environmental modifications for lighting, flooring, modification of work area

Training in mobility skills on the bed; transfers to and from the floor, in the home, and in the external environment for falls prevention (e.g., use of a ladder, elevator, escalator, stairs, opening door, transfers to and from automobile, and functional mobility through visually challenging environments and environments with challenging support surfaces)

Knowledge of community and online resources for patient information

Patient education about condition, symptoms

Specific to Ménierè's disease patients: in coordination with nursing, work on meal-planning skills if dietary restriction is recommended by the physician

In coordination with audiology, for patients with hearing loss, recommend communication and functional devices for telephone, alarm clock, and other devices for which sound is important; recommendations for modification of work and other tasks, as needed, for hearing loss

Recommendation of assistive devices for balance and safety during standing, walking, carrying objects, and other activities of daily living

Task modification to reduce cognitive load during dual- and multitask performance; dual-task performance training

Glossary

Benign paroxysmal positional vertigo
A common disorder of the vestibular system characterized by vertigo elicited by head movements in the pitch plane and characterized by a positive response on the Dix–Hallpike maneuver.

Disequilibrium
Poor balance.

Labyrinthitis
Inflammation or disease of the vestibular labyrinth of the inner ear.

Ménière's disease
A disorder of the inner ear affecting both the auditory and vestibular systems. It is characterized by sensorineural hearing loss on at least one occasion, two or more spontaneous episodes of vertigo lasting at least 20 minutes, and tinnitus or aural fullness in the affected ear. Nystagmus is present during an attack (Committee on Hearing and Equilibrium, American Academy of Otolaryngology—Head and Neck Surgery, 1995).

Neurotologist
An otolaryngologist who specializes in ear and inner-ear disorders, including vestibular disorders.

Nystagmus
A stereotyped combination of repetitive slow- and fast-phase eye movements. The slow phase, usually difficult to observe with the naked eye, represents compensatory vestibulo-ocular or optokinetic responses; the fast phase represents rapid saccades that reset the position of the globe in the eye socket.

Optokinetic responses
Conjugate eye movements used to follow a full-field moving visual stimulus (i.e., when the entire visual scene moves around the person).

Oscillopsia
The illusion of object motion during head movement.

Otolaryngologist
A physician who specializes in ear, nose, and throat disorders.

Otoneurologist
A neurologist who specializes in vestibular and auditory disorders.

Presbystasis
Disequilibrium of aging. This diagnosis excludes known causes of balance problems, such as central neurologic conditions, peripheral vestibular impairments, or peripheral neuropathies that affect the lower extremities (e.g., diabetic neuropathies).

Pursuit
Also known as *smooth pursuit*. Conjugate eye movements are used to follow a discrete moving visual stimulus.

Saccades
Conjugate eye movements in which the eyes move for one of three reasons: (1) as the quick phase of nystagmus, to reset the position of the globe in the eye socket; (2) for gaze error correction (i.e., to catch up with a visual stimulus that is moving too fast for pursuit movements); and (3) volitional movements to look around a stationary visual environment. Saccades are the only volitional eye movements that we are able to generate. (You are using saccades to read this page.)

Spatial orientation

Awareness of one's position relative to gravity and the environment.

Vergence

Disconjugate eye movements used to make the eyes move toward or away from each other, in order to focus on an object.

Vertigo

The illusion of self-motion (e.g., spinning, falling).

Vestibular rehabilitation

The use of activities and exercise to treat vertigo, balance problems, functional limitations, and disability caused by impairments in the vestibular system.

Vestibular system

The sensory system with receptors in the vestibular labyrinth of the inner ear. It detects head motion and contributes to control of posture, eye movements, and spatial orientation. The brain pathways include the vestibular portion of Cranial Nerve VIII; the vestibular nuclei; the parts of the cerebellum that receive and process vestibular signals; the projections from the vestibular nuclei that descend in the spinal cord via the vestibulospinal tracts; the projections from the vestibular nuclei that ascend in the medial longitudinal fasciculus to Cranial Nerves III, IV, and VI to control the vestibulo-ocular reflex; and the smaller projections that ascend from the vestibular nuclei to the thalamus and related nuclei with further small projections to the vestibular cortex.

References

American Medical Association. (2006). *Current procedural terminology* (2006 ed.). Chicago: Author.

American Occupational Therapy Association. (2002). Occupational therapy practice framework: Domain and process. *American Journal of Occupational Therapy, 56,* 609–639.

American Occupational Therapy Association. (2004). Guidelines for supervision, roles, and responsibilities during the delivery of occupational therapy services. *American Journal of Occupational Therapy, 58,* 663–667.

Cawthorne, T. (1944). The physiological basis for head exercises. *Journal of the Chartered Society of Physiotherapy, 29,* 106–107.

Cohen, H. (1992). Vestibular rehabilitation reduces functional disability. *Otolaryngology—Head and Neck Surgery, 107,* 638–643.

Cohen, H. S. (2006). Disability and rehabilitation in the dizzy patient. *Current Opinion in Neurology, 19,* 49–54.

Cohen, H., Ewell, L. R., & Jenkins, H. A. (1995). Disability in Ménière's disease. *Archives of Otolaryngology, 121,* 29–33.

Cohen, H. S., & Jerabek, J. (1999). Effectiveness of liberatory maneuvers for benign paroxysmal positional vertigo of the posterior canal. *Laryngoscope, 109,* 584–590.

Cohen, H., Kane-Wineland, M., Miller, L. V., & Hatfield, C. L. (1995). Occupation and visual/vestibular interaction in vestibular rehabilitation. *Otolaryngology—Head and Neck Surgery, 112,* 526–532.

Cohen, H. S., & Kimball, K. T. (2000). Development of the Vestibular Disorders Activities of Daily Living Scale. *Archives of Otolaryngology, 126,* 881–887.

Cohen, H. S., & Kimball, K. T. (2002). Improvements in path integration after vestibular rehabilitation. *Journal of Vestibular Research, 12,* 47–51.

Cohen, H. S., & Kimball, K. T. (2003). Increased independence and decreased vertigo after vestibular rehabilitation. *Otolaryngology—Head and Neck Surgery, 128,* 560–566.

Cohen, H. S., & Kimball, K. T. (2004a). Treatment variations on the Epley maneuver for benign paroxysmal positional vertigo. *American Journal of Otolaryngology, 25,* 33–37.

Cohen, H. S., & Kimball, K. T. (2004b). Changes in a repetitive head movement task after vestibular rehabilitation. *Clinical Rehabilitation, 18,* 125–131.

Cohen, H. S., & Kimball, K. T. (2004c). Decreased ataxia and improved balance after vestibular rehabilitation. *Otolaryngology—Head and Neck Surgery, 130,* 418–425.

Cohen, H. S., & Kimball, K. T. (2005). Effectiveness of treatments for benign paroxysmal positional vertigo of the posterior canal. *Otology and Neurotology, 26,* 1034–1040.

Cohen, H. S., Kimball, K. T., & Adams, A. (2000). Application of the Vestibular Disorders Activities of Daily Living Scale. *Laryngoscope, 110,* 1204–1209.

Cohen, H., Miller, L. V., Kane-Wineland, M., & Hatfield, C. L. (1995). Case Report—Vestibular rehabilitation with graded occupations. *American Journal of Occupational Therapy, 49,* 362–367.

Cohen, H. S., Wells, J., Kimball, K. T., & Owsley, C. (2003). Driving disability in dizziness. *Journal of Safety Research, 34*(4), 361–369.

Committee on Hearing and Equilibrium, American Academy of Otolaryngology—Head and Neck Surgery. (1995). Guidelines for the diagnosis and evaluation of therapy in Ménierè's disease. *Otolaryngology—Head and Neck Surgery, 113,* 181–185.

Cooksey, F. S. (1945). Physical medicine. *Practitioner, 155,* 300–305.

Cooksey, F. S. (1946). Rehabilitation in vestibular injuries. *Proceedings of the Royal Society of Medicine, 39,* 273–278.

Eagger, S., Luxon, L. M., Davies, R. A., Coelho, A., & Ron, M. A. (1992). Psychiatric morbidity in clients with peripheral vestibular disorder: A clinical and neuro-otological study. *Journal of Neurology, Neurosurgery, and Psychiatry, 55,* 383–387.

Farber, S. D. (1989). Living with Ménière's disease: An occupational therapist's perspective. *American Journal of Occupational Therapy, 43,* 341–343.

Macias, J. D., Lambert, K. M., Massingale, S., Ellensohn, A., & Fritz, J. A. (2000). Variables affecting treatment in benign paroxysmal positional vertigo. *Laryngoscope, 110,* 1921–1924.

Morris, P. A. (1991). A habituation approach to treating vertigo in occupational therapy. *American Journal of Occupational Therapy, 45,* 556–558.

Steenerson, R. L., & Cronin, G. W. (1996). Comparison of the canalith repositioning procedure and vestibular habituation training in forty patients with benign paroxysmal positional vertigo. *Otolaryngology—Head and Neck Surgery, 1214,* 61–64.

Steenerson, R. L., Cronin, G. W., & Marbach, P. M. (2005). Effectiveness of treatment techniques in 932 cases of benign paroxysmal positional vertigo. *Laryngoscope, 115,* 226–231.

Yardley, L., & Hallam, R. S. (1996). Psychosocial aspects of balance and gait disorders. In A. M. Bronstein, T. Brandt, & M. Woollacott (Eds.), *Clinical disorders of balance, posture and gait* (pp. 251–267). London: Arnold.

Yardley, L., Luxon, L. M., & Haacke, N. P. (1994). A longitudinal study of symptoms, anxiety, and subjective well-being in clients with vertigo. *Clinical Otolaryngology and Allied Sciences, 19,* 109–116.

Yardley, L., & Putman, J. (1992). Quantitative analysis of factors contributing to handicap and distress in vertiginous clients: A questionnaire study. *Clinical Otolaryngology and Allied Sciences, 17,* 231–236.

Additional Reading

Aw, S. T., Halmagyi, G. M., Black, R. A., Curthoys, I. S., Yavor, R. A., & Todd, M. J. (1999). Head impulses reveal loss of individual semicircular canal function. *Journal of Vestibular Research, 9,* 173–180.

Baloh, R. W., Furman, J. M. R., Halmagyi, M., & Allum, J. H. J. (1995). Recent advances in clinical neurotology. *Journal of Vestibular Research, 5,* 231–252.

Baloh, R. W., & Halmagyi, G. M. (Eds.). (1996). *Disorders of the vestibular system.* New York: Oxford University Press.

Baloh, R. W., & Honrubia, V. (1990). *Clinical neurophysiology of the vestibular system* (2nd ed.). Philadelphia: F. A. Davis.

Black, R. A., Halmagyi, G. M., Thurtell, M. J., Todd, M. J., & Curthoys, I. S. (2005). The active head-impulse test in unilateral peripheral vestibulopathy. *Annals of Neurology, 62,* 290–293.

Brandt, T. (1998). *Vertigo: Its multisensory syndromes.* Berlin: Springer-Verlag.

Brandt, T., Steddin, S., & Daroff, R. B. (1994). Therapy for benign paroxysmal positioning vertigo, revisited. *Neurology, 44,* 796–800.

Bronstein, A. M., Brandt, T., & Woollacott, M. (Eds.). (1996). *Clinical disorders of balance, posture and gait.* London: Arnold/Hodder Headline PLC.

Campbell, A. J., Robertson, M. C., La Grow, S. J., Kerse, N. M., Sanderson, G. F., Jacobs, R. J., et al. (2005, October). Randomised controlled trial of prevention of falls in people aged 75 with severe visual impairment: The VIP trial. *British Medical Journal, 331*(7520), 817. Retrieved March 21, 2006, from http://bmj.bmjjournals.com/cgi/reprint_abr/331/7520/817

Cawthorne, T. (1946). Vestibular injuries. *Proceedings of the Royal Society of Medicine, 39,* 270–273.

Chronister, K. M. (2003). Divided attention: The role that cognition plays in fall prevention programs has been overlooked. *Rehab Management, 16,* 30, 32–33.

Chronister, K. (2004). Cognition: The missing link in fall-prevention programs. *Rehab Management, 9,* 11–14.

Clemson, L., Cumming, R. G., Kendig, H., Swann, M., Heard, R., & Taylor, K. (2004). The effectiveness of a community-based program for reducing the incidence of falls in the elderly: A randomized trial. *Journal of the American Geriatric Society, 52,* 1487–1494.

Cohen, H. (1994). Vestibular rehabilitation improves daily life function. *American Journal of Occupational Therapy, 48,* 919–925.

Cohen, H. (1998). *Special senses 2: The vestibular system. Neuroscience for rehabilitation.* Philadelphia: Lippincott Williams & Wilkins.

Cohen, H. S. (2000). Vertigo and balance disorders: Vestibular rehabilitation. *Occupational Therapy Practice, 5,* 14–18.

Cohen, H. S. (2004). Vestibular rehabilitation and stroke. In G. Gillen & A. Burkhardt (Eds.), *Stroke rehabilitation: A function-based approach* (2nd ed., pp. 164–171). St. Louis, MO: Mosby.

Cohen, H. S. (in press). Disability in vestibular disorders. In S. J. Herdman (Ed.), *Vestibular rehabilitation* (3rd ed). Philadelphia: F. A. Davis.

Cohen, H., Blatchly, C. A., & Gombash, L. L. (1993). A study of the clinical test of sensory interaction and balance. *Physical Therapy, 73,* 346–351.

Cohen, H., Friedman, E. M., Lai, D., Duncan, N., Pellicer, M., & Sulek, M. (1997). Balance in children with otitis media with effusion. *International Journal of Pediatric Oto-Rhino-Laryngology, 42,* 107–115.

Cohen, H. S., & Gavia, J. A. (1998). A task for assessing vertigo elicited by repetitive head movements. *American Journal of Occupational Therapy, 52,* 644–649.

Cohen, H., Heaton, L. G., Congdon, S. L., & Jenkins, H. A. (1996). Changes in sensory organization test scores with age. *Age and Ageing, 25,* 39–44.

Cohen, H. S., Kimball, K. T., & Stewart, M. G. (2004). Benign paroxysmal positional vertigo and co-morbid conditions. *ORL—Journal of Oto-Rhino-Laryngology and Related Specialties, 66,* 11–15.

Cohen, H., Rubin, A. M., & Gombash, L. L. (1991). The team approach to intervention of the dizzy client. *Archives of Physical Medicine and Rehabilitation, 73,* 703–708.

Colebatch, J. G. (2001). Vestibular evoked potentials. *Current Opinion in Neurology, 14,* 21–26.

Colebatch, J. G., Halmagyi, G. M., & Skuse, N. F. (1994). Myogenic potentials generated by a click-evoked vestibulocollic reflex. *Journal of Neurology, Neurosurgery, and Psychiatry, 57,* 190–107.

Cronin, G. W. (1990). Vestibular rehab enhances patient's quality of life. *Advance for Occupational Therapists, 6*(43), 2.

Crowe, T. K., Deitz, J. C., Richardson, P. K., & Atwater, S. W. (1990). Interrater reliability of the Pediatric Clinical Test of Sensory Interaction for Balance. *Physical and Occupational Therapy in Pediatrics, 10,* 1–27.

Cumming, R. G., Thomas, M., Szonyi, G., Frampton, G., Salkeld, G., & Clemson, L. (2001). Adherence to occupational therapist recommendations for home modifications for falls prevention. *American Journal of Occupational Therapy, 55,* 641–648.

Davison, J., Bond, J., Dawson, P., Steen, I. N., & Kenny, R. A. (2005). Patients with recurrent falls attending accident and emergency benefit from multifactorial intervention—A randomized controlled trial. *Age and Ageing, 34,* 162–168.

De la Meilleure, G., Dehaene, I., Depondt, M., Damman, W., Crevits, L., & Vanhooren, G. (1996). Benign paroxysmal positional vertigo of the horizontal canal. *Journal of Neurology, Neurosurgery, and Psychiatry, 60,* 68–71.

Dix, M. R. (1974). Intervention of vertigo. *Physiotherapy, 60,* 380–384.

Dix, M. R. (1976). The physiological basis and practical value of head exercises in the intervention of vertigo. *Practitioner, 217,* 919–924.

Dix, M. R. (1984). Rehabilitation of vertigo. In M. R. Dix & J. D. Hood (Eds.), *Vertigo* (pp. 467–479). Chichester, NY: Wiley.

Fife, T. D., Tusa, R. J., Furman, J. M., Zee, D. S., Frohman, E., Baloh, R. W., et al. (2000). Assessment: Vestibular testing techniques in adults and children. Report of the Therapeutics and Technology Assessment Subcommittee of the American Academy of Neurology. *Neurology, 55,* 1431–1441.

Gottshall, K., Gray, N., & Drake, A. I. (2005). A unique collaboration of female medical providers within the United States Armed Forces: Rehabilitation of a marine with post-concussive vestibulopathy. *Work, 24,* 381–386.

Halmagyi, G. M., & Curthoys, I. A. (1988). A clinical sign of canal paresis. *Archives of Neurology, 45,* 737–739.

Hecker, H. C., Haug, C. O., & Herndon, J. W. (1974). Intervention of the vertiginous client using Cawthorne's vestibular exercises. *Laryngoscope, 84,* 2065–2072.

Hillman, E. J., Bloomberg, J. J., McDonald, V. P., & Cohen, H. S. (1999). Dynamic visual acuity while walking in normal and labyrinthine-deficient clients. *Journal of Vestibular Research, 9,* 49–57.

Honrubia, V., Bell, T. S., Harris, M. R., Baloh, R. W., & Fisher, L. M. (1996). Quantitative evaluation of dizziness characteristics and impact on quality of life. *American Journal of Otology, 17,* 595–602.

Horak, F. B., Shumway-Cook, A., Crowe, T. K., & Black, F. O. (1988). Vestibular function and motor proficiency of children with impaired hearing, or with learning disability and motor impairments. *Developmental Medicine and Child Neurology, 30,* 64–79.

Jacobson, G. P., & Newman, C. W. (1990). The development of the Dizziness Handicap Inventory. *Archives of Otolaryngology, 116,* 424–427.

Jacobson, G. P., Newman, C. W., & Kartush, J. M. (1993). *Handbook of balance function testing.* St. Louis, MO: Mosby/YearBook.

Konnur, M. K. (2000). Vertigo and vestibular rehabilitation. *Postgraduate Medicine, 46,* 222–223.

McCabe, B. F. (1970). Labyrinthine exercises in the intervention of diseases characterized by vertigo: Their physiologic basis and methodology. *Laryngoscope, 80,* 1429–1433.

Medeiros, I. R. T., Bittar, R. S. M., Pedalini, E. B., Lorenzi, M. C., Formigoni, L. G., et al. (2005). Vestibular rehabilitation therapy in children. *Otology and Neurotology, 26,* 699–703.

Myers, A. M., Powell, L. E., Maki, B. E., Holliday, P. J., Brawley, L. R., & Sherk, W. (1996). Psychological indicators of balance confidence: Relationship to actual and perceived abilities. *Journal of Gerontology: Medical Science, 51A,* M37–M43.

Norré, M. E., & De Weerdt, W. (1979). Vestibular habituation training: Technique and first results—Preliminary report. *Acta Oto-Rhino-Laryngologica Belgica, 33,* 347–364.

Parnes, L. S., & Sindwani, R. (1997). Impact of vestibular disorders on fitness to drive: A consensus of the American Neurotology Society. *American Journal of Otology, 18,* 79–85.

Rine, R. M., Braswell, J., Fisher, D., Joyce, K., Kalar, K., & Shaffer, M. (2004). Improvement of motor development and postural control following intervention in children with sensorineural hearing loss and vestibular impairment. *International Journal of Pediatric Oto-Rhino-Laryngology, 68,* 1141–1148.

Sherlock, J. (1996). Getting into balance. *Rehab Management, 9,* 33–38.

Shumway-Cook, A., & Horak, F. B. (1986). Assessing the influence of sensory interaction on balance. *Physical Therapy, 66,* 1548–1550.

Shumway-Cook, A., & Horak, F. B. (1989). Vestibular rehabilitation: An exercise approach to managing symptoms of vestibular dysfunction. *Seminars in Hearing, 10,* 196–208.

Sindwani, R., & Parnes, L. S. (1997). Reporting of vestibular clients who are unfit to drive: Survey of Canadian otolaryngologists. *Journal of Otolaryngology, 26,* 104–111.

Steultjens, E. M. J., Dekker, J., Bouter, L. M., Jellma, S., Bakker, E. B., & van den Ende, C. H. M. (2004). Occupational therapy for community dwelling elderly people: A systematic review. *Age and Ageing, 33,* 453–460.

Uneri, A., & Turkdogan, D. (2003). Evaluation of vestibular functions in children with vertigo attacks. *Archives of Disease in Childhood, 88*, 510–511.

Whitney, S. L., Poole, J. L., & Cass, S. P. (1998). A review of balance instruments for older adults. *American Journal of Occupational Therapy, 52*, 666–671.

Wilson, V. J., & Melvill Jones, G. (1979). *Mammalian vestibular physiology*. New York: Plenum.

Wilson, V. J., & Melvill Jones, G. (1985). *Adaptive mechanisms of gaze control*. New York: Plenum.

Yardley, L. (1994). Prediction of handicap and emotional distress in clients with recurrent vertigo: Symptoms, coping strategies, control beliefs, and reciprocal causation. *Social Science and Medicine, 39*, 573–581.

Yardley, L., Burgneau, J., Nazareth, I., & Luxon, L. (1998). Neuro-otological and psychiatric abnormalities in a community sample of people with dizziness: A blind, controlled investigation. *Journal of Neurology, Neurosurgery and Psychiatry, 65*, 679–684.

Other Information Resources

American Academy of Otolaryngology—Head and Neck Surgery
One Prince Street
Alexandria, VA 22314-3357
703-836-4444
www.entnet.org
This group is the professional organization for otolaryngologists, including neurotologists. To find a neurotologist in your area, see the "Find an ENT" link. See also useful patient information brochures.

Anatomical Chart Company
Lippincott Williams & Wilkins
www.lww.com/anatomicalchart/
They produce good charts and three-dimensional models of the vestibular labyrinth.

Journal of Vestibular Research
Eye and Ear Institute
203 Lothrop Street, Suite 500
Pittsburgh, PA 15213
e-mail: jvr@upmc.edu
Web address: www.jvr-web.org
This journal specializes in publishing research on basic and clinical vestibular sciences, including research on vestibular rehabilitation and balance disorders.

National Institute on Deafness and Other Communication Disorders (NIDCD)
National Institutes of Health
31 Center Drive, MSC 2320
Bethesda, MD 20892-2320
800-241-1044
www.nidcd.nih.gov
The NIH funds much of the biomedical and biobehavioral research in this country. The NIDCD, an institute of the NIH, funds research on balance and vestibular function, including research on vestibular rehabilitation. See their Web page for free patient information brochures and a tutorial for patients with balance problems.

Vestibular Disorders Association
PO Box 4467
Portland OR 97208
Telephone: 800-837-8428
Telephone in Oregon: 503-229-7705
e-mail: veda@vestibular.org
Web address: www.vestibular.org
This patient advocacy group has useful information for patients about a variety of vestibular disorders. They also maintain a resource list of health care professionals who specialize in care of people with vestibular disorders.

Authors
Helen S. Cohen, EdD, OTR, FAOTA, *Chairperson*
Ann Burkhardt, OTD, OTR/L, BCN, FAOTA
Gaye W. Cronin, OTD, OTR
Mary Jo McGuire, MS, OTR, FAOTA

for

The Commission on Practice
Susanne Smith Roley, MS, OTR/L, FAOTA, *Chairperson*

Adopted by the Representative Assembly 2006C405

Reviewed by the Commission on Practice September 2010

This replaces the 2000 document "Specialized Knowledge and Skills in Adult Vestibular Rehabilitation for Occupational Therapy Practice" (*American Journal of Occupational Therapy, 55,* 661–665).

Specialized Knowledge and Skills in Feeding, Eating, and Swallowing for Occupational Therapy Practice

Introduction

Occupational therapy's long-standing expertise in activities of daily living includes involvement in the feeding, eating, and swallowing performance of individuals across the life span (American Occupational Therapy Association [AOTA], 2002). Both occupational therapists and occupational therapy assistants[1] provide essential services in the comprehensive management of feeding, eating, and swallowing problems. These problems can be wide ranging and may include physical difficulty (e.g., bringing food to the mouth), processing food in the mouth (e.g., motor or sensory deficits), dysphagia, psychosocially based eating disorders (e.g., food obsessions, maladaptive eating habits), dysfunction related to cognitive impairments (e.g., understanding nutrition or food preparation), surgical intervention, and neurological impairments, as well as positioning problems that affect feeding, eating, and swallowing. Interventions focused on occupations of daily living include facilitating an individual's ability to participate in feeding and eating activities that are valued and meaningful to that person, such as learning to eat independently, joining friends for lunch, or feeding a child. Occupational therapists and occupational therapy assistants possess the education, experience, knowledge, and skills necessary in the evaluation and intervention of feeding, eating, and swallowing problems. Physical, cognitive, social, emotional, and cultural elements of feeding, eating, and swallowing are considered in evaluation and intervention.

The purpose of this document is to describe the knowledge and skills that are necessary for occupational therapists and occupational therapy assistants to provide comprehensive feeding, eating, and swallowing management and services. It provides information on occupational therapists' and occupational therapy assistants' roles in feeding, eating, and swallowing; outlines advanced-level knowledge and skills; and defines feeding-, eating-, and swallowing-related terms.

Occupational Therapy's Role in Feeding, Eating, and Swallowing Management

Feeding, Eating, and Swallowing

Feeding and eating occur within the social environment and often include family members and caregivers as part of the process. Thus, when occupational therapy practitioners address feeding, eating, and swallowing concerns, the collaboration with and involvement of family members and caregivers as well as other professionals is paramount.

Feeding, eating, and swallowing are complex activities that require effective, coordinated function of the motor, sensory, and cognitive systems. In recent years, the complexity of occupational therapy services to address these issues has grown. Feeding, eating, and swallowing services now are often provided to clients who have complicated, specialized problems and who may be medically fragile. In addition, new

---

[1]*Occupational therapists* are responsible for all aspects of occupational therapy service delivery and are accountable for the safety and effectiveness of the occupational therapy service delivery process. *Occupational therapy assistants* deliver occupational therapy services under the supervision of and in partnership with an occupational therapist (AOTA, 2004).

technologies are increasingly available for evaluation and intervention of swallowing or dysphagia management. Thus, in a variety of situations, occupational therapists and occupational therapy assistants demonstrate baseline knowledge in feeding, eating, and swallowing and may provide advanced-level knowledge and skills in the field of dysphagia management.

Feeding, eating, and swallowing are interdependent activities, and definitions of each term overlap in literature sources. For purposes of this paper, broad definitions are noted. *Feeding* is the term used to describe "the process of setting up, arranging, and bringing food [or fluid] from the plate or cup to the mouth; sometimes called self-feeding" (AOTA, 2006a). *Eating* is defined as "the ability to keep and manipulate food or fluid in the mouth and swallow it; eating and swallowing are often used interchangeably" (AOTA, 2006a). Feeding and eating, essential to human functioning for nourishment of the body, is a form of social interaction and is involved in many facets of a person's culture—from leisure to professional activities. *Swallowing* involves a complicated act in which food, fluid, medication, or saliva is moved from the mouth through the pharynx and esophagus into the stomach (AOTA, 2006a). Thus, feeding, eating, and swallowing are strongly influenced by psychosocial, cultural, and environmental factors. As part of the evaluation and intervention process, occupational therapists and occupational therapy assistants under the supervision of an occupational therapist consider comprehensive management of feeding, eating, and swallowing problems; adaptive feeding equipment ranging from modified utensils to sophisticated feeding equipment (e.g., the Winsford Feeder); the physical and sensory difficulty of bringing food, liquid, or medication to the mouth; sensory processing issues in the mouth (e.g., oral defensiveness); management of mechanical devices for feeding; dysphagia; psychosocially based eating disorders (e.g., anorexia, bulimia); behaviorally based eating disorders (e.g., selective eating); dysfunction related to cognitive impairments, neurological impairments, or surgical intervention; and positioning problems that affect feeding, eating, and swallowing.

Feeding, eating, and swallowing are within the domain and scope of practice for occupational therapy. Occupational therapists and occupational therapy assistants have the knowledge and skills necessary to take a lead role in the evaluation and intervention of feeding, eating, and swallowing problems. Further, occupational therapists have the entry-level knowledge and skills to evaluate oral and pharyngeal swallowing function.

Occupational Therapy Services

Occupational therapy practitioners[2] use their knowledge and skills to provide services over a broad range of ages, medical conditions, and social or cultural situations. For many clients, feeding, eating, and swallowing issues are quite complex. For instance, in populations with complicated feeding problems such as post-surgical cancer patients, patients in intensive care units, or young infants, the interplay of medical and developmental factors is complex and requires advanced-level knowledge to provide safe and effective service. As foundational skills in understanding impairments in feeding, eating, and swallowing, occupational therapists and occupational therapy assistants receive education in the structure and function of the human body, including the biological and physical sciences (e.g., anatomy, physiology, neuroanatomy, kinesiology), human development throughout the life span, and human behavior, including the behavioral and social sciences (Accreditation Council for Occupational Therapy Education, 2006). They develop clinical-reasoning skills to consider the interplay of physical, cognitive, environmental, and sociocultural factors in providing effective services for feeding, eating, and swallowing dysfunction.

As part of therapeutic services, occupational therapists are trained to conduct comprehensive evaluations, which include selecting, administering, and interpreting assessment measures. They also develop specific intervention plans and provide therapeutic interventions.

---

[2]When the term *occupational therapy practitioner* is used in this document, it refers to both occupational therapists and occupational therapy assistants (AOTA, 2006b).

The occupational therapist assumes the ultimate responsibility for the delivery of occupational therapy services. Occupational therapy assistants are trained to provide services under the supervision of and in collaboration with an occupational therapist (AOTA, 2004). During the evaluation process, occupational therapy assistants may gather data and administer selected assessment tools or measures for which they have demonstrated competence.

During intervention, both occupational therapists and occupational therapy assistants select, administer, and adapt activities that support the intervention plan developed by the occupational therapist. Practitioners must always adhere to state and agency regulatory laws when providing services across these continua of care. Reimbursement for services may be available through various sources, including legislation (e.g., Individuals With Disabilities Education Act, Medicare), private insurance, Medicaid, and private pay. Information on specific entry-level knowledge and skills occupational therapists and occupational therapy assistants should have to serve clients with feeding, eating, and swallowing dysfunction can be found in Appendix A.

For both occupational therapists and occupational therapy assistants, the progression from entry-level knowledge and skills to advanced-level knowledge and skills is individualized. Although practitioners exit their academic program with the basic knowledge and skills to provide occupational therapy services to clients with feeding, eating, and swallowing dysfunction, over time they may develop additional individualized expertise such as in the area of dysphagia. Occupational therapy practitioners ensure advanced competence in feeding, eating, and swallowing by maintaining and documenting competence in practice, education, and research and by participating in professional development, educational activities, and critical examination of available evidence (AOTA, 2005a). In addition, higher level knowledge, skills, and clinical reasoning are developed through experience.

The practitioner's acquisition of advanced-level knowledge and skills as related to intervention with people with feeding, eating, and swallowing difficulties is individualized; thus, a practitioner may possess differing levels of expertise in a wide variety of skill areas and populations served by occupational therapy. For example, an occupational therapist with advanced-level skills in feeding with premature infants may possess only entry-level skills in assessing swallowing function in a client who has had a cerebral vascular accident resulting in hemiplegic weakness. It is the ethical responsibility of occupational therapists and occupational therapy assistants to ensure that they are competent in the services they provide and that they continually seek out new knowledge and techniques that apply to their clinical practice (AOTA, 2005a).

Supervision Considerations

The amount of supervision provided to an occupational therapist or occupational therapy assistant in the area of feeding, eating, and swallowing should directly relate to their training and experience and state practice acts. Occupational therapy assistants and entry-level occupational therapists should seek supervision and mentoring from a more experienced occupational therapist or an occupational therapist with advanced knowledge and skills in feeding, eating, and swallowing. The occupational therapist and occupational therapy assistant also may supervise other nonlicensed health care aides providing feeding and eating assistance to clients (AOTA, 2004). Most state practice acts mandate the frequency and duration for supervision for entry-level occupational therapists, occupational therapy assistants, and nonlicensed health care aides. The occupational therapist has the primary role in evaluation and intervention planning; the occupational therapy assistant collaborates with the occupational therapist in the provision of specific interventions (AOTA, 2004, 2005b). Occupational therapy assistants who hold an AOTA specialty certification in feeding, eating, and swallowing may have a more active role in collaborating in the evaluation process and in making intervention decisions. However, it is implicit that these tasks are carried out under the supervision of an occupational therapist. The supervising occupational therapist must be experienced in feeding, eating, and swallowing disorders or seek consultation from an occupational therapist who has such experience.

Knowledge and Skills

The progression from entry-level knowledge and skills to advanced-level knowledge and skills is individualized for each occupational therapist and occupational therapy assistant. Although practitioners exit their academic program with the basic knowledge and skills to provide occupational therapy services to clients with feeding, eating, and swallowing dysfunction, over time they may develop additional individualized expertise, such as in the area of dysphagia. Entry-level knowledge and skills for both occupational therapists and occupational therapy assistants, as supported by the 2006 Standards (Accreditation Council of Occupational Therapy Education, 2006), are delineated in Appendix A. The advanced-level knowledge and skills necessary to provide a continuum of services in the area of feeding, eating, and swallowing are delineated in Appendix B. These advanced-level skills build on existing knowledge, performance skills, critical reasoning, interpersonal abilities, and ethical reasoning.

Appendix A.
Entry-Level Knowledge and Skills Assessment

Occupational Therapists and Occupational Therapy Assistants Will Have Entry-Level Knowledge and Skills to Assess:

Context	Occupational Therapist	Occupational Therapy Assistant *(Based on the Establishment of Service Competency and Supervision by an Occupational Therapist)*
Cultural components that affect feeding: utensils, food types, meanings/symbolism of food, mealtime practices and rituals, dietary restrictions	✓	✓
Attitudes and values of client, family or caregivers, and friends toward feeding and mealtime	✓	✓
Settings where feeding/eating take place	✓	✓
Social opportunities during mealtime that support or interfere with social interaction	✓	✓
Aspects of the client's developmental status/life phase that support or interfere with eating/feeding	✓	—
Effect of medical condition/disability status on feeding performance	✓	—
Factors in the environment that support or interfere with feeding/eating (e.g., foods, seating, time, feeders)	✓	—
Pre-Oral Phase		
Role of appetite and hunger sensation	✓	✓
Tactile and proprioceptive qualities of food and equipment in both the hands and the mouth	✓	✓
Ability to see/locate food/drink/utensils	✓	✓
Ability to appreciate smell—pleasant/noxious	✓	✓
Need for use of auditory cues (verbal cues, utensils hitting plate)	✓	✓
Ability to achieve a position of proximal postural control that allows upper-extremity and oral function for eating	✓	✓
Nature of communication during feeding/mealtime	✓	✓
Feeding experience as satisfactory to self	✓	✓

✓ = able to perform the task
— = does not perform the task

(continued)

Appendix A.
Entry-Level Knowledge and Skills Assessment *(cont.)*

Occupational Therapists and Occupational Therapy Assistants Will Have Entry-Level Knowledge and Skills to Assess:

	Occupational Therapist	Occupational Therapy Assistant *(Based on the Establishment of Service Competency and Supervision by an Occupational Therapist)*
Pre-Oral Phase *(continued)*		
Ability to bring food to mouth as supported or prevented by factors such as figure ground, depth perception, spatial relations, and motor planning	✓	—
Neuromotor components that support or interfere with adequate positioning	✓	—
Upper-extremity function and hand manipulation adequate for self-feeding	✓	—
Influence of motor activity involved in bringing food to mouth	✓	—
Ability to orient mouth to receive food (timing, positioning of structures)	✓	—
Initiation of eating as supported/prevented by level of alertness/arousal, orientation to task, recognition, and memory	✓	—
Persistence with feeding that is supported/prevented by level of arousal, attention span, initiation of activity, memory, and sequencing	✓	—
Carryover of skill to future feeding tasks is supported/prevented by level of memory, learning, and generalization	✓	—
Factors that influence the willingness or unwillingness to eat (self-image, self-esteem, caregiver, family, feeder interaction, eating history, dying)	✓	—
Oral Phase		
Behaviors or reports that indicate pain or discomfort in the oral area	✓	✓
Behaviors that interfere with the oral phase (spitting foods, pocketing foods, refusing to swallow)	✓	✓
Level of awareness/sensation in the oral–motor area	✓	—
Level of reception and perception of tactile (texture), temperature, proprioception, and gustatory qualities of food and utensils	✓	—
Factors supporting/interfering with secretion management	✓	—

Appendix A.
Entry-Level Knowledge and Skills Assessment *(cont.)*

Occupational Therapists and Occupational Therapy Assistants Will Have Entry-Level Knowledge and Skills to Assess:

	Occupational Therapist	Occupational Therapy Assistant *(Based on the Establishment of Service Competency and Supervision by an Occupational Therapist)*
Oral Phase *(continued)*		
Respiratory control factors that permit safe and efficient bolus manipulation (mouth breathers, Adult Respiratory Distress Syndrome, bronchopulmonary dysplasia), chronic obstructive pulmonary disease, cardiopulmonary compromise	✓	—
Structural or neuromotor factors (reflexes, range of motion, muscle tone, strength, endurance) that support or interfere with oral–motor function	✓	—
Level of coordinated movements (praxis) of oral structures (cheeks, lips, jaw, tongue, palate, teeth) with or without foods	✓	—
Oral structures' ability to work together to contain, form, and propel the bolus	✓	—
Bolus manipulation supported/compromised by memory, attention span, orientation, and problem solving	✓	—
Speed of the oral phase adequate to support sufficient oral intake	✓	—
Pharyngeal Phase		
Behaviors, reports, or symptoms that indicate pain or discomfort localized to the pharyngeal area	✓	—
Presence of signs and symptoms indicating possible pharyngeal dysfunction or clinical signs indicating possible aspiration (e.g., coughing, choking, tachypnea)	✓	—
Esophageal Phase		
Behaviors, reports, or symptoms that indicate pain or discomfort in the esophageal area	✓	—
Presence of refluxed material from the stomach into the esophagus, pharynx, or oral cavity	✓	—

Occupational Therapists and Occupational Therapy Assistants Will Have Entry-Level Knowledge and Skills to:

	Occupational Therapist	Occupational Therapy Assistant
Instrumentation		
Understand formal instrumentation used by therapists or other professionals to evaluate the oral, pharyngeal, and esophageal phase of the swallow, including, but not limited to, videofluoroscopy, ultrasonography, fiberoptic endoscopy, scintigraphy, and manometry	✓	—

(continued)

Appendix A.
Entry-Level Knowledge and Skills Assessment *(cont.)*

Occupational Therapists and Occupational Therapy Assistants Will Have Entry-Level Knowledge and Skills to:

	Occupational Therapist	Occupational Therapy Assistant *(Based on the Establishment of Service Competency and Supervision by an Occupational Therapist)*
Discharge Planning *(Discharge Planning is Addressed Throughout the Intervention Process)*		
Collaborate with client, family, caregivers, and team members to formulate discharge needs	✓	—
Provide appropriate referrals, follow-up plans, and reevaluation related to discharge needs	✓	—
Develop and document discharge and follow-up programs and resources in accordance with discharge environment	✓	—
Provide for educational needs related to feeding, eating, and swallowing management and establishment of proficiency of recommendations with client and family	✓	—
Implement discharge and follow-up plan with client, family, caregivers, and team members to promote transition to discharge environment and integration of intervention management techniques	✓	—
Terminate intervention when client has achieved maximum benefit from services	✓	—

Entry-Level Knowledge and Skills Intervention

Occupational Therapists and Occupational Therapy Assistants Will Have Entry-Level Knowledge and Skills to:

	Occupational Therapist	Occupational Therapy Assistant *(Based on the Establishment of Service Competency and Supervision by an Occupational Therapist)*
Context		
Consider cultural practices in selecting foods, utensils, and mealtime setting	✓	✓
Provide environmental modifications to promote appetite and feeding/eating performance (e.g., location, timing, seating, lighting)	✓	✓
Use eating/feeding activities appropriate for developmental status/life phase	✓	✓
Facilitate social interactions that support feeding performance	✓	✓
Plan intervention within the context of person's medical condition, particularly considering specific restrictions and limitations, expected progression, and outcome	✓	—

Appendix A.
Entry-Level Knowledge and Skills Intervention *(cont.)*

Occupational Therapists and Occupational Therapy Assistants Will Have Entry-Level Knowledge and Skills to:

Pre-Oral Phase	Occupational Therapist	Occupational Therapy Assistant (Based on the Establishment of Service Competency and Supervision by an Occupational Therapist)
Facilitate olfactory stimulation	✓	✓
Provide verbal or physical cues	✓	✓
Use sensitization and desensitization techniques	✓	✓
Facilitate oral hygiene	✓	✓
Facilitate visual–perceptual activity and body schema awareness	✓	✓
Increase awareness on affected/neglected side	✓	✓
Facilitate strategies to minimize visual field deficits and enhance acuity	✓	✓
Modify environment to enhance attention	✓	✓
Help client/caregiver to develop problem-solving methods	✓	✓
Use communicative strategies to increase participation in feeding	✓	✓
Use techniques to attain and maintain optimal level of arousal	✓	✓
Provide appropriate positioning and seating equipment	✓	✓
Provide nonnutritive oral stimulation, techniques, and/or exercises	✓	✓
Facilitate upper-extremity control and hand function (dexterity, strength, coordination)	✓	✓
Facilitate oral–motor control through exercises, play, and games	✓	✓
Improve self-esteem to increase engagement in self-feeding	✓	✓
Structure mealtime habits	✓	✓
Implement nutritional recommendations	✓	✓
Manipulate feeding schedule to facilitate hunger	✓	—
Select, modify, and establish set-up of mealtime equipment	✓	—
Facilitate postural control	✓	—
Fabricate upper-extremity orthotics	✓	—
Use behavior modification	✓	—

(continued)

293

Appendix A.
Entry-Level Knowledge and Skills Intervention *(cont.)*

Occupational Therapists and Occupational Therapy Assistants Will Have Entry-Level Knowledge and Skills to:

	Occupational Therapist	Occupational Therapy Assistant *(Based on the Establishment of Service Competency and Supervision by an Occupational Therapist)*
Oral Phase		
Provide nonnutritive oral stimulation and exercises (jaw, lip, cheeks, tongue)	✓	✓
Use desensitization techniques	✓	✓
Maintain appropriate position during mealtime (facilitate stability or movement)	✓	✓
Time the introduction of food to facilitate coordinated respiration	✓	✓
Facilitate placement of food in mouth and use of utensils	✓	✓
Use verbal, written, tactile cues to initiate, maintain, and follow through (chew, swallow) with feeding/eating task	✓	✓
Provide an environmental modification program	✓	✓
Facilitate oral compensatory strategies for altered sensation, structure, or function	✓	—
Select and modify equipment for feeding	✓	—
Grade or alter qualities of bolus (e.g., texture, taste, temperature)	✓	—
Provide a behavior modification program	✓	—
Pharyngeal Phase		
Facilitate head and neck positioning for swallowing (e.g., chin tuck, head turns)	✓	—
Facilitate compensatory swallow techniques	✓	—
Esophageal Phase		
Modify position before, during, and after feeding task	✓	—
Refer to gastrointestinal service when appropriate	✓	—

Appendix B.
Advanced-Level Knowledge and Skills

Occupational Therapist	Occupational Therapy Assistant
I. *Eating function*—The occupational therapist with advanced-level knowledge and skills has built upon foundational knowledge of the eating process, thus enhancing the depth and specificity of evaluation and intervention. The occupational therapist has developed	I. *Eating function*—The occupational therapy assistant with advanced-level knowledge and skills has built upon foundational knowledge of the eating process for the purpose of providing more comprehensive intervention. The occupational therapy assistant has developed
A. Extensive knowledge of anatomy and physiology of the phases of eating for the purpose of assessing structural, neuromotor, and sensory factors that support or interfere with function and of determining intervention strategies	A. Advanced knowledge of anatomy and physiology of the phases of eating
1. Pre-oral phase	1. Pre-oral phase
2. Oral phase	2. Oral phase
3. Pharyngeal phase	3. Pharyngeal phase
4. Esophageal phase	4. Esophageal phase
B. Extensive knowledge of airway functions, including protective responses and respiratory control factors that affect swallowing and eating.	B. Advanced knowledge of airway functions, including protective responses and respiratory control factors that affect swallowing and eating.
II. *Specialized client populations and settings*—The occupational therapist with advanced-level knowledge and skills has gained extensive knowledge and experience in the feeding, eating, and swallowing needs of specific client populations or clients in specific settings. The increased depth of knowledge allows the occupational therapist to provide services to clients who are more medically fragile or whose problems/ needs are more complex than those addressed by entry-level therapists. By developing expertise with specific client populations, occupational therapists with advanced-level knowledge and skills not only provide services that represent "best practice" but also contribute to the development of new and innovative approaches to evaluation and intervention for that population. Areas of expertise that may be developed include	II. *Specialized client populations and settings*—The occupational therapy assistant with advanced-level knowledge and skills has gained extensive knowledge and experience in the feeding, eating, and swallowing needs of specific client populations or clients in specific settings. The increased depth of knowledge allows the occupational therapy assistant with advanced-level knowledge and skills to provide services to clients who are more medically fragile or whose problems/ needs are more complex than those addressed by the occupational therapy assistant with entry-level knowledge and skills. Areas of expertise that may be developed include
A. Specific medical diagnoses	A. Specific medical diagnoses
1. In-depth knowledge of diagnosis, including potential impact on feeding, eating, and swallowing	1. In-depth knowledge of diagnosis, including potential impact on feeding, eating, and swallowing
2. Common medications used and their interaction with the feeding, eating, and swallowing process; advising regarding oral administration of medications (e.g., crushing meds, through nasogastric tube, changing to liquid suspension)	2. Common medications used and their interaction with the feeding, eating, and swallowing process
3. Dietary needs or restrictions	3. Dietary needs or restrictions
4. Specialized equipment that may be used and can affect feeding, eating, and swallowing (e.g., tracheostomy tubes, ventilators, feeding tubes)	4. Specialized equipment that may be used and can affect feeding, eating, and swallowing (e.g., tracheostomy tubes, ventilators, feeding tubes)
B. Specialized settings such as general intensive care units and neonatal intensive care units (AOTA, 1993)	B. Specialized settings such as intensive care units (AOTA, 1993)

(continued)

Appendix B.
Advanced-Level Knowledge and Skills *(cont.)*

Occupational Therapist	Occupational Therapy Assistant
C. Specific developmental, social, or cultural factors	C. Specific developmental, social, or cultural factors
1. In-depth knowledge of age-related expectations, such as feeding processes in infants and children and the effects of aging on feeding	1. In-depth knowledge of age-related expectations, such as feeding processes in children and the effects of aging on feeding
2. Extensive knowledge of particular cultural groups and the influence of their custom on eating, particularly for persons with feeding, eating, and swallowing problems	2. Extensive knowledge of particular cultural groups and the influence of their custom on eating, particularly for persons with feeding, eating, and swallowing problems
3. Extensive knowledge of social or emotional factors that can influence feeding	3. Extensive knowledge of social or emotional factors that can influence feeding
III. *Instrumental evaluation*—The occupational therapists with advanced-level knowledge and skills may develop the following skills for instrumental evaluations relevant to their area of practice. These assessment techniques require specialized formal training and equipment. They may include, but are not limited to, videofluoroscopy, cervical auscultation, ultrasonography, fiberoptic endoscopy, scintigraphy, manometry, electromyography, and manofluorography.	III. *Instrumental evaluation*—The occupational therapy assistants with advanced-level knowledge and skills may develop the following skills for those instrumental evaluations relevant to their area of practice.
A. Knowledge and application of instrumental techniques, including purpose, indications for use, limitations, reliability, and validity	A. Knowledge of the instrumentation techniques, including purpose, indications for use, limitations, reliability, and validity
B. Ability to recommend appropriate instrumental evaluation	B. Ability to assist the occupational therapist in carrying out the assessment
C. Collaboration with other professionals in carrying out the instrumental evaluation and interpretation of data	
D. Ability to independently carry out the assessment, including interpretation of data and implementation of recommendations	
E. Ability to use results effectively in evaluation and intervention	
IV. *Specialized interventions*—Occupational therapists with advanced-level knowledge and skills have knowledge and skills of all existing intervention procedures in their specialty area and can provide the clinical judgment and rationale for selection of any procedure being used. They are aware of new interventions and potential applications from other fields. Skills may be developed in using specialized interventions that include, but are not limited to	IV. *Specialized interventions*—Occupational therapy assistants who have advanced-level knowledge and skills of specialized intervention procedures in their specialty area in order to implement intervention recommendations made by the occupational therapist. Skills may be developed in implementing specialized interventions that include, but are not limited to
A. Interventions to facilitate oral performance, improve pharyngeal swallow, and potentially reduce the risk of aspiration, if present. Use of these interventions is based on the results of instrumental evaluation of function, with safety to the client as a primary concern. Examples include	A. Interventions to improve pharyngeal swallow and esophageal function. Use of these interventions is based on results of instrumental evaluation of function by the occupational therapist. Examples Include
1. Compensatory swallowing techniques/strategies	1. Compensatory swallowing techniques
2. Thermal or tactile stimulation	2. Thermal or tactile stimulation
3. Grading or altering the bolus size/texture/changing consistency of liquids/route of administering medications orally	3. Grading or altering the bolus size/texture
4. Specialized positioning	4. Specialized positioning

Appendix B.
Advanced-Level Knowledge and Skills *(cont.)*

Occupational Therapist	Occupational Therapy Assistant

B. Enteral feeding
 	
   1. Knowledge of purpose, types, indications, limitations, and precautions
 	
   2. Ability to integrate enteral feeding systems into occupational therapy intervention plan
 	
   3. Ability to make recommendations regarding use of or need for enteral feeding systems
	B. Enteral feeding
	
	   1. Knowledge of purpose, types, indications, limitations, and precautions

C. Oral appliances (prosthodontics)
 	
   1. Knowledge of purpose, indications, limitations, and precautions
 	
   2. Ability to fabricate or collaborate on fabrication
 	
   3. Client training and education
	C. Oral appliances (prosthodontics)
	
	   1. Knowledge of purpose, indications, limitations, and precautions

V. *Training and education*—Occupational therapists who have advanced-level knowledge and skills that should be disseminated to others. Through formal and informal methods, occupational therapists with advanced-level knowledge and skills should provide training and education to other occupational therapists, occupational therapy assistants, students, staff members, and professionals from related fields.	V. *Training and education*—Occupational therapy assistants with advanced-level knowledge and skills provide training and education to clients, family, and staff members, in collaboration with an occupational therapist.

Definitions—Common Terminology

Adaptive feeding equipment

Equipment used to support optimal feeding performance and to compensate for associated deficits related to coordination, strength, praxis, range of motion, or positioning.

Airway protection

Methods designed to prevent accidental loss of food, medications, or liquids into the airway while eating or drinking.

Aspiration

The entry of secretions, fluids, food, or any foreign substance below the vocal cords and into the lungs; may result in aspiration pneumonia, which may be fatal.

Bolus

The mass of food or liquid that is orally processed and swallowed.

Cervical auscultation

A method of assessing the pharyngeal swallow by listening to stereotypical sounds using the stethoscope.

Chin tuck

An intervention strategy where the head is flexed (chin tucked downward toward the chest) during the swallow allowing the anterior structures of the pharynx posteriorly resulting in a smaller entrance to the larynx; this strategy reduces the chance of food or liquid to fall into the airway.

Clearing techniques

Strategies used to clear the mouth or pharynx of food or liquid residue.

Clinical evaluation

The observation of feeding, eating, and swallowing, including client/caregiver interaction, positioning, food consistencies, method of intake, food preferences, oral structures, oral–motor patterns, tone, tactile responses, strength, fatigue, time required for mealtime activities, oral reflexes, sucking, coordination, labial, lingual, velar, facial, mandibular, dentition.

Clinical feeding, eating, and swallowing evaluation

A comprehensive evaluation, not including instrumentation, that examines the client's ability to feed, eat, and initiate the swallowing process; also referred to as "bedside dysphagia evaluation."

Cranial nerves

Nerves that provide motor and sensory innervation to the head and neck.

Diet liberalization

The relaxation of standards of accepted diets as ways to treat illness or decrease symptoms related to dsyphagia.

Double/multiple swallows

A swallow strategy whereby two or more attempts are used to swallow the food, medications, or liquid.

Dysphagia

Difficulty with any stage of swallowing (oral, pharyngeal, esophageal); dysfunction in any stage or process of eating; includes any difficulty in the passage of food, liquid, or medicine during any stage of swallowing that impairs the client's ability to swallow independently or safely.

Eating

"…the ability to keep and manipulate food or fluid in the mouth and swallow it; eating and swallowing are often used interchangeably" (AOTA, 2006a).

Eating disorders

Dysfunction in eating and nutrition related to complex biological, psychological, and sociocultural factors that may result in a life-threatening illness, such as anorexia and bulimia nervosa.

Effortful/hard swallows

A swallow strategy whereby the tongue muscles are volitionally contracted with increased effort while swallowing; results in the base of the tongue moving posteriorly during the pharyngeal swallow, which helps to clear food material from the valleculae during swallow.

Electromyography (EMG)

A procedure by which skeletal muscles are electrically stimulated and changes in electrical activity are recorded. Paralysis of the pharyngeal constrictors and vocal cords can be determined.

Enteral feeding

Feedings that use the intestinal tract for absorption of nutrients; often called gastrostomy tube feedings.

Esophageal phase

The phase of swallowing in which the bolus travels through the esophagus into the stomach.

Esophageal state function

Includes upper esophagus/cricopharyngeal function, esophageal motility.

Feeding

"…the process of setting up, arranging, and bringing food [or fluid] from the plate or cup to the mouth; sometimes called self-feeding" (AOTA, 2006a).

Feeding, eating, and swallowing history

Includes medical diagnoses, past medical history, food allergies, gastrointestinal disorders, current medications, developmental level (as appropriate), nutritional status, neurological status, respiratory status, pertinent diagnostic studies, feeding history including progression of solids and liquids, alternate/supplemental feeding interventions, positioning, cognition, behavior, communication, eating habits/patterns, methods of feeding, dietary restrictions.

Fiberoptic endoscopic evaluation of swallowing (FEES)
Process of passing a flexible fiberoptic endoscope through the nose and positioning it to observe structures and function of the swallowing mechanism to include the nasopharynx, oropharynx, and hypopharynx. The procedure is also known as fiberoptic endoscopic examination of swallowing and videoendoscopic swallowing study.

Food and liquid consistencies
Includes thin liquids, nectar-thick liquids, honey-thick liquids, puree, chopped, soft, solid food consistencies.

Gastrostomy tube
A tube placed surgically or endoscopically into the stomach through which fluids and nutrition are provided.

Graded tactile pressure
Includes deep touch, light touch, sustained touch, pulsing touch, symmetrical touch, asymmetrical touch.

Grading/altering bolus
Manipulation of the food or liquid to change its properties related to temperature, size, or texture.

Instrumental assessment
An assessment of swallowing using radiological or imaging procedures; may include but is not limited to modified barium swallow, fiberoptic endoscopy, ultrasound, scintigraphy, electromyography, and manometry.

Jejunostomy tube
A tube placed into the jejunum of the small intestine during surgery through which enteral feedings are provided.

Manofluorography
Simultaneous videofluoroscopy and manometry by which oropharyngeal and esophageal pressure and bolus information are recorded. This procedure is also known as pharyngeal manofluorography and videomanometry.

Manometry
A procedure by which the strength, timing, and sequencing of pressure events in the esophagus are measured by a catheter with pressure transducers. Alone, it is an ineffective tool for the diagnosis of oropharyngeal dysphagia (Bastian, 1998).

Mendelsohn maneuver
A swallowing technique to facilitate prolonged laryngeal elevation during the swallow; results in keeping the upper esophageal sphincter open longer to allow passage of the bolus.

Nasogastric tube
A tube used to provide feedings directly into the stomach through a tube inserted in the nose into the stomach.

National Dysphagia Diet (NDD)
From the National Dysphagia Diet Task Force (2000) of the American Dietetic Association, these diet levels aim to establish standard terminology and practice applications of dietary texture modification in dysphagia management. Diet levels include the following:

> *NDD Level I:* Dysphagia–Pureed (homogenous, very cohesive, pudding-like, requiring very little chewing ability)

NDD Level II: Dysphagia–Mechanical Altered (cohesive, moist, semisolid foods, requiring some chewing)

NDD Level III: Dysphagia–Advanced (soft foods that require more chewing ability)
- Regular: All foods allowed
- Proposed levels of liquid viscosity are:
  –Thin
  –Nectar-like
  –Honey-like
  –Spoon-thick

Oral phase
The phase of swallow in which the bolus of food or liquid is propelled to the pharynx by the tongue.

Oral preparatory phase
The phase of swallowing during which the bolus of food or liquid is masticated by the teeth and gums and manipulated by the lips, cheek, and tongue to create a bolus of appropriate texture for swallowing; this phase also allows for sensory appreciation of bolus qualities.

Oral reflexes
Abnormal and primitive reflexes include hyperactive gag, tonic bite, tongue thrust, jaw jerk, rooting, sucking.

Oral stage function
Includes bolus intake and containment, bolus formation, bolus transit and clearing time, velar function, behavioral components, base of tongue contact to pharyngeal wall, residue post swallow.

Orogastric tube
Used to lavage or decompress the stomach; it must be removed prior to assessment.

Penetration
The entry of secretions, fluids, food, medications, or any foreign substance into the laryngeal vestibule at or above the level of the true vocal cords.

Pharyngeal phase
The phase of swallow when the swallowing response is initiated.

Pharyngeal state function
Includes nasopharyngeal insufficiency and reflux, vallecular function, pyriform sinus function, epiglottal function, timing of swallow response, initiation of pharyngeal swallow, timing of clearance, pharyngeal competence, pharyngeal wall residue, laryngeal elevation, laryngeal penetration, or aspiration risk.

Pleasure/recreational feedings
Meals or snacks that provide enjoyment and stimulation but that are not depended on to provide nutrition.

Pocketing
Retention of food between the teeth and cheek.

Pre-oral phase
The process in which food, medication, or drink is brought to the mouth either by the person engaged in eating or by the feeder.

Presentation
Includes temperature, texture, size, placement, utensil choice, flavor, rate, method of delivery.

Prosthodontics

Prosthetic appliances used to facilitate oral and/or pharyngeal function either inside or outside of the oral cavity. May also be used for cosmesis.

Reflux

Reflux of food, medication, liquids, and gastric juice from the stomach into the esophagus; also called gastroesophageal reflux disease (GERD).

Scintigraphy

A procedure by which a radioactive bolus is monitored during and after ingestion to assess and measure bolus transit and aspiration (Bastian, 1998).

Secretion management

The ability to retain, manipulate, and swallow one's own saliva.

Self-feeding

The process of setting up, arranging, and bringing food from the plate or cup to the mouth; sometimes just referred to as feeding.

Silent aspiration

Aspiration that occurs without coughing or overt choking, indicating motor and/or sensory deficits (if present) that inhibit protective responses.

Supraglottic swallow

A swallowing technique used for airway protection where the client is told to take a breath and hold it while swallowing and then coughs after the swallow; results in the voluntary closure of the vocal folds before, during, and after the swallow.

Swallowing

A complicated act where food, fluid, medication, or saliva is moved from the mouth through the pharynx and esophagus into the stomach (AOTA, 2006a).

Therapeutic feedings

Controlled delivery of food, medication, or liquid used to facilitate therapeutic outcomes to improve feeding, eating, and swallowing ability; not used as a primary source of nutrition or hydration.

Thickening agent

Substances used to increase the viscosity of liquids.

Total parenteral nutrition

A formula providing nutrients through an intravenous tube.

Ultrasonography

The use of high frequency sound waves to provide ultrasonic images of the upper digestive tract structures and motilities, bolus transit, and vallecular stasis. It is not effective to detect penetration or aspiration (Bastian, 1998).

Upper aerodigestive tract

The combined organs and tissues of the respiratory tract and the upper part of the digestive tract (including the lips, nose, mouth, tongue, pharynx, larynx, upper trachea, and upper esophagus).

VitalStim

A Food and Drug Administration (FDA)–cleared method to promote swallowing through the application of neuromuscular electrical stimulation to the swallowing muscles to strengthen and re-educate muscles and to facilitate motor control/function of the swallowing mechanism.

References

Accreditation Council for Occupational Therapy Education. (2006). *ACOTE standards and interpretive guidelines.* Retrieved September 19, 2006, from http://www.aota.org/nonmembers/area13/docs/acotestandards806.pdf

American Occupational Therapy Association. (1993). Occupational therapy roles. *American Journal of Occupational Therapy, 47,* 1087–1099.

American Occupational Therapy Association. (2002). Occupational therapy practice framework: Domain and process. *American Journal of Occupational Therapy, 56,* 609–639.

American Occupational Therapy Association. (2004). Guidelines for supervision, roles, and responsibilities during the delivery of occupational therapy services. *American Journal of Occupational Therapy, 58,* 663–667.

American Occupational Therapy Association. (2005a). Occupational therapy code of ethics. *American Journal of Occupational Therapy, 59,* 639–642.

American Occupational Therapy Association. (2005b). Standards of practice for occupational therapy. *American Journal of Occupational Therapy, 59,* 663–665.

American Occupational Therapy Association. (2006a). *AOTA specialty certification in feeding, eating, and swallowing: 2007 candidate handbook—Occupational therapists* [PDF, available from http://www.aota.org/memservices/certappprogram/cr_login.aspx]. Bethesda, MD: Author.

American Occupational Therapy Association. (2006b). Policy 1.44: Categories of occupational therapy personnel. *American Journal of Occupational Therapy, 60,* 683–684.

Bastian, R. W. (1998). Contemporary diagnosis of the dysphagic patient. In R. L. Plant & G. L. Schectiter (Eds.), The otolaryngologic clinics of North America. *Dysphagia in Children, Adults, and Geriatrics, 31,* 489–506.

National Dysphagia Diet Task Force. (2000). *National dysphagia diet: Standardization for optimal care.* Washington, DC: American Dietetic Association.

World Health Organization. (2001). *International classification of functioning, disability and health (ICF).* Geneva, Switzerland: Author.

Selected Readings

Adult Eating and Dysphagia Treatment

Bastian, R. W. (1998). Contemporary diagnosis of the dysphagic patient. In R. L. Plant & G. L. Schectiter (Eds.), The otolaryngologic clinics of North America. *Dysphagia in Children, Adults, and Geriatrics, 31,* 489–506.

Groher, M. E. (1997). *Dysphagia: Diagnosis and management* (3rd ed.). Boston: Butterworth-Heinemann.

Healthy People 2010. Retrieved March 5, 2007, from http://www.cdc.gov/nchs/datawh/nchsdefs/healthypeople2010.htm

Joint Commission on Accreditation of Healthcare Organizations. (2007). Retrieved March 5, 2007, from www.jointcommission.org

Note. This list of selected readings is not meant to be exhaustive but to suggest current resources for library building pertinent to eating and dysphagia treatment. Key words that are helpful in accomplishing a literature review search of this topic may include *dysphagia, feeding, eating, swallowing disorders, deglutition disorders,* and *dysphagia rehabilitation.*

Langmore, S. E., & Miller, R. M. (1994). Behavioral treatment for adults with oropharyngeal dysphagia. *Archives of Physical Medicine and Rehabilitation, 75,* 1154–1159.

Logemann, J. A. (1998). *Evaluation and treatment of swallowing disorders* (2nd ed.). Austin, TX: Pro-Ed.

Logsdon, B. (2002). Cultivating competence. *Advance for Directors in Rehabilitation, 11*(10), 71–73.

Neumann, S. (1993). Swallowing therapy with neurologic clients: Results of direct and indirect therapy methods in 66 clients suffering from neurological disorders. *Dysphagia, 8,* 150–153.

Neumann, S., Bartolome, D., Buchholz, D., & Prosiegal, M. (1995). Swallowing therapy of neurologic patients: Correlation of outcome with pretreatment variables and therapeutic methods. *Dysphagia, 10,* 1–5.

Clinical Dysphagia Assessment

Avery-Smith, W., Dellarosa, D. M., & Rosen, A. B. (1992). Clinical assessment of dysphagia in adults. *Occupational Therapy Practice, 3*(2), 51–58.

Avery-Smith, W., Rosen, A. B., & Dellarosa, D. (1997). *Dysphagia evaluation protocol.* San Antonio, TX: Therapy Skill Builders.

Depippo, K. L., Holas, M. A., & Reding, M. J. (1994). The Burke Dysphagia Screening Test: Validation of its use in patients with stroke. *Archives of Physical Medicine and Rehabilitation, 75,* 1284–1286.

Fleming, S. M., & Weaver, A. W. (1986). Index of dysphagia: A tool for identifying deglutition problems. *Dysphagia, 1,* 206–208.

Hardy, E. (1995). *Bedside evaluation of dysphagia.* Bisbee, AZ: Imaginart.

Hopper, P., & Holme, S. (1999). The role of fiberoptic endoscopy in dysphagia rehabilitation. *Journal of Head Trauma Rehabilitation, 5,* 475–485.

Leopold, N. A., & Kagel, M. C. (1997). Dysphagia—Ingestion or deglutition: A proposed paradigm. *Dysphagia, 12,* 202–206.

Shanley, C., & O'Loughlin, G. (2000). Dysphagia among nursing home residents: An assessment and management protocol. *Journal of Gerontology in Nursing, 26*(8), 35–48.

Eating Disorders

Bouley, B., & Sadik, C. (1992). Inpatient treatment of eating disorders within a cognitive–behavioral framework. *Occupational Therapy Practice, 3*(2), 1–11.

Giles, G. M. (1985). Anorexia nervosa and bulimia: An activity-oriented approach. *American Journal of Occupational Therapy, 39,* 510–517.

Martin, J. E. (1998). *Eating disorders, food, and occupational therapy.* London: Whurr.

Instrumental Dysphagia Assessment

Bastian, R. (1993). The videoendoscopic swallowing study: An alternative and partner to the videofluoroscopic swallowing study. *Dysphagia, 8,* 359–367.

Broniatowski, M. (1998). Fiberoptic endoscopic evaluation of dysphagia and videofluoroscopy. *Dysphagia, 13,* 22–23.

Langmore, S. E., Schatz, K., & Olsen, N. (1988). Fiberoptic endoscopic examination of swallowing safety: A new procedure. *Dysphagia, 2,* 216–219.

Leder, S. B., Sasaki, C. T., & Burrell, M. I. (1998). Fiberoptic endoscopic evaluation of dysphagia to identify silent aspiration. *Dysphagia, 13*, 19–21.

Logemann, J. A. (1993). *Manual for the videofluoroscopic study of swallowing* (2nd ed.). Austin, TX: Pro-Ed.

Perlman, A. L. (1993). Electromyography and the study of oropharyngeal swallowing. *Dysphagia, 8*, 351–355.

Silverman, K. H. (1994). The use of scintigraphy in the management of patients with pulmonary aspiration. *Dysphagia, 9*, 107–115.

Pediatric Eating and Dysphagia Treatment

Arvedson, J. C., & Brodsky, L. (1993). *Pediatric swallowing and feeding: Assessment and management*. San Diego, CA: Singular.

Backes, L., Deitz, J., Price, R., Glass, R., & Hays, R. (1994). The effect of oral support on sucking efficiency in pre-term infants. *American Journal of Occupational Therapy, 48*, 490–498.

Carruth, B. R., & Skinner, J. D. (2002). Feeding behaviors and other motor development in healthy children (2–24 months). *Journal of the American College of Nutrition, 21*(2), 88–96.

Clark, G. (1993). Oral–motor and feeding issues. In C. Royeen (Ed.), *AOTA Self-Study Series: Classroom applications for school-based practice*. Bethesda, MD: American Occupational Therapy Association.

Glass, R. P., & Wolf, L. S. (1994). Global perspective on feeding assessment in the neonatal intensive care unit. *American Journal of Occupational Therapy, 48*, 487–489.

Mathisen, B., Worrall, L., Masel, J., Wall, C., & Shepherd, R.W. (1999). Feeding problems in infants with gastro-oesophageal reflux disease: A controlled study. *Journal of Paediatrics and Child Health, 35*(2), 163–169.

Morris, S., & Klein, M. (2000). *Pre-feeding skills* (2nd ed.). San Antonio, TX: Therapy Skill Builders.

Nelson, C. A., Meek, M. M., & Moore, J. C. (1994). *Head–neck treatment issues as a base for oral–motor function*. Albuquerque, NM: Clinician's View.

Rogers, B. (2004). Feeding method and health outcomes of children with cerebral palsy. *Journal of Pediatrics, 145*(Suppl.2).

Schwarz, S. M. (2003). Feeding disorders in children with developmental disabilities. *Infants and Young Children, 16*, 317–330.

Sullivan, P. B., & Rosenbloom, L. (1996). *Feeding the disabled child*. London: Mac Keith Press.

Tuchman, D. N., & Walter, R. S. (1994). *Disorders of feeding and swallowing in infants and children: Pathophysiology, diagnosis, and treatment*. San Diego, CA: Singular.

Waterman, E. T., Koltai, P. J., Downey, J. C., & Cacace, A. T. (1992). Swallowing disorders in a population of children with cerebral palsy. *International Journal of Pediatric Otorhinolaryngology, 24*, 63–71.

Wolf, L. S., & Glass, R. P. (1992). *Feeding and swallowing disorders in infancy: Assessment and management*. San Antonio, TX: Therapy Skill Builders.

Miscellaneous

Mody, M., & Nagai, J. (1990). A multidisciplinary approach to the development of competency standards and appropriate allocation for patients with dysphagia. *American Journal of Occupational Therapy, 44*, 369–372.

Authors

This paper was originally authored in 2000 by the Eating and Feeding Task Force: Gloria Frolek Clark, MS, OTR/L, FAOTA *(Chairperson)*; Wendy Avery-Smith, MS, OTR; Lynn S. Wold, MA, OTR; Paige Anthony, COTA; and Suzanne E. Holm, MA, OTR, BCN.

In 2005–2006, the paper was revised and updated by Gloria Frolek Clark, MS, OTR/L, FAOTA *(Coordinator)* and

The AOTASB Feeding & Swallowing Specialty Certification Panel:

Pam Roberts, MSHA, OTR/L, CPHQ, FAOTA, *Chairperson*
Marcia S. Cox, MHS, OTR/L
Suzanne E. Holm, MA, OTR, BCN
Sharon T. Kurfuerst, MEd, OTR/L
Amy K. Lynch, MS, OTR/L
Linda Miller Schuberth, MA, OTR/L

for

The Commission on Practice
Susanne Smith Roley, MS, OTR/L, FAOTA, *Chairperson*

Adopted by the Representative Assembly 2007C76

Note. This document replaces the 2000 document, *Specialized Knowledge and Skills for Eating and Feeding in Occupational Therapy Practice.* Previously published and copyrighted in 2000 by the American Occupational Therapy Association and reprinted in 2003 (*American Journal of Occupational Therapy, 57,* 660–678).

Specialized Knowledge and Skills of Occupational Therapy Educators of the Future

Introduction

In 2006, the American Occupational Therapy Association (AOTA) articulated a *Centennial Vision* statement for the profession as it nears its 100th anniversary. This statement affirms that

> We envision that occupational therapy is a powerful, widely recognized, science-driven, and evidence-based profession with a globally connected and diverse workforce meeting society's occupational needs. (AOTA, 2007)

This vision reflects the long-standing commitment of the profession to serve society in ways that are relevant and forward-thinking. As social concerns evolve, occupational therapy practitioners must understand the occupational implications of broad contextual issues that affect health and well-being directly and indirectly. Global effort to deal with climate change, for example, are causing downward economic pressures on middle-class living standards, thus altering daily routines, limiting occupational opportunities, increasing chronic health conditions, and reducing access to health care (Kawachi & Wamala, 2006). Occupational therapy practitioners need not only know how to respond to evolving social needs; they need to do so quickly, creatively, and proactively.

Occupational therapy education is critical to the achievement of this vision in 2017 and beyond. The constellation of skills and attitudes occupational therapy practitioners must possess are the result of their inherent abilities and motivations refined into long-standing dispositions through a deliberate educational process. Indeed, occupational therapy education embodies the aspirations for the kind of society we wish to see. To talk about the purpose of the profession is also to talk about the purpose of occupational therapy education, as it is here where these aspirations are nurtured and shaped.

Use of This Document

Occupational therapy is essentially an educative profession. Occupational therapy practitioners are skilled at analyzing limitations that may result in diminished occupational participation and designing therapeutic programs through which people learn new skills or re-learn skills lost to illness, injury, or contextual constraints. While to some degree all occupational therapy practitioners are educators, this document focuses on recognized roles related to education in the profession (Academic Program Director, Academic Faculty, Academic Fieldwork Coordinator, and Fieldwork Educator). The purpose is to articulate the attributes practitioners should possess in such roles in order to have an enduring legacy in the fulfillment of the *Centennial Vision* and beyond. These attributes are described in the language of possibility, including the characteristics of innovator/visionary, scholar/explorer, leader, integrator, and mentor. Because the embodiment of these attributes is developmental, they are described in a continuum of experience from novice, intermediate, and advanced practitioner.

The context surrounding the educator will determine which attributes are most needed and/or appropriate. While all professionals will demonstrate some aspects of the attributes, not everyone is expected to achieve the advanced level in all the attributes. Indeed, because of experience, available opportunities, and personal curiosities and strengths, an educator will likely demonstrate some attributes at the novice level while demonstrating others at the intermediate and advanced levels. Therefore, the purpose of this document is not to identify rigid standards of performance but rather to serve as a guide of desired attributes toward which an educator may aspire in order to contribute to the fulfillment of the *Centennial Vision* and beyond.

It is recommended that this document be used as an aid in the articulation of the professional development plans of faculty. Such plans are essential in their growth and are required by the Accreditation Council for Occupational Therapy Education (ACOTE) for all program directors and faculty who teach two or more courses (ACOTE, 2006, Standard A.5.2).

Desired attributes include the following:

- *Innovator/Visionary:* Someone who embraces new directions, is forward-thinking, projecting into the future. This person thinks outside of the traditional confines of the profession to predict and propose how to meet future societal needs. A visionary can see past traditional boundaries to new possibilities at all levels of personal and societal life.

- *Scholar/Explorer:* A scholar/explorer is someone who seeks, uses, and produces knowledge and effectively disseminates new findings to internal and external audiences. These individuals use a critical, theoretically grounded, and systematic approach in their scholarly endeavors to produce outcomes that inform and address societal needs.

- *Leader:* Someone who analyzes past, present, and future trends and develops solutions to problems or strategies for taking advantage of opportunities by collaborating, inspiring, and influencing people to create a desired future.

- *Integrator:* Someone who seeks and finds divergent information, perceives meaningful relationships, and makes connections through analysis to create a new, more coherent understanding.

- *Mentor:* A trusted role model who inspires, encourages, influences, challenges, and facilitates the growth and development of others' goals and aspirations. This involves a collaborative process that may be between peers, colleagues, experienced and inexperienced individuals, practitioners and academicians, and others. The mentor may function in various roles such as educator, tutor, coach, counselor, encourager, consultant, etc.

As stated earlier, the embodiment of these attributes is developmental, and not all tributes are likely to be developed at the same time nor needed equally. An educator can demonstrate an attribute at a novice level while demonstrating another at an advanced level. In this document, *novice* performance is understood as beginning expertise, as when a person has had limited experience in an area and therefore has limited familiarity with the associated knowledge or its application. *Intermediate* performance is understood as consistent demonstration of and attribute in specific situations as a result of prior experience in those situations. Finally, *advanced* performance is understood as the ability to demonstrate an attribute in multiple situations, including some in which a person has no prior experience. Advanced performance denotes a high level of expertise.

In Tables 1–5, each attribute is represented, summarizing how it might be demonstrated in each educator role. It is assumed that the incumbent in a role has met or exceeded occupational therapy practitioner competencies described in the *Standards for Continuing Competence* (AOTA, 2005). The attributes are general statements and specific characteristics may not apply to all situations.

References

Accreditation Council for Occupational Therapy Education. (2006). *Standards and interpretive guidelines.* Available at http://www.aota.org/Educate/Accredit/StandardsReview/guide/42369.aspx

American Occupational Therapy Association. (2005). Standards for continuing competence. *American Journal of Occupational Therapy, 59,* 661–662.

American Occupational Therapy Association. (2007). AOTA's *Centennial Vision* and executive summary. *American Journal of Occupational Therapy, 61,* 613–614.

Kawachi, I., & Wamala, S. (2006). *Globalization and health.* New York: Oxford University Press.

Authors
Commission on Education

René Padilla, PhD, OTR/L, FAOTA, *Chairperson*
Andrea Bilics, PhD, OTR/L
Judith C. Blum, MS, OTR/L
Paula C. Bohr, PhD, OTR/L, FAOTA
Jennifer C. Coyne, COTA/L
Jyothi Gupta, PhD, OTR/L
Linda Musselman, PhD, OTR, FAOTA
Linda Orr, MPA, OTR/L
Abbey Sipp, *ASD Liaison*
Patricia Stutz-Tanenbaum, MS, OTR
Neil Harvison, PhD, OTR/L , *AOTA Staff Liaison*

Adopted by the Representative Assembly 2009FebCS112

Note: This document replaces the following documents: *Role Competencies for a Professional-Level Program Director in an Academic Setting, 2003M167; Role Competencies for a Program Director in an Occupational Therapy Assistant Academic Setting, 2005C239; Role Competencies for a Professional-Level Occupational Therapist Faculty Member in an Academic Setting, 2003M168; Role Competencies for a Faculty Member in an Occupational Therapy Assistant Academic Setting, 2005C240; Role Competencies for an Academic Fieldwork Coordinator, 2003M169;* and *Role Competencies for a Fieldwork Educator, 2005M284.*

Table 1.
Innovator/Visionary

Experience	Academic Program Director	OT/OTA Faculty Member	Academic Fieldwork Coordinator	Fieldwork Educator
Novice	1. Analyzes the current curriculum to reflect the future needs of the program, profession, and society. 2. Analyzes institutional needs in order to identify new ways that the program can fulfill the institution's mission. 3. Develops curriculum that challenges and prepares students to identify and fulfill innovative practice roles.	1. Demonstrates the ability to prepare ethical and competent practitioners for both traditional and emerging practice settings. 2. Develops plan to maintain self abreast of the breadth and depth of knowledge of the profession in order to incorporate such knowledge in student learning. 3. Assists with the development of new learning processes that can enhance learning opportunities for students in the program. 4. Develops a plan of continued proficiency in emerging pedagogy through investigation, and formal and informal education.	1. Embraces new approaches for fieldwork, including in non-OT practice settings, international fieldwork, diverse settings. 2. Projects an exemplary curricular model representing the OT/OTA academic program.	1. Embraces new approaches for fieldwork in traditional or emerging practice settings. 2. Implements a model fieldwork program that reflects the curricular design of the academic program. 3. Uses innovation within own fieldwork setting to enhance student learning experience during fieldwork.
Intermediate	1. Projects future trends and societal needs of the profession and appropriately adapts the curriculum, including both the academic and fieldwork components. 2. Establishes a management plan that guides student development in the OT program and facilitates faculty development within the OT unit and the college/university community.	1. Proposes and implements nontraditional learning environments that facilitate development of competent and ethical professionals. 2. Participates in college-/university-wide committees and assists in propelling the institution forward in the future in order to meet projected societal needs. 3. Embraces the use and development of course materials and experiences that are innovative and non-traditional.	1. Proposes strategies that facilitate linkages between academic program curriculum and fieldwork practice opportunities. 2. Proposes strategies to support client centered, meaningful, occupation-based, and evidence-based outcomes of the OT process during fieldwork experiences.	1. Proposes strategies that facilitate collaborative partnerships between academic program curricula and fieldwork practice opportunities. 2. Proposes strategies to support client-centered, meaningful, occupation-based, and evidence-based outcomes of the OT process during fieldwork experiences.

Table 1.
Innovator/Visionary *(cont.)*

Experience	Academic Program Director	OT/OTA Faculty Member	Academic Fieldwork Coordinator	Fieldwork Educator
Intermediate		4. Assesses and predicts the effectiveness of new learning processes to enhance learning opportunities for students in the program.		3. Promotes innovation among fieldwork educators in OT as well as other disciplines in own and other related settings to enhance student learning experiences and interdisciplinary collaboration.
Advanced	1. Anticipates future directions of the profession in meeting societal needs by exploring new possibilities for strategic planning and identifying factors related to funding, resources, etc. 2. Identifies opportunities to engage with the community to promote OT as a profession in order to serve society's evolving needs. 3. Identifies new ways of applying the use of occupation that will lead to societal growth, prosperity and social justice.	1. Proposes innovative solutions and designs innovative strategies to address predicted future trends in education, practice, and research. 2. Proposes, builds, and sustains novel integrative collaborations across disciplines.	1. Predicts future directions for fieldwork environments in emerging practice areas and propose fieldwork opportunities for students. 2. Innovates strategies for providing fieldwork in emerging practice areas 3. Anticipates and prepares for the direction of legal and health care policy that influences fieldwork and designs strategies for compliance.	1. Predicts future directions of practice and fieldwork in emerging environments and develops fieldwork opportunities for students. 2. Consults with other fieldwork educators and sites to develop creative learning experiences for students. 3. Innovates strategies for providing fieldwork in emerging practice areas. 4. Anticipates and prepares for the direction of legal and health care policy that influences fieldwork and designs strategies for compliance.

(continued)

Table 2.
Scholar/Explorer

Experience	Academic Program Director	OT/OTA Faculty Member	Academic Fieldwork Coordinator	Fieldwork Educator
Novice	1. Possesses requisite knowledge and skills to design and conduct independent research relevant to OT practice and education and to disseminate results. 2. Recognizes the importance of scholarship within the academic community in general and within own educational institution in particular. 3. Designs a curriculum that meets accreditation standards relating to the scholarly role and skills of entry-level practitioners. 4. Actively engages in scholarly activities within area of expertise. 5. Creates a scholarly environment in which faculty and students have substantive resources and infrastructure necessary for productive scholarship.	1. Effectively critiques and uses new research literature and educational materials that will promote critical thinking, evidence-based practice, and lifelong learning in preparing future practitioners. 2. Critically integrates theory and research evidence into practice and facilitates that process in learners. 3. Models behaviors that demonstrate the importance of scholarship to learners and practitioners. 4. Initiates research inquiry within contextually determined expectations, either independently or with a mentor.* 5. Initiates the processes to develop a line of inquiry for research.* *May not always be possible for faculty in an OTA program.*	1. Effectively critiques and utilizes new research literature and educational materials that will promote critical thinking, evidence-based practice, and lifelong learning in preparing future practitioners. 2. Facilitates fieldwork educators' ability to effectively critique and use new research literature and educational materials that will promote critical thinking, evidence-based practice, and lifelong learning in preparing future practitioners. 3. Critically integrates theory and research evidence into practice and facilitates that process in fieldwork educators. 4. Facilitates integration and agreement of the academic philosophy and curriculum design within the fieldwork site. 5. Identifies questions about the fieldwork learning experiences for future research. 6. Facilitates best practices in using scholarship of teaching and learning in practice settings.	1. Critically evaluates current research to reflect best practice in teaching and practice. 2. Engages in systematic literature reviews to support and enhance practice. 3. Recognizes scholarly role in client service provision and program evaluation. 4. Models engagement in evidence-based practice specific to setting and populations served. 5. Seeks current evidence and information regarding effective fieldwork education and educational methodologies. 6. Translates practice knowledge into learning modes appropriate for fieldwork students. 7. Identifies questions about the fieldwork learning experiences for future research. 8. Monitors and interprets fieldwork student learning outcomes and effectiveness of student fieldwork program. 9. Coordinates with the Academic Fieldwork Coordinator to monitor and interpret student fieldwork learning outcomes.

Table 2.
Scholar/Explorer *(cont.)*

Experience	Academic Program Director	OT/OTA Faculty Member	Academic Fieldwork Coordinator	Fieldwork Educator
Intermediate	1. Coordinates active research agenda within the occupational therapy program. 2. Facilitates interdisciplinary collaboration and cooperation in research.	1. Contributes to the production of new findings and educational materials that add to the knowledge base of the profession. 2. Actively cultivates knowledge, skills, and interests in students by incorporating evidence from research into practice. 3. Conducts scholarship independently and begins to identify a coherent line(s) of inquiry.* 4. Successfully advises and guides students and practitioners in research.* 5. Disseminates findings in a public format such as presentations and publications. 6. Seeks opportunities to serve as a reviewer, editor, or publisher of scholarly work to internal and external audiences. *May not always be possible for faculty in an OTA program.*	1. Synthesizes new research literature and educational materials that will promote critical thinking, evidence-based practice, and lifelong learning in preparing future practitioners. 2. Conducts workshops and training programs to facilitate fieldwork educators' ability to use evidence in fieldwork education. 3. Plans and engages in the scholarship of teaching and learning regarding fieldwork education. 4. Collaborates with fieldwork educators and faculty to conduct research regarding fieldwork.	1. Designs evidence-based practice learning opportunities for fieldwork students to enhance understanding of the OT process. 2. Contributes to the breadth and body of knowledge through collaborative research projects. 3. Generates a clinical research agenda in collaboration with clinical and academic colleagues. 4. Collaborates with Academic Fieldwork Coordinator and faculty to conduct research regarding fieldwork.
Advanced	1. Provides national leadership in the development of and/or implementation of scholarship that further establishes foundational knowledge and efficacy of occupational therapy interventions.	1. Develops collaborative opportunities in research and scholarly work with other faculty. 2. Effectively produces and disseminates new findings within and outside of the profession.	1. Creates and disseminates new resources for fieldwork educators and Academic Fieldwork Coordinators to incorporate best practices in fieldwork education through student–fieldwork educator collaboration.	1. Models for students the importance of practitioner scholarship by engaging in independent and/or collaborative research projects and program evaluation.

(continued)

Table 2.
Scholar/Explorer *(cont.)*

Experience	Academic Program Director	OT/OTA Faculty Member	Academic Fieldwork Coordinator	Fieldwork Educator
Advanced	2. Contributes to and/or leads national dialogue concerning the advancement of OT theory and practice through research and scholarship.	3. Establishes a well-defined scholarly agenda or lines of inquiry. 4. Provides leadership in advancing the profession's knowledge base. 5. Uses innovative methodologies to identify, analyze, and effectively address the changing needs of society at the local, national, or global levels. 6. Establishes a national or international reputation or recognition as an expert in their area of inquiry.	2. Conducts research with other Academic Fieldwork Coordinator and fieldwork educators 3. Uses research evidence to inform professional educational policy.	2. Engages in multi-site research.

Table 3.
Leader

Experience	Academic Program Director	OT/OTA Faculty Member	Academic Fieldwork Coordinator	Fieldwork Educator
Novice	1. Uses management and leadership skills related to finance, planning, policy, marketing, public relations, and legal issues in order to meet accreditation standards and fulfill the program and institutional missions within an increasingly challenging educational environment. 2. Uses excellent interpersonal skills and demonstrates the ability to relate to diverse groups, constituencies, and organizations. 3. Takes responsibility for the assessment process for specific and overall program evaluation to enable the individual faculty to assess, diagnose, and apply interventions necessary to ensure quality.	1. Facilitates student development toward leadership roles. 2. Models ethical and professional behavior to facilitate the transition from student to clinician, advocate, and future fieldwork educator. 3. Assesses course materials, objectives, and educational experiences to promote optimal learning for students. 4. Develops plan of continued competency in leadership skills as related to role of teaching. 5. Participates with faculty in identifying trends that may influence future student learning and preparation.	1. Takes responsibility to develop systems to manage data for record keeping, fieldwork contract agreements, confidential student health records, and so on to ensure compliance with standards and legal requirements of local, state, and federal jurisdictions. 2. Develops a working relationship between the institution and fieldwork sites to facilitate ongoing collaborative partnerships to support education and practice. 3. Assists and monitors students in the development of their successful transition from the academic to the fieldwork portion of the educational program. 4. Evaluates the ongoing effectiveness of the fieldwork program, including student performance and fieldwork site integration of academic curricular design.	1. Critically reviews site-specific fieldwork program to ensure that quality learning experiences reflect best practice. 2. Advocates for department-wide participation in fieldwork education. 3. Facilitates student's transition into practice.
Intermediate	1. Forms strategic alliances with critical constituent groups within and outside the program's organization that can assist and promote the program's	1. Seeks and obtains leadership role as representative from OTA/OT/OS department on institution-wide committees and organizations where collaboration occurs between various disciplines of study.	1. Analyzes current and future trends in OT practice to develop fieldwork settings to reflect emerging practice.	1. Modifies site-specific fieldwork objectives to ensure that high-quality learning experiences reflect best practice.

(continued)

Table 3.

Leader *(cont.)*

Experience	Academic Program Director	OT/OTA Faculty Member	Academic Fieldwork Coordinator	Fieldwork Educator
	goals. 2. Builds and maintains systems that ensure that the program operates in concert with the mission of the institution and the mission of the academic unit in which the program is housed. 3. Seeks and accepts institutional leadership roles.	2. Analyzes past, present, and future trends to integrate practice, theory, literature, and research for instruction in evidence-based practice. 3. Collaborates with other faculty members on scholarship/research activities related to the advancement of occupational therapy, occupational science, teaching, and outcomes assessment.	2. Develops or explores innovative strategies of supervision for students in emerging practice areas. 3. Collaborates with other clinical coordinators within the institution to streamline policies and procedures with regard to student placements in fieldwork.	2. Educates colleagues and develops networks and programs to ensure fieldwork excellence. 3. Participates in knowledge generation by contributing to local, regional, and/or national fieldwork discussion/dialogues. 4. Participates in national initiatives that are collaborative efforts between educational institutions and fieldwork sites (e.s. backpack awareness month).
Advanced	1. Applies the processes of advancement (philanthropy), including identifying, cultivating, and securing gifts through the matching of potential donors with well-articulated needs. 2. Seeks and accepts leadership roles within the community as well as within state, national, and international associations.	1. Proposes innovative solutions and designs innovative strategies to address predicted future trends in education, practice, and research. 2. Proposes, builds, and sustains novel integrative collaborations across disciplines.	1. Develops national and international fieldwork student exchanges, placements, and programs. 2. Provides national and global leadership in the development of fieldwork education. 3. Develops and evaluates the ongoing effectiveness and quality of national and international fieldwork education. 4. Seeks and fully embraces the leadership role in the education of regional fieldwork consortiums.	1. Develops national models for fieldwork education in collaboration with other Fieldwork Educators and Academic Feildwork Coordinators across disciplines. 2. Shares innovative models of fieldwork supervision on a state, national, and international levels. 3. Seeks leadership roles in regional, national, and international fieldwork education.

Table 4.
Integrator

Experience	Academic Program Director	OT/OTA Faculty Member	Academic Fieldwork Coordinator	Fieldwork Educator
Novice	1. Forms strategic alliances with critical constituent groups within and outside the program's organization that can assist and promote the program's goals.	1. Develops a plan to continue proficiency in teaching through investigation, continuing education, and self-investigation. 2. Meets diverse learning needs of students and faculty. 3. Creates learning environments that facilitate the development of culturally sensitive, competent, and ethical professionals. 4. Independently seeks, selectively chooses relevant resources from OT and other disciplines, and disseminates information to promote advanced understanding in a variety of areas. 5. Develops a strategic plan for professional development that combines teaching, scholarship, and service.	1. Seeks close collaboration with fieldwork educators to facilitate student fieldwork learning and align clinical fieldwork program with curriculum design/outcomes. 2. Facilitates partnerships between program faculty and fieldwork educators. 3. Supports communication, collaboration, and connections between students and fieldwork educators to support the selection, matching, and scheduling of appropriate fieldwork experiences. 4. Designs culturally sensitive fieldwork programs and fieldwork objectives. Advocates for interdisciplinary fieldwork learning opportunities. 5. Collaborates with fieldwork educators and faculty to facilitate congruence of curriculum design and best practice.	1. Seeks close collaboration with academic programs to facilitate student fieldwork learning and align clinical fieldwork program with curriculum design/outcome. 2. Develops and/or modifies clinical fieldwork manual/ objectives to reflect national standards and academic fieldwork objectives. 3. Collaborates with Academic Fieldwork Coordinator to ensure integration of curriculum design into the practice setting. 4. Designs culturally sensitive fieldwork programs and fieldwork objectives. 5. Facilitates collaborative learning among fieldwork students within the profession and across disciplines.
Intermediate	1. Integrates increasingly diverse sources of information in order to define problems, explore solutions, and formulate appropriate decisions that result in effective management of the academic unit to meet its mission.	1. Develops a framework from which to practice using divergent resources. 2. Demonstrates progress of professional development plan that combines teaching, scholarship, and service.	1. Analyzes current trends to create new fieldwork opportunities. 2. Facilitates development of Academic Fieldwork Advisory Panels that integrate diverse perspectives from the community.	1. Serves on Academic Fieldwork Advisory Panels. 2. Actively facilitates interdisciplinary fieldwork learning opportunities.

(continued)

Table 4.
Integrator *(cont.)*

Experience	Academic Program Director	OT/OTA Faculty Member	Academic Fieldwork Coordinator	Fieldwork Educator
Intermediate		3. Forms strategic alliances across disciplines to advance the profession.		3. Develops and/or modifies fieldwork student manual/objectives to reflect national standards and academic fieldwork objectives. 4. Functions as a practice resource for Academic Fieldwork Coordinators to enhance fieldwork collaboration and academic outcomes. 5. Models cultural sensitivity when designing fieldwork programs and fieldwork objectives.
Advanced	1. Fosters ongoing relationships among educators, researchers, and practitioners that address the needs of both the profession and society. 2. Creatively collaborates with consumers, interdisciplinary educators, and researchers to meet the increasingly complex needs of national and global communities. 3. Effectively utilizes various venues, such as regulatory bodies, nongovernmental organizations, legislatures, and other bodies such as the World Health Organization or the Centers for Disease Control and Prevention in order to promote the health and well-being of people through occupation.	1. Collaborates with diverse disciplines for information synthesis and dissemination. 2. Articulates and represents the role of OT in emerging areas of practice at the local, national, and international levels. 3. Creatively collaborates with consumers, interdisciplinary educators, and researchers to meet the increasingly complex needs of national and global communities. 4. Effectively uses various venues, such as regulatory bodies, nongovernmental organizations, legislatures, and other internationally recognized agencies in order to promote the health and well-being through occupation.	1. Bridges the gap between OT/OTA practitioner needs (evidence-based practice) and resources available through OT/OTA academic program and student fieldwork experiences. 2. Enhances relationships with regional/national/international fieldwork committees. 3. Creatively contributes to a national/ international understanding of the importance of fieldwork education by facilitating meaningful relationships and networking among practitioners, students, and educators.	1. Contributes to a more coherent understanding of health care service provision and a national fieldwork student network. 2. Develops/contributes to interdisciplinary experimental learning modules. 3. Serves on regional/national/international fieldwork committees. 4. Creatively contributes to a national and International understanding of the importance of fieldwork education by facilitating meaningful relationships and networking among practitioners, students, and educators.

Table 5.
Mentor

Experience	Academic Program Director	OT/OTA Faculty Member	Academic Fieldwork Coordinator	Fieldwork Educator
Novice	1. Serves as a model to mentor diverse faculty, students, alumni, and occupational therapy practitioners in their area of expertise. 2. Facilitates mentoring relationships within the academic institution. 3. Models professional and ethical behavior within the academic setting. 4. Instills in students the professional responsibility of seeking and offering mentoring relationships. 5. Analyzes personal and professional goals and acquires resources necessary to attain professional growth.	1. Demonstrates a competent and positive attitude that results in the mentoring of students in professional development in scholarship, research, and/or service. 2. Develops and fosters trusting relationships with practitioners interested in transitioning from practice into academia. 3. Identifies a variety of tangible and intangible resources that can enhance the professional growth of self and others. 4. Analyzes personal and professional goals and acquires resources necessary to attain professional growth. 5. Encourages potential students to develop relationships with OT/OTA practitioners, alumni, students, and faculty prior to entering the profession. 6. Facilitates the inclusion of a diverse community of faculty and students through the mentoring process.	1. Coaches and guides students to engage in appropriate professional and fieldwork education activities. 2. Creates a collaborative process between academic faculty and fieldwork educators. 3. Serves as a model and consultant for fieldwork educators to facilitate development of quality fieldwork programs. 4. Facilitates the growth of practitioners and fieldwork educators for implementing best practice principles during fieldwork education. 5. Analyzes personal and professional goals and acquires resources necessary to attain professional growth. 6. Encourages potential students to develop relationships with occupational therapy practitioners, students, alumni, and faculty prior to entering the profession. 7. Facilitates the inclusion of a diverse community of faculty and students through the mentoring process. 8. Serves as a model representative of the academic program locally and regionally.	1. Mentors students prior to and during fieldwork by functioning as a model. 2. Serves as a model to mentor diverse individuals and occupational therapy practitioners in their area of expertise. 3. Encourages potential students to develop relationships with occupational therapy practitioners, students, and faculty prior to entering the profession. 4. Analyzes personal and professional goals and acquires resources necessary to attain professional growth.

(continued)

Table 5.
Mentor *(cont.)*

Experience	Academic Program Director	OT/OTA Faculty Member	Academic Fieldwork Coordinator	Fieldwork Educator
Intermediate	1. Develops innovative strategies for negotiating creative, constructive, and ethical solutions to address interpersonal and academic issues within a complex environment. 2. Develops resources, policies and procedures/guidelines for faculty that can be used to facilitate progressively higher levels of responsibility at the department, university, community, and professional levels. 3. Uses a variety of methods and technology to expand mentoring relationships beyond the academic institution and the community it serves.	1. Identifies individuals or groups in need of mentoring who would otherwise not seek mentorship and encourages them to develop mentoring relationships to maximize their potential. 2. Participates in mentoring or coaching of junior faculty through constructive feedback and role modeling of work with students, practitioners, and peers. 3. Effectively mentors and functions as faculty advisor for student organizations. 4. Inspires others to serve as mentor to students, alumni, practitioners, and faculty. 5. Actively contributes to the accomplishment of long-term expectations and outcomes of mentor relationships necessary for own personal and professional growth. 6. Uses a variety of methods and technology to expand mentoring relationships beyond the academic institution and the community it serves.	1. Collaborates with fieldwork educators to promote effective and innovative learning opportunities for students. 2. Tutors and coaches non-OT fieldwork educators in their development as supervisors and their implementation of fieldwork experiences reflecting OT practice. 3. Models and facilitates development of innovative strategies to obtain excellence within the constraints of the fieldwork practice environment. 4. Coaches students, fieldwork educators, and Academic Fieldwork Coordinators to negotiate and problem solve challenging fieldwork dilemmas. 5. Creates effective resources reflecting current trends and emerging practice areas to sustain excellence in fieldwork education. 6. Influences the development of innovative programs to bridge the gap between fieldwork and didactic content into a cohesive curriculum design. 7. Uses a variety of methods and technology to expand mentoring relationships beyond existing fieldwork education network.	1. Identifies a variety of tangible and intangible resources that can be used to enhance the professional growth of self and others. 2. Recruits and guides inexperienced OT/OTA staff to develop in the role as a fieldwork educator. 3. Models excellence as a fieldwork educator and fieldwork site coordinator. 4. Models excellence and commitment to the tenets of the profession using occupational-based and evidence-based practice during the OT process. 5. Develops mentorship programs within the facility that reflect and promote interdisciplinary and intradisciplinary fieldwork excellence. 6. Uses a variety of methods and technology to expand mentoring relationships beyond the fieldwork site. 7. Develops innovative strategies for negotiating creative, constructive, and ethical solutions to address interpersonal and practice issues within a complex environment. 8. Serves as role model for other fieldwork educators.

Table 5.
Mentor *(cont.)*

Experience	Academic Program Director	OT/OTA Faculty Member	Academic Fieldwork Coordinator	Fieldwork Educator
Advanced	1. Anticipates and facilitates the development of future mentoring relationships within and outside the educational program to meet the needs of the profession and society. 2. Facilitates intra- and interdisciplinary mentoring relationships for faculty, students, alumni, and practitioners. 3. Models advocacy and acts as a change agent to fulfill the occupational and social justice vision of the profession both nationally and globally. 4. Identifies and addresses professional and societal trends that may present new ethical challenges for the profession and society. 5. Inspires others to develop new strategies and paradigms in response to societal issues.	1. Creates and shares networks, resources, and opportunities for growth of mentees at the national and international levels. 2. Develops and sustains programs across disciplines and geographical regions to foster mentees' successful performance in scholarship, teaching, and practice. 3. Models advocacy and acts as a change agent to fulfill the occupational and social justice vision of the profession both nationally and globally. 4. Develops innovative strategies for facilitating connections among students, educators, alumni, practitioners, and other colleagues for unusual, challenging, and/ or complex mentee needs or situations. 5. Anticipates and develops mentoring opportunities and programs designed to address disparities in health care, social injustices, issues within the profession, and society. 6. Develops innovative strategies for negotiating creative, constructive, and ethical solutions to address interpersonal and academic issues within a complex environment.	1. Models the creation of innovative fieldwork training programs globally to anticipate and meet the needs of the profession in the future. 2. Facilitates national and international networks among academic fieldwork coordinators to collectively and systematically address fieldwork issues. 3. Develops innovative strategies for negotiating creative, constructive, and ethical solutions that address interpersonal and academic issues within a complex environment. 4. Develops and sustains programs across disciplines and geographical regions to foster mentees' successful performance in scholarship, teaching, and practice. 5. Anticipates and develops mentoring opportunities and programs designed to address disparities in health care, social injustices, issues within the profession, and society. 6. Models advocacy and acts as a change agent to fulfill the occupational and social justice vision of the profession both nationally and globally.	1. Consults on the development of new fieldwork programs, supporting at other fieldwork sites, settings, and practice areas. 2. Develops national and international programs of mentorship excellence that connect students, practitioners, fieldwork educators, and academic fieldwork coordinators. 3. Anticipates and develops mentoring opportunities and programs designed to address disparities in health care, social injustices, issues within the profession, and society. 4. Models advocacy and act as a change agent to fulfill the occupational and social justice vision of the profession both nationally and globally.

Specialized Knowledge and Skills for Occupational Therapy Practice in the Neonatal Intensive Care Unit

Purpose

The purpose of this paper is to provide a reference for occupational therapists on the advanced knowledge and skills necessary to practice in a neonatal intensive care unit (NICU). Occupational therapy practice with infants in the NICU and their families is high risk and specialized, only appropriate for occupational therapists with advanced knowledge and skills in neonatal care.

Introduction

Occupational therapy philosophy and education provide the foundation for this profession to make a valuable contribution to neonatal practice (American Occupational Therapy Association [AOTA], 2004b). Specialized knowledge of neonatal medical conditions and developmental variability and abnormality in infants cared for in the NICU is essential to safe, effective practice. The therapist must recognize the complex medical needs and vulnerabilities of acutely ill or premature infants. These infants frequently are physiologically fragile and easily compromised by environmental conditions. Interactions and therapeutic interventions that may appear innocuous can trigger physiologic instability in an infant and can be life threatening. In fact, protecting the fragile neonate from excessive or inappropriate sensory aspects of the environment is often a more urgent priority than direct interventions or interactions with the infant. Occupational therapy approaches, such as sensory integration and neurodevelopmental intervention, are applicable within the NICU setting. However, these approaches may need to be modified according to the infant's medical status, physiological homeostasis, and developmental and family needs.

The special needs of families whose infants are in the NICU also must be recognized. The infant's medical status and uncertain outcome, the highly technical environment of the NICU, separation from parents, and potential maternal complications after labor and delivery may contribute to family stress or crisis. These situations often alter the parent–infant attachment process, which is essential to optimal infant developmental outcomes. Families are best served by an occupational therapist who is not only knowledgeable about infant needs, but also sensitive to family circumstances, priorities, concerns, and cultural beliefs. The occupational therapist must seek ways to establish supportive, collaborative, and therapeutic relationships with family members in order to foster the infant's optimal development.

The social and physical aspects of the environment can be stressful to both the infant and the family. All persons who interact with the infant constitute the social environment. The physical environment is composed of inanimate elements and properties (e.g., lighting, sound, bedding, equipment). The occupational therapist must understand the interplay of the social and physical features of the NICU and the way in which this interplay influences the infant, family, and staff members. This knowledge is used as a basis for the occupational therapy evaluation and contributes to effective intervention strategies.

Working within the social and physical bounds of the NICU environment, an important role of the occupational therapist is to assist each family to foster optimal infant development, including the encouragement of developmentally appropriate occupations, sensorimotor processes, and neurobehavioral organization. This must occur while considering the often fragile medical and physiological status of the infant. Through direct observation, intervention, consultation, education, and research, the occupational therapist collaborates with others to provide the infant with the most effective and appropriate social and physical environment.

The occupational therapist working in the NICU must have a basic knowledge of occupational therapy, pediatric experience, and specialized knowledge and skills related to the complex needs of high-risk infants, their families, and the NICU environment. Basic occupational therapy education includes knowledge of biological sciences, disease processes, mental health, and typical and atypical child and adult family development. Occupational therapy's domain of concern, encompassing the interaction among the biological, developmental, and social–emotional aspects of human function as expressed in daily activities and occupations, makes it particularly suited to address the needs of the developing infant and family (AOTA, 2002). The occupational therapy method of activity analysis and adaptation to achieve a functional outcome is valuable in promoting "goodness of fit" (i.e., the match between the infant's capabilities and the physical and social environment), as there is often a mismatch between the NICU environment, parental expectations, and the infant's capabilities.

Experience in pediatric occupational therapy is essential for practice in the NICU. This experience provides a perspective on the continuum of typical and atypical child development and on the significance of the family in the child's life. Experience in pediatric occupational therapy affords the practitioner opportunities for development of the critical thinking skills necessary for evaluation and intervention to promote competent occupational performance and emotional well-being of children and their families. Therefore, the therapist interested in practicing in the NICU should have experience in the following areas: pediatric occupational therapy with infants and young children, longitudinal follow-up of infants treated in the NICU, and collaboration with families.

In addition to basic occupational therapy education and pediatric experience, the occupational therapist working in the NICU requires advanced knowledge and skills to provide complex interventions to critically ill neonates and their families. These interventions require continuous evaluation and a dynamic approach to intervention planning. They also require knowledge of grief reactions, social structures, attachment, medical procedures, and other issues relating to the health and well-being of the family unit. Intervention in the NICU context is not a recommended area of practice for occupational therapy assistants because such knowledge and skills are beyond the scope of their practice. Since practice in the NICU requires advanced-level expertise and clinical reasoning, this area of practice also is not recommended for entry-level occupational therapists or occupational therapists who do not have the pediatric experience described above. Extensive continuing education; mentoring by an occupational therapist experienced in neonatal care; and graded, closely supervised, mentored practice are recommended for any occupational therapist entering neonatal practice. Supervision often is required until the therapist demonstrates competency in working with infants and their families in the NICU environment (AOTA, 2004a).

The specialized knowledge required for practice in the NICU includes familiarity with relevant medical conditions, procedures, and equipment; an understanding of the individualized developmental abilities and vulnerabilities of infants; an understanding of theories of neonatal neurobehavioral organization; working knowledge of family systems, early social–emotional development, infant mental health, and NICU ecology; and an understanding of multidisciplinary team collaboration. Most importantly, the NICU therapist must have a clear understanding of the manner in which these factors interact to influence behavior. The occupational therapist develops the necessary skills through continuing education and supervised mentored clinical experience in evaluation and intervention specific to the NICU. Neonatal practice requires advanced clinical reasoning skills. These skills include the flexibility to recognize and respond to unfamiliar situations and nuances of behavior, the ability to anticipate future directions of intervention, and the ability to perceive the clinical condition as a whole. The occupational therapist in the NICU applies these competencies with regard to the infant; the infant's family and caregivers; and the NICU environment, including staff. Specifically, the occupational therapist in the NICU designs an individualized intervention plan in collaboration with the family and others that incorporates the family's priorities and NICU contexts along with the individualized needs of the infant. This requires understanding the occupations and activities valued by families and the NICU culture; defining what factors limit each infant's participation or engagement in those occupations and activities; identifying factors that would constitute readiness for engagement in occupations and activities; and finally, delineating what physical and/or social environmental supports will maximize participation for both the infant and the family in the short term and in the long term.

Maintenance of clinical competency and an evidence-based approach to practice are both vitally important in the rapidly changing field of neonatology. Clinical competence can be sustained through regular supervision or a mentoring relationship, participation in peer study groups, reflective process, and formal and informal continuing education. An evidence-based approach to practice necessitates ongoing critical review of the relevant research, literature, and clinical tools available in this rapidly changing field of practice. An occupational therapy practitioner is knowledgeable about evidence-based research and applies it ethically and appropriately to the occupational therapy process (AOTA, 2005b).

Knowledge and Skills: The Infant, Family, and NICU Environment

The following information identifies the knowledge and skills needed to function as an occupational therapist in the NICU. This information is organized under the three main areas of occupational therapy concern described previously: the infant, the family, and the NICU environment.

The Infant

To be competent, the occupational therapist has to have an in-depth understanding of approaches to evaluation and intervention, including use of a developmentally supportive consultative model of service delivery. These approaches are presented in the literature specific to occupational therapy, neonatology, psychology, and infant and family studies. In addition, the therapist has to have a thorough understanding of medical factors and the potential risks they pose to normal fetal and infant growth and development. The therapist must understand and critically analyze this information within the context of occupational therapy practice and the specific philosophy of the NICU in which the occupational therapist works. The therapist develops an evaluation plan that includes use of appropriate standardized tools, parent or caregiver interviews, and observations of infant adaptation to the social and physical environments. The occupational therapist, in conjunction with the family and medical caregivers, then develops appropriate intervention strategies, individually suited to each infant and family.

For clarity in this paper, infant behavior is discussed separately from family and environmental concerns. However, in program implementation, the infant is assessed and treated within the context of the family and the NICU environment.

The following is a comprehensive outline of the essential knowledge base that an occupational therapist must possess for working with NICU infants.

I. Medical knowledge base as the foundation for understanding infant behavior

    A. General information

        1. Medical terminology and abbreviations used in the NICU

        2. Basic principles, uses, and potential complications of the medical equipment and procedures, including precautions and implications for the therapist and infant

        3. Medical complications frequently encountered, including pathophysiology, risks, precautions, and prognoses associated with specific conditions.

B. Specific knowledge

1. NICU equipment

2. Diagnostic procedures

3. Medical procedures

4. Nursing procedures and routines

5. Respiratory support

6. Thermoregulatory support

7. Nutritional support

8. Medication effects

9. Infection control

10. Institution-specific policies and procedures.

II. Factors that may influence infant and child development

A. Prenatal

1. Maternal and fetal complications during pregnancy

2. Genetic disorders, congenital anomalies, syndromes, isolated defects

3. Teratogens (e.g., licit and illicit drug exposure, radiation, environmental contaminates)

4. Infectious diseases (e.g., rubella, cytomegalovirus, herpes, toxoplasmosis, HIV)

5. Social risk factors (e.g., poverty, inadequate support, stress, environmental toxins).

B. Perinatal

1. Maternal complications during delivery

2. Neonatal complications during delivery

3. Gestational age and birth weight.

C. Postnatal conditions and complications

1. Respiratory

2. Cardiovascular

3. Neurologic

4. Sensory

5. Orthopedic

6. Gastrointestinal

7. Metabolic

8. Hemolytic

9. Dermatologic

10. Infectious disease

11. Iatrogenic complications.

III. Knowledge of the developmental course, abilities, and vulnerabilities of infants in the NICU

    A. Differences in body structure and body functions, developmental progression, variations, deviations, and abnormalities in infants in relation to preterm, term, or postterm birth and/or prenatal, perinatal, or postnatal factors

        1. Infant neurobehavioral organization

            a. Physiologic (e.g., cardiorespiratory)

            b. States of arousal

            c. Regulatory abilities
                Sleep and waking states
                Circadian rhythms
                Typical and atypical patterns
                Self-regulation
                External regulation
                Medication effects/side effects

            d. Neurosocial (e.g., attention, interaction).

        2. Sensory development and processing of sensory information

            a. Sequential developmental progression in utero and adaptations to the extra-uterine environment

            b. Thresholds for stimulation within the sensory systems: tactile, vestibular, proprioceptive, visual, auditory, olfactory, gustatory

            c. Responses: arousal, attention, modulation, transition, range, decompensation

            d. Sensory acuity.

        3. Motor function

            a. Neuromotor development, including, but not limited to, muscle tone, posture, quality of movement, reflexes and reactions, and motor control

            b. Biomechanical factors, including, but not limited to, active and passive range of motion, strength, and orthopedic status.

        4. Social–emotional development

            a. Early communicative cues

            b. Self-regulation of interaction

            c. Initial formation of attachment relationships

            d. Temperament.

    B. Emerging competencies in infant occupation

        1. General factors that influence participation in daily life activities

            a. Postconceptional age and weight

            b. Physical and developmental maturation

            c. Physiological status and medical conditions

            d. Neurobehavioral organization

      e. Sensory processing

      f. Biomechanical and neuromotor function

      g. Social interaction

      h. Physical environment

      i. Social environment.

  2. Specific activities

      a. Ability to cope with and participate in caregiving

         (1) Feeding process

            (a) Modes (e.g., breast, bottle, tube)

            (b) Function (e.g., ability to meet nutritional needs, physiologic cost, endurance)

            (c) Oral–motor mechanism (e.g., structure, function, quality)

            (d) Maturation of mechanical and neural control of sucking, swallowing, and breathing

            (e) Relationship among nutritive and non-nutritive sucking, respiration, and oxygenation

            (f) Positioning and handling

            (g) Feeding readiness cues

            (h) Physiologic issues, such as metabolic and neurologic

            (i) Competency of the infant as a partner

            (j) Relationship with primary caregivers

            (k) Tolerance of oral–facial and intraoral sensations.

         (2) Bathing

         (3) Dressing and diapering

         (4) Medical routines and procedures.

      b. Engaging in nurturing interactions

         (1) Skin-to-skin holding (kangaroo care)

         (2) Physical and social dialogue

         (3) Feeding.

      c. Interrelationship between medical and developmental domains

         (1) Present conditions

         (2) Future implications.

IV. Knowledge of evolving developmental approaches in the NICU

  A. Historical and current perspectives

    1. Supplemental stimulation

    2. Reduced stimulation

    3. Environmental neonatology

4. Individualized developmental care

5. Family-centered care

6. Relationship-based approach.

B. Modification and integration of current pediatric occupational therapy frames of reference (e.g., sensory integration, neurodevelopmental therapy, coping, dynamic systems).

V. Specific skills related to occupational therapy with infants in the NICU, including the ability to

A. Instruct, consult, and communicate with caregivers

B. Use NICU equipment appropriately and safely, including understanding of the purpose, basic operation, settings, and precautions of all relevant equipment

C. Conduct appropriate assessments

1. Determine appropriate timing of infant assessments on the basis of the infant's medical and physiological status, postconceptional age, and NICU and family routines

2. Select and administer formal and informal assessment procedures that are appropriate for postconceptional age and medical condition and that identify developmental abilities, vulnerabilities, and limitations in daily life activities and occupations as they are influenced by medical status and

   a. Neurobehavioral organization

   b. Sensory development and processing

   c. Motor function

   d. Pain

   e. Daily activity (e.g., feeding)

   f. Social–emotional development.

3. Assess the effects of physical environment, caregiving practices, positioning, and nurturance on the infant's neurobehavioral organization, sensory, motor, and medical status.

D. Formulate an individualized therapeutic intervention plan that supports the infant's current level of function and facilitates optimal social–emotional, physical, cognitive, and sensory development of the infant within the context of the family and the NICU

1. Determine appropriate timing of infant interventions on the basis of the infant's medical and physiological status, postconceptional age, and NICU and family bedside routines

2. Modify sensory aspects of physical environment according to infant sensory threshold

3. Participate with the infant and caregivers in occupational therapy interventions that reinforce the role of the family as the constant in the life of the infant and support the individual infant's medical and physiological status in order to

   a. Enhance infant neurobehavioral organization

   b. Facilitate social participation

   c. Promote optimal infant neuromotor functioning and engagement in daily life activities

   d. Promote developmentally appropriate motor function and engagement in daily life activities through the use of biomechanical techniques, when appropriate

   e. Facilitate well-organized infant behavior through adaptation of infant daily life activities.

E. Continuously observe and critically analyze subtle infant responses to the intervention program and modify as needed

F. Collaborate with family, NICU staff, and other persons who potentially may have an impact on infant well-being to

1. Create and maintain individualized developmental care plans

2. Incorporate the occupational therapy program into NICU routines

3. Modify intervention and discharge plans considering anticipated infant outcome.

G. Provide documentation that is objective, interpretive, thorough, and concise

H. Formulate discharge and follow-up plans in coordination with the interdisciplinary team and community resources to meet the developmental needs of the infant and family.

The Family

Parents and other family members are acknowledged to be the most important and consistent influence in the infant's life. Their occupational roles as primary caregivers and nurturers constantly need to be recognized and reaffirmed. Typically, parents are mediators of the infant's affective, sensory, and motor experiences. When an infant is hospitalized in the NICU immediately after birth, parents are not always able to play this mediation role. The bi-directional attachment process, which begins at delivery and in which both infant and parent play a part, can be disrupted. Since attachment provides a foundation for the infant's future development and independent function, its promotion is an important consideration for the occupational therapist. Therefore, the occupational therapist collaborates with family members, on-site and off-site, to facilitate the infant's optimal development, promote the parents' occupational roles, support parent–infant attachment, and ensure a successful transition from hospital to home and community.

The following outline summarizes the knowledge base that would enable an occupational therapist to provide services in the NICU from a family-centered perspective.

I. Knowledge of the family as a basis for collaboration

A. Family systems

1. Family structure, occupational roles, cultural identification, beliefs, values, and practices

2. Family resources: Sources and allocation (e.g., time, money, energy, social–emotional support)

3. Family adaptation: Adjustment to adding a new family member, adjustment to stressful situations

4. Needs, culture, and roles of family members, including siblings.

B. Adult learning styles

1. Individual differences in learning

2. Relationship between emotional state and learning capacities

3. Changes in parental focus during NICU course.

C. Parent–infant interactions: progression and individual differences

1. Parents' role in the infant's early social–emotional development

2. Attachment as an ongoing two-way process between parents and infant, including the importance of attachment to later developmental function and the influence of hospitalization on parents and infants on the attachment process

3. Development of synchronous interactions

4. Importance of parents' learning to accurately observe, interpret, and respond to their infant's unique cues.

D. The transition of the infant from hospital to home and community

1. Possible stresses and difficulties inherent in the transition process for the infant and each family member

2. Knowledge of community resources and local, state, and federal guidelines and services.

II. Specific skills related to occupational therapy with families of infants in the NICU. The occupational therapist

A. Identifies family hopes, dreams, expectations, attitudes, knowledge, strengths, priorities, preferred communication styles, and skills regarding daily care, play, and other interactions with the infant

B. Identifies family members' learning styles

C. Assists parents in feeling comfortable with their infant and as parents to a new family member

D. Guides family members in observing and interpreting their infant's behavior and in adapting their own behaviors in response to the infant's cues to elicit appropriate sensory, motor, and social responses

1. During daily life activities

2. During interactions involving exploration, attention, and orientation

3. While engaged in nurturing interactions.

E. Recognizes and acknowledges the infant's contribution and strengths in others' lives

F. Fosters successful parent–infant interactions via mutual problem solving, anticipatory guidance, modeling of behaviors, didactic and experiential education, and modification of the infant's environment

G. Integrates family observations and priorities in formulating occupational therapy intervention recommendations

H. Interprets and discusses occupational therapy evaluation findings in collaboration with the family

I. Adapts intervention approaches according to family culture, changing emotions, needs, and resources that may be influenced by the infant's changing medical status or other circumstances

J. Formulates and implements a discharge and follow-up plan with the family and other team members to ensure a smooth transition to the community, integrating occupational therapy goals into the overall goals and priorities of the family.

The NICU Environment

The neonate who is born prematurely or acutely ill is not well-adapted to the stressful and technologically complex environment of the NICU. This mismatch between the infant and the environment may have a deleterious effect on the infant's medical and developmental outcomes. Therefore, a primary intervention goal in the NICU is to provide the best match or fit between the infant and the NICU environment. Adapting or structuring the environment to enhance function is a well-accepted occupational therapy approach. However, this first requires knowledge of the various components of the environment as well as their interplay. The occupational therapist assesses the environment and collaborates with others to shape the infant's physical and social environment to provide a milieu of developmentally supportive care. The following competencies are essential:

I. Knowledge of the unique sensory properties of the NICU and their relationship to each infant's neurobehavioral organization

   A. *Tactile:* Timing, intensity, texture, handling for medical and nursing procedures, parent interaction

   B. *Proprioceptive–vestibular:* Timing, intensity, handling for medical and nursing procedures, parent interaction

   C. *Olfactory and gustatory experiences specific to the NICU* (timing, quality, intensity)

   D. *Auditory:* Intensity, duration, timing, animate versus inanimate

   E. *Visual:* Timing, ambient and focal light intensity, contents of visual field.

II. Knowledge of the social environment and its relationship to each infant's neurobehavioral organization, including interactions and relationships among

   A. Parents and infant

   B. Extended family members and infant

   C. Staff members and infant

   D. Parents and staff members

   E. Occupational therapist, parents, staff, and infant.

III. Knowledge of the physical environment and its relationship to each infant's maturation and behavioral organization

   A. Medical equipment and procedures as described under the medical knowledge base section

   B. Frequency, timing, duration, quality, and intensity of sensory input from medical equipment and procedures

   C. Sensory input from equipment, procedures, and staff activities that is disruptive to the infant's neurobehavioral organization.

IV. Knowledge of the NICU culture

   A. The NICU's specific philosophy of care, including its particular orientation toward acute and chronic care of infants

   B. The team members' roles, functions, attitudes, and positions in the organizational structure of the individual NICU

   C. The influence of NICU stressors (e.g., census changes and subsequent staffing patterns)

   D. Communication patterns and structure, both formal and informal, among staff members and between family and staff members

   E. Spoken and unspoken rules of behavior

   F. The effect of the physical and social environments on staff performance and morale

   G. Hospital administrative policies (e.g., confidentiality).

V. Specific skills related to occupational therapy in assessing and adapting the environment. The occupational therapist

   A. Assesses the sensory aspects of the NICU physical and social environments and its effect on infant well-being

B. Develops intervention strategies in collaboration with the family, NICU staff, and other team members to adapt the environment in order to foster optimal infant development and family interactions

1. Communicates with all levels of staff to establish rapport and develop team commitment to developmental and family goals

2. Integrates occupational therapy goals into the infant's medical priorities and the NICU setting.

C. Develops and implements strategies to influence philosophy and practice of developmental and family-centered care within the NICU

D. Assesses the effect of intervention strategies and revises the plan accordingly.

VI. Knowledge of structures that support occupational therapy practice in the NICU

The occupational therapist position exists within the NICU structure. The following knowledge and skills are needed to ensure integration of occupational therapy services into the NICU setting for optimal infant-family outcomes:

A. Ability to articulate the role and function of occupational therapists in the NICU to demonstrate their value and effectiveness

B. Ability to use relevant research literature to support occupational therapy practice in the NICU

C. Knowledge of the hospital's structure, mission, strategic plan, and fiscal priorities as they relate to both NICU and occupational therapy programs

D. Ability to identify and access sources of administrative and fiscal support to maintain occupational therapy services in the NICU

E. Knowledge of the larger local, state, and national health and social service systems as they influence policy and fiscal support for occupational therapy services in the NICU and early intervention services

F. Ability to identify sources of administrative and fiscal support for the practice of occupational therapy within the NICU from the community and the health care system at large

G. Knowledge of confidentiality guidelines (e.g., HIPAA).

Professional and Personal Characteristics Necessary for Occupational Therapists Practicing in the NICU

The NICU, as a critical care area, necessitates certain professional and personal characteristics. These characteristics include the following:

1. Ability to synthesize information from multiple sources, including research findings, and judiciously apply it to the NICU

2. Ability to observe the infant and environment for prolonged periods, without intervening, and to identify and understand subtle nuances of behavior and physiology

3. Interest in and ability to bring about changes in the infant's social and physical environments through direct intervention with the infant and family, consultation and collaboration with other team members, and implementation of policies and procedures at the organizational level

4. Understanding of one's interpersonal communication skills and style and the ability to modify them in response to family and staff behavior, learning styles, and needs

5. Commitment to seek ongoing knowledge, education, and peer consultation in this field

6. Ability to provide formal and informal educational programs for the hospital and the community

7. Insight into one's professional knowledge and skills

8. Ability to value, communicate, and collaborate with other NICU team members, community-based early intervention programs, and other resources

9. Understanding of and ability to articulate one's values and attitudes about

   a. The rights and responsibilities of families

   b. Relationships between cultural or religious beliefs and medical management decisions

   c. Working with infants who ultimately may not survive

   d. Working with infants who may have severe and permanent disabilities

   e. Working with families whose values, attitudes, behaviors, and life circumstances differ from one's own

   f. Allocating limited fiscal, personnel, and technological resources to sustain life.

10. Understanding of the *AOTA Code of Ethics* (2005a) as it applies to the NICU.

Definitions

Activity
"[T]he performance of a task or action by an individual" (World Health Organization [WHO], 2001, p. 10).

Activity Limitations
"[D]ifficulties an individual may have in executing activities" (WHO, 2001, p. 10).

Attachment
"A bond between an infant and a caregiver, usually its mother. Attachment is generally formed within the context of a family, providing the child with the necessary feelings of safety and nurturing at a time when the infant is growing and developing. This relationship between the infant and his caregiver serves as a model for all future relationships" (Gale, 2005).

Body Functions
"[T]he physiological or psychological functions of body systems" (including psychological functions; WHO, 2001, p. 10).

Body Structures
"[A]natomical parts of the body, such as organs, limbs, and their components" (WHO, 2001, p. 10).

Bonding
See *Attachment*.

Clinical Reasoning Skills in Occupational Therapy
The process by which occupational therapists individualize and modify treatment. It includes not only the application of theory to practice, but also the treatment of the meaning of illness as experienced by the individual and family (Mattingly, 1991).

Environmental Factors
"[T]he physical, social, and attitudinal environment in which people live and conduct their lives" (WHO, 2001, p. 10).

Environmental Neonatology

The study of environment of newborn special care facilities and its impact on the medical and developmental status of at-risk infants (Gottfried & Gaiter, 1985).

Family

A unit composed of individuals who are linked by shared kinship, function, and/or responsibilities and who identify themselves in a common relationship (Crockenberg, Lyons-Ruth, & Dickson, 1993).

Family-Centered Care

A constellation of philosophies, attitudes, and approaches to the care of children with special health and developmental needs that recognizes that the family is the constant in the child's life and that parent–professional partnerships are essential to effective and high-quality service delivery (Dunst, Trivette, & Deal, 1988; Institute for Family-Centered Care, 1990).

Goodness-of-Fit

"When the properties of the environment and its expectations and demands are in accord with the organism's own capacities, characteristics, and style of behaving" (Chess & Thomas, 1999, p. 3).

Impairments

"[P]roblems in body function or structure such as a significant deviation or loss" (WHO, 2001, p. 10).

Infant Mental Health

"Infant" refers to children under 3 years of age. "Mental" includes social–emotional and cognitive domains. "Health" refers to the well-being of young children and families (Fraiberg, 1980). A multidisciplinary intervention approach for the "early identification of risk and treatment to reduce the likelihood of serious developmental failure and relationship disturbance" (Weatherston, 2002, p. 1).

Medical Caregivers

House staff involved in the care of infants in the NICU. Although personnel may vary between institutions, medical caregivers typically include nurses, physicians (e.g., neonatologists, attending physicians, residents, interns), therapists, pharmacists, nutritionists, and other personnel (adapted from U. S. National Library of Medicine, 2005).

Neurobehavioral Organization

An interrelationship among infant central nervous system integrity and maturation, behaviors, and the caregiving environment. The interrelationship is expressed in terms of self-regulation and mutual regulation of autonomic, motoric, state, and interactional functions (Als, 1982).

Neurosocial

The ability to interact as the nervous system matures in preterm infants. There are three developmental stages of neurosocial development: turning in, coming out, and reciprocity (Gorski, Davidson, & Brazelton, 1979).

NICU

Neonatal intensive care unit. Newborn Nurseries are designated as Basic (Level I), Specialty (Level II), or Subspecialty (Level III) on the basis of their responsibilities and the availability of special service. Basic Neonatal Care Nurseries (*Level I*) provide postnatal care to healthy newborn infants and are equipped to provide resuscitation and to stabilize ill newborn infants until they can be transferred to a neonatal intensive care facility. Specialty Care Nurseries (*Level II*) "provide care to infants who are moderately ill with problems that are expected to resolve rapidly or who are recovering from serious illness" after receiving subspecialty care. Subspecialty Nurseries (*Level III*) provide care to infants who are extremely premature, are critically ill, or require surgical management (American Academy of Pediatrics & American College of Obstetricians and Gynecologists, 2004, p. 134).

Participation
"[I]nvolvement in a life situation" (WHO, 2001, p. 10).

Participation Restrictions
"[P]roblems an individual may experience in involvement in life situations" (WHO, 2001, p. 10).

Physiologic Instability
Refers to a lack of balance or equilibrium within the autonomic nervous system. Signs of physiologic instability may include changes in cardiorespiratory status (heart rate, respiratory rate, decreased oxygen saturation), color changes (pale, dusky, mottled, flushed), or visceral cues (yawning, sneezing, gagging, spitting up, hiccupping, having bowel movement). Conversely, an infant with physiologic stability will be calm with stable color and vital signs (Als, 1986).

Regulatory Abilities
The infant's capacity to modulate or modify his or her own state of arousal and neurobehavioral organization (Als, 1982).

Relationship-Based Approach
An approach that is "guided by a neurodevelopmental framework for understanding preterm infants and depends on the capacities of professionals to collaborate with one another and with families in support of the infants medical, developmental, and emotional well being" (Als & Gilkerson, 1997, p. 178).

References

Als, H. (1982). Toward a synactive theory of development: Promise for the assessment of infant individuality. *Infant Mental Health Journal, 3*, 229–243.

Als, H. (1986). A synactive model of neonatal behavioral organization: Framework for the assessment of neurobehavioral development in the premature infant and for the support of infants and parents in the neonatal intensive care environment. *Physical and Occupational Therapy in Pediatrics, 6*(3/4), 3–53.

Als, H., & Gilkerson, L. (1997). The role of relationship-based developmentally supportive newborn intensive care in strengthening outcome of preterm infants. *Seminars in Perinatology, 21*, 178–189.

American Academy of Pediatrics, & American College of Obstetricians and Gynecologists. (2004). *Guidelines for perinatal care* (5th ed.). Elk Grove Village, IL: Author

American Occupational Therapy Association. (2002). Occupational therapy practice framework: Domain and process. *American Journal of Occupational Therapy, 56*, 609–639.

American Occupational Therapy Association. (2004a). Guidelines for supervision, roles, and responsibilities during the delivery of occupational therapy services. *American Journal of Occupational Therapy, 58*, 663–677.

American Occupational Therapy Association. (2004b). Scope of practice. *American Journal of Occupational Therapy, 58*, 673–677.

American Occupational Therapy Association. (2005a). Occupational therapy code of ethics (2005). *American Journal of Occupational Therapy, 59*, 639–642.

American Occupational Therapy Association. (2005b). Standards of practice for occupational therapy. *American Journal of Occupational Therapy, 59*, 663–665.

Chess, F., & Thomas, A. (1999). *Goodness of fit: Clinical applications from infancy through adult life*. Philadelphia: Brunner/Mazel.

Crockenberg, S., Lyons-Ruth, K., & Dickson, S. (1993). The family context of infant mental health: II. Infant development in multiple family relationships. In C. H. Zeanah (Ed.), *Handbook of infant mental health* (pp. 38–55). New York: Guilford.

Dunst, C. J., Trivette, C. M., & Deal, A. G. (1988). *Enabling and empowering families: Principles and guidelines for practice.* Cambridge, MA: Brookline Books.

Fraiberg, S. (1980). *Clinical studies in infant mental health.* New York: Basic Books.

Gale, T. (2005). *The Gale encyclopedia of children's health: Infancy through adolescence.* Farmington Hills, MI: Thomson Gale.

Gorski, P., Davidson, M. E., & Brazelton, T. B. (1979). Stages of behavioral organization in the high-risk neonate: Theoretical–clinical considerations. *Seminars in Perinatology, 3,* 61–73.

Gottfried, A. W., & Gaiter, J. L. (1985). *Infant stress under intensive care.* Baltimore: University Park Press.

Institute for Family-Centered Care. (1990). *Association for the care of children's health.* Washington, DC: Author.

Mattingly, C. (1991). What is clinical reasoning? *American Journal of Occupational Therapy, 45,* 979–996.

U.S. National Library of Medicine. (2005, December 13). *MedlinePlus medical encyclopedia.* Retrieved January 11, 2006, from http://www.nlm.nih.gov/medlineplus/ency/article/007241.htm

Weatherston, D. J. (2002). Introduction to the infant mental health program. In J. J. Shirilla & D. J. Weatherston (Eds.), *Case studies in infant mental health: Risk, resiliency, and relationships* (pp. 1–13). Washington, DC: ZERO to THREE.

World Health Organization. (2001). *International classification of functioning, disability, and health (ICF).* Geneva, Switzerland: Author.

Related Readings

Als, H., Duffy, F. H., McAnulty, G. B., Rivkin, M. J., Vajapeyam, S., Mulkern, R. V., et al. (2004). Early experience alters brain function and structure. *Pediatrics, 113,* 846–857.

Als, H., Gilkerson, L., Duffy, F. H., McAnulty, G. B., Buehler, D. M., VanderBerg, K., et al. (2003). A three-center randomized controlled trial of individualized developmental care for very low birth weight infants: Medical, neurodevelomental, parenting, and caregiving effects. *Journal of Developmental and Behavioral Pediatrics, 24,* 399–408.

Anzalone, M. E. (1994). Occupational therapy in neonatology: What is our ethical responsibility? *American Journal of Occupational Therapy, 48,* 563–566.

Browne, J. V. (2003). New perspectives on premature infants and their parents. *ZERO to THREE, 24*(2), 4–12.

Buehler, D., Als, H., Duffy, F., McAnulty, G., & Liederman, J. (1995). Effectiveness of individualized developmental care for low-risk preterm infants: Behavioral and electrophysiologic evidence. *Pediatrics, 96,* 923–932.

Carter, B. S. (2003). Collaborative decision making in the NICU: When life is uncertain, satisfice. *ZERO to THREE, 24*(2), 21–25.

Holloway, E. (1998). Relationship-based occupational therapy in the neonatal intensive care unit. In J. Case-Smith (Ed.), *Pediatric occupational therapy and intervention* (pp. 111–126). Boston: Butterworth-Heinemann.

Holloway, E. (in press). Fostering early parent–infant playfulness in the neonatal intensive care unit. In L. D. Parham & L. S. Fazio (Eds.), *Play in occupational therapy for children* (2nd ed.). St. Louis, MO: Mosby.

Hunter, J. G. (2005). Neonatal intensive care unit. In J. Case-Smith, (Ed.), *Occupational therapy with children* (5th ed., pp. 688–770). St. Louis, MO: Elsevier/Mosby.

Johnson, B. H., Abraham, M. R., & Parrish, R. N. (2004). Designing the neonatal intensive care until for optimal family involvement. *Clinics in Perinatology, 31,* 353–383.

McGrath, J. M., & Conliffe-Torres, S. (1996). Integrating family-centered developmental assessment and intervention into routine care in the neonatal intensive care unit. *Nursing Clinics of North America, 31,* 367–368.

Meyer, E. C., Lester, B. M., Boukydis, C. F. Z., & Bigsby, R. (1998). Family-based intervention with high-risk infants and their families. *Journal of Clinical Psychology in Medical Settings, 5,* 49–69.

Talmi, A., & Harmon, R. J. (2003). Relationships between preterm infants and their parents: Disruption and development. *ZERO to THREE, 24*(2), 13–20.

Vergara, E., & Bigsby, R. (2004). *Developmental and therapeutic interventions in the NICU.* Baltimore: Paul H. Brookes.

Authors
Revised by the 2005 Neonatal Intensive Care Unit Task Force
Elsie Vergara, ScD, OTR, FAOTA, *Chairperson*
Marie Anzalone, ScD, OTR, FAOTA
Rosemarie Bigsby, ScD, OTR, FAOTA
Delia Gorga, PhD, OTR, FAOTA
Elise Holloway, MPH, OTR
Jan Hunter, MA, OTR
Ginny Laadt, PhD, OTR/L
Susan Strzyzewski, MEd, OTR

for

The Commission on Practice
Susanne Smith Roley, MS, OTR/L, FAOTA, *Chairperson*

Adopted by the Representative Assembly 2006C404

Reviewed by the Commission on Practice July 2010

This replaces the 2000 document "Specialized Knowledge and Skills for Occupational Therapy Practice in the Neonatal Intensive Care Unit" (*American Journal of Occupational Therapy, 54,* 641–648).

Specialized Knowledge and Skills in Mental Health Promotion, Prevention, and Intervention in Occupational Therapy Practice

Purpose

The purpose of this document is to describe the specialized knowledge and skills for entry-level occupational therapy practice in the promotion of mental health and the prevention and intervention of mental health problems, including mental illness. The foundations of occupational therapy are rooted firmly in psychiatry. The profession brings a habilitation and rehabilitation perspective to mental health services in keeping with increased emphasis on recovery and functionality directed toward participation in daily life occupations. The American Occupational Therapy Association (AOTA) supports the inclusion of the profession of occupational therapy as a core mental health profession in the U.S. *Code of Federal Regulations* and as a qualified mental health profession as defined by state statute and regulation (AOTA, 2006a).

In addition to intervention for persons with mental illness, occupational therapy practitioners contribute to the promotion of *mental health,* which refers to a positive state of functioning reflected in the presence of four characteristics: (1) positive affective or emotional state (e.g., subjective sense of well-being, feeling happy); (2) positive psychological and social function (e.g., self-acceptance, fulfilling relationships, self control); (3) productive activities; and (4) resilience in the face of adversity and the ability to cope with life stressors (U.S. Department of Health and Human Services, 1999; World Health Organization [WHO], 2004). A public health approach to mental health has been advocated by WHO (2001), which emphasizes the promotion of mental health as well as the prevention of and intervention for mental illness. As such, this document focuses on the knowledge and skills that substantiate occupational therapy's role in mental health promotion, prevention, and intervention.

Both occupational therapists and occupational therapy assistants are educated to provide services that support mental and physical health, rehabilitation, and recovery-oriented approaches. Occupational therapy practitioners[1] serve people throughout their life course in institutional, outpatient, home, school, and other community settings. Entry-level occupational therapists must have at least a master's degree but also may enter the profession with a clinical doctorate degree. Occupational therapy assistants enter the field at the associate's-degree level.

Intended for internal and external audiences, this document specifies the knowledge, reasoning, and performance skills necessary for competent and ethical occupational therapy practice in mental health promotion, prevention and intervention.

---

[1]When the term *occupational therapy practitioner* is used in this document, it refers to both occupational therapists and occupational therapy assistants (AOTA, 2006b). *Occupational therapists* are responsible for all aspects of occupational therapy service delivery and are accountable for the safety and effectiveness of the occupational therapy service delivery process. *Occupational therapy assistants* deliver occupational therapy services under the supervision of and in partnership with an occupational therapist (AOTA, 2009).

Introduction

The roots of occupational therapy are grounded in psychiatry. The moral treatment movement sought to replace the brutality and idleness of earlier treatment for disorders of the mind with kindness and "occupation" (Gordon, 2009, p. 203). In the early 20th century, the founders and early writers in occupational therapy created a body of literature that supported the value of occupation in the healing of mind and body (Gordon, 2009, p. 205). In 1922, Adolph Meyer acknowledged the importance of "work and play and rest and sleep" in his desire to address a therapeutic approach that healed the mind and improved the human condition for those with mental illness (as cited in Gordon, 2009, p. 207).

"Occupational therapy is founded on the understanding that engaging in occupations structures everyday life and contributes to health and well-being" (AOTA, 2008, p. 628). The term *occupation* is defined as "activities that people engage in throughout their daily lives to fulfill their time and give life meaning" (p. 672). The goals of occupational therapy are twofold: (1) to promote mental health and well-being in all persons with and without disabilities and (2) to restore, maintain, and improve function and quality of life for people at risk for or affected by mental illness. Occupational therapy practitioners support "health and participation in life through engagement in occupation" (p. 627).

Through the use of everyday activities, occupational therapy practitioners promote mental health and support functioning in people with or at risk of experiencing a range of mental health disorders, including psychiatric, behavioral, and substance abuse. Occupational therapy facilitates full participation in valued occupations in one's home, school, workplace, and community. As in all occupational therapy practice, services in mental health are client-centered. The client may be an individual or group of individuals, an organization, or a population. Occupational therapists work with clients to determine their wants and needs. Together, they determine the factors that are either barriers or supports to healthy participation in daily life activities. Occupational therapy assistants work under the supervision of and in partnership with occupational therapists (AOTA, 2009) to implement the plan and to assist the team with ongoing evaluation of success and need for change in the intervention strategies.

Through the clinical reasoning process, occupational therapy practitioners select and apply different theoretical perspectives and approaches informed by evidence. These perspectives and approaches are drawn primarily from occupational therapy and occupational science but also from other fields and areas of practice such as physical and psychiatric rehabilitation, psychology, school mental health, sociology, psychiatry, neuropsychiatry, and anthropology. This clinical reasoning process guides occupational therapy evaluation and intervention.

Although there is overlap in knowledge, skills, and attitudes with other professions, occupational therapy offers a unique contribution to mental health service provision. The profession holds a firm belief in the inherent need of all humans to engage in occupations, which are central to fulfilling meaningful life roles, engaging with one's environment, improving and sustaining health and well-being, and allowing full participation in society (Wilcock, 2007). Occupational therapy practitioners are educated to select and use evaluations and interventions that not only promote mental health but also address physical, sensory, and cognitive function affecting clients' abilities to participate in daily life while considering their interests, values, habits, and roles.

The profession recognizes and emphasizes the complex interplay among the individual variables, the activity demands, and the environmental demands. Occupational therapy practitioners are skilled in analyzing, adapting, or modifying the task or environment to support goal attainment and optimal engagement in occupation so that clients can develop and maintain healthy ways of living in their home, workplace, and community.

Using This Document

Health care, education, community, and mental health services stakeholders (e.g., clients, family members, policymakers, mental health practitioners of all disciplines) may use the document

- As a resource to advocate for inclusion of and coverage for occupational therapy as a core mental health service,

- To assist in articulating occupational therapy's contribution to the promotion of mental health in all persons, and

- To assist in articulating occupational therapy's contribution to mental illness prevention and intervention by promoting successful participation in a meaningful array of occupations that foster emotional well-being.

Occupational therapy practitioners and educators may use the document to

- Guide mental health curriculum and fieldwork development;

- Educate others on the mental health practice knowledge and skills that occupational therapy practitioners have in common with other core mental health practitioners;

- Educate others on occupational therapy's vital and unique contribution to mental health services; and

- Engage clients and family members in discussions about how occupational therapy practice supports mental health promotion, prevention, and intervention to assist individuals and groups in developing and meeting their goals that promote health and participation in daily life.

To facilitate its usefulness, this document is organized into two sections. Section 1, "Core Mental Health Professional Knowledge and Skills," describes knowledge and skills that occupational therapy practitioners share with other core mental health professionals. A deeper understanding of occupational therapy's approach to mental health services can be gleaned by reviewing Section 2, "Specific Occupational Therapy Knowledge and Skills Applied to Mental Health Promotion, Prevention, and Intervention," which describes mental health knowledge and skills specific to occupational therapy practice. Both sections help readers differentiate entry-level occupational therapy and occupational therapy assistant knowledge and skills.

The core mental health knowledge and skills of occupational therapy practitioners have been organized into four domains: (1) Foundations, (2) Evaluation and Intervention, (3) Professional Role and Service Outcomes, and (4) Mental Health Systems. Occupational therapists use and apply skills and knowledge from each domain to promote mental health and help persons with or at risk for psychiatric, substance abuse, and behavior disorders develop and maintain successful and satisfying ways of living in their home, work, and community. Occupational therapy assistants possess knowledge and skills to deliver services in each domain under the supervision of and in partnership with occupational therapists.

- *Foundations*—Occupational therapy practitioners are knowledgeable about how mental illnesses affect the ability to successfully participate in everyday occupations and what skills, compensatory strategies, or accommodations are needed to mitigate this impact. The are knowledgeable about (1) the promotion of positive mental health through competency enhancement (e.g., skill development, task adaptations, environmental supports, participation in meaningful occupations); (2) prevention of mental illness using risk reduction efforts (e.g., relaxation strategies with early signs of anxiety; establishing habits and routines that support adequate sleep, time for relationships, physical activity, and task accomplishment); and (3) intervention strategies to minimize symptoms experienced with the presence of mental illness (e.g., therapeutic task groups, relaxation strategies) provide an essential contribution to mental health services systems. Occupational therapy interventions promote successful participation in everyday occupations, allowing people to remain engaged and to re-engage in fulfilling, meaningful, and contributory roles. The foundation for this knowledge comes from occupational therapy; occupational science; and other fields of study such as physical and psychiatric rehabilitation, psychology, school mental health, sociology, psychiatry, neuropsychiatry, and anthropology.

- *Evaluation and intervention*—Occupational therapists are qualified to use relevant screening and assessment procedures to identify strengths, needs, problems, and concerns regarding a person's occupational engagement and successful performance of their daily life tasks. Further, therapists determine specific occupational performance issues and selected environmental and contextual factors that support and hinder performance. Occupational therapy assistants can assist with this evaluation process. Occupational therapy mental health interventions are based on assessment/evaluation results, developmental and life stage knowledge, and theoretical concepts of occupation. Interventions can be provided on an individual or group basis as in direct care or education or can be provided via consultation to populations of people to promote mental health and to address mental ill health.

- *Professional role and service outcomes*—Occupational therapy practitioners are educated to partner with consumers of mental health services, families and other natural support persons, individual practitioners, interdisciplinary teams, and community stakeholders to enhance service outcomes. To do this, practitioners learn to value multiple perspectives in addition to that of occupational therapy. In addition, occupational therapists are trained in the process of program evaluation, the knowledge and tools necessary to measure outcomes of occupational therapy intervention, and the context of the application of outcome measurement to mental health practice. They also are responsible for developing mechanisms to ensure the quality and effectiveness of service provision along with client satisfaction.

- *Mental health systems*—Occupational therapists have an understanding of how systems influence mental health services delivery, support mental health and the prevention of mental illness, and facilitate or inhibit people's ability to be full participants in their communities. Disability, health care, education, workforce, welfare, shelter, legal, criminal justice, housing, and social and familial systems all affect people with or at risk for psychiatric conditions. Occupational therapists are educated to analyze the interaction between and among systems, contexts, persons, populations, and occupations. Therapists use this knowledge to meet the participation needs of individuals as well as others within their communities (e.g., schools, employers, landlords, families).

References

American Occupational Therapy Association. (2006a). AOTA's statement on mental health practice. FAQ: *School mental health.* Retrieved January 10, 2010, from http://www.aota.org/Practitioners/Practice Areas/MentalHealth/Highlights/36364.aspx

American Occupational Therapy Association. (2006b). Policy 1.44: Categories of occupational therapy personnel. In *Policy manual* (2007 ed., pp. 33–34). Bethesda, MD: Author.

American Occupational Therapy Association. (2008). Occupational therapy practice framework: Domain and process (2nd ed.). *American Journal of Occupational Therapy, 62,* 625–683.

American Occupational Therapy Association. (2009). Guidelines for supervision, roles, and responsibilities during the delivery of occupational therapy services. *American Journal of Occupational Therapy, 63,* 797–803.

American Psychiatric Association. (2000). *Diagnostic and statistical manual of mental disorders* (4th ed., text. rev.). Washington, DC: American Psychiatric Association.

Gordon, D. M. (2009). The history of occupational therapy. In E. Crepeau, E. Cohn, & B. Schell (Eds.), *Willard and Spackman's occupational therapy* (11th ed., pp. 202–215). Philadelphia: Lippincott Williams & Wilkins.

U.S. Department of Health and Human Services. (1999). *Mental health: A report of the Surgeon General—Executive summary.* Rockville, MD: Author.

Wilcock, A. (2007). *An occupational perspective on health* (2nd ed.). Thorofare, NJ: Slack.

World Health Organization. (2001). *International classification of functioning, disability, and health (ICF).* Geneva, Switzerland: Author.

World Health Organization. (2004). *Promoting mental health: Concepts, emerging evidence, practice* (Summary report). Geneva, Switzerland: Author.

Authors

This document is based on a charge from the 2007 Representative Assembly and the work of the Mental Health Competencies Ad Hoc Committee. The Ad Hoc Committee along with the COP developed this work into a Knowledge and Skills Paper.

Katherine A. Burson, MS, OTR/L, CPRP, *Ad Hoc Committee Chairperson*
Cynthia Barrows, MS, OTR/L, CPRP
Cathy Clark, MS, OTR/L
Jyothi Gupta, PhD, OT(C), OTR/L
Jamie Geraci, MS, OTR/L
Lisa Mahaffey, MS, OTR/L
Penelope Moyers Cleveland, EdD, OTR/L, BCMH, FAOTA, *AOTA Board Liaison to the Ad Hoc Committee*

for

The Commission on Practice
Janet DeLany, DEd, OTR/L, FAOTA, *Chairperson*

Adopted by the Representative Assembly 2010CApr15

Section 1. Core Mental Health Professional Knowledge and Skills

The entry-level occupational therapy practitioners in mental health have these knowledge and skills in common with all other core mental health professionals:

X = competent at entry level

A = able to assist at entry level

KX = competent at entry level to analyze and integrate knowledge to make judgments about occupational therapy service provision

KA = competent at entry level to demonstrate knowledge and apply it to occupational therapy practice

		OT	OTA
Evaluation and Intervention			
Knowledge of			
1.	Influence of neurophysiological changes, environmental factors, and contexts on mental health and the development of psychiatric conditions.	KX	KA
2.	Historical and current perspectives on mental health and its promotion, mental illness and its treatments, including the consumer/survivor/ex-patient movement and concepts of recovery.	KX	KA
3.	Current *Diagnostic and Statistical Manual of Mental Disorders* taxonomy (American Psychiatric Association, 2000) with regard to psychiatric diagnosis, etiology, symptoms, impairments, clinical course, and prognosis.	KX	KA
4.	Common comorbidities with mental illnesses (e.g., diabetes, COPD, obesity, substance abuse, ADHD, autism spectrum disorders).	KX	KA
5.	Psychiatric medications and their actions and side effects.	KX	KA
6.	Non-discipline-specific, evidence-based practices and service delivery models (e.g., assertive community treatment, illness management and recovery, supported employment, permanent supportive housing, school mental health, cognitive–behavioral therapy, social and emotional learning (SEL), positive behavioral interventions and supports (PBIS).	KX	KA
Performance Skills			
7.	Assess mental health status (e.g., affect, cognitive competency, insight, comprehension, impulse control, suicide risk) and factor findings in all phases of evaluation and intervention.	X	A
8.	Establish rapport and promote behavioral change in clients by selecting therapeutic counseling and communication strategies (e.g., therapeutic use of self, communication of hope, ethical and interpersonal boundaries, motivational interviewing, active listening, limit setting, group process, conflict resolution).	X	A
9.	Prevent, manage, and/or facilitate the resolution of crisis for individuals and groups by comparing and selecting effective counseling techniques and interventions (e.g., crisis prevention and management, conflict resolution, strategies for dealing with problem behaviors, psychopathological behaviors, psychiatric emergencies).	X	A
10.	Perform comprehensive and targeted functional assessments using evidence-informed approaches and tools.	X	A
11.	Establish medical necessity for rehabilitation services directed toward functional impairments associated with psychiatric conditions by articulating how symptoms and underlying neuropsychiatric conditions interfere with performance of daily life tasks.	X	A

	OT	OTA
12. Design and execute individual and group intervention approaches used in mental health practice, including but not limited to those below: I. Cognitive–behavior therapy II. Psychoeducation III. Psychodynamic approach IV. Behavioral approaches V. Social and emotional learning VI. Recovery models VII. Resiliency models VIII. Psychosocial rehabilitation IX. Skills training X. Biopsychosocial XI. Dialectic behavioral therapy XII. Motivational stages of change.	X	A

Reasoning Skills

	OT	OTA
13. Evaluate human development and behaviors throughout the life course, including how the time and/or the life stage of the emergence of mental illness influence development and the capacity to function as a member of society.	X	A
14. Integrate client-centered and recovery-oriented approaches in collaborating with clients to facilitate goal development and attainment.	X	X
15. Identify and evaluate one's own values, attitudes, and beliefs toward individuals with psychiatric conditions and their potential impact on a person's potential for recovery.	X	X
16. Evaluate the influence of culture, diversity, socioeconomics, and values on a person's experience of mental health challenges, their view of mental health treatment, and their experience of and potential for recovery.	X	A
17. Critique current medical and psychological intervention approaches associated with common psychiatric diagnoses, including the impact of medication side effects on functioning.	X	A
18. Synthesize relevant theories and models that guide intervention and delivery of mental health services, in different settings.	X	A

Professional Role and Service Outcomes

Knowledge of

	OT	OTA
19. Mental health practice roles that an occupational therapist or occupational therapy assistant can assume, such as case manager, group facilitator, community support worker, qualified mental health professional, consultant, program developer, and advocate.	KX	KA
20. Mental health disciplines and professions (e.g., psychology, social work, nursing, psychiatry, mental health technicians, therapeutic recreation, art therapy, music therapy, peer support, rehabilitation counseling, occupational therapy) and the issues involved in both role differentiation and role collaboration.	KX	KA
21. Methodologies for measuring individual, program, and systems outcomes in mental health practice.	KX	KA
22. Methods and principles used to conduct needs assessments and generate practical recommendations.	KX	KA

Performance Skills

	OT	OTA
23. Demonstrate skill in writing medical documentation and behavioral objectives.	X	X
24. Demonstrate basic skills in program development and consultation, supervision, management, administration, quality improvement, outcome measurement, and advocacy related to mental health services.	X	A

(continued)

(cont.)

		OT	OTA
Reasoning Skills			
25.	Synthesize and evaluate perspectives of collaborating disciplines to maximize client outcomes.	X	A
26.	Synthesize and incorporate key factors into consultation and program planning and development, including determining client expectations, understanding the purpose of the organization, understanding of systems, desired and expected outcomes, culture and willingness to change, resources available to client or organization, and regulations and laws governing the organization.	X	A
27.	Critique barriers to implementation of programs and interventions.	X	A
Mental Health Systems			
Knowledge of			
28.	Legislation, policies, procedures, and related legal and ethical issues that influence mental health service delivery (e.g., involuntary treatment, insurance parity, advance directives, confidentiality, school mental health).	KX	KA
29.	Payment systems relevant to mental health practice settings.	KX	KX
30.	Diverse mental health service delivery contexts (e.g., schools, hospitals, community-based centers, shelters, prisons, institutes for mental disease).	KX	KA
31.	Mental health stakeholder groups (e.g., consumers, family members, at-risk populations, employers, mental health care providers, community programs, advocacy groups, legislators, third-party payers).	KX	KA
32.	Agencies and standards that influence mental health and rehabilitation service delivery (e.g., SAMHSA, RSA, CMS, state Medicaid agency, Center for School Mental Health, state mental health authority, state vocational rehabilitation agency, private insurance, standards of practice, state licensure, certification, JCAHO, CARF, confidentiality).	KX	KA
Performance Skills			
33.	Access relevant information to ensure service delivery and documentation complies with current applicable standards (e.g., state mental health acts, HIPAA, confidentiality acts, licensure laws, CARF, JCAHO, President's New Freedom Commission Report, criminal justice acts).	X	A
34.	Engage in activities to transform mental health service delivery systems to be consumer-driven, family-driven, and community-focused.	X	X
Reasoning Skills			
35.	Critique social, economic, policy, and system factors that affect the health, well-being, and participation of persons with serious mental illnesses (e.g., poverty, housing, education, unemployment, estrangement from family, inadequate insurance, lack of integration between/among service systems).	X	A
36.	Evaluate the dynamic interactions between/among an individual, family, community, and social systems and their impact on a person's mental health.	X	A
37.	Integrate the consumer/survivor/ex-patient movement and its implications for mental health services and systems of care.	X	X

Note. CARF = Commission on Accreditation of Rehabilitation Facilities. CMS = Centers for Medicare and Medicaid Services. COPD = chronic obstructive pulmonary disease. HIPAA = Health Insurance Portability and Accountability Act of 1996 (P.L. 104-191). JCAHO = Joint Commission on the Accreditation of Healthcare Organizations. OT = occupational therapist. OTA = occupational therapy assistant. RSA = Rehabilitation Services Administration. SAMHSA = Substance Abuse and Mental Health Services Administration.

Section 2. Specific Occupational Therapy Knowledge and Skills Applied to Mental Health Promotion, Prevention, and Intervention Practice

Led by their firm belief in the inherent drive of all humans to engage in meaningful and purposeful occupations and also the influence of occupational engagement on health and recovery from psychiatric conditions, occupational therapy practitioners use occupation and an understanding of the variables that influence a person's ability to successfully engage in occupations (everyday activities) to engage clients in achieving their occupational participation recovery goals.

X = competent at entry level

A = able to assist at entry level

KX = competent at entry level to analyze and integrate knowledge to make judgments about occupational therapy service provision

KA = competent at entry level to demonstrate knowledge and apply it to occupational therapy practice

	OT	OTA
Foundations		
Knowledge of		
38. Occupational therapy practices for medical, physical/somatic, intellectual, learning, and other nonpsychiatric disabling conditions.	KX	KA
Performance Skills		
39. Evaluate the relationship between/among health, well-being, and participation in daily life activities throughout the life course for individuals at risk for or with mental health challenges.	KX	KA
40. Analyze activities, occupations, contexts, and environmental characteristics to determine those that challenge or support the client's interests, skills, and performance.	KX	KA
Reasoning Skills		
41. Evaluate and select occupational therapy theories, frames of references, and intervention models of practice to design and deliver occupational therapy services in various practice settings in order to promote mental health, prevent mental illness, and intervene with the presence of diagnosed psychiatric conditions.	X	A
42. Assess and determine how to guide the transactional interactions among persons with or at risk for psychiatric conditions, environment, and activity to influence engagement in occupations, participation, and health of clients.	X	A
Evaluation and Intervention		
Knowledge of		
43. Role of occupational therapy in the evaluation and intervention processes persons with or at risk for psychiatric conditions and the promotion of mental health in all individuals with or without disabilities.	KX	KA
44. Impact of mental health on the ability to engage in everyday occupations (e.g., ADLs, IADLs, education, work, play, leisure and social participation, sleep/rest).	KX	KA
45. Impact of psychiatric conditions and medication side effects on performance skills (e.g., sensory–perceptual, motor and praxis, emotional regulation, cognitive, communication and social skills) and performance patterns (e.g., habits, routines, roles, rituals) within relevant contexts and environments.	KX	KA
46. Influence of a client's values, beliefs, spirituality, sense of efficacy, and experience of mental health challenges on the meaningfulness of occupations.	KX	KA
47. Assessment tools and methods to evaluate occupational engagement and the impact of mental and physical impairments on performance skills (e.g., sensory–perceptual, motor and praxis, emotional regulation, cognitive, communication and social skills) and performance patterns (e.g., habits, routines, roles, rituals).	KX	KA

(continued)

(cont.)

		OT	OTA
48.	Environmental supports for and barriers to occupational performance and environmental modification strategies to enable participation at home, school, community, and work.	KX	KA
49.	Cognitive skills training and adaptive strategies.	KX	KA
50.	Sensory processing and modulation skill development and adaptive strategies.	KX	KA
51.	Strategies and environmental accommodations used to compensate for performance skill and pattern challenges commonly associated with psychiatric conditions.	KX	KA
52.	Learning styles and a variety of teaching methods that can be adapted to accommodate challenges commonly associated with psychiatric conditions.	KX	KA

Performance Skills

		OT	OTA
53.	Develop an occupational profile using client-centered strategies to gather information about a client's occupational history and experiences, life roles, interests, needs, and concerns about performance in areas of occupation and identifying strengths and limitations.	X	A
54.	Incorporate knowledge of co-occurring medical and somatic conditions into the evaluation and intervention process to facilitate engagement in meaningful and necessary occupations.	X	A
55.	Evaluate client's performance in ADLs, IADLs, sleep and rest, education, work, play/leisure, and social participation using standardized and nonstandardized procedures.	X	A
56.	Evaluate client's performance skills that support and interfere with participation in meaningful life roles using standardized and nonstandardized procedures. Performance skills include • Motor and praxis skills • Sensory–perceptual skills • Emotional regulation skills • Cognitive skills • Communication and social skills.	X	A
57.	Evaluate a client's performance patterns that support and interfere with participation in meaningful life roles using standardized and nonstandardized procedures. Performance patterns include habits, routines, roles, and rituals.	X	A
58.	Evaluate client factors that may affect performance in areas of occupation using standardized and nonstandardized procedures. Client factors include a client's values, beliefs, and spirituality; body functions (e.g., cardiovascular, pulmonary) and body structures (e.g., bones, organs).	X	A
59.	Observe, measure, and inquire about the physical and social/interpersonal environmental influences on engagement in occupation through formal and informal evaluation procedures.	X	A
60.	Establish medical necessity for rehabilitation services directed toward functional impairments associated with psychiatric conditions by discerning and articulating the relationship between/among functional impairments, occupational engagement, and the performance skills and patterns affected by the mental health challenges.	X	A
61.	Collaborate with clients to determine targeted outcomes specific to that individual's personal vision of recovery.	X	X
62.	In collaboration with clients, develop intervention plans to help clients complete tasks related to life roles such as developing of skills, habits, and routines for work or school; obtaining and preparing meals for self or others; maintaining home or apartment; and participating in healthy social and leisure occupations as determined from the evaluation.	X	A
63.	Apply a variety of approaches used in mental health practice, such as but not limited to, those listed in Item 12 above, in individual and group interventions to enable occupational performance and participation.	X	A
64.	Enable clients to explore a variety of interests and begin to develop competencies to support increased participation in meaningful occupations.	X	X
65.	Develop intervention sessions using activities to teach and practice new skills and when possible develop actual opportunity to engage in needed tasks such as work or school tasks.	X	X

	OT	OTA
66. Design and implement individual and group interventions that support development of cognitive, sensory regulation, social, and communication skills requisite for role performance.	X	A
67. Teach clients to understand the role of their sensory system in regulating their level of alertness and how to use different sensory tools to increase or decrease their level of alertness so they can focus on and participate successfully in their chosen activities.	X	A
68. Teach clients to understand their cognitive strengths and challenges and to make use of strategies and treatments that optimize occupational performance.	X	A
69. Develop modifications to tasks and environments to compensate for cognitive, sensory, interpersonal, and communication challenges, and increase successful/effective participation in life roles.	X	A
70. Select and communicate to clients, relevant support systems, and other professionals best evidence that supports intervention choices.	X	A
71. Select appropriate teaching methods (e.g., handouts; schedules; organizational charts; visual, auditory, and tactile cueing systems; grading of activity; chunking) to address client needs with respect to culture, learning style, and current abilities.	X	A
Reasoning Skills		
72. Synthesize information from different theoretical perspectives, models of practice, frames of reference, and evidenced-based practices from occupational therapy, physical and psychiatric rehabilitation, psychology, sociology, psychiatry, school mental health, and neuropsychiatry to select relevant assessment tools and guide the evaluation and intervention processes.	X	A
73. Determine need to refer clients for additional evaluation or services to specialists internal and external to the profession.	X	X
74. Analyze the environmental and contextual factors that support or hinder a person's ability to participate in meaningful and productive roles and occupations.	X	A
75. Determine the effects of medical treatment side effects (e.g., psychiatric medications, ECT) on participation in occupation: ADLs, IADLs, rest and sleep, education, work, play and leisure, and social participation.	X	A
76. Identify and analyze historical barriers to occupational participation that result in inability to develop an occupational identity or in loss of occupational identity.	X	A
77. Synthesize information gathered from the evaluation of a person's strengths, skills, abilities, preferences, goals, challenges, needs, and environments, as well as information from activity analysis to create effective interventions to enable occupational performance at home, school, and workplace.	X	A
78. Anticipate barriers to participation due to aging, physical disabilities, medical conditions and illnesses, and problem solve to maximize participation.	X	A
79. Synthesize intervention and support needs with appropriate resources to maximize participation in desired occupations.	X	A
80. Formulate most effective intervention to enable occupational participation (e.g., skills training, adaptation of task, modification of environment).	X	A
81. Determine how environmental supports and barriers influence participation in meaningful and productive roles in one's community and facilitate reducing barriers.	X	A
82. Explain the clinical reasoning process behind the occupational therapy procedures or care processes in a way that is understandable and usable for the client, other professionals, and funding sources.	X	A

(continued)

(cont.)

	OT	OTA
83. Select appropriate means to explain the importance of participation and its relationship to recovery for people with or at risk for psychiatric conditions in a way that is understandable and relevant to clients, team members, and third-party payers.	X	X

Professional Role and Service Outcomes

Knowledge of

	OT	OTA
84. AOTA Code of Ethics, applicable licensure laws, AOTA Scope of Practice, and AOTA Standards of Practice as they pertain to mental health practice.	KX	KX

85. Different practice roles that occupational therapy practitioners may assume in mental health practice.
  i. Direct intervention aimed at changing the functional participation of a client using a variety of approaches such as promoting health, restoring or maintaining function, modifying the environment or activity, or preventing disability
  ii. Education of caregivers and staff aimed at imparting knowledge and information that results in improved health and improved ability to perform and participate in desired occupations
  iii. Consultation aimed at improving occupational participation goals for the client.
	KX	KA

86. Practice scopes of occupational therapy and other mental health disciplines and professions (e.g., psychology, social work, nursing, psychiatry, mental health technicians, therapeutic recreation, art therapy, music therapy, peer support, rehabilitation counseling).	KX	KA
87. Funding sources for occupational therapy services in different mental health service delivery systems.	KX	KX
88. Strategies to evaluate occupation-based outcomes in mental health service delivery systems and client satisfaction with occupational therapy services.	KX	KA

Performance Skills

	OT	OTA
89. Build respectful relationships and select effective strategies to work with persons with a variety of skills, abilities, and experiences (e.g., paraprofessionals, professionals, consumers, family members) to make successful changes in the organization.	X	X
90. Clarify how occupational therapy interventions support and compliment interventions of other providers.	X	X
91. Conduct needs assessment to determine when OT services may benefit a partial or full mental health system that does not currently utilize occupational therapy.	X	A
92. Partner with consumers, family members, and other mental health professionals/disciplines in the development, implementation, and evaluation of mental health and occupational therapy services.	X	A
93. Select and use standardized procedures and tools to organize, collect, compile, analyze, synthesize, and interpret quantitative and qualitative occupational performance practice outcomes and client satisfaction data, summarizing findings into comprehensive, objective reports.	X	A
94. Design ongoing processes for quality improvement based on functional outcomes.	X	A
95. Design and implement needs assessments that determine best occupation-based practices for individuals with or at risk for psychiatric conditions, factoring in setting, population characteristics, and funding.	X	A
96. Frame consultation within the regulations and structure of the organization.	X	A
97. Operationalize administrative and occupational therapy process changes that target improved outcomes for occupational therapy intervention and client satisfaction in mental health practice settings.	X	A

	OT	OTA
Reasoning Skills		
98. Appraise the priority outcomes for an individual or groups of individuals receiving occupational therapy services in a mental health context.	X	A
99. Infer the role of recovery in promoting occupational engagement for people with psychiatric conditions.	X	X
100. Critique, discern, and interpret the applicability of qualitative and/or quantitative outcome and satisfaction measurements and methods when evaluating services directed toward persons with or at risk for psychiatric conditions.	X	A
101. Choose interventions that fit the values and abilities of those providing and receiving care.	X	A
102. Discern and critique factors that affect change for clients with or at risk for psychiatric conditions.	X	A
103. Discern and critique factors that facilitate/hinder provision of occupational therapy services in settings that serve people with or at risk for psychiatric conditions.	X	A
104. Justify administrative changes in the provision of occupational therapy services that will promote positive outcomes for clients in settings that serve people with or at risk for psychiatric conditions.	X	A
105. Compare and contrast occupational therapy outcome measures with outcome measures related to the recovery model in mental health practice.	X	A
106. Integrate health insurance language and mental health recovery language with *Occupational Therapy Practice Framework* (AOTA, 2008).	X	A
Mental Health Systems		
Knowledge of		
107. Different environments and contexts in which occupational therapy practitioners have a role in mental health promotion, prevention, and intervention (e.g., psychiatric settings, schools, residential facilities, jails).	KX	KA
108. Systems (e.g., organizations, entitlements, community programs) to be accessed that enable occupational participation and performance.	KX	KA
Performance Skills		
109. Use relationships with advocacy organizations and persons with the lived experience of mental illness to understand challenges with occupational engagement and performance, such as what these persons have identified as most and least helpful in regaining, maintaining, and improving their ability to engage fully and meaningfully in desired occupations (e.g., roles, activities).	X	X
110. Facilitate clients' access to support systems (e.g., family, associations, friends, organizations) to enhance recovery.	X	X
111. Recommend reasonable changes/accommodations that can be made to policies, procedures, and practices to improve occupational engagement, participation, and performance of populations served.	X	A
112. Locate and access information about a system's goals, priorities, or needs.	X	X
113. Choose methods to explain the role of occupational therapy to various mental health stakeholder groups that relate to stakeholders' system, goals, priorities, or needs (see Item 31 for example stakeholder groups).	X	A
114. Discern actual and potential consumer and family member leadership roles within mental health service systems (e.g., programs, agencies, organizations, private and public payer systems).	X	A

(continued)

(cont.)

		OT	OTA
115.	Use evidence to help organizations understand how the regulations with which they must comply influence occupational participation of persons with or at risk for psychiatric conditions.	X	A
116.	Obtain and synthesize information about third-party payer coverage for occupational therapy services directed toward the remediation and restoration of functional impairments caused by mental illnesses (example payers include private insurance, Medicaid, Medicare, vocational rehabilitation, state board of education).	X	A
Reasoning Skills			
117.	Differentiate and critique mental health services and service delivery systems that are consumer-driven and community-focused from those that are more staff-driven and mental health setting–focused.	X	X
118.	Differentiate and critique "recovery," "resiliency," and "strengths-based" planning, interventions, and programs from those that are problem-based or deficit-based.	X	X
119.	Discern and create means by which occupational therapy practitioners partner with consumers and family members to develop consumer-driven and family-driven care for individuals and programs.	X	A
120.	Evaluate the interactions between/among individuals, family, community, and other social systems (e.g., schools, faith-based organizations, police, long-term-care facilities, group homes, one-stop centers, vocational rehabilitation systems) and their impact on occupational participation and mental health.	X	A
121.	Discern how changes in policies, procedures, and practices in various systems may enhance or deter occupational performance and participation for persons with or at risk for mental health challenges/conditions (example systems include family, community agency or program, mental health care, medical care, education/schools, employment/employer, social security, disability).	X	A

Note. ADLs = activities of daily living. AOTA = American Occupational Therapy Association. ECT = electroconvulsive therapy. IADLs = instrumental activities of daily living. OT = occupational therapist. OTA = occupational therapy assistant.

Specialized Knowledge and Skills in Technology and Environmental Interventions for Occupational Therapy Practice

Purpose

The purpose of this document is to describe the knowledge and skills that are necessary for occupational therapists and occupational therapy assistants[1] to provide ethical, competent occupational therapy services related to technology and environmental interventions. Intended for internal and external audiences, it provides information about occupational therapy practitioners' roles and collaborative partnerships with other professionals in technology and environmental interventions, outlines professional development and supervision guidelines, defines terms related to technology and environmental interventions, and describes entry- and advanced-level knowledge and skills. In this document, the phrase *technology and environmental interventions* represents the broad range and combination of technology, environmental interventions, and reasonable accommodation strategies. The emphasis is on technology and environmental interventions that support the ability of people with or without disabilities to fully participate in their daily lives in accessible environments and livable communities and through engagement in occupations.

Introduction

Occupational therapy practitioners have long-standing expertise in providing occupational therapy services to clients that incorporate technology and environmental modification, often in collaboration with other professionals. Clients include individuals, organizations, and populations (American Occupational Therapy Association [AOTA], 2008). When addressing technology and environmental interventions, occupational therapy practitioners consider the context in which people engage in daily life occupations that support their participation, health, and wellness. On the basis of their understanding of their clients' occupational engagement desires and needs, capacities, and contexts, occupational therapy practitioners collaborate with the client and with other professionals in the evaluation, design, fabrication, customization, modification, and application of new or existing technologies and environmental interventions. They also conduct outcome studies, support advocacy initiatives, offer guidance regarding funding resources and referrals, and provide training and consultation (Hammel & Angelo, 1996). Occupational therapy practitioners deliver technology and environmental-related services in a variety of settings, such as hospitals, rehabilitation centers, skilled nursing facilities, outpatient facilities, home health agencies, schools, work sites, industry, homes, and communities and in a variety of roles such as the primary service provider, team member, advocate, and expert consultant.

---

[1]*Occupational therapists* are responsible for all aspects of occupational therapy service delivery and are accountable for the safety and effectiveness of the occupational therapy service delivery process. *Occupational therapy assistants* deliver occupational therapy services under the supervision of and in partnership with an occupational therapist (AOTA, 2004a). When the term *occupational therapy practitioner* is used in this document, it refers to both occupational therapists and occupational therapy assistants (AOTA, 2006).

Occupational Therapy's Role in Technology and Environmental Modification

Technology and environmental interventions can support people's participation in occupations which, by definition, hold purpose and meaning for them. This is especially beneficial when the activities are otherwise too difficult or challenging. Occupational therapy practitioners collaborate with the client and other professionals to create a successful match among the client, the technology, and environmental interventions and the context for their use. As part of therapeutic services, occupational therapists are trained to conduct comprehensive evaluations to identify the skills and abilities of the client and to guide the recommendation for services. The evaluation includes the development of an occupational profile and selecting, administering, and interpreting assessments to analyze the occupational performance of individuals, organizations, and populations. This includes consideration of the client's performance skills, capacities, and performance patterns, the characteristics of the technology and the environmental interventions, the activity demands, and the contexts for the technology and environmental interventions. Occupational therapy assistants contribute to the evaluation process by gathering data and administering selected assessment tools or measures for which they have demonstrated competence (AOTA, 2004a).

During intervention, both occupational therapists and occupational therapy assistants select, administer, and adapt technologies and environments that support the intervention plan developed by the occupational therapist. The goal is to promote, improve, or maintain the ability of people to engage in basic and instrumental activities of daily living: work, education, leisure, play, social participation, and sleep occupations that are meaningful and necessary (AOTA, 2008). Examples include the selection and adaptation of computers and software to support education and work; the positioning and modification of speech and communication devices to facilitate social participation; the design and customization of seating devices, mobility equipment, and physical environments to promote play and leisure participation; the selection and training in the use of environmental controls and of vision and hearing technologies to support involvement in instrumental activities of daily living; and the fabrication and modification of assistive devices for self-care tasks. Interventions also may focus on advocacy initiatives, educational and training programs for organizations and populations, and policy development that promote accessible environments and livable communities.

When measuring the outcomes of interventions, occupational therapy practitioners focus on how the technology and environmental interventions support the client's health, participation (World Health Organization, 2001), and engagement in occupation (AOTA, 2008). The selected outcomes need to be measurable, reliable, and valid; sensitive to measuring change; reflective of clients' goals; and consistent with payer needs. Outcomes include subjective impressions such as improved competence, well-being, self-efficacy, hope, and quality of life (AOTA, 2008). Outcomes also include objective measurements such as improved efficiency, accessibility, task completion, independence or interdependence, and the ability of the client to assume or regain valued life roles and occupations.

Occupational therapy practitioners must adhere to state and agency regulatory laws when providing services across practice setting and the continua of care. Reimbursement for services may be available through various sources, including legislation (e.g., Individuals with Disabilities Education Improvement Act, Medicare), private insurance, Medicaid, and private pay.

Professional Development

For both occupational therapists and occupational therapy assistants, the progression from entry-level to advanced-level knowledge and skills related to technology and environmental interventions evolves through education and experience. At a level commensurate with their respective academic programs, occupational therapy and occupational therapy assistant students receive education in the structure and function of the human body, including the biological and physical sciences; human development throughout the life span and human behavior, including the behavioral and social sciences; and effects of mental and physical health, disease processes, genetic conditions, trauma, and context on occupational perform-ance. They acquire foundational knowledge and skills regarding technology and environmental interven-tions, and they develop clinical-reasoning skills to consider the interplay of physical, cognitive, environmental, and sociocultural factors in providing effective services (AOTA, 2007a, 2007b, 2007c). Over time, as they advance in their education and arena of practice, occupational therapy practitioners may develop additional expertise in technology and environmental interventions. They ensure advanced knowledge and skills in technology and environmental interventions by maintaining and documenting competence in practice, education, and research and by participating in professional development, educa-tional activities, and critical examination of available evidence (AOTA, 2004c). Examples include participat-ing in local and national continuing education conferences such as those sponsored by AOTA, the Assistive Technology Industry Association (ATIA), Closing the Gap (CTG), the California State University National Conference (CSUN), and the Rehabilitation Engineering and Assistive Technology Society of North Amer-ica (RESNA); completing postsecondary courses; and seeking advanced competency and specialty certifi-cation through AOTA or external organizations such as RESNA. In addition, they gain higher level knowledge, skills, and clinical reasoning through experience and mentoring opportunities.

The occupational therapy practitioner's acquisition of advanced-level knowledge and skills related to tech-nology and environmental interventions is individualized; thus, a practitioner may possess differing lev-els of expertise in a wide variety of skill areas and populations served by occupational therapy. For example, an occupational therapy practitioner may have advanced-level skills in computer and informa-tion technologies for students in school systems but only entry-level knowledge in vehicle modification and transportation for older adult populations. It is the ethical responsibility of occupational therapy practition-ers to ensure that they are competent in the services they provide and routinely seek out new knowledge and techniques that apply to their practice (AOTA, 2004c).

Supervision Considerations

The amount of supervision provided to occupational therapy practitioners in the area of technology and environmental interventions directly relates to their training and experience and state practice acts. Occu-pational therapy assistants and entry-level occupational therapists should seek supervision and mentoring from a more experienced occupational therapist or an occupational therapist with advanced knowledge and skills in technology and environmental interventions. The occupational therapist and occupational therapy assistant also may supervise other non-licensed personnel when providing technology and envi-ronmental modification to clients (AOTA, 2004a). Most state practice acts mandate the frequency and dura-tion for supervision of entry-level occupational therapists, occupational therapy assistants, and non-licensed personnel. The occupational therapist has the primary role in evaluation and intervention planning; the occupational therapy assistant collaborates with the occupational therapist in the provision of specific interventions (AOTA, 2004a, 2004b, 2004c).

Terminology and Definitions

- *Assistive technology device (ATD):* "Any item, piece of equipment, or product system, whether acquired commercially, modified, or customized, that is used to increase, maintain, or improve functional capabil-ities of individuals with disabilities." *Assistive technology service* means "any service that directly assists an individual with a disability in the selection, acquisition, or use of an assistive technology device" (Assistive Technology Act of 2004, P.L. 108-364), including evaluation, fitting and customization, coor-dination of services, and training.

- *Basic technology:* Commonly used technologies or environmental interventions such as activities of daily living equipment and basic home modifications (Hammel & Angelo, 1996).

- *Complex technology:* "Technology and environmental interventions that require advanced or specialized knowledge, training, and experience to evaluate, provide interventions, and measure outcomes such as custom seating and mobility and integrated systems (e.g., mobility + environmental control + computer access) (Hammel & Angelo, 1996).

- *Electronic and information technology:* Information technology, equipment, and interconnected systems or subsystems of equipment that are used in the creation, conversion, or duplication of data or information. It includes, but is not limited to, telecommunications products (e.g., telephones), information kiosks and transaction machines, Internet sites, multimedia, and office equipment such as copiers and fax machines (U.S. Access Board, 2000).

- *Rehabilitative and educational technologies:* Technology that is "used as a tool for remediation or rehabilitation," such as visual perception or cognitive training, improvement in motor control, or identification of letters and numbers. Depending on the client contexts, rehabilitation and educational technologies have the role of remediation, restoration, or acquisition of foundational skills (Cook & Polgar, 2008, p. 6).

- *Technology:* The combination of assistive, basic, complex, electronic and information, and rehabilitative and educational technologies.

- *Technology and environmental competency (TEC):* The combination of technology (e.g., assistive, electronic and information, rehabilitative), environmental interventions, and reasonable accommodation strategies used to increase, maintain, or improve functional capabilities of individuals with disabilities and/or create accessible environments (e.g., home, work, school, community, virtual).

- *Universal design:* The design of products and environments to be usable by all people, to the greatest extent possible, without the need for adaptation or specialized design (Center for Universal Design, 1997).

Entry- and Advanced-Level Knowledge and Skills

The appendix provides a matrix that outlines the entry- or advanced-level knowledge and skills that occupational therapists and occupational therapy assistants should demonstrate when providing occupational therapy services related to technology and environmental interventions. An *X* denotes the minimum knowledge and skills that the occupational therapist or occupational therapy assistant should demonstrate to practice competently at that level; an *A* denotes that the occupational therapist or the occupational therapy assistant may assist or contribute information but is not able to perform the task alone and requires supervision. Occupational therapy practitioners have a professional responsibility to work within their own level of competency, as well as within the scope of practice as defined and regulated by state licensure and *Occupational Therapy Code of Ethics,* including the duty to maintain high standards of competency within a practice area and to seek out supervision and continuing education in those areas of practice that are above their level of competency (AOTA, 2004b, 2005).

References

American Occupational Therapy Association. (2004a). Guidelines for supervision, roles, and responsibilities during the delivery of occupational therapy services. *American Journal of Occupational Therapy, 58,* 663–667.

American Occupational Therapy Association. (2004b). Scope of practice. *American Journal of Occupational Therapy, 58,* 673–677.

American Occupational Therapy Association. (2004c). Standards of practice for occupational therapy. *American Journal of Occupational Therapy, 52,* 866–869.

American Occupational Therapy Association. (2005). Occupational therapy code of ethics (2005). *American Journal of Occupational Therapy, 59,* 639–642.

American Occupational Therapy Association. (2006). Policy 1.44: Categories of occupational therapy personnel. In *Policy manual* (2007 ed., pp. 33–34). Bethesda, MD: Author.

American Occupational Therapy Association. (2007a). Accreditation standards for a doctoral-degree-level educational program for the occupational therapist. *American Journal of Occupational Therapy, 61,* 641–651.

American Occupational Therapy Association. (2007b). Accreditation standards for a master's-degree-level educational program for the occupational therapist. *American Journal of Occupational Therapy, 61,* 652–661.

American Occupational Therapy Association. (2007c). Accreditation standards for an educational program for the occupational therapy assistant. *American Journal of Occupational Therapy, 61,* 652–661.

American Occupational Therapy Association. (2008). Occupational therapy practice framework: Domain and process (2nd ed.). *American Journal of Occupational Therapy, 62,* 625–683.

Assistive Technology Act of 2004, P.L. 108-364, 108 Cong., 118 SAT. 1707(2004).

Center for Universal Design. (1997). *Principles of universal design.* Raleigh, NC: Author.

Cook, A. M., & Polgar, S. M. (2008). *Cook and Hussey's assistive technologies principles and practice.* St. Louis, MO: Mosby/Elsevier.

Hammel, J., & Angelo, J. (1996). Technology competencies for occupational therapy practitioners. *Assistive Technology, 8*(1), 34–42.

U. S. Access Board. (2000, December 21). Electronic and Information Technology Accessibility Standards (Section 508). *Federal Register.* Retrieved September 5, 2008, from http://www/access-board.gov/508

World Health Organization. (2001). *International classification of functioning, disability and health (ICF).* Geneva, Switzerland: Author.

Authors

This document is based on the work of Hammel and Angelo (1996) and on a motion from the April 2006 Representative Assembly. The knowledge and skills were revised by the Technology Special Interest Section Standing Committee with consultation from a panel of international experts from external organizations with occupational therapy and technology expertise and developed into a Knowledge and Skills Paper.

This 2008 paper was revised by
    Joy Hammel, PhD, OTR/L, FAOTA, *Chairperson*
    Daniel Knowland, OTR/L
    Roger Smith, PhD, OT, FAOTA
    Lynn Gitlow, PhD, OTR/L, ATP
    Robin Jones, COTA, ROH
    Susan Leech, EdD, OTR, ATP
    Beth Goodrich, MEd, MS, OTR, ATP
    Brent Braveman, PhD, OTR/L, FAOTA

    With contributions from

Janet V. DeLany, DEd, OTR/L, FAOTA
Kim Hartmann, PhD, OTR/L, FAOTA

for

The Commission on Practice
Susanne Smith Roley, MS, OTR/L, FAOTA, *Chairperson*

Adopted by the Representative Assembly 2008CO107

Note: This document replaces the 2004 Statement *Assistive Technology Within Occupational Therapy Practice.*

Appendix.

Specialized Knowledge and Skills in Technology and Environmental Interventions

X = able to perform the task. A = assists with the task. ■ = does not perform the task.

		Entry-Level		Advanced	
	Knowledge and Skills	**OTA**	**OT**	**OTA**	**OT**
	All knowledge and skills assume active collaboration with the client, consumer, or user of the technology and environmental solutions, significant others relevant to the situation (e.g., family, caregivers), service delivery team members, and other relevant stakeholders (e.g., case managers, funders, advocates) throughout the process.				
A.	**Evaluation**				
A.1	*Upon referral for services, screen for occupational performance capacities and limitations, screen for environmental supports and barriers, and identify if the need for a comprehensive OT evaluation exists.*	A	X	A	X
A.2	*Determine technology and environmental needs as part of a comprehensive OT evaluation that includes occupational profile and an analysis of occupational performance.*				
A.2.a	Evaluate the client's occupational and participation needs in areas of occupation (e.g., basic and instrumental activities of daily living, education, work, play, leisure, social participation, sleep) and the potential need for technology and environment applications to support these needs.	A	X	A	X
A.2.b	Evaluate the client's contexts, including cultural, virtual, temporal (e.g., chronological, developmental, life cycle, disability status), and environments (physical, social) for their influence on technology and environmental access, application, and use.	A	X	A	X
A.2.c	Assess prior and current use of technology and environmental interventions across existing roles, occupations, activities, and contexts.	A	X	A	X
A.2.d	Evaluate and analyze the activity demands, the client's performance skills and performance patterns, and client factors across contexts of potential technology and environmental use, including transitions between contexts.	A	X	A	X
A.2.e	Screen and identify the level of technology and environmental intervention needed, ranging from none to basic to advanced/complex.	A	X	A	X
A.2.f	Communicate range of relevant and related interventions that could be considered (e.g., technology, environmental modification, training, pharmacology, surgery, therapy).	A	X	A	X

(continued)

Appendix.

Specialized Knowledge and Skills in Technology and Environmental Interventions *(cont.)*

X = able to perform the task. A = assists with the task.　■ = does not perform the task.

		Entry-Level		Advanced	
	Knowledge and Skills	**OTA**	**OT**	**OTA**	**OT**
A.2.g	Refer clients to appropriate professionals for technology and environmental resources when the services the client needs or seeks are beyond the scope of practice and competency level of the OT practitioner.	X	X	X	X
A.3	*Conduct a BASIC technology and environmental evaluation.*				
A.3.a	Evaluate basic technology and environmental needs within areas of occupation (e.g., basic and instrumental activities of daily living, work, education, play, leisure, social participation, sleep).	A	X	A	X
A.3.b	Compare and contrast different basic technology and environmental features and access methods in relation to the client, activity and environmental needs, supports, demands, and constraints.	A	X	X	X
A.3.c	Integrate basic theoretical information from OT, occupational science, and other disciplines into the plan (e.g., physical therapy, speech and language pathology, audiology, disability studies, engineering, rehabilitation engineering, education, ergonomics, psychology, public health, sociology, anthropology, architecture, urban planning).	A	X	A	X
A.3.d	Interpret and integrate basic technology and environmental evaluation results into intervention or service delivery plan and also outcome measures, reevaluating as needed.	A	X	A	X
A.3.e	Develop occupational goals, anticipated outcomes, and intervention plans, incorporating basic technology and environmental applications as appropriate.	A	X	A	X
A.3.f.	Coordinate evaluation of OT-related needs within interdisciplinary basic technology and environmental services.	A	X	A	X
A.4	*Conduct specialized or complex technology and environmental evaluations (assumes A.1–A.3 met).*				
A.4.a	Conduct advanced evaluation of complex or specialized technology and environmental applications (e.g., those related to computer access, seating and positioning needs, mobility and driving programs, sensory needs, environmental control, communication alternatives).	A	A	A	X
A.4.b	Utilize information resources on specialized or complex technology and environmental applications within decision making.	A	A	X	X

Appendix.
Specialized Knowledge and Skills in Technology and Environmental Interventions *(cont.)*

X = able to perform the task. A = assists with the task.　■ = does not perform the task.

		Entry-Level		Advanced	
	Knowledge and Skills	**OTA**	**OT**	**OTA**	**OT**
A.4.c	Compare and contrast different complex, specialized, or integrated technology and environmental features and access methods in relation to the client, contexts, activity, and environmental needs, supports, demands, and constraints.	A	A	X	X
A.4.d	Integrate advanced technology and environmental theoretical information from OT, occupational science, and other disciplines into the intervention or service delivery plan and also outcome measures.	A	A	A	X
A.4.e	Evaluate relationship of materials and different design choices, including advantages, trade-offs, and constraints within complex technology and environmental plans.	A	A	X	X
A.4.f	Interpret and integrate results of complex technology and environmental evaluation into intervention or service delivery plans and also outcome measures, reevaluating as needed.	A	A	A	X
A.4.g	Develop advanced technology and environmental goals, anticipated outcomes, and intervention plans, with incorporation in OT intervention plan and outcome measures, as relevant.	A	A	A	X
B.	**Intervention**				
B.1	*Provide technology and environmental interventions as part of a comprehensive OT plan.*				
B.1.a	Provide basic interventions that optimize the client's performance skills, performance patterns, and body functions. Examples include daily living skills training, cognitive rehabilitation, strengthening, ergonomic practice, visual/perceptual rehabilitation, and energy conservation.	X	X	X	X
B.1.b	Provide basic interventions that optimize the client's engagement in areas of occupation within the home, work, school, and community contexts. Examples include environmental interventions, ergonomic design, ADA training, and disability awareness training to promote participation and accessibility.	X	X	X	X
B.1.c	Design, alter, and/or adapt tasks to meet the occupational and activity demands of the context. Examples include rewriting job descriptions, rearranging class schedules, sharing job duties, and comparing level of assistance to do task (attendant vs. technology).	X	X	X	X

(continued)

Appendix.

Specialized Knowledge and Skills in Technology and Environmental Interventions *(cont.)*

X = able to perform the task. A = assists with the task.　■ = does not perform the task.

		Entry-Level		Advanced	
	Knowledge and Skills	**OTA**	**OT**	**OTA**	**OT**
B.2	*Provide access to, delivery of, and training in basic technology and environmental applications.*				
B.2.a	Utilize design and fabrication principles within basic technology and environment applications, including consideration of mechanics/strength of materials, mechanical components, systems, and electrical circuits and components.	A	X	X	X
B.2.b	Incorporate universal design principles within technology and environmental applications (e.g., simplicity, ease of use, equitable access).	A	X	X	X
B.2.c	Address issues of repair and maintenance in basic technology and environmental applications, including basic repair, preventative maintenance training and schedules, and limitations and violations of warranty for mechanical, electrical, and electronic equipment.	X	X	X	X
B.2.d	Address factors related to cost and benefit/impact of custom versus commercial technology and environment applications.	A	X	A	X
B.2.e	Perform product trials, recommend product specifications, order technologies and environmental solutions, and install and train individuals in use, maintenance, and repair.	A	X	X	X
B.2.f	Utilize fabrication tools, materials, and machines as needed to match basic technology and environmental applications to user's needs.	X	X	X	X
B.2.g	Participate in the design, fabrication, and customization of basic technology and environmental applications within a defensible level of competence as appropriate to the case and the level of expertise required, with referral to advanced expertise as indicated.	X	X	X	X
B.2.h	Periodically reevaluate basic technology and environmental use, needs, and integration into everyday life.	A	X	A	X
B.3	*Provide access to, delivery of, and training in complex or specialized technology and environmental applications (assumes B.1–B.2 met).*				
B.3.a	Utilize advanced design and fabrication principles (e.g., design to address issues of corrosion, temperature, pressure over time, compatibility or integration of multiple technologies).	A	A	A	X
B.3.b	Utilize advanced environmental and universal design principles to match client needs and specific environmental demands (e.g., school, work, community, home).	A	A	A	X

Appendix.
Specialized Knowledge and Skills in Technology and Environmental Interventions *(cont.)*

X = able to perform the task. A = assists with the task.   ■ = does not perform the task.

		Entry-Level		Advanced	
	Knowledge and Skills	**OTA**	**OT**	**OTA**	**OT**
B.3.c	Address issues of compatibility and integration of technologies (e.g., hardware and software interface) across different environments and systems/equipment.	A	A	X	X
B.3.e	Utilize fabrication tools, materials, and machines as needed to match user's needs.	A	X	X	X
B.3.f	Perform product trials and feature analyses; coordinate delivery and installation of technology and environmental interventions; and train technology and environmental user and important others in the use, repair, and maintenance of complex, specialized, and integrated technology and environmental applications (e.g., wheelchair, environmental control, augmentative communication for education and work).	A	X	A	X
B.3.g	Collaborate in the design, fabrication, and customization of complex or specialized technology and environmental applications within a defensible level of competence as appropriate to the case and the level of expertise required, with referral to specialized expertise as needed.	A	A	A	X
B.3.h	Periodically reevaluate complex technology and environmental use, needs, and integration into everyday life.	A	X	A	X
C.	**Evidence-Based Practice and Outcomes**				
C.1	*Participate in and apply results from evidence-based practice within OT and basic technology and environmental service delivery.*				
C.1.a	Identify and document the outcomes of OT and basic technology and environmental interventions, including those related to occupational performance, participation in daily life, emotional and physical health and wellness, prevention, quality of life, and consumer use and satisfaction.	X	X	X	X
C.1.b	Participate in OT and basic technology and environmental program evaluations and continuous quality improvement initiatives to improve the effectiveness and efficiency of service delivery.	X	X	X	X
C.1.c	Participate in OT, occupational science, and basic technology and environmental research.	X	X	X	X
C.1.d	Critically analyze and apply evidence-based research within OT and basic technology and environmental practice.	A	X	A	X

(continued)

Appendix.
Specialized Knowledge and Skills in Technology and Environmental Interventions *(cont.)*

X = able to perform the task. A = assists with the task.　■ = does not perform the task.

		Entry-Level		Advanced	
	Knowledge and Skills	**OTA**	**OT**	**OTA**	**OT**
C.2	*Participate in evidence-based practice within OT and complex or specialized technology and environmental delivery (assumes D.1 knowledge and skills met).*				
C.2.a	Identify and document the outcomes of OT and advanced technology and environmental interventions, including those related to occupational performance, participation in daily life, emotional and physical health and wellness, prevention, quality of life, and consumer use and satisfaction.	A	A	A	X
C.2.b	Participate in OT and advanced technology and environmental quality improvement and program evaluation activities.	A	A	A	X
C.2.c	Participate in OT, occupational science, and advanced technology and environmental research.	A	A	X	X
C.2.d	Critically analyze and apply evidence-based research within OT, occupational science, and advanced technology and environmental practice.	A	A	A	X
D.	**Resource Coordination and Advocacy**				
D.1	*Provide and coordinate OT and basic technology and environmental resources, services, and supports.*				
D.1.a	Understand and apply technology and environmental-related legislation and policies across the delivery process (e.g., ADA, IDEA, Technology Act).	X	X	X	X
D.1.b	Utilize and link clients and consumers to basic technology and environmental information resources (e.g., product databases, vendors, legislation and policies, funding/reimbursement sources, additional services, user groups, conferences, continuing education, advocacy organizations, legal).	X	X	X	X
D.1.c	Effectively communicate the role of OT practitioners in providing a global, occupation-based perspective encompassing technology and environmental use and delivery.	X	X	X	X
D.1.d	Describe the contributions of other disciplines and their roles within technology and environmental service delivery (e.g., rehabilitation engineering, physical therapy, speech and language pathology, audiology, engineering, education, vocational rehabilitation, case management).	X	X	X	X
D.1.e	Describe the role of distributors, vendors, suppliers, manufacturers, designers, and fabricators within technology	X	X	X	X

Appendix.
Specialized Knowledge and Skills in Technology and Environmental Interventions *(cont.)*

X = able to perform the task. A = assists with the task.   ■ = does not perform the task.

		Entry-Level		Advanced	
	Knowledge and Skills	**OTA**	**OT**	**OTA**	**OT**
	and environmental delivery.				
D.1.f	Describe mechanisms, regulations, and policies regarding delivery and funding/ reimbursement of basic OT and technology and environmental applications.	X	X	X	X
D.1.g	Strategize different sources of funding (e.g., government funding, foundation grants, loan programs, private resources) within different settings (e.g., inpatient, community, schools, worksite) to improve access, including shared or matched funding strategies.	X	X	X	X
D.1.h	Justify and document the provision of OT and basic technology and environmental services and solutions for reimbursement.	X	X	X	X
D.1.i	Participate in advocacy activities related to technology and environment on an individual case level, and collaborate with consumer to become an informed self advocate for his or her own needs.	X	X	X	X
D.1.j	Participate in advocacy activities related to technology and environmental on a systems change level, and collaborate with the disability community in technology and environmental activism.	X	X	X	X
D.1.k	Maintain the *Occupational Therapy Code of Ethics* and *Standards of Practice* in primary discipline or field (e.g., therapy, engineering, education) and within technology and environmental service delivery.	X	X	X	X
D.2	*Provide and coordinate complex or specialized technology and environmental resources (assumes D.1 met).*				
D.2.a	Utilize and link clients and consumers to complex or specialized technology and environmental information resources (e.g., product databases, vendors, legislation and policies, funding/reimbursement sources, additional services, user groups, conferences, continuing education, advocacy organizations, legal assistance).	X	X	X	X
D.2.b	Describe mechanisms for obtaining reimbursement of OT and complex or specialized technology and environmental services.	A	A	A	X
D.2.c	Justify and document the provision of OT and complex or specialized technology and environmental services.	A	A	A	X
D.2.d	Maintain the *Occupational Therapy Code of Ethics* and *Standards of Practice* in specialized fields of technology and environmental service delivery (e.g., seating and mobility, computer access).	X	X	X	X

Position Papers

Complementary and Alternative Medicine

The American Occupational Therapy Association (AOTA) asserts that complementary and alternative medicine (CAM) may be used responsibly by occupational therapists and occupational therapy assistants as part of a comprehensive approach to enhance engagement in occupation by people, organizations, and populations to promote their health and participation in life (AOTA, 2005; Giese, Parker, Lech-Boura, Burkhardt, & Cook, 2003). Occupational therapy is a holistic, client-centered practice that acknowledges the importance of context and environment in framing a client's occupational needs, desires, and priorities (AOTA, 2008). Because CAM is a culturally sensitive system used by nearly 40% of adults and 12% of children in the United States (Barnes, Bloom, & Nahin, 2008), it is important to acknowledge the ethical and pragmatic issues surrounding the use of CAM in occupational therapy practice. This position paper defines the appropriate use of CAM by occupational therapy practitioners[1] within the scope of occupational therapy practice.

Use

The U.S. Department of Health and Human Services reports that CAM is used in the United States by persons who are "seeking ways to improve their health and well-being or to relieve symptoms associated with chronic, even terminal, illnesses or the side effects of conventional treatments for them" (Barnes et al., 2008). CAM interventions most often are used for treatment of pain conditions by non-poor women ages 30–69 with significant levels of education beyond high school (Barnes et al., 2008). Similar to the holistic nature of occupational therapy practice, practitioners who use CAM also address the influence of the contexts on health status and collaborate with clients who demonstrate a desire for personal control over health outcomes (Cheung, Wyman, & Halcon, 2007). Clients who are living with and adjusting to life with chronic conditions such as back pain or a traumatic event such as domestic abuse may combine the holistic nature of CAM approaches with other intervention approaches to improve their ability to participate in occupations they need and want to perform.

Definition

The National Center for Complementary and Alternative Medicine (NCCAM) of the National Institutes of Health has identified five domains of CAM practice and defines *complementary and alternative medicine* as "a group of diverse medical and health care systems, practices, and products that are not presently considered to be part of conventional medicine" (NCCAM, 2010). The five domains of CAM practice are (1) alternative medical systems, (2) mind–body interventions, (3) biologically based treatments, (4) manipulative and body-based methods, and (5) energy therapies. By definition, *alternative medicine* is practiced *in place of* conventional medicine, while *complementary interventions* are accessed *in conjunction with* allopathic medical practices.

---

[1]When the term *occupational therapy practitioner* is used in this document, it refers to both occupational therapists and occupational therapy assistants (AOTA, 2006). *Occupational therapists* are responsible for all aspects of occupational therapy service delivery and are accountable for the safety and effectiveness of the occupational therapy service delivery process. *Occupational therapy assistants* deliver occupational therapy services under the supervision of and in partnership with an occupational therapist (AOTA, 2009).

The definition of CAM is dynamic. Practices contained within the definition of CAM change as clinical evidence supports their inclusion with conventional health practices, and novel approaches emerge (AOTA, 2005; Giese et al., 2003). The term *integrative medicine* is used for combined treatments from conventional medicine and CAM for which there is high-quality scientific evidence of safety and effectiveness (NCCAM, 2008).

Research

The NCCAM was established by Congress in 1998 through Title VI, Section 601, of the Omnibus Consolidated and Emergency Appropriations Act of 1999 (P.L. 105-277) as the federal government's lead agency for scientific research on CAM. The NCCAM mission is to investigate promising CAM products and practices with neutrality and scientific rigor to determine their safety and effectiveness, to train CAM researchers, and to provide information about CAM to professionals and the general public (NCCAM, 2008). Since its inception, the NCCAM has funded more than 1,200 research projects at scientific institutions across the United States and internationally.

The NCCAM has proposed a framework for setting research priorities that consists of four pillars: (1) scientific promise, (2) extent and nature of practice and use, (3) amenability to rigorous scientific inquiry, and (4) potential to change health practices (NCCAM, 2009). Key priority areas are currently non-mineral, non-vitamin, natural products and mind–body interventions such as yoga, tai chi, qi gong, guided imagery, meditation, deep-breathing exercises, and progressive relaxation (NCCAM, 2009). Studies to support the integration of CAM and conventional medicine, to encourage insurance coverage for CAM therapies, and to develop practice and referral guidelines are needed in addition to research about the safety and efficacy of CAM practices (Coulter & Khorsan, 2008; Herman, D'Huyvetter, & Mohler, 2006).

Access to information about CAM practices has been enhanced by a collaborative project between the National Library of Medicine and the NCCAM. These two government agencies have created *CAM on PubMed* (see http://nccam.nih.gov/research/camonpubmed/), a search option that automatically limits research citations to a CAM subset from the MEDLINE database and additional life science journals.

Use Within the Scope of Occupational Therapy Practice

Occupational therapy values engagement in occupations and promotes the health and participation of people, organizations, and populations through engagement in occupation (AOTA, 2008). *Occupations* are "activities...of everyday life, named, organized, and given value and meaning by individuals and a culture" (Law, Polatajko, Baptiste, & Townsend, 1997, p. 29). Occupations encompass activities of daily living (ADLs), instrumental activities of daily living, rest and sleep, education, work, play, leisure, and social participation (AOTA, 2008).

Occupational therapy practitioners may utilize CAM in the delivery of occupational therapy services when they are used as preparatory methods or purposeful activities to facilitate the ability of clients to engage in their daily life occupations. CAM approaches have been utilized in occupational therapy for several years and include but are not limited to guided imagery, massage, myofascial release, meditation, and behavioral relaxation training (AOTA, 1998; Brachtesende, 2005; Lindsay, Fee, Michie, & Heap, 1994; Scott, 1999). Yoga postures also have been used prior to engagement in ADLs to reduce reliance on pain medication and to promote relaxation for restorative sleep (Brachtesende, 2005).

Occupational therapy practitioners need to respect the use of CAM as part of the client's occupational performance habits, routines, or rituals and to understand that CAM practices may be embedded within particular cultures (Cassidy, 1998a, 1998b). In a study of patients with cardiac conditions in Hong Kong, the use of qi gong as a method for reducing stress added psychological benefit to the reduction of blood pressure when compared to progressive relaxation training alone (Hui, Wan, Chan,

& Yung, 2006). By collaborating with the client in the selection and application of specific CAM interventions, the occupational therapy practitioner supports and respects the client's autonomy and reasoned participation in decision-making. Outcome studies about engagement in occupation continue to be a priority for determining the efficacy and effectiveness of using CAM techniques during occupational therapy intervention.

To determine whether to use CAM in the delivery of occupational therapy services, occupational therapists must evaluate the client, develop an intervention based on the client's needs and priorities, and conduct outcomes measurement. The evaluation contributes to the understanding of the client's strengths, priorities, and current limitations in carrying out daily occupations. Evaluation and intervention address factors that influence the client's occupational performance, including how the client performs the daily life occupations, the demands of those occupations, and the contexts and environments within which those occupations are performed. As part of the evaluation and the intervention, the occupational therapy practitioner must determine whether the use of CAM is consistent with the client's cultural practices, priorities, and needs; is safe to use; and is an appropriate approach to facilitate the ability of the client to participate in daily life occupations and to promote health and participation. Selected assessments are used to measure the effectiveness of the outcomes of occupational therapy services and guide future therapeutic interventions with the client. The occupational therapy practitioner must measure whether the use of CAM results in positive outcomes for improving occupational performance.

Ethical Considerations, Continuing Competency, and Standards of Practice

The *Occupational Therapy Code of Ethics and Ethics Standards (2010)* (AOTA, 2010a) mandates safe and competent practice, holding occupational therapy practitioners responsible for maintenance of high standards of competence. Occupational therapy practitioners need to maintain continuing competency in CAM approaches just as they do with other areas of practice. Using CAM approaches may require additional training, competency examinations, certification, and regulatory knowledge (AOTA, 2010b). The use of specific CAM approaches may be subject to federal, state, and often local municipal regulations that govern practice, advertising, ethics, professional terminology, and training (AOTA, 2010c). It is the responsibility of occupational therapy practitioners to know and comply with applicable laws and regulations associated with the use of CAM approaches during occupational therapy intervention. Occupational therapy practitioners must abide by state regulations when billing for occupational therapy services that incorporate the use of CAM. Practitioners must distinguish between the incorporation of CAM techniques into occupational therapy practice and the use of CAM as a salutatory method that is separate from occupational therapy practice (AOTA, 2007, 2008).

Issues of client safety and health care worker safety are salient to all areas of occupational therapy practice. The use of CAM requires attention to client safety in consumer decision-making, client interventions, and professional education and training. The risks and benefits of CAM used in occupational therapy should be communicated to clients as standard practice in a client-centered, evidence-based approach to service provision.

Payment for Services

The NCCAM (2008) reports that U.S. adults annually spend $34 billion out-of-pocket on CAM products and services. CAM services, although often paid for privately, increasingly are covered by insurance companies and health maintenance organizations (Astin, Pelletier, Marie, & Haskell, 2000; Cleary-Guida, Okvat, Oz, & Ting, 2001; Wolsko, Eisenberg, Davis, Ettner, & Phillips, 2002). Factors that influence third-party payers to include selected CAM in health care policies include cost-effectiveness, consumer demand, demonstrated clinical efficacy, and state mandate (Pelletier & Astin, 2002; Pelletier, Astin, & Haskell, 1999).

Summary

Occupational therapy practitioners facilitate proficient and meaningful engagement in the significant occupations of life. CAM practices, systems, and products may be appropriately incorporated into occupational therapy practice to encourage a client's engagement in meaningful occupations. Scientific studies are needed to validate the safety and efficacy of CAM methods within occupational therapy practice. Advanced-level training and continuing education are important to acquire the knowledge and skill to utilize CAM methods, to address the concerns for patient safety and informed consent, and to meet the rigors of regulatory requirements.

References

American Occupational Therapy Association. (1998). OT perspective: Complementary care survey results. *OT Week, 12*(48), 4.

American Occupational Therapy Association. (2005). Complimentary and alternative medicine (CAM). *American Journal of Occupational Therapy, 59,* 653–655.

American Occupational Therapy Association. (2006). Policy 1.41. Categories of occupational therapy personnel. In *Policy manual* (2009 ed.). Bethesda, MD: Author.

American Occupational Therapy Association. (2007). *Definition of occupational therapy practice for the AOTA Model Practice Act.* (Available from the State Affairs Group, American Occupational Therapy Association, 4720 Montgomery Lane, Bethesda, MD 20814)

American Occupational Therapy Association. (2008). Occupational therapy practice framework: Domain and process (2nd ed.). *American Journal of Occupational Therapy, 62,* 625–683.

American Occupational Therapy Association. (2009). Guidelines for supervision, roles, and responsibilities during the delivery of occupational therapy services. *American Journal of Occupational Therapy, 63,* 173–179.

American Occupational Therapy Association. (2010a). Occupational therapy code of ethics and ethics standards (2010). *American Journal of Occupational Therapy, 64*(Suppl.), S17–S26.

American Occupational Therapy Association. (2010b). Standards for continuing competence. *American Journal of Occupational Therapy, 64*(Suppl.), S103–S105.

American Occupational Therapy Association. (2010c). Standards of practice for occupational therapy. *American Journal of Occupational Therapy, 64*(Suppl.), S106–S111.

Astin, J. A., Pelletier, K. R., Marie, A., & Haskell, W. L. (2000). Complementary and alternative medicine use among elderly persons: One-year analysis of a Blue Shield Medicare supplement. *Journals of Gerontology Series A: Biological Sciences and Medical Sciences, 55*(1), M4–M9.

Barnes, P. M., Bloom, B., & Nahin, R. (2008, December 10). Complementary and alternative medicine use among adults and children: United States, 2007. *CDC National Health Statistics Report.* Retrieved January 6, 2010, from, http://nccam.nih.gov/news/camstats/2007/

Brachtesende, A. (2005). Using complementary and alternative medicine in occupational therapy. *OT Practice, 10*(11), 9–13.

Cassidy, C. M. (1998a). Chinese medicine users in the United States. Part I: Utilization, satisfaction, medical plurality. *Journal of Alternative and Complementary Medicine, 4*(1), 17–27.

Cassidy, C. M. (1998b). Chinese medicine users in the United States. Part II: Preferred aspects of care. *Journal of Alternative and Complementary Medicine, 4*(2), 189–202.

Cheung, C. K., Wyman, J. F., & Halcon, L. L. (2007). Use of complementary and alternative therapies in community-dwelling older adults. *Journal of Alternative and Complementary Medicine, 13*(9), 997–1006.

Cleary-Guida, M. B., Okvat, H. A., Oz, M. C., & Ting, W. (2001). A regional survey of health insurance coverage for complementary and alternative medicine: Current status and future ramifications. *Journal of Alternative and Complementary Medicine, 7,* 269–273.

Coulter, I. D., & Khorsan, R. (2008). Is health services research the Holy Grail of complementary and alternative medicine research? *Alternative Therapies in Health and Medicine, 14*(4), 40–45.

Giese, T., Parker, J. A., Lech-Boura, J., Burkhardt, A., & Cook, A. (2003). *The role of occupational therapy in complementary and alternative medicine* [White Paper, adopted by the AOTA Board of Directors June 22, 2003]. (Available from American Occupational Therapy Association, 4720 Montgomery Lane, Bethesda, MD 20814)

Herman, P. M., D'Huyvetter, K., & Mohler, M. J. (2006). Are health services research methods a match for CAM? *Alternative Therapies in Health and Medicine, 12*(3), 78–83.

Hui, P. M., Wan, M., Chan, W. K., & Yung, P. M. (2006). An evaluation of two behavioral rehabilitation programs, qigong versus progressive relaxation, in improving the quality of life in cardiac patients. *Journal of Alternative and Complementary Medicine, 12*(4), 373–378.

Law, M., Polatajko, H., Baptiste, W., & Townsend, E. (1997). Core concepts of occupational therapy. In E. Townsend (Ed.), *Enabling occupation: An occupational therapy perspective* (pp. 29–56). Ottawa, ON: Canadian Association of Occupational Therapists.

Lindsay, W. R., Fee, M., Michie, A., & Heap, I. (1994). The effects of cue control relaxation on adults with severe mental retardation. *Research in Developmental Disabilities, 15,* 425–437.

National Center for Complementary and Alternative Medicine. (2008). *Overview of NCCAM.* Retrieved January 6, 2010, from http://nccam.nih.gov/news/events/grants08/slides2.htm

National Center for Complementary and Alternative Medicine. (2009). *NCCAM priority setting—Framework and other considerations.* Retrieved January 6, 2010, from http://plan.nccam.nih.gov/index.cfm?module=paper2

National Center for Complementary and Alternative Medicine. (2010). *What is complementary and alternative medicine?* Retrieved January 6, 2010, from http://www.nccam.nih.gov/health/whatiscam/

Omnibus Consolidated and Emergency Appropriations Act of 1999, P.L. 105-277, Title VI, Section 601.

Pelletier, K. R., & Astin, J. A. (2002). Integration and reimbursement of complementary and alternative medicine by managed care and insurance providers: 2000 update and cohort analysis. *Alternative Therapies in Health and Medicine, 8*(1), 38–39, 42, 44.

Pelletier, K. R., Astin, J. A., & Haskell, W. L. (1999). Current trends in the integration and reimbursement of complementary and alternative medicine by managed care organizations (MCOs) and insurance providers: 1998 update and cohort analysis. *American Journal of Health Promotion, 4,* 125–133.

Scott, A. H. (1999). Wellness works: Community service health promotion groups led by occupational therapy students. *American Journal of Occupational Therapy, 53,* 566–574.

Wolsko, P. M., Eisenberg, D. M., Davis, R. B., Ettner, S. L., & Phillips, R. S. (2002). Insurance coverage, medical conditions, and visits to alternative medicine providers: Results of a national survey. *Archives of Internal Medicine, 162,* 281–287.

Additional Reading

Bausell, R. B., Lee, W. L., & Berman, B. M. (2001). Demographic and health-related correlates to visits to complementary and alternative medical providers. *Medical Care, 9,* 190–196.

Burkhardt, A., & Parker, J. (1998, November 26). OT perspective: Complementary care survey results. *OT Week, 12*(48), 4.

Carlson, J. (2003). *Complementary therapies and wellness: Practice essentials for holistic healthcare.* Upper Saddle River, NJ: Prentice Hall.

Eisenberg, D. M., Davis, R. B., Ettner, S. L., Appel, S., Wilkey, S., Van Rompay, M., et al. (1998). Trends in alternative medicine use in the United States, 1990–1997: Results of a follow-up national survey. *JAMA, 280,* 1569–1575.

Eisenberg, D. M., Kessler, R. C., Van Rompay, M. I., Kaptchuk, T. J., Wilkey, S. A., Appel, S., et al. (2001). Perceptions about complementary therapies relative to conventional therapies among adults who use both: Results from a national survey. *Annals of Internal Medicine, 13,* 344–351.

Kaboli, P. J., Doebbeling, B. N., Saag, K. G., & Rosenthal, G. E. (2001). Use of complementary and alternative medicine by older patients with arthritis: A population-based study. *Arthritis and Rheumatology, 45,* 398–403.

Ni, H., Simile, C., & Hardy, A. M. (2002). Utilization of complementary and alternative medicine by United States adults: Results from the 1999 National Health Interview Survey. *Medical Care, 40,* 353–358.

Rakel, D. P., Guerrera, M. P., Bayles, B. P., Desai, F. J., & Ferrara, E. (2008). CAM education: Promoting a salutogenic focus in health care. *Journal of Alternative and Complementary Medicine, 14*(1), 87–93.

Author
Terry Giese, MBA, OT/L, FAOTA

for

The Commission on Practice
Janet V. DeLany, DEd, MSA, OTR/L, FAOTA, *Chairperson*

Adopted by the Representative Assembly Coordinating Council (RACC) for the Representative Assembly. Revised by the Commission on Practice 2011.

This revision replaces the 2005 document *Complimentary and Alternative Medicine* (previously published and copyrighted in 2005 by the American Occupational Therapy Association in the *American Journal of Occupational Therapy, 59,* 653–655).

The Importance of Occupational Therapy Assistant Education to the Profession

The American Occupational Therapy Association (AOTA) recognizes the value, necessity, and viability of occupational therapy assistant (OTA) education at the associate degree and certificate levels. Occupational therapy assistants are collaborative partners in the profession's pursuit to achieve its *Centennial Vision*. OTA education provides a sound foundation for practice for the development of competent skill sets to fulfill various professional roles. These roles include direct client care, collaboration with all levels of practice, and advocacy in both traditional and non-traditional care settings.

Meeting the *Centennial Vision* relies on the profession to help enable people "to improve their physical and mental health, secure well-being, and enjoy higher quality of life" (AOTA, 2007, p. 613). OTA education provides the knowledge base for occupational therapy assistant practitioners to successfully provide occupation-based intervention across the life span and the skills to promote healthy occupational choices in the communities they serve. The collaboration of occupational therapists and occupational therapy assistants in service delivery ensures greater affordability and accessibility of occupational therapy services for all populations so that more of society's occupational needs can be met effectively.

In addition, meeting the *Centennial Vision* relies on the profession's ability to "ensure a diverse workforce for multiple roles" (AOTA, 2007, p. 613). OTA programs are designed to meet the needs of a diverse student body, which often are representative of the surrounding community in which the graduates ultimately become employed and serve. OTA graduates are poised to practice within the challenges of traditional and emerging areas of practice with an entrepreneurial spirit that further augments the *Centennial Vision* statement.

OTA education cultivates leadership and mentorship skills in students, preparing them to assume leadership roles within the profession and their communities. OTA education includes the dissemination of knowledge and development of skills needed for occupational therapy assistant practitioners to participate in research and scientific inquiry. Collaboration in research aids the profession in its efforts to be science-driven and promotes the wider use of evidence-based practice in traditional and emerging areas of practice.

The Commission on Education recognizes that OTA education adds an important and valued dimension to the provision of occupational therapy services. The Commission on Education is committed to the support of OTA education by seeking role clarification and promoting collaboration between associate degree/certificate and professional levels of education in occupational therapy to ensure the profession meets the *Centennial Vision* and society's occupational needs.

Reference

American Occupational Therapy Association. (2007). AOTA's *Centennial Vision* and executive summary. *American Journal of Occupational Therapy, 61*, 613–614.

Prepared by

Judith C. Blum, MS, OTR/L

Jennifer C. Coyne, COTA/L

Linda Orr, MPA, OTR/L

for

The Commission on Education
René Padilla, PhD, OTR/L, FAOTA, *Chairperson*

Adopted by the Representative Assembly 2008CC40

Note: This paper replaces the 2002 position paper *The Viability of Occupational Therapy Assistant Education.*

Fieldwork Level II and Occupational Therapy Students: A Position Paper

The purpose of this paper is to define the Level II fieldwork experience and to clarify the appropriate conditions and principles that must exist to ensure that interventions completed by Level II fieldwork students are of the quality and sophistication necessary to be clinically beneficial to the client. When appropriately supervised, adhering to professional and practice principles, and in conjunction with other regulatory and payer requirements, the American Occupational Therapy Association (AOTA) considers that students at this level of education are providing occupational therapy interventions that are skilled according to their professional education level of practice.

AOTA asserts that Level II occupational therapy fieldwork students may provide occupational therapy services under the supervision of a qualified occupational therapist in compliance with state and federal regulations. Occupational therapy assistant fieldwork students may provide occupational therapy services under the supervision of a qualified occupational therapist or occupational therapy assistant under the supervision of an occupational therapist in compliance with state and federal regulations.

Occupational therapy Level II fieldwork students are those individuals who are currently enrolled in an occupational therapy or occupational therapy assistant program accredited, approved, or pending accreditation by the Accreditation Council for Occupational Therapy Education (ACOTE®; 2012). At this point in their professional education, students have completed necessary and relevant didactic coursework that has prepared them for the field experience.

The fieldwork Level II experience is an integral and crucial part of the overall educational experience that allows the student an opportunity to apply theory and techniques acquired through the classroom and Level I fieldwork learning. Level II fieldwork provides an in-depth experience in delivering occupational therapy services to clients, focusing on the application of evidence-based purposeful and meaningful occupations, administration, and management of occupational therapy services. The experience provides the student with the opportunity to carry out professional responsibilities under supervision and to observe professional role models in the field (ACOTE, 2012).

The academic program and the supervising occupational therapy practitioner[1] are responsible for ensuring that the type and amount of supervision meet the needs of the student and ensure the safety of all stakeholders. The following General Principles represent the minimum criteria that must be present during a Level II fieldwork experience to ensure the quality of services being provided by the Level II student practitioner:

a. The student is supervised by a currently licensed or credentialed occupational therapy practitioner who has a minimum of 1 year of practice experience subsequent to initial certification and is adequately prepared to serve as a fieldwork educator.

---

[1]When the term *occupational therapy practitioner* is used in this document, it refers to both occupational therapists and occupational therapy assistants (AOTA, 2006).

b. Occupational therapy students will be supervised by an occupational therapist. Occupational therapy assistant students will be supervised by an occupational therapist or an occupational therapy assistant in partnership with the occupational therapist who is supervising the occupational therapy assistant (AOTA, 2009).

c. Supervision of occupational therapy and occupational therapy assistant students in fieldwork Level II settings will be of the quality and scope to ensure protection of consumers and provide opportunities for appropriate role modeling of occupational therapy practice.

d. The supervising occupational therapist and/or occupational therapy assistant must recognize when direct versus indirect supervision is needed and ensure that supervision supports the student's current and developing levels of competence with the occupational therapy process.

e. Supervision should initially be direct and in line of sight and gradually decrease to less direct supervision as is appropriate depending on the

- Competence and confidence of the student,

- Complexity of client needs,

- Number and diversity of clients,

- Role of occupational therapy and related services,

- Type of practice setting,

- Requirements of the practice setting, and

- Other regulatory requirements (ACOTE, 2012).

f. In all cases, the occupational therapist assumes ultimate responsibility for all aspects of occupational therapy service delivery and is accountable for the safety and effectiveness of the occupational therapy service delivery process involving the student. This also includes provision of services provided by an occupational therapy assistant student under the supervision of an occupational therapy assistant (AOTA, 2009).

g. In settings where occupational therapy practitioners are not employed,

1. Students should be supervised daily on site by another professional familiar with the role of occupational therapy in collaboration with an occupational therapy practitioner (see b above).

2. Occupational therapy practitioners must provide direct supervision for a minimum of 8 hours per week and be available through a variety of other contact measures throughout the workday. The occupational therapist or occupational therapy assistant (under the supervision of an occupational therapist) must have 3 years of practice experience to provide this type of supervision (ACOTE, 2012).

h. All state licensure policies and regulations regarding student supervision will be followed, including the ability of the occupational therapy assistant to serve as fieldwork educator.

i. Student supervision and reimbursement policies and regulations set forth by third-party payers will be followed.

j. If allowed by payment policies and applicable state and federal laws, occupational therapy services provided by students under the supervision of a qualified practitioner will be billed as services provided by the supervising licensed occupational therapy practitioner.

It is the professional and ethical responsibility of occupational therapy practitioners to be knowledgeable of and adhere to applicable state and federal laws and payer rules and regulations related to fieldwork education.

References

Accreditation Council for Occupational Therapy Education. (2012). Accreditation Council for Occupational Therapy Education (ACOTE®) standards. *American Journal of Occupational Therapy, 66*(6 Suppl.).

American Occupational Therapy Association. (2006). Policy 1.44: Categories of occupational therapy personnel. In *Policy manual* (2011 ed., pp. 33–34). Bethesda, MD: Author.

American Occupational Therapy Association. (2009). Guidelines for supervision, roles, and responsibilities during the delivery of occupational therapy services. *American Journal of Occupational Therapy, 63,* 797–803.

Authors

Debbie Amini, EdD, OTR/L, CHT, *Chairperson, Commission on Practice*
Jyothi Gupta, PhD, OTR/L, OT, *Chairperson, Commission on Education*

for

The Commission on Practice
Debbie Amini, EdD, OTR/L, CHT, *Chairperson*

and

The Commission on Education
Jyothi Gupta, PhD, OTR/L, OT, *Chairperson*

Adopted by the Representative Assembly Coordinating Council (RACC) for the Representative Assembly, 2012, in response to RA Charge # 2011AprC26.

Note. This document is based on a 2010 Practice Advisory, "Services Provided by Students in Fieldwork Level II Settings." Prepared by a Commission on Practice and Commission on Education Joint Task Force:
Debbie Amini, EdD, OTR/L, CHT
Janet V. DeLany, DEd, OTR/L, FAOTA
Debra J. Hanson, PhD, OTR
Susan M. Higgins, MA, OTR/L
Jeanette M. Justice, COTA/L
Linda Orr, MPA, OTR/L

Obesity and Occupational Therapy

Obesity is a significant and wide-ranging health and social problem in the United States. Occupational therapy is a health care profession that is qualified to provide interventions with individuals, groups, and society to effect change to promote optimum health. Occupational therapy services often are used directly and indirectly to influence weight management and related health concerns through attention to healthy lifestyle choices and engagement in fulfilling occupations. The purpose of this paper is to explain the position of the American Occupational Therapy Association (AOTA) to persons within and outside the profession on the role of occupational therapists and occupational therapy assistants[1] in addressing the impact of obesity on people's ability to engage in daily activities.

Overview of Occupational Therapy's Domain and Process

Since its founding, occupational therapy has been a healing profession of practitioners who "assist clients (people, organizations, and populations) to engage in everyday activities or occupations that they want and need to do in a manner that supports health and participation" (AOTA, 2008, p. 626). Occupational therapy practitioners[2] apply their knowledge about engagement in occupation—that is, "everyday activity" (AOTA, 2008, p. 628)—to help clients who may be experiencing disease, impairment, disability, dissatisfaction, or adverse circumstances participate in their daily life in a manner that supports their health and wellbeing. By working with clients from this perspective, occupational therapy practitioners use everyday activities therapeutically to improve the health and quality of life of consumers and to prevent future disease or disability.

AOTA and its members are committed to improving individual quality of life; promoting community health; and supporting primary, secondary, and tertiary care for the management of obesity (AOTA, 2012). This position paper explores the growing dangers of the obesity epidemic for health and describes specific and effective services provided by occupational therapy practitioners in a variety of practice settings for clients at risk for or experiencing the negative health effects of obesity throughout the life course. It also explains how the occupational therapy profession provides expertise and leadership in working with the problem of obesity in U.S. society as it affects individuals, families, groups, and populations across the life course.

Obesity in the United States

Definitions and Prevalence

Being *overweight* (defined as having a body mass index [BMI] of 25 to 29.9) or *obese* (defined as having a BMI of 30 or greater; Centers for Disease Control and Prevention [CDC], 2012b) reduces the likelihood of a

---

[1]*Occupational therapists* are responsible for all aspects of occupational therapy service delivery and are accountable for the safety and effectiveness of the occupational therapy service delivery process. *Occupational therapy assistants* deliver occupational therapy services under the supervision of and in collaboration with an occupational therapist (AOTA, 2009).

[2]When the term *occupational therapy practitioner* is used in this document, it refers to both occupational therapists and occupational therapy assistants (AOTA, 2006).

person's participation in physical activity, including leisure activity (Trost, Owen, Bauman, Sallis, & Brown, 2002). Although only 9% of Americans believe that they have a weight problem (Lee & Oliver, 2002) and fewer than 45% of overweight and obese patients receive weight counseling from their physicians (Rose, Frank, & Carrera, 2011), an all-time high 35.5% of adult American men and 35.8% of women are considered obese (Flegal, Carroll, Kit, & Ogden, 2012). The prevalence of *Grade 3 obesity*, also commonly referred to as *severe* or *morbid obesity* (defined as having a BMI over 40; Flegal et al., 2012; National Center for Health Statistics, 2007) is rising substantially faster than obesity (Sturm, 2003); the current prevalence of Grade 3 obesity is 6.3% for the population (Flegal et al., 2012).

These figures translate to more than 72 million Americans considered obese (CDC, 2011). Although statistics show that the prevalence of obesity among adults, adolescents, and children plateaued in 2009–2010 compared with 2007–2008 (Flegal et al., 2012; Ogden, Carroll, Kit, & Flegal, 2012), rates are not yet declining.

Risk for obesity is elevated for individuals who have physical disabilities such as spinal cord injuries (Krause & Broderick, 2004); persons diagnosed with schizophrenia and other forms of mental illness (Bacon, Farnworth, & Boyd, 2012; Chwastiak et al., 2009; Northey & Barnett, 2012); persons with fewer years of education or poorer economic or job status; and Latino and African American individuals (Blanchard, 2009; CDC, 2006, 2011; Cousins et al., 1992; Flegal et al., 2012; Friedman & Brownell, 1996; Institute of Medicine [IOM], 2012; Wardle, Waller, & Jarvis, 2002). As a result of increased need across all populations, the field of *bariatrics* (defined as the medical investigation, prevention, and treatment of obesity with interventions including diet and nutrition, exercise, behavior modification, lifestyle changes, surgical alternatives, and appropriate medications) is continuing to expand (Foti, 2004, 2005).

Risks and Costs

Several studies have demonstrated that obesity appears to be correlated with increased risk of both acute and chronic diseases, including Type 2 diabetes, sleep apnea, chronic low back pain, hypertension, hyperlipidemia, multiple forms of cancer, cardiovascular disease, stroke, liver and gall bladder disease, osteoarthritis, activity limitations, reproductive health complications including infertility, psychological distress, discrimination, and an increased mortality rate that is responsible for a remarkable 95.7 million years of life lost across the overweight and obese population (CDC, 2011; Expert Panel on the Identification, Evaluation, and Treatment of Overweight in Adults, 1998; Finkelstein, Brown, Wrage, Allaire, & Hoerger, 2010; Forhan, Law, Vrkljan, & Taylor, 2011; Hemminki, Li, Sundquist, & Sundquist, 2011).

The related medical costs are estimated at $147 billion annually, representing nearly 10% of all medical spending in the United States (Finkelstein, Trogdon, Cohen, & Dietz, 2009). About half of the total is paid by Medicare and Medicaid, creating a significant financial burden for taxpayers (Finkelstein & Strombotne, 2010). Job absenteeism due directly or indirectly to obesity-related illness results in costs of $12.8 billion per year and an additional $30.3 billion in medical costs for employers (Finkelstein, DiBonaventura, Burgess, & Hale, 2010; McKinnon et al., 2009). In addition, reduced productivity by obese workers while on the job, referred to as *presenteeism*, results in another $30.0 billion in losses to businesses annually (Finkelstein, DiBonaventura, et al., 2010).

Studies show that more than one-third of children aged 6 to 19 years are considered at risk for overweight or are overweight, defined as being at or above the 85th percentile of the sex-specific BMI-for-age growth chart (CDC, 2012a; Center for Health and Health Care in Schools [CHHCS], 2005; Janicke, Harman, Kelleher, & Zhang, 2009); the current prevalence of obesity among children and adolescents is 16.9% (Ogden et al., 2012). These young people are at risk for a variety of health-related concerns, including a trajectory toward obesity as an adult and the health risks associated with it (CHHCS, 2005; Nonnemaker, Morgan-Lopez, Pais, & Finkelstein, 2009; Waters et al., 2011). In addition, a bidirectional relationship between obesity and psychiatric diagnoses has been observed among children (Janicke et al., 2009).

Societal issues—such as easy access to inexpensive junk food and overexposure to junk food marketing; steadily increasing food portion sizes; decreased provision of healthy food choices and physical education in schools; lack of safety for outdoor activities in lower income areas; and the growing popularity of sedentary activities, including viewing television, playing seated video games, and using the computer—have contributed to the rapid rise of overweight and obesity in childhood (Finkelstein & Strombotne, 2010; IOM, 2012; McKinnon et al., 2009; Miller, Rosenbloom, & Silverstein, 2004). As a result, today's children are the first American generation in modern times who will not have as long a life expectancy as their parents (Nonnemaker et al., 2009).

On a societal level, obesity has been called the "last acceptable form of prejudice" (Chambliss, Finley, & Blair, 2004), one that often results in reduced education, housing, and employment opportunities (Puhl & Brownell, 2001); decreased access to and use of health care and wellness services (Wallis, 2004); exposure to stigmatization, discrimination, and bullying (IOM, 2012); and restricted social participation as a result of negative portrayals in popular media (Greenberg, Eastin, Hofschire, Lachlan, & Brownell, 2003; Moloney, 2000). Such negative consequences can have a devastating impact on individuals throughout their life, limiting their opportunities for or access to participation in their desired occupations.

Positive Results of Weight Loss

Weight loss of as little as 5% to 10% of initial body weight can result in significant improvements in measures of blood pressure, cholesterol levels, and glycemic control as well as other improved health outcomes (Expert Panel, 1998; Fabricatore & Wadden, 2003; Manson, Skerrett, Greenland, & VanItallie, 2004; Trogdon, Finkelstein, Reyes, & Dietz, 2009). Conversely, while long-term and appropriate weight loss has been shown to improve health conditions, short-term loss and rebounding with increased weight gain, inappropriate dieting methods, or extreme weight loss may have damaging effects. Typical methods used by consumers who wish to lose weight consist of adhering to a short-term calorie-restricted diet; engaging in a regular, not intense, or irregularly active exercise program; and/or a quick fix of fad diets or weight-loss drugs followed by a return to unhealthy eating habits and a sedentary lifestyle (Andrus, 2011; Heshka et al., 2003: Lowe, Miller-Kovach, Frye, & Phelan, 1999; Manson et al., 2004; Mokdad et al., 2001; Moloney, 2000; Smith & Fremouw, 1987; Willet, 2001). With millions of Americans of all ages struggling—and failing—to achieve and maintain a healthy lifestyle using current methods for weight management, it is clear that health care consumers need to implement successful approaches to attaining effective and sustainable changes in lifestyle that influence weight and, more important, produce related improvements in overall health.

Occupational Therapy's Role in Lifestyle Change

Through a knowledge of psychosocial, physical, environmental, and spiritual factors, as well as of cultural traditions and perspectives that influence performance (AOTA, 2008), occupational therapy practitioners are uniquely qualified to help consumers develop and implement an individualized, structured approach to lifestyle change. A randomized trial published in *JAMA* (Heshka et al., 2003) indicated that weight loss is more effectively achieved when a health care consumer is assisted through a structured program than when a client relies on self-help methods. Using analysis and understanding of performance patterns related to daily life activities (AOTA, 2008; Clark, 2000; Quiroga, 1995; Wilcock, 1998; Yerxa, 2002), occupational therapy practitioners provide meaningful and effective interventions that facilitate participation by the client in modifying daily life habits, roles, and patterns that contribute to chronic conditions, including obesity (Forhan et al., 2011).

For example, occupational therapy interventions are effective in fostering use of virtual reality technology to increase physical activity for patients living in a mental health residential facility (Bacon et al., 2012), engaging adolescents in increased physical activity (Ketteridge & Boshoff, 2008), adapting physical activity for children who are obese (Gill, 2011), and educating children about optimal nutritional choices (Munguba, Valdés, & da Silva, 2008).

When assessing needs, setting goals, and developing and implementing interventions to assist clients who are overweight or obese, the occupational therapy practitioner works closely with the client to design specific plans or programs to meet individual goals and desires in whatever areas of occupation are affected. Occupational therapy intervention may focus on prevention, remediation/restoration, adaptation/ compensation, and maintenance programs in either long-term or short-term settings (AOTA, 2008).

Occupational therapy programs incorporate the client's personal preferences, circumstances, context, and needs into a customized healthy living regimen that takes into account any preexisting medical conditions (AOTA, 2008). Through education, strategies, and intervention planning, occupational therapy practitioners can help clients build habits, including engagement in health-promoting activities, that allow them to maintain targeted changes that influence their weight within the complex dynamic of their everyday lives. Occupational therapists provide interventions for people of diverse populations across the life course, in settings ranging from clinical to community environments.

Occupational therapy interventions in the area of weight management may include community programs of health promotion through lifestyle change; education programs; facilitation of the development of new habits and routines; Lifestyle Redesign® programs; recommendation of home modifications; adaptations/equipment; use of assistive and/or virtual technologies; compensatory training in activities of daily living and instrumental activities of daily living; wellness programs for children, teens, and adults; play and physical education in the schools; safe patient-handling programs in hospitals and skilled nursing facilities; and bariatric and postsurgical acute care interventions (Foti, 2004, 2005). Other relevant resources that can be provided by occupational therapy practitioners include adaptive equipment evaluation, home modification planning, task modification solutions, durable medical equipment considerations, compensatory strategies, caregiver training, and client resource development and advocacy (AOTA, 2008).

These and other occupational therapy services addressing obesity and related conditions may be covered by major health care payers, including Medicare, Medicaid, and private health insurance (Finkelstein & Strombotne, 2010). With the high expenses generated by obesity-related health conditions (Finkelstein et al., 2009; Finkelstein, DiBonaventura, et al., 2010; McKinnon et al., 2009), the need to reduce spending is an economic necessity. Preventing illness is consistently more cost-effective than treating it, and occupational therapy has demonstrated in past research both cost-effectiveness and success in preventing declines in health, for example, among community-dwelling older adults and other populations (Clark et al., 1997, 2012).

A study by Trogdon et al. (2009) using a return-on-investment model found that, in workplaces, a weight loss of 5% among all overweight and obese employees would result in an annual savings in medical and absenteeism costs of $90 per person. Low-cost interventions, such as a group led by an occupational therapist, could reduce costs for businesses, with even more savings realized if substantial weight loss is achieved. Thus, occupational therapy is positioned to become an ever more valuable component of the growing public health imperative to reverse obesity trends in a cost-effective manner.

Conclusion

Occupational therapy addresses the prevention and concerns of obesity through a holistic and client-centered approach to lifestyle through participation in activities that promote health. Occupational therapy interventions can facilitate weight loss and enable clients to make healthy changes in daily life, including incorporating productive and social activity as well as informed choices about eating habits and physical activity, to address obesity, thus improving health outcomes and maintaining long-term wellness.

References

American Occupational Therapy Association. (2006). Policy 1.44: Categories of occupational therapy personnel. In *Policy manual* (2011 ed., pp. 33–34). Bethesda, MD: Author.

American Occupational Therapy Association. (2008). Occupational therapy practice framework: Domain and process (2nd ed.). *American Journal of Occupational Therapy, 62*, 625–683. http://dx.doi.org/10.5014/ajot.62.6.625

American Occupational Therapy Association. (2009). Guidelines for supervision, roles, and responsibilities during the delivery of occupational therapy services. *American Journal of Occupational Therapy, 63*, 797–803. http://dx.doi.org/10.5014/ajot.63.6.797

American Occupational Therapy Association. (2012). AOTA's societal statement on obesity. *American Journal of Occupational Therapy, 66*(6, Suppl.), S81–S82. http://dx.doi.org/10.5014/ajot.2012.66S81

Andrus, J. (2011). Helping patients with weight loss. *American Journal of Nursing, 111*, e1–e3. Retrieved February 12, 2012, from http://journals.lww.com/ajnonline/Fulltext/2011/07000/Helping_Patients_with_Weight_Loss.28.aspx

Bacon, N., Farnworth, L., & Boyd, R. (2012). The use of the Wii Fit in forensic mental health: Exercise for people at risk of obesity. *British Journal of Occupational Therapy, 75*, 61–68. http://dx.doi.org/10.4276/030802212X13286281650992

Blanchard, S. A. (2009). Variables associated with obesity among African-American women in Omaha. *American Journal of Occupational Therapy, 63*, 58–68. http://dx.doi.org/10.5014/ajot.63.1.58

Center for Health and Health Care in Schools. (2005, March). *Childhood overweight: What the research tells us.* Retrieved August 4, 2006, from www.healthinschools.org/sh/obesityfacts.asp

Centers for Disease Control and Prevention. (2006, September 12). *People with disabilities are less healthy than those without disabilities.* Retrieved October 19, 2006, from www.cdc.gov/Media/pressrel/r060912.htm

Centers for Disease Control and Prevention. (2011, May 26). *Obesity: Halting the epidemic by making health easier—At a glance 2011.* Retrieved February 13, 2012, from www.cdc.gov/chronicdisease/resources/publications/aag/pdf/2011/Obesity_AAG_WEB_508.pdf

Centers for Disease Control and Prevention. (2012a, April 27). *Basics about childhood obesity.* Retrieved September 6, 2012, from www.cdc.gov/obesity/childhood/basics.html

Centers for Disease Control and Prevention. (2012b, April 27). *Defining overweight and obesity.* Retrieved September 6, 2012, from www.cdc.gov/obesity/adult/defining.html

Chambliss, H. O., Finley, C. E., & Blair, S. N. (2004). Attitudes toward obese individuals among exercise science students. *Medicine and Science in Sports and Exercise, 36*, 468–474. http://dx.doi.org/10.1249/01.MSS.0000117115.94062.E4

Chwastiak, L. A., Rosenheck, R. A., McEvoy, J. P., Stroup, T. S., Swartz, M. S., Davis, S. M., & Lieberman, J. A. (2009). The impact of obesity on health care costs among persons with schizophrenia. *General Hospital Psychiatry, 31*, 1–7. http://dx.doi.org/10.1016/j.genhosppsych.2008.09.012

Clark, F. A. (2000). The concepts of habit and routine: A preliminary theoretical synthesis. *OTJR: Occupation, Participation and Health, 20*(Suppl. 1), 123–137.

Clark, F., Azen, S. P., Zemke, R., Jackson, J., Carlson, M., Mandel, D., . . . Lipson, L. (1997). Occupational therapy for independent-living older adults: A randomized controlled trial. *JAMA, 278*, 1321–1326. http://dx.doi.org/10.1001/jama.1997.03550160041036

Clark, F., Jackson, J., Carlson, M., Chou, C.-P., Cherry, B. J., Jordan-Marsh, M., . . . Azen, S. P. (2012). Effectiveness of a lifestyle intervention in promoting the well-being of independently living older people: Results of the Well Elderly 2 Randomised Controlled Trial. *Journal of Epidemiology and Community Health,*

66, 782–790. Retrieved February 14, 2012, from http://jech.bmj.com/content/early/2011/06/01/jech.2009.099754.full.pdf+html

Cousins, J. H., Rubovits, D. S., Dunn, J. K., Reeves, R. S., Ramirez, A. G., & Foreyt, J. P. (1992). Family versus individually oriented intervention for weight loss in Mexican American women. *Public Health Reports, 107*, 549–555.

Expert Panel on the Identification, Evaluation, and Treatment of Overweight in Adults. (1998). Clinical guidelines on the identification, evaluation, and treatment of overweight and obesity in adults. *American Journal of Clinical Nutrition, 68*, 899–917.

Fabricatore, A. N., & Wadden, T. A. (2003). Treatment of obesity: An overview. *Clinical Diabetes, 21*, 67–72. http://dx.doi.org/10.2337/diaclin.21.2.67

Finkelstein, E. A., Brown, D. S., Wrage, L. A., Allaire, B. T., & Hoerger, T. J. (2010). Individual and aggregate years-of-life-lost associated with overweight and obesity. *Obesity, 18*, 333–339. http://dx.doi.org/10.1038/oby.2009.253

Finkelstein, E. A., DiBonaventura, M., Burgess, S. M., & Hale, B. C. (2010). The costs of obesity in the workplace. *Journal of Occupational and Environmental Medicine, 52*, 971–976. http://dx.doi.org/10.1097/JOM.0b013e3181f274d2

Finkelstein, E. A., & Strombotne, K. L. (2010). The economics of obesity. *American Journal of Clinical Nutrition, 91*(5, Suppl.), 1520S–1524S. http://dx.doi.org/10.3945/ajcn.2010.28701E

Finkelstein, E. A., Trogdon, J. G., Cohen, J. W., & Dietz, W. (2009). Annual medical spending attributable to obesity: Payer-and service-specific estimates. *Health Affairs, 28*, w822–w831. http://dx.doi.org/10.1377/hlthaff.28.5.w822

Flegal, K. M., Carroll, M. D., Kit, B. K., & Ogden, C. L. (2012). Prevalence of obesity and trends in the distribution of body mass index among US adults, 1999–2010. *JAMA, 307*, 491–497. http://dx.doi.org/10.1001/jama.2012.39

Forhan, M., Law, M., Vrkljan, B. H., & Taylor, V. H. (2011). Participation profile of adults with class III obesity. *OTJR: Occupation, Participation and Health, 31*, 135–142. http://dx.doi.org/10.3928/15394492-20101025-02

Foti, D. (2004). Bariatric care: Practical problem solving and interventions. *Physical Disabilities Special Interest Section Quarterly, 27*(4), 1–3.

Foti, D. (2005, February 7). Caring for the person of size. *OT Practice, 10*, 9–14.

Friedman, M. A., & Brownell, K. D. (1996). A comprehensive treatment manual for the management of obesity. In V. Van Hasselt & M. Hersen (Eds.). *Sourcebook of psychological treatment manuals for adult disorders* (pp. 375–422). New York: Plenum Press.

Gill, S. V. (2011). Optimising motor adaptation in childhood obesity. *Australian Occupational Therapy Journal, 58*, 386–389. http://dx.doi.org/10.1111/j.1440-1630.2011.00957.x

Greenberg, B. S., Eastin, M., Hofschire, L., Lachlan, K., & Brownell, K. D. (2003). Portrayals of overweight and obese individuals on commercial television. *American Journal of Public Health, 93*, 1342–1348. http://dx.doi.org/10.2105/AJPH.93.8.1342

Hemminki, K., Li, X., Sundquist, J., & Sundquist, K. (2011). Obesity and familial obesity and risk of cancer. *European Journal of Cancer Prevention, 20*, 438–443. http://dx.doi.org/10.1097/CEJ.0b013e32834761c0

Heshka, S., Anderson, J. W., Atkinson, R. L., Greenway, F. L., Hill, J. O., Phinney, S. D., . . . Pi-Sunyer, F. X. (2003). Weight loss with self-help compared with a structured commercial program: A randomized trial. *JAMA, 289,* 1792–1798. http://dx.doi.org/10.1001/jama.289.14.1792

Institute of Medicine. (2012). *Measuring progress in obesity prevention: Workshop report.* Washington, DC: National Academies Press.

Janicke, D. M., Harman, J. S., Kelleher, K. J., & Zhang, J. (2009). The association of psychiatric diagnoses, health service use, and expenditures in children with obesity-related health conditions. *Journal of Pediatric Psychology, 34,* 79–88. http://dx.doi.org/10.1093/jpepsy/jsn051

Ketteridge, A., & Boshoff, K. (2008). Exploring the reasons why adolescents participate in physical activity and identifying strategies that facilitate their involvement in such activity. *Australian Occupational Therapy Journal, 55,* 273–282. http://dx.doi.org/10.1111/j.1440-1630.2007.00704.x

Krause, J. S., & Broderick, L. (2004). Patterns of recurrent pressure ulcers after spinal cord injury: Identification of risk and protective factors 5 or more years after onset. *Archives of Physical Medicine and Rehabilitation, 85,* 1257–1264. http://dx.doi.org/10.1016/j.apmr.2003.08.108

Lee, T., & Oliver, J. E. (2002). *Public opinion and the politics of America's obesity epidemic* (KSG Working Paper No. RWP02-017). Boston: John F. Kennedy School of Government, Harvard University.

Lowe, M. R., Miller-Kovach, K., Frye, N., & Phelan, S. (1999). An initial evaluation of a commercial weight loss program: Short-term effects on weight, eating behavior, and mood. *Obesity Research, 7,* 51–59.

Manson, J. E., Skerrett, P. J., Greenland, P., & VanItallie, T. B. (2004). The escalating pandemics of obesity and sedentary lifestyle. A call to action for clinicians. *Archives of Internal Medicine, 164,* 249–258. http://dx.doi.org/10.1001/archinte.164.3.249

McKinnon, R. A., Orleans, C. T., Kumanyika, S. K., Haire-Joshu, D., Krebs-Smith, S. M., Finkelstein, E. A., . . . Ballard-Barbash, R. (2009). Considerations for an obesity policy research agenda. *American Journal of Preventive Medicine, 36,* 351–357. http://dx.doi.org/10.1016/j.amepre.2008.11.017

Miller, J., Rosenbloom, A., & Silverstein, J. (2004). Childhood obesity. *Journal of Clinical Endocrinology and Metabolism, 89,* 4211–4218. http://dx.doi.org/10.1210/jc.2004-0284

Mokdad, A. H., Bowman, B. A., Ford, E. S., Vinicor, F., Marks, J. S., & Koplan, J. P. (2001). The continuing epidemics of obesity and diabetes in the United States. *JAMA, 286,* 1195–1200. http://dx.doi.org/10.1001/jama.286.10.1195

Moloney, M. (2000). Dietary treatments of obesity. *Proceedings of the Nutrition Society, 59,* 601–608. http://dx.doi.org/10.1017/S0029665100000859

Munguba, M. C., Valdés, M. T. M., & da Silva, C. A. B. (2008). The application of an occupational therapy nutrition education programme for children who are obese. *Occupational Therapy International, 15,* 56–70. http://dx.doi.org/10.1002/oti.244

National Center for Health Statistics (2007, June 13). *Morbid obesity.* Retrieved September 6, 2012, from http://nchspressroom.wordpress.com/2007/06/13/morbid-obesity/

Nonnemaker, J. M., Morgan-Lopez, A. A., Pais, J. M., & Finkelstein, E. A. (2009). Youth BMI trajectories: Evidence from the NLSY97. *Obesity, 17,* 1274–1280.

Northey, A., & Barnett, F. (2012). Physical health parameters: Comparison of people with severe mental illness with the general population. *British Journal of Occupational Therapy, 75,* 100–105. http://dx.doi.org/10.4276/030802212X13286281651199

Ogden, C. L., Carroll, M. D., Kit, B. K., & Flegal, K. M. (2012). Prevalence of obesity and trends in body mass index among U.S. children and adolescents, 1999–2010. *JAMA, 307,* 483–490. http://dx.doi.org/10.1001/jama.2012.40

Puhl, R., & Brownell, K. D. (2001). Bias, discrimination, and obesity. *Obesity Research, 9,* 788–805. http://dx.doi.org/10.1038/oby.2001.108

Quiroga, V. (1995). *Occupational therapy: The first 30 years 1900–1930.* Bethesda, MD: AOTA Press.

Rose, A. E., Frank, E., & Carrera, J. S. (2011). Factors affecting weight counseling attitudes and behaviors among U.S. medical students. *Academic Medicine, 86,* 1463–1472. http://dx.doi.org/10.1097/ACM.0b013e3182312471

Smith, M. E., & Fremouw, W. J. (1987). A realistic approach to treating obesity. *Clinical Psychology Review, 7,* 449–465. http://dx.doi.org/10.1016/0272-7358(87)90022-5

Sturm, R. (2003). Increases in clinically severe obesity in the United States, 1986–2000. *Archives of Internal Medicine, 163,* 2146–2148. http://dx.doi.org/10.1001/archinte.163.18.2146

Trogdon, J., Finkelstein, E. A., Reyes, M., & Dietz, W. H. (2009). A return-on-investment simulation model of workplace obesity interventions. *Journal of Occupational and Environmental Medicine, 51,* 751–758. http://dx.doi.org/10.1097/JOM.0b013e3181a86656

Trost, S. G., Owen, N., Bauman, A. E., Sallis, J. F., & Brown, W. (2002). Correlates of adults' participation in physical activity: Review and update. *Medicine and Science in Sports and Exercise, 34,* 1996–2001. http://dx.doi.org/10.1097/00005768-200202000-00025

Wallis, L. (2004). Overweight patients face prejudice in health care. *Nursing Standard, 18,* 6.

Wardle, J., Waller, J., & Jarvis, M. J. (2002). Sex differences in the association of socioeconomic status with obesity. *American Journal of Public Health, 92,* 1299–1304. http://dx.doi.org/10.2105/AJPH.92.8.1299

Waters, E., de Silva-Sanigorski, A., Hall, B. J., Brown, T., Campbell, K. J., Gao, Y., . . . Summerbell, C. D. (2011). Interventions for preventing obesity in children. *Cochrane Database of Systematic Reviews, 2011*(12), Art. No.: CD001871. http://dx.doi.org/10.1002/14651858.CD001871.pub3

Wilcock, A. A. (1998). *An occupational perspective on health.* Thorofare, NJ: Slack.

Willet, W. C. (2001). *Eat, drink, and be healthy.* New York: Free Press.

Yerxa, E. J. (2002). Habits in context: A synthesis, with implications for research in occupational science. *OTJR: Occupation, Participation and Health, 22,* 104–110.

Authors
Faryl Saliman Reingold, OTD, OTR/L
Katie Jordan, OTD, OTR/L

for

The Commission on Practice
Debbie Amini, EdD, OTR/L, CHT, *Chairperson*

Adopted by the Representative Assembly Coordinating Council (RACC) for the Representative Assembly, 2012.

Note: This revision replaces the 2007 document previously published and copyrighted 2007, by the American Occupational Therapy Association in the *American Journal of Occupational Therapy, 61,* 701–703.

To be published and copyrighted in 2013 by the American Occupational Therapy Association in the *American Journal of Occupational Therapy, 67*(Suppl.).

Occupational Therapy's Commitment to Nondiscrimination and Inclusion

The occupational therapy profession affirms the right of every individual to access and fully participate in society. This paper states the profession's stance on nondiscrimination and inclusion.

Nondiscrimination exists when we accept and treat all people equally. In doing so, we avoid differentiating between people because of biases or prejudices. The principle of equality as defined and supported in the core values of occupational therapy requires that "all individuals be perceived as having the same fundamental human rights and opportunities" (American Occupational Therapy Association [AOTA], 1993, p. 1085). We value individuals and respect their culture, ethnicity, race, age, religion, gender, sexual orientation, and capacities, consistent with the principles defined and described in the *Occupational Therapy Code of Ethics* (AOTA, 2005). Nondiscrimination is a necessary prerequisite for inclusion. *Inclusion* requires that we ensure not only that everyone is treated fairly and equitably but also that all individuals have the same opportunities to participate in the naturally occurring activities of society, such as attending social events, having access to public transportation, and participating in professional organizations. We also believe that when we do not discriminate against others and when we include all members of society in our daily lives, we reap the benefits of being with individuals who have different perspectives, opinions, and talents from our own.

We support nondiscrimination and inclusion throughout our profession. Our concerns are twofold—for the persons who receive occupational therapy services and for our professional colleagues. In professional practice, our evaluations and interventions are designed to facilitate our clients' engagement in occupations to support their health and participation in the various contexts and environments of their lives. This includes, but is not limited to, the individuals' cultural, personal, temporal, virtual, physical, and social contexts as described in the *Occupational Therapy Practice Framework* (AOTA, 2008). As occupational therapists and occupational therapy assistants, we assume a collaborative partnership with clients and their significant others to support the individual's right to self-direction.

We believe that inclusion is achieved through the combined efforts of clients, their families, and significant others; health, education, and social services professionals; legislators; community members; and others. We support all individuals and their significant others' rights to fully participate in making decisions that concern their daily occupations: activities of daily living, instrumental activities of daily living, rest and sleep, work, education, play, leisure, and social participation.

AOTA and its members recognize the legal mandates concerning nondiscriminatory practices. However, the concept of nondiscrimination is not limited to that which is dictated by law. This professional association, through its members, boards, commissions, committees, officers, and staff, supports the belief that all members of the occupational therapy professional community are entitled to maximum opportunities to develop and use their abilities. These individuals also have the right to achieve productive and satisfying professional and personal lives.

We are committed to nondiscrimination and inclusion as an affirmation of our belief that the interests of all members of the profession are best served when the inherent worth of every individual is recognized and valued. We maintain that society has an obligation to provide the reasonable accommodations necessary to allow individuals access to social, educational, recreational, and vocational opportunities. By embracing the concepts of nondiscrimination and inclusion, we will all benefit from the opportunities afforded in a diverse society.

References

American Occupational Therapy Association. (1993). Core values and attitudes of occupational therapy practice. *American Journal of Occupational Therapy, 47,* 1085–1086.

American Occupational Therapy Association. (2005). Occupational therapy code of ethics. *American Journal of Occupational Therapy, 59,* 639–642.

American Occupational Therapy Association. (2008). Occupational therapy practice framework: Domain and process (2nd ed.). *American Journal of Occupational Therapy, 62,* 625–688.

Authors
Ruth H. Hansen, PhD, FAOTA
Jim Hinojosa, PhD, OT, FAOTA

for

The Commission on Practice
Mary Jane Youngstrom, MS, OTR, *Chairperson*

Adopted by the Representative Assembly 1999M4

Edited by the Commission on Practice 2004

Received by the Representative Assembly 2004C28

Edited by the Commission on Practice 2009

Note: This document replaces the 1995 Position Paper *Occupational Therapy: A Profession in Support of Full Inclusion,* the accompanying 1996 White Paper *The Role of the Occupational Therapy Practitioner in the Implementation of Full Inclusion,* and the 1999 and 2004 Position Paper *Occupational Therapy's Commitment to Nondiscrimination and Inclusion.*

Occupational Therapy's Perspective on the Use of Environments and Contexts to Support Health and Participation in Occupations

Purpose

This paper articulates the position of the American Occupational Therapy Association (AOTA) regarding how, across all areas of practice, occupational therapy practitioners[1] select, create, and use environments and contexts to support clients' health and participation in desired occupations.

Introduction

The value and purpose of occupational therapy is to support the health and participation of clients by engaging them in their desired occupations (AOTA, 2008). *Occupations* are activities that "reflect cultural values, provide structure to living and meaning to individuals; these activities meet human needs for self-care, enjoyment, and participation in society" (Crepeau, Cohn, & Schell, 2003, p. 1031). Where and how occupational therapy services are provided is based on the notion that clients' engagement in occupation is inextricably situated in environments and contexts. The *environment* refers to external physical and social aspects that surround clients while engaging in the occupation. *Contexts* are the cultural, personal, temporal, and virtual aspects of this engagement; some contexts are external to the client (e.g., virtual), some are internal to the client (e.g., personal), and some may have both external features and internalized beliefs and values (e.g., cultural) (AOTA, 2008). Occupational therapy practitioners view human performance as a transactive relationship among people, their occupations, and environments and contexts.

Using their expertise in analyzing these complex and reciprocal relationships, occupational therapy practitioners make recommendations to structure, modify, or adapt the environment and context to enhance and support performance. Both environment and context influence clients' success in desired occupations and therefore are critical aspects of any occupational therapy assessment, intervention, and outcome. This assumption is consistent with current educational and health care laws and policies that stipulate that assessment and intervention by providers take place in the natural and least restrictive environments that support the client's successful participation (Americans with Disabilities Act of 1990; Individuals with Disabilities Education Improvement Act Amendments of 2004; *Olmstead v. L.C. and E.W.*, 1999).

Occupational Therapy Process

Occupational therapy practitioners support people where life is lived. To support people to live meaningful lives in environments and contexts that best meet their needs and desires, practitioners interpret a wide range of laws, regulations, and standards as they seek to maintain the integrity and values of the profession to benefit clients. Table 1 reviews key legislation related to occupational therapy intervention and how these laws apply to practice.

---

[1]When the term *occupational therapy practitioner* is used in this document, it refers to both occupational therapists and occupational therapy assistants (AOTA, 2006). *Occupational therapists* are responsible for all aspects of occupational therapy service delivery and are accountable for the safety and effectiveness of the occupational therapy service delivery process. *Occupational therapy assistants* deliver occupational therapy services under the supervision of and in partnership with an occupational therapist (AOTA, 2010).

Table 1. Legislation and Court Cases Related to Occupational Therapy Practice

Federal Law/Court Case/Movement	Key Constructs	Application to OT Practice
Rehabilitation Act of 1973, Section 504	• Creates an obligation not to discriminate on the basis of special education needs for individuals with disabilities • Helps ensure students with disabilities receive the services, supports, and accommodations necessary to meet their needs • Specifically states "SEC. 504. No otherwise qualified handicapped individual in the United States, as defined in section 7(6), shall, solely by reason of his handicap, be excluded from the participation in, be denied the benefits of, or be subjected to discrimination under any program or activity receiving Federal financial assistance"	• Has implications for providing services to all individuals with disabilities in any program funded with federal funds • Addresses services for students with disabilities to ensure participation and access to the general education curriculum
No Child Left Behind Act (NCLB, 2001)	• Is the most recent re-authorization of ESEA (see below). • Expands accountability standards for public education • Includes children with disabilities in the accountability models developed to gauge student and school success	• Creates increased motivation for schools to use all existing resources to improve student achievement • Along with IDEA 2004, gives rise and momentum to models of schoolwide support such as response to intervention and positive behavioral supports • Creates broader opportunities for OT to benefit students with and without disabilities
Individuals with Disabilities Education Improvement Act (IDEA, 2004)	• Follows up on the Elementary and Secondary Education Act (ESEA) of 1965, which authorized grants to state institutions and state-operated schools devoted to the education of children with disabilities • Expands and renames the Education of All Handicapped Children Act of 1975 and the successor Individuals with Disabilities Education Act of 1997. • Reauthorizes and expands the discretionary programs, mandates transition services, defines assistive technology devices and services, and adds autism and traumatic brain injury to the list of categories of children and youth eligible for special education and related services • Requires that "removal of children with disabilities from the regular educational environment occurs only if the nature or severity of the disability is such that education in regular classes can not be achieved satisfactorily" [34 C.F.R. 300.114(a)(ii)].	• Clearly establishes OT as a primary service in early intervention and specifically identifies OT as a related service under Part B for school-age children • Changes how society views children with disabilities; opens doors for participation; and raises expectations of productivity, dignity, and independence

Table 1. Legislation and Court Cases Related to Occupational Therapy Practice *(cont.)*

Federal Law/Court Case/Movement	Key Constructs	Application to OT Practice
Social Security Amendments of 1965 (Medicare)	• Establishes a national public health care program to meet the needs of older Americans and people with disabilities (Social Security Disability Insurance) who qualify for service on the basis of disability status and a sufficient work history • Under Part A, covers expenses associated with inpatient hospital stays, skilled nursing facilities, and some home health care • Under Part B, covers approved outpatient physician services, outpatient hospital services, certain home health services, and durable medical supplies and equipment	• Creates a system of health care financing and insurance for older Americans • Creates a steady funding stream for health care, including OT • Focuses mainly on specific health care issues and is not as involved in providing social supports and services as is Medicaid
Older Americans Act (OAA, 1965)	• Establishes a system and network for social, health, and community support for older Americans • Creates a network of local, regional, and state Area Agencies on Aging (AAAs) and provides broad federal grants to meet identified needs • Allows local AAAs to use funding to best meet the needs within their communities	• Provides flexible funding options that support OT services in community health and social services programs for seniors • Increases focus and desire for community-based living resources and aging in place
Omnibus Budget Reconciliation Act of 1987 (Federal Nursing Home Reform Act)	• Creates a set of national minimum standards of care and rights for people living in certified nursing facilities • Requires nursing homes to develop individualized care plans for residents that focus on maintaining or improving the ability to walk, bathe, and complete other ADLs absent of medical reasons • Requires nursing homes to develop individualized care plans for residents and training of paraprofessional staff • Protects residents' right be free of unnecessary and inappropriate physical and chemical restraints	• Creates opportunities for OT practitioners to facilitate balanced lifestyles and healthy routines in institutional care settings often in partnership with Nursing (Restorative Nursing Programs), Activities staff, and other departments • OT practitioners may advocate to support the needs of older adults and their families and caregivers by addressing environmental modifications and adaptations needed for maximum performance and safety, both in personal environments (e.g., wheelchairs, beds) as well as bedrooms, bathrooms, and common areas.
Americans with Disabilities Act (ADA) of 1990	• Extends previous civil rights legislation • Provides a clear mandate to end discrimination against people with disabilities in all areas of life • Includes five titles that address employment, state and local government services, transportation, public accommodations (i.e., public places and services), and telecommunications	• Supports initiatives and interventions that promote function and participation for people with disabilities across the life span • Supports independent living, accessibility, environmental modifications, and other reasonable accommodations

(continued)

Table 1. Legislation and Court Cases Related to Occupational Therapy Practice *(cont.)*

Federal Law/Court Case/Movement	Key Constructs	Application to OT Practice
Independent Living Movement (Batavia, 1999) 1972—First independent living center opens	• Is an important part of the broader movement for disability rights • Supports the premise that people with even the most severe disabilities should have the choice of living in the community • Supports an individual to use personal assistance services to manage his or her personal care, to keep a home, to have a job, to attend school, to worship, and to otherwise participate in the life of the community • Advocates for the removal of architectural and transportation barriers that prevent people with disabilities from sharing fully in all aspects of society	• Supports OT evaluation and intervention to be provided in natural environments where people live, work, and play and to adapt to and encounter the realities of the physical, social, attitudinal, and political contexts • Intervention includes consultation, program development, and advocacy with teachers in schools, supervisors in jobs, citizens' organizations, local governments, businesses, local media, and advocacy organizations
Olmstead v. L.C. and E. W. (1999)	• Affirms the right of individuals with disabilities to live in their community in 6–3 ruling by the U.S. Supreme Court against the State of Georgia • Requires states to place people with mental disabilities in community settings rather than in institutions • Dictates that the community placement must be appropriate; that the transfer from institutional care to a less restrictive setting is not opposed by the affected individual; and that the placement can be reasonably accommodated, taking into account the resources available to the state and the needs of others with mental disabilities	• Establishes precedent for an enforcement of a federal mandate for services to be provided in the least restrictive environment and in settings of choice for people with disabilities • Creates opportunities and obligations for OT practitioners to comply with the letter and spirit of the decision by designing intervention to support community living for people with disabilities and remove barriers such as attitudinal, physical, social, and policy related

Note. OT = occupational therapy; ADLs = activities of daily living.

Occupational therapy practitioners engage in a collaborative process with clients to identify clients' strengths and barriers to health and participation in society. As part of this process, practitioners consider a variety of personal, environmental, and contextual factors that guide the evaluation, intervention, and expected outcomes of occupational therapy services. Personal factors such as clients' age, time of intervention during the life course, service delivery environments, clients' or caregivers' goals, clients' occupational performance, and the services available can guide the decision-making process.

Occupational therapy practitioners "engineer" the environment as they consider the occupational needs of clients in their lived environments. They analyze performance in relation to how features of the environment and context support learning and performance and generate practical solutions to solve problems. For example, practitioners recommend modifications to improve the physical accessibility of kitchens for clients who desire to engage in the occupation of cooking while using their wheelchairs. Practitioners also may add visual cues around the kitchen to structure cooking tasks to increase safety for people with cognitive limitations.

Occupational therapy practitioners recognize that the provision of service in environments and contexts are linked to the purpose of the intervention. Depending on the needs of clients, practitioners understand that environments and contexts will vary from natural to a modified environment that has a more planned structure. For example, a client with difficulty organizing his or her daily routine initially may function better in a structured social program. The intervention goal then is to diminish the need for structured programming to gain self-sufficiency in organizing and planning daily life.

The dilemma in decision-making about what type of environment and context best supports clients' participation in life along a continuum of natural to more structured directly relates to clients' occupational performance. With the value of participation and health, there is a drive toward customizing interventions to suit the person, population, or organization's desired abilities. For example, when someone needs to learn or relearn safety and emergency maintenance, it is optimal to teach him or her with the specific emergency alert system that he or she will actually use.

However, sometimes the natural environment and context initially may pose too many demands or not provide enough support. In such circumstances, it may be more advantageous for people to gain specific skills in occupational competence in a more structured environment and, with practice and feedback, incrementally learn to apply these skills and occupations to the natural environment. Occupational therapy practitioners are sensitive to how the structured or natural environments provide supports or barriers and continuously monitor and adjust these environments to support clients' occupational performance.

It is the intent that these structures be reduced as clients gain competence. For example, during inpatient rehabilitation, an adult with a spinal cord injury would practice community mobility and upon discharge to home would be able to use public transportation. In contrast, some individuals may be better able to participate in daily life occupations when they move from a natural to a more structured environment. For example, an adult with serious mental illness initially may experience enhanced occupational performance in a community group home rather than in a private home.

To narrowly define natural environment and structured environments may risk limiting clients' engagement or participation in meaningful occupations. Ultimately, interventions support clients where life is lived: in their homes, classrooms, playgrounds, work, and recreation or community centers, wherever their occupations take place. Providing intevention in these settings is consistent with the values and purpose of occupational therapy. Practitioners provide services in the natural enviroment and least restrictive environment whenever possible. They also realize that many factors such as limited financial, organizational, and personnel resources and the complexity of the client's condition may constrain this service delivery option. When this occurs, they make recommendations for continuing interventions beyond the immediate setting.

Providing opportunities for all members of society to engage in health-promoting occupations, flexibility in the analysis of the environment and context in which clients thrive is essential. Table 2 provides examples of how occupational therapy practitioners use and modify environments to support health and participation in occupations.

Table 2. Case Studies: Environmental Considerations and Interventions for Specific Populations

Case Description	Environmental Considerations for OT Service Delivery	Selected Examples of OT Interventions Addressing Environments and Contexts	Research Evidence and Related Resources Guiding Practice
A **15-month-old boy** was born at 29 weeks' gestation. He has had difficulty sitting up, particularly during feeding, and achieving other developmental milestones. He is living at home with his family.	The focus of intervention is to support the entire family system to sustain their family life while addressing the developmental needs of the child. Intervention is provided in the home with recommendations as to how to adapt the natural environment to support the child's occupational performance and development.	• After discharge from the NICU, provide direct intervention in home to promote safety and establish child's developmental skills. • Collaborate with family to structure and modify the physical and social environments within the home to support occupational performance. • Educate caregiver in developmental principles, positioning, and activities to facilitate feeding and development. • Consult with family and other members of transdisciplinary team related to supporting family goals.	• Performing everyday activities in the natural setting provides reinforcement and support to achieve and enhance performance and competence (Dunst et al., 2001; Dunst, Trivette, Hamby, & Bruder, 2006). • Helping families accommodate to demands of daily life with a child with delays helps families develop appropriate and sustainable routines congruent with their values and child's developmental needs (Keogh, Bernheimer, Gallimore, & Weisner, 1998).
A **3-year-old boy** with social and emotional regulation challenges attends a center-based pre-school program.	The focus of intervention is to provide early childhood services in an inclusive classroom to enhance the child's opportunities for play with peers in naturally occurring situations that arise in the classroom. OT intervention is integrated into the classroom activities.	• Structure play group to promote peer social interaction skills. • Direct intervention with child and parents to promote self-regulation and establish routines to enable child's transitions throughout the day. • Consult with early childhood team to analyze demands of pre-school class and make recommendations for adaptations to support performance.	• Center-based early intervention services have a positive effect on children's social functioning (Blok, Fukkink, Gebhardt, & Leseman, 2005). • Preschoolers with disabilities perform as well, if not better, when placed in quality inclusive classroom settings and playgroups (Bailey, Aytch, Odom, Symons, & Wolery, 1999; Odom, 2000). • Parents of children with disabilities commonly report that they perceive inclusive classroom practices as contributing to their child's self-esteem, confidence, and happiness as well as reshaping their own expectations of their child's ability to develop and learn with others (Buysse, Skinner, & Grant, 2001).

Table 2. Case Studies: Environmental Considerations and Interventions for Specific Populations *(cont.)*

Case Description	Environmental Considerations for OT Service Delivery	Selected Examples of OT Interventions Addressing Environments and Contexts	Research Evidence and Related Resources Guiding Practice
A **7-year-old student** with cognitive, motor, and speech delays participates in a special day class in a public school. He has difficulty processing sensory information, interacting with peers, focusing on academic tasks, using his hands for tasks, and maneuvering on equipment on the playground.	Guided by the child's needs, the IEP team, which includes the OT and the parents, determines that the child is having difficulty participating with typical peers and benefits from a special day class for students with behavioral challenges. Although such placements are viewed as more "restrictive," the regular classroom environment currently is overwhelming for the child. The goal of the tailored environment is to provide the structure necessary for the child to learn specific skills for participation in a less-restrictive environment in the future.	• Educate IEP team about the effect of the environment on sensory processing and the relationship to behavior in school setting. • Consult with IEP team and teachers to structure, adapt, and modify the classroom and playground environments so that the child has opportunities to meet sensory needs by participating in vestibular-, tactile-, and proprioceptive-based activities throughout school day. • Collaborate with student to help him establish strategies and routines for sensory regulation, emotional and behavioral de-escalation, and appropriate coping skills. • Develop a peer buddy system to promote appropriate social interactions with modeling and role play during social group. • Provide direct intervention to facilitate integration of sensory systems in an environment rich in sensory experiences and equipment.	• Student may attend to classroom instruction for longer periods of time when sensory needs are addressed (Schilling, Washington, Billingsley, & Deitz, 2003). • Teaching children self-regulation strategies (a cognitive approach to manage sensory needs) helps children manage their behavior (Barnes, Vogel, Beck, Schoenfeld, & Owen, 2008; Vaughn et al., 2003). • Supporting occupational performance and behavior in a school-age child improves participation at school (Schaaf & Nightlinger, 2007). • Suspended equipment and opportunities to carefully monitor various and safe sensory experiences is a hallmark of sensory integration intervention. These opportunities may be available only in a carefully designed environment (Parham et al., 2007).
A **28-year-old man** with schizoaffective disorder lives alone. He has difficulty organizing his daily routines to manage his medications. He was recently admitted to the hospital due to an acute exacerbation of his illness. He wants to be discharged home.	The intervention focuses on developing medication routines to help the client return to his apartment. If unable to manage his medications, he might need to move to a group home with more structured supervision. By analyzing the social and physical environment within the client's home and community, OT practitioners can identify external cues and resources to optimize client's occupational performance.	• Educate medical team and case manager about performance deficits that affect medication routines. • Request pharmacist/nurse to teach client how to read labels and practice filling medication box correctly. • Advocate for reminder calls for refills from pharmacy or others. • Teach client skills for medication management to establish habits and routines such as regular sleep/wake times; use of an alarm clock and calendar to track when to take and refill medication; or keeping of medication in a consistent location, such as on a nightstand.	Environmental supports are more likely to improve functional behavior for people with schizophrenia when the supports are customized for the person and situated in the person's home (Velligan, et al., 2000, 2006).

(continued)

Table 2. Case Studies: Environmental Considerations and Interventions for Specific Populations *(cont.)*

Case Description	Environmental Considerations for OT Service Delivery	Selected Examples of OT Interventions Addressing Environments and Contexts	Research Evidence and Related Resources Guiding Practice
		• Provide visual cues such as list of medications with pictures and purpose or reminder signs. • Establish connection with mental health support groups.	
Clients living in a shelter for homeless people desire to meet basic needs, remain safe, and reduce the potential for harm.	Using a consultative model, the intervention focuses on modifying the physical and social environment to promote safety and meet basic needs of the clients.	• Establish defined areas and organize schedules within the shelter to enable individuals to engage in self-care, education, work preparation, and play–leisure activities. • Design physically accessible spaces and equipment to enable individuals to complete basic activities of daily living. • Educate clients in life skills interventions to address the environment demands of homelessness. • Establish a self-governance and grievance committee to address safety within the shelter. • Post emergency procedures and community resources.	Life skills interventions have the potential to support the complex needs of individuals situated within the homeless context (Helfrich, Aviles, Badiani, Walens, & Sabol, 2006).
A **52-year-old successful businessman** had a right middle cerebral artery stroke with resulting left-sided weakness and decreased balance 1 year ago. He lives at home and has tried to return to his job as a financial consultant but struggled to maintain his productivity at work.	Because this client may not regain all performance skills, intervention focuses on designing environmental modifications in the home, work, and community settings that will support his heath and participation in occupations.	• Adapt activity demands for participation in necessary and desired occupations. • Modify home environment to optimize safety and reduce the impact of weakness and fatigue (Fange & Iwarsson, 2005; Stark, 2004; Stearns et al., 2000). • Consult with employer to modify the work environment by using assistive technology to change the task demands. • Set up an ergonomically advantageous setting by adjusting work routines and schedule to support work performance (Whiteneck, Gerhardt, & Cusick, 2004). • Consult with community agencies regarding access (e.g., transportation, public bathrooms, timing of crosswalk lights, safe railings).	• Specific strategies are effective to improve performance skills and participation in roles and routines after stroke (Ma & Trombly, 2002; Trombly & Ma, 2002). • OTs evaluate contextual factors of work environments (e.g., work tasks, routines, tools, equipment) and use this information to plan interventions that facilitate work performance (AOTA, 2005). • OT practitioners consult with community agencies, business owners, and building contractors, among others, to create environments that promote occupational performance for all (AOTA, 2000).

(continued)

Table 2. Case Studies: Environmental Considerations and Interventions for Specific Populations *(cont.)*

Case Description	Environmental Considerations for OT Service Delivery	Selected Examples of OT Interventions Addressing Environments and Contexts	Research Evidence and Related Resources Guiding Practice
Older adults living in an assisted-living facility are at high risk for balance and falls.	The focus of intervention is to maintain the clients' occupational engagement through a multifactorial approach such as strength and balance training; education; modifying activity demands; and creating a safe and supportive environment, including falls prevention.	Consult with facility administrators, architects, and facility staff to design environment that • Reflects a non-institutional character • Eliminates barriers to physical mobility • Provides lighting without glare • Clusters small activity areas together.	• The design of the social and physical environment influences the function and well being for older adults (Day, Carreron, & Stump, 2000). • OT practitioners advocate for and contribute to the creation of an environment where the demands do not exceed the capabilities of the client (Cooper & Day, 2003). • OT practitioners identify and modify environmental barriers (Davison, Bond, Dawson, Steen, & Kenny, 2005).
A **74-year-old woman** lives in an apartment in the inner city with her husband of 45 years. She has a moderate Alzheimer's disease. She has become lethargic and no longer initiates activities. Her husband now does all the shopping, cooking, and cleaning. He is overwhelmed with the demands of caregiving.	The intervention focuses on supporting the caregiver's and the care recipient's health and participation in desired occupations and activities and enabling them to remain in their home as they age.	• Educate caregiver about the disease process and the impact of the environment on the care recipient's occupational performance. • Recommend modifications to the home environment to manage daily care activities. • Provide emotional support as well as information on coping strategies and stress management to caregivers. • Facilitate use of community and family support. • Provide support and education for the uses of adaptive equipment in the home.	• Persons with dementia or Alzheimer's disease can live at home, remaining in their roles and contexts for a longer period of time, if given enough support from caregivers (Haley & Bailey, 1999). • An in-home skills training and environmental adaptation program (Gitlin et al., 2003) improves the quality of life for both the caregiver and the care recipient, with fewer declines in occupational performance of care recipients and less need for care giving (Gitlin, Hauck, Dennis, & Winter, 2005). Home-based OT is effective and cost efficient for community-dwelling elders and their caregivers (Graff et al., 2008). • Persons with Alzheimer's disease perform better at home than in unfamiliar environments; it is harder for them to adapt to new environments (Hoppes, Davis, & Thompson, 2003).

Note. OT = occupational therapy; NICU = neonatal intensive care unit; IEP = individualized education program.

Summary

Occupational therapy practitioners work with a wide variety of clients across the life span. The goal of occupational therapy is to support health and participation in life through engagement in occupation (AOTA, 2008). Occupational therapists consider current educational and health care laws and policies as they make recommendations to modify, adapt, or change environments and contexts to support or improve occupational performance. On the basis of theory, evidence, knowledge, client preferences and values, and occupational performance, occupational therapists assess the intervention settings and environmental and contextual factors influencing clients' occupational performance. Interventions and recommendations focus on selecting and using environments and contexts that are congruent with clients' needs and maximize participation in daily life occupations. Practitioners' expertise is essential to support clients' health and participation in meaningful occupations.

References

American Occupational Therapy Association. (2000). Occupational therapy and the Americans With Disabilities Act (ADA). *American Journal of Occupational Therapy, 54,* 622–625.

American Occupational Therapy Association. (2005). Occupational therapy services in facilitating work performance. *American Journal of Occupational Therapy, 59,* 676–679.

American Occupational Therapy Association. (2006). Policy 1.44: Categories of occupational therapy personnel. In *Policy manual* (2007 ed., pp. 33–34). Bethesda, MD: Author.

American Occupational Therapy Association. (2008). Occupational therapy practice framework: Domain and process (2nd ed.). *American Journal of Occupational Therapy, 62,* 625–683.

American Occupational Therapy Association. (2010). Guidelines for supervision, roles, and responsibilities during the delivery of occupational therapy services. *American Journal of Occupational Therapy, 64.*

Americans with Disabilities Act of 1990, P.L. 101-336, 104 Stat. 327-378.

Bailey, D. B., Aytch, L. S., Odom, S. L., Symons, F., & Wolery, M. (1999). Early intervention as we know it. *Mental Retardation and Developmental Disabilities Research Reviews, 5,* 11–20.

Barnes, K. J., Vogel, K. A., Beck, A. J., Schoenfeld, H. B., & Owen, S. V. (2008). Self-regulation strategies of children with emotional disturbance. *Physical and Occupational Therapy in Pediatrics, 28,* 369–386.

Batavia, A. I. (1999). Independent living centers, medical rehabilitation centers, and managed care for people with disabilities. *Archives of Physical Medicine and Rehabilitation, 80,* 1357–1360.

Blok, H., Fukkink, R., Gebhardt, E., & Leseman, P. (2005). The relevance of delivery mode and other programme characteristics for the effectiveness of early childhood intervention. *International Journal of Behavioral Development, 29*(1), 35–47.

Buysse, V., Skinner, D., & Grant, S. (2001). Toward a definition of quality inclusion: Perspectives of parents and practitioners. *Topics in Early Childhood Special Education, 24,* 146–161.

Cooper, B. A., & Day, K. (2003). Therapeutic design of environments for people with dementia. In L. Letts, P. Rigby, & D. Stewart (Eds.), *Using environments to enable occupational performance* (pp. 253–268). Thorofare, NJ: Slack.

Crepeau, E. B., Cohn, E. S., & Schell, B. A. (Eds.). (2003). *Willard and Spackman's occupational therapy* (10th ed.). Philadelphia: Lippincott Williams & Wilkins.

Davison, J., Bond, J., Dawson, P., Steen, I. N., & Kenny, R. A. (2005). Patients with recurrent falls attending accident and emergency benefit from multifactorial intervention: A randomized controlled trial. *Age and Aging, 34,* 162–168.

Dunst, C., Bruder, M., Trivette, C., Hamby, D., Raab, M., & McLean, M. (2001). Characteristics and consequences of everyday natural learning opportunities. *Topics in Early Childhood Special Education, 21*(2), 68–92.

Dunst, C., Trivette, C., Hamby, D., & Bruder, M. (2006). Influences of contrasting natural learning environment experiences on child, parent, and family well-being. *Journal of Developmental and Physical Disabilities, 18,* 235–250.

Day, K., Carreon, D., & Stump, C. (2000). The therapeutic design of environments for people with dementia: A review of the empirical research. *Gerontologist, 40,* 397–421.

Education of All Handicapped Children Act of 1975, P. L. 94-142, 20 U.S.C., § 1400 et seq.

Elementary and Secondary Education Act of 1965, P. L. 89-10, 20 U.S.C.

Fange, A., & Iwarsson, S. (2005). Changes in ADL dependence and aspects of usability following housing adaptation: A longitudinal perspective. *American Journal of Occupational Therapy, 59,* 296–304.

Gitlin, L., Hauck, W., Dennis, M., & Winter, L. (2005). Maintenance of effects of the Home Environmental Skill-Building Program for family caregivers and individuals with Alzheimer's disease and related disorders. *Journals of Gerontology: Series A: Biological Sciences and Medical Sciences, 60,* 368–374.

Gitlin, L. N., Winter, L., Corcoran, M., Dennis, M. P., Schinfeld, S., & Hauck, W. W. (2003). Effects of the Home Environmental Skill-Building Program on the caregiver–care recipient dyad: 6-month outcomes from the Philadelphia REACH initiative. *Gerontologist, 43,* 532–546.

Graff, M., Adang, E., Vernooij-Dassen, M., Dekker, J., Jomsson, L., Thijssen, M., et al. (2008). Community occupational therapy for older patients with dementia and their care givers: Cost effectiveness study. *British Medical Journal, 336,* 134–138.

Haley, W., & Bailey, S. (1999). Research on family caregiving in Alzheimer's disease: Implications for practice and policy. In B. Vellas & J. Fitten (Eds.), *Research and practice in Alzheimer's disease* (Vol. 2, pp. 321–332). Paris: Serdi.

Helfrich, C., Aviles, A., Badiani, C., Walens, D., & Sabol, P. (2006). Life skills interventions with homeless youth, domestic violence victims, and adults with mental illness. In K. S. Miller, G. L. Herzberg, & S. A. Ray (Eds.), *Homeless in America* (pp. 189–207). New York: Haworth Press.

Hoppes, S., Davis, L. A., & Thompson, D. (2003). Environmental effects on the assessment of people with dementia. A pilot study. *American Journal of Occupational Therapy, 57,* 396–402.

Individuals with Disabilities Education Act Amendments of 1997, P. L. 105-17, 20 U.S.C. § 1400 et seq.

Individuals with Disabilities Education Improvement Act, P.L. 108-446, 20 USC Chapter 33 (2004).

Keogh, B. K., Bernheimer, L. P., Gallimore, R., & Weisner, T. S. (1998). Child and family outcomes over time: A longitudinal perspective on developmental delays. In M. Lewis & C. Feiring (Eds.), *Families, risk, and competence* (pp. 269–287). Mahwah, NJ: Lawrence Erlbaum.

Ma, H., & Trombly, C. A. (2002). Synthesis of the effects of occupational therapy for persons with stroke, part II: Remediation of impairments. *American Journal of Occupational Therapy, 56,* 260–274.

No Child Left Behind Act of 2001, P. L. 107-110, 20 U.S.C. § 6301.

Odom, A. L. (2000). Preschool inclusion: What we know and where we go from here. *Topics in Early Childhood Special Education, 20,* 20–27.

Older Americans Act of 1965, P. L. 89-73 42 U.S.C. 3056 et seq. (amended 2006, P. L. 109-365, 42 U.S.C. 3001).

Olmstead v. L.C. and E.W., U.S.C. 98–536 (1999).

Omnibus Budget Reconciliation Act of 1987 (Federal Nursing Home Reform Act), 42 U.S.C. 1396r, 42 U.S.C., 1395i-3, 42, CFR 483.

Parham, L. D., Cohn, E. S., Spitzer, S., Koomar, J. A., Miller, L. J., Burke, J. P., et al. (2007). Fidelity in sensory integration intervention research. *American Journal of Occupational Therapy, 61,* 216–227.

Rehabilitation Act of 1973, Section 504, P. L. 93-112, 29 USC § 794.

Schaaf, R. C., & Nightlinger, K. M. (2007). Occupational therapy using a sensory integrative approach: A case study of effectiveness. *American Journal of Occupational Therapy, 61,* 239–246.

Schilling, D. L., Washington, K., Billingsley, F. F., & Deitz, J. (2003). Classroom seating for children with attention deficit hyperactivity disorder: Therapy balls versus chairs. *American Journal of Occupational Therapy, 57,* 534–541.

Social Security Amendments of 1965, P. L. 89-97, § 332, 79 Stat. 403.

Stark, S. (2004). Removing environmental barriers in the homes of older adults with disabilities improves occupational performance. *Occupational Therapy Journal of Research: Occupation, Participation, and Health, 24*(1), 32–40.

Stearns, S. C., Bernard, S. L., Fasick, S. B., Schwartz, R., Konrad, R. T., Ory, M. G., et al. (2000). The economic implications of self-care: The effect of lifestyle, functional adaptations, and medical self-care among a national sample of Medicare beneficiaries. *American Journal of Public Health, 90,* 1608–1612.

Trombly, C. A., & Ma, H. (2002). A synthesis of the effects of occupational therapy for persons with stroke, part I: Restoration of roles, tasks, and activities. *American Journal of Occupational Therapy, 56,* 250–259.

Vaughn, S., Kim, A.-H., Sloan, C. V. M., Hughes, M. T., Elbaum, B., & Sridhar, D. (2003). Social skills interventions for young children with disabilities. *Remedial and Special Education, 24,* 2–15.

Velligan, D. I., Bow-Thomas, C. C., Huntzinger, C., Ritch, J., Ledbetter, N., Prihoda, T. J., et al. (2000). Randomized controlled trial of the use of compensatory strategies to enhance adaptive functioning in outpatients with schizophrenia. *American Journal of Psychiatry, 157*(8), 1317–1323.

Velligan, D. I., Mueller, J., Wang, M., Dicocco, M., Diamond, P. M., Maples, N.J., et al. (2006). Use of environmental supports among patients with schizophrenia. *Psychiatric Services, 57*(2), 219–224.

Whiteneck, G. G., Gerhardt, K. A., & Cusick, C. P. (2004). Identifying environmental factors that influence the outcomes of people with traumatic brain injury. *Journal of Head Trauma Rehabilitation, 19,* 191–204.

Authors
Ellen S. Cohn, ScD, OTR/L, FAOTA
Cherylin Lew, OTD, OTR/L

With contributions from
Kate Hanauer, OTS
DeLana Honaker, PhD, OTR/L, BCP
Susanne Smith Roley, MS, OTR/L, FAOTA

for

The Commission on Education
Janet V. DeLany, DEd, OTR/L, FAOTA, *Chairperson*

Adopted by the Representative Assembly 2009CONov149

Occupational Therapy Services in the Promotion of Psychological and Social Aspects of Mental Health

Introduction and Purpose

The purpose of this statement is to describe the role of occupational therapists and occupational therapy assistants[1] in addressing the psychological and social aspects of human performance as they influence mental health and participation in occupations. Psychological and social well-being are necessary for positive mental health functioning and transcend a specific diagnosis or practice setting. These aspects are addressed in all occupational therapy interventions and are primary influences on health and recovery and the ability to learn or resume meaningful occupations. Although challenges to occupational performance related to psychological and social factors may not be the primary reason why some clients (e.g., people, organizations, populations) receive occupational therapy services, the relationship between these factors and occupational performance is central to their successful engagement in desired and needed occupations (Fidler, 1997). The World Health Organization (WHO) described *mental health* not merely as the absence of mental illness but the presence of "a state of well-being in which the individual realizes his or her own abilities, can cope with the normal stresses of life, can work productively and fruitfully, and is able to make a contribution to his or her community" (WHO, 2004, p. 12).

Audience

This statement is intended for occupational therapists and occupational therapy assistants in practice, academia, research, advocacy, and administrative positions. Other audiences for this paper include regulatory and policymaking bodies, provider groups, accreditation agencies, other professionals, and the general public who may be seeking clarification about occupational therapy's scope of practice and domain of concern related to this topic.

Definition

Psychological and social well-being contribute to mental health and to successful engagement in meaningful occupations and roles. *Psychological factors* are those mental functions that are internal to the client and allow for interest in and sustained engagement with meaningful activities and occupations. Psychological factors influence thought, emotion, behavior, and personality that are experienced within the context of everyday living (Bonder, 1993). As described within the *International Classification of Functioning, Disability and Health* (WHO, 2001), they are global mental functions related to the experience of self, time, and emotion; they also include energy, drive, temperament, and personality. Psychological factors also can be described as motivation for personal growth, impulse control, emotional stability, body image, self-concept, self-esteem, coping, sense of life purpose, sense of autonomy over personal choices and environmental demands, and behavioral regulation (Keyes, 2009).

---

[1]*Occupational therapists* are responsible for all aspects of occupational therapy service delivery and are accountable for the safety and effectiveness of the occupational therapy service delivery process. *Occupational therapy assistants* deliver occupational therapy services under the supervision of and in partnership with an occupational therapist (AOTA, 2009).

Social factors occur at both the personal and environmental levels. At the personal level, they include the ability of the client to communicate and interact with others. People exhibiting social well-being will demonstrate empathy, affection, and intimacy, as well as the ability to maintain caring relationships. Having a positive worldview, caring about society, having a sense of belonging, accepting the contributions of others, and valuing one's efforts to support the greater good contribute to one's mental health (Keyes, 2009).

At the environmental level, social factors are external to the individual and reflect the connection to the surrounding world. Factors include the availability, attitudes, and values of social support systems at the family, community, and societal levels. Social environments that allow for successful engagement in life may include supportive families and friends, spiritual activities, support groups, clubs, available housing, fiscal resources, and inclusive policies and regulations (Bonder, 1993; WHO, 2001).

Positive psychological and social factors of mental health such as intact self-concept, motivation, and resilience can assist a client who is experiencing challenges with daily life by providing the internal foundation necessary for coping, goal setting, and behaviors leading to personal and environmental/contextual adaptations. The ability to acknowledge, accept, and ultimately adapt to real or perceived challenges enhances a client's sense of self-worth and self-efficacy, which in turn contributes to the maintenance, restoration, or creation of intact psychosocial functioning (Bandura, 1994; Drench, Noonan, Sharby, & Ventura, 2007; Livneh & Antonak, 1997).

Clients demonstrate positive mental health through the performance of skills, particularly those related to emotional regulation, communication, and social interaction (American Occupational Therapy Association [AOTA], 2008). Clients demonstrate their psychological abilities through their display of affect and behavior and description of their thoughts, feelings, and concerns (Bonder, 1993). They demonstrate their social abilities through how they initiate and maintain relationships, interpret and respond to verbal and non-verbal forms of communication, respond to the thoughts and emotions of others, communicate their needs, and choose socially appropriate responses.

Both psychological and social factors and performance skills influence and are influenced by the supports and challenges that clients experience in day-to-day living. Clients who exhibit self-efficacy, hopefulness, and motivation are able to successfully adapt to change and engage appropriately in desired socially constructed activities and situations. In contrast, clients struggling to successfully engage in their daily occupations may be experiencing psychosocial difficulties.

Rationale and Significance

Occupational therapy practitioners[2] recognize that positive mental health is an integral part of the ability of all people to engage in desired and necessary life occupations regardless of physical and social situation or context. Practitioners also understand that challenges to subjective well-being can occur because of a variety of circumstances such as when clients face major life changes due to acquired illness or disability; face unique functional challenges due to congenital or developmental disabilities; or cope with anticipated change in habits, routines, and roles resulting from a move or loss of a significant other (Livneh & Antonak, 1997).

Occupational therapy practitioners understand that a client's ongoing occupational performance is sustained by the interrelationship of patterns of daily living, personal history, experiences, interests, values, beliefs, and needs. Taking the time to understand what is currently important and meaningful to the client as well as understanding past roles, experiences, strengths, and patterns of coping sheds light on

---

[2]When the term *occupational therapy practitioner* is used in this document, it refers to both occupational therapists and occupational therapy assistants (AOTA, 2006).

how current issues and problems are affecting the client's health and participation in desired occupations (Bonder, 1997).

Occupational therapy practitioners collaborate with the client in achieving adaptation to actual or potential life changes through (1) provision of activities and occupations that assist with future goal setting; (2) occupational engagements that allow the client to demonstrate abilities, recognize assets, and understand continuing challenges; and (3) adaptations to the physical and social environment.

Background and Historical Perspective

Attention to the psychological and social factors influencing mental health and occupational performance is grounded in the historical roots of the occupational therapy profession. Its founders were concerned with the negative effects of inactivity on individuals. They envisioned occupational therapy as a holistic profession, focusing on the mind–body interrelationship and the importance of occupations in helping those with physical, psychological, and social challenges maintain a positive life orientation (Mosey, 1996). The founders believed that humans brought to their occupations a complex mix of personal, physical, psychological, and social factors and also were influenced by cultural, social, environmental, and political variables (Kielhofner, 1997). "This founding vision had at its center a profound belief in the value of therapeutic occupations as a way to remediate illness and maintain health." (Slagle, 1924, as cited in AOTA, 2008, p. 664). It emphasized the importance of establishing a therapeutic relationship and designing interventions from a holistic perspective incorporating all aspects of the client and environment (AOTA, 2008; Meyer, 1922).

Today occupational therapy remains a holistic profession, committed to supporting client's health and participation in life through addressing the constellation of contextual, environmental, physical, psychological, and social factors that support engagement in desired occupation.

Significance to Occupational Therapy: Relationship to Domain and Process

"Engagement in occupation as the focus of occupational therapy intervention involves addressing both subjective (emotional and psychological) and objective (physically observable) aspects of performance" (AOTA, 2008, p. 628; see also Wilcock & Townsend, 2008). During the evaluation and intervention process, occupational therapy practitioners collaborate with the client to consider the interrelated personal, contextual, and environmental factors that support performance and are pertinent to the client's occupational needs (Smith Roley & DeLany, 2008). Identifying the psychological attributes and social capacities supports a holistic view of the client and contributes to the design of interventions that promote health and successful engagement in desired and meaningful.

Description of Practice, Practice Settings, and Related Issues

Interventions

The overarching goal of occupational therapy is to support the client's "health and participation in life through engagement in occupation" (AOTA, 2008, p. 652). Clients include individuals, organizations, and populations. Their engagement in occupations can occur in any setting in which clients participate in work, play, education, leisure, rest and sleep, activities of daily living, and instrumental activities of daily living. Examples of settings include home, work, community, hospitals and rehabilitation settings, and schools.

Clients receive occupational therapy services when they have experienced a disruption in their ability to participate in meaningful occupations or may receive occupational therapy services as part of an early intervention or health promotion program. Addressing psychological and social factors of mental health through interventions designed to enhance or restore well-being, occupational balance, and occupational engagement are critical components of the therapeutic process.

Occupational therapy practitioners are educated to utilize occupations and therapeutic relationships. Occupational therapy practitioners may use conditional and interactive reasoning (Schell & Schell, 2008), communicate within and through occupation, and administer standardized and non-standardized assessments to evaluate the impact of psychological and social factors on the client's engagement in occupation. Specific strategies used to elicit strengths and needs may include therapeutic use of self, active listening, developing opportunities for choices and personal narratives, facilitating problem solving, modeling, and supporting effective communication strategies (Keyes, 2009; Taylor, 2008).

Therapeutic use of self is defined as an "occupational therapy practitioner's understanding and planned use of his or her personality, insights, perceptions, feelings, and judgments as part of the therapeutic process" (adapted from Punwar & Peloquin, 2000, p. 285, as cited in AOTA, 2008). Therapeutic use of self includes methods for responding to clients; skills necessary to respond to a client; characteristics to model for the client; levels of active engagement with a client; effective use of personal attributes; and approaches that motivate, guide, and promote confidence in the client. Therapeutic use of self contributes to client-centered collaboration, caring, and empathy and the integration of multiple methods of clinical reasoning, in particular narrative reasoning. The integration of the elements of a therapeutic use of self within occupational engagement provide for a dynamic and powerful therapeutic process (Taylor, 2008).

Occupational therapy practitioners also may provide additional interventions for clients struggling with psychological and social challenges through the therapeutic use of occupations and activities, education, consultation, and advocacy initiatives. Occupational therapy practitioners use *occupations and activities* as a means of enhancing psychological and social aspects of the client's mental health and for improving engagement in satisfying life experiences (AOTA, 2008). Occupational therapy practitioners recognize the interrelated nature of the client's mental health and occupational engagement and seek to improve both while addressing them simultaneously. The therapeutic use of occupations includes opportunities for

- *Mastery experiences,* in which occupational engagement allows the client to demonstrate abilities, recognize assets, and understand and adapt to continuing challenges

- *Role modeling,* in which the client learns to effectively problem solve and engage in occupations by observing the occupational therapy practitioner.

Occupational therapy practitioners also may adapt the physical and social environment and the demands of the activity to support the client's successful engagement in the desired activities and occupations. Occupational therapy practitioners may recommend strategies and resources for the client to minimize physical and psychological challenges that affect occupational engagement.

The occupational therapy practitioner also may *educate* the client about goal setting and communication strategies (AOTA, 2008). Goal setting can enhance a sense of hopefulness and motivation to work for positive future outcomes. Occupational therapy practitioners facilitate the goal-setting process through assisting with values clarification, identification and acknowledgment of future desires, and the process of self-reflection (Drench et al., 2007). Communication and adaptation to the social environment involves educating the client about interpersonal communication, including verbal and non-verbal behaviors and socially appropriate behaviors when in various life contexts such as on-on-one situations with friends and significant individuals within the home, school, work, social situations, and public places.

Occupational therapy practitioners can provide *consultation* to caregivers and others who work with clients experiencing psychological and social difficulties to address how to use occupations to promote positive self-concept, motivation, and mood and to assist the client in developing resiliency and in adapting to challenges (AOTA, 2008; Brodaty, Green, & Koschera, 2003; Graff et al., 2006).

Occupational therapy practitioners can be advocates, working on behalf of individuals or populations who may be experiencing occupational deprivation or injustices that limit their ability to engage in meaningful and relevant activities. *Advocacy* also can include practitioners working within organizations to address policies and practices that promote positive mental health that otherwise would adversely affect occupational performance. Addressing these concerns can lead to enhanced self-efficacy and success of the individual facing challenges (AOTA, 2008). Table 1 provides selected case examples of occupational therapy interventions for the promotion of psychological and social aspects of mental health.

Table 1. Selected Case Examples

Case Description	Challenges to Occupational Performance and Mental Health	Occupational Therapy Interventions, With Focus on Mental Health
Niraida, age 9, has juvenile rheumatoid arthritis (JRA) and lives with her mother and maternal grandparents. Niraida uses wrist splints on both hands after school and at night to prevent wrist deformity. She currently uses a simple voice-to-text program to expedite the completion of classroom assignments and homework. She is independent in splint usage and other joint care routines. Niraida's teacher describes her as studious and cooperative. However, her teacher and mother report that she seems to be comfortable communicating only with adults and is quiet and reserved in the classroom. She engages in many solitary activities despite invitations by other children to play various board games and low-impact playground games.	• Niraida participates socially with peers and engages in play and leisure activities on only a limited basis. She seldom raises her hand to ask questions and participate in classroom activities and discussions. • Niraida's teacher and mother are concerned with her limited social participation with her peers. • Niraida's mother reports that she is challenged by her need to temper her protective instincts with encouraging Niraida to participate in age-appropriate activities that will also protect her joints.	• The OT analyzes and generates a list of activities that were physically safe for Niraida. The OT works with the classroom teacher to incorporate those activities that Niraida selects from the list into classroom activities that require peer interaction. The OT collaborates with Niraida and her family to create a variety of low-impact activities that Niraida can play at home with a few classmates. The OT assists Niraida in the design of a card to invite classmates to her home. • The OT meets with Niraida's mother to discuss the latest information about JRA and pertinent information regarding child development and changes in social factors that will soon be facing Niraida and her family as she enters adolescence.
Each year, the **2nd through 8th graders** undergo statewide end-of-grade testing. Testing is standardized and occurs for several days in two 1.5-hour blocks per day. Typically this school system provides time for recess each day, thus allowing children an opportunity to engage in activities that support emotional regulation, stress reduction, and social participation. During testing season, recess is cancelled, thus limiting the ability of children to break from the structure and routines of the day. School system OT practitioners have noted a high rate of referrals following the March testing period. In a proactive measure, the OT department decides to meet with teachers and school organization officials to determine what factors are leading to this phenomenon and how to deal with it from an organizational, group, and individual perspective.	• Many children have difficulty coping with and adapting to this change in daily schedule and react by being disruptive in the classroom. Teacher responses to this change in behavior typically include behavioral management approaches such as time out and detention. • The change in routine sensory inputs, decreased time for typical communications, and decrease in recess as a result of detentions and time outs have limited the ability of the children to engage in needed sensory modulation activities and possibly has contributed to the increase of disruptive behavior.	• The OT practitioners work with the school principal and the curriculum director to assess how the changes in the children's routines and rituals and in the temporal aspects of the school day may have contributed to the increase of disruptive behaviors. • After consulting with the state examination department to determine what changes in the examination schedule would be allowed, the OT practitioners collaborate with the school personnel to develop a system to address the children's increased stress and sensory needs. This includes incorporating stretch breaks into the testing schedule, teaching mental imaging relaxation techniques, providing nourishing snacks and hand-held tactile toys such as koosh balls, and offering alternative seating arrangements.

(continued)

Table 1. Selected Case Examples *(cont.)*

Case Description	Challenges to Occupational Performance and Mental Health	Occupational Therapy Interventions, With Focus on Mental Health
Jayla, age 16, has a 6-week-old infant. Her daughter was several weeks early and of low birthweight; she is currently having difficulty with bottle feeding due to sucking difficulties. The baby is receiving consultive OT and birth to 3 services while in the high school–run day care facility. Jayla and her daughter live with Jayla's parents in the suburban home; both parents are currently employed and financially support their daughter and grandchild.	• Jayla currently is struggling with re-establishing peer relationships since the birth of her baby. Despite the child's special needs, she is reluctant to feed the baby in front of her peers or adults at the day care center. • Jayla's parents are insistent that she become responsible for all aspects of the baby's care while resuming her high school responsibilities. She is not completing school work, has not been concerned with her personal appearance, and often asks her mother to watch the baby while she retreats to her room. Jayla states that she feels unsuccessful in all of her occupations and demonstrates some resentment toward others in her life. • Jayla states that she is happy some days and then sad, mostly because she is missing her friends and social activities. Despite her struggles, Jayla reports that she loves her infant and is willing to do what it takes to get her life back on track.	• The OT and client collaborate to identify areas of occupation, the performance patterns associated with each occupation, the activity demands of each occupation, and Jayla's personal priorities. • The OT works with Jayla to identify present and future goals, understand her new and emerging roles, and reappraise what occupations she needs and wants to accomplish. The OT helps Jayla prioritize her responsibilities and develop time management skills so that she can care for her child and complete her school work. The OT also helps Jayla and her parents develop a schedule that allows Jayla to socialize with her friends and participate in high school activities thus, integrating her roles of mother and student.
Several **new residents of a senior assisted-living facility** face the potential for social isolation. The seniors hail from diverse cultural backgrounds and have lived in communities with others who shared their culture and speak their native language.	• The occupational therapist conducts a focus group, using interpreters as needed to obtain an occupational profile of the residents' valued routines, habits, roles, and meaningful occupations as well as their challenges in their new environment. Some residents identify feeling anxious about their new living environment and express sadness at leaving their previous communities. Some report difficulty sleeping and feeling isolated and lonely. • During the group, the residents are asked about the occupational needs, and their daily routines in their home country and the assisted-living facility. Participants emphasize values related to leisure and social relationships. • The residents also are asked about any fears or barriers that might limit involvement in planned activities. Residents express uncertainty about speaking up, because they are fearful of losing housing. They also are concerned about costs of leisure activities, as most are on a limited budget. They identify exercise and increased opportunities to get out of the facility as important goals.	• The OT practitioner meets with the organizational leaders and facility staff to identify what resources and supports are available. Although initially concerned about the cost of leisure and exercise groups, the facility administrators become supportive once the preventative benefits for reducing health problems secondary to social isolation are explained. • On the basis of the needs assessment, the OT practitioner establishes a daily exercise/movement to music group and facilitates development of an information board that highlights roles, values, and unique attributes about the countries of the residents. Interested residents are asked to develop a poster with unique and important facts about their countries, and in a follow-up group, residents discuss commonalities and differences. • A resident council is developed to identify goals and monitor progress and to be a liaison with the organization's administrators.

Table 1. Selected Case Examples *(cont.)*

Case Description	Challenges to Occupational Performance and Mental Health	Occupational Therapy Interventions, With Focus on Mental Health
		• Because food, socialization, and children were identified as important cultural values, the OT practitioner supports the council in organizing a monthly ethnic food potluck and developing a program that pairs residents with local high school students to present social events about their native cultures. • The OT conducts a program evaluation that indicates the residents are proud of their heritage and are excited and motivated to participate in their new community and share their culture with others.
Marta, age 25, has a diagnosis of schizoaffective disorder. She lives with her mother, who is supportive but works two jobs to care for the family and is not able to spend much time with her. Marta has been going to the community mental health center once a month to see her psychiatrist.	• The OT uses the Canadian Occupational Performance Measure (COPM; Law et al., 2005) to help identify Marta's priorities in occupational performance. Marta identifies that she is dissatisfied with performance in productivity and leisure occupations. She reports feeling isolated, bored, and lonely at home. • One of Marta's desired roles is to get her GED so that she can work toward finding a part-time job to help with home expenses. She feels responsible that her mother has to work so hard. She also wants to develop friendships and spend leisure time with people her own age. • Marta lacks self-confidence, stating that she feels "stupid" and is unsure if she can really accomplish her goals. She feels anxious that people will ask her why she still lives with her mother and is fearful of people finding out she has a mental illness because of the social stigma. She talks about how her serious mental illness has taken away the life she had planned (e.g., college, career, family). She expresses anxiety about navigating the college campus as well as signing up for classes. She is unsure what is involved in getting a GED and is worried she won't be able to do the homework, as concentrating is difficult for her, and her medications make it hard for her to get up in the morning. Although she is interested in meeting people her own age in the class, she doesn't know what to talk about around people she doesn't know.	• Using active listening skills, the OT practitioner spends time talking to a tearful Marta about her fears and goals. To assist her as she works toward managing and adjusting to her chronic health issues, Marta is asked to complete a list of what she does well and what is difficult. Marta and the OT practitioner collaborate on setting priorities and weekly goals. The OT practitioner talks with Marta about how she has handled stressful situations in the past and asks her to identify successful strategies. • The OT practitioner facilitates Marta's involvement with the disabilities office at the community college, where she meets a peer specialist who shows her around the college and answers questions about the GED class. They also get a copy of the course curriculum and work together to plan how Marta can structure her time at home to get homework completed. They discuss her fears about meeting new people and identify conversational strategies she can use when in the classroom and on campus. They identify possible questions about her life that she might get from classmates and practice responses. • The OT practitioner advises Marta about how to connect with a National Alliance on Mental Illness group for young adults for further support. • The OT practitioner continues to use the COPM on an ongoing basis to identify Marta's areas of improved performance and satisfaction as well as to identify new goals.

(continued)

411

Table 1. Selected Case Examples (cont.)

Case Description	Challenges to Occupational Performance and Mental Health	Occupational Therapy Interventions, With Focus on Mental Health
	• Despite these fears, Marta has a positive attitude and is motivated to work toward her goals. She also has learned some coping strategies she has found to be helpful in dealing with stressful situations.	
Alia, age 36, is employed as a comptroller at a local community college who sustained a right dominant humeral fracture with radial nerve injury in a motor vehicle accident 3 weeks ago. Alia is married and is the mother of four young children. Her husband manages a local sandwich franchise.	• During the initial OT assessment, Alia shared that since graduating from college 12 years ago, she has been employed in her current position. She takes pride in her work and is well respected by her co-workers. When home, Alia enjoys spending time with her children and keeping a tidy home. • According to Alia, she is unable to engage in her roles as worker, mother, and homemaker since her injury. • She cannot return to work or care for her children and home as she would like due to impaired function of dominant hand and arm. • Results of the COPM indicate that Alia is not satisfied with her performance as a homemaker or worker. She reports becoming increasingly anxious and beginning to experience a depressed mood due to her concerns for family finances, social isolation, and need to rely on husband to complete all child care and household chores. • Results of the Adult Self-Perception Profile (Messer & Harter, 1986) indicate that Alia is experiencing a diminished sense of competence in those areas that she feels are very important. The score of the General Self-Efficacy Scale (Jerusalem & Schwarzer, 1992) was 18, indicating a moderate degree of self-efficacy/self-concept.	• The OT allows Alia the opportunity to share her concerns about her future use of her arm and discusses prognosis of condition. The OT then encourages Alia to problem solve about her goals for work, home, and child care. They collaborate on plans for environmental modifications and alternate strategies, techniques, and adaptive equipment/splints that enable Alia to engage in desired activities. • In addition, the OT and Alia contact with worksite to inquire about potential to return to work in a part-time, light-duty capacity.
Qasim, age 29, sustained a spinal cord injury in a diving accident 5 months ago. Qasim works as a carpenter specializing in roofing. He is a husband and the father of two young children. He has recently returned home after spending 3 months in a spinal cord rehabilitation facility.	• The OT assessment includes use of the following tools: the General Self-Efficacy Scale and the Adult Self-Perception Profile. According to the results, Qasim is angry and resentful about his disability status. He is fearful that he will not be able to function in his roles as father and husband and is unsure how he will support himself and his family financially as a person with a disability.	• The OT and Qasim collaborate to identify goals, which include addressing the areas of occupation of child care, social participation, and work. The OT offers Qasim the opportunity to express his concerns for his future roles and invites him to join a spinal cord injury support group.

Table 1. Selected Case Examples *(cont.)*

Case Description	Challenges to Occupational Performance and Mental Health	Occupational Therapy Interventions, With Focus on Mental Health
	• Qasim is experiencing feelings and concerns that are typical to individuals who are facing a permanent change in function due to a major injury. Due to his loss of body functions and roles as family supporter and worker, Qasim acknowledges that he is experiencing a diminished sense of self (concept and confidence) and a depressed and anxious mood. He is losing the ability to engage with others (e.g., peers, customers) in social situations on a daily basis and expresses helplessness and hopelessness about the future. However, he is having difficulty communicating these concerns to family members.	• When Qasim is ready, the OT works with him on several activities, including adapting his environment, setting realistic future goals, and planning and executing many activities to re-build his sense of self-efficacy and reshape his self-concept. One such activity is planning and executing an afternoon outing with his 6-year-old daughter and wife. • The OT also works with Qasim to explore program offerings at the local community college and to set up appointments with the local vocational rehabilitation office and college disabilities counselors.
Bill, age 81, is a retired accountant with severe rheumatoid arthritis who has been moved from an independent-living facility to a skilled-nursing facility. Bill is no longer able to drive and has had to give up the majority of his personal property.	• The occupational profile that included the Rosenberg Self-Esteem Scale (Rosenberg, 1965), reveals that Bill is experiencing a significant loss of self-efficacy due to his inability to be an autonomous individual who freely transports himself to the homes of friends and family. He also is experiencing sadness related to the loss of his treasured family heirlooms, including an antique bed and credenza that could not be taken to the nursing home; these items currently are being kept in a local storage facility. • He has expressed that feelings of loss and a diminished sense of self, confidence, and self-efficacy are causing him to have difficulty engaging in sleep and obtaining adequate rest. He has begun isolating himself in his room and is not socially participating with others. He is experiencing change in social context and loss of daily engagement with friends from previous living situation. The Activity Card Sort, (Baum & Edwards, 2008) revealed that Bill has given up several activities and occupations of interest since he has moved and still has a desire to return to several of them.	The OT collaborates with Bill to identify activities of interest that are offered within the facility. The OT also introduces assistive devices that allow Bill to resume a favorite hobby by compensating for his arthritic impairments and organizes a schedule of events that he can attend at the facility and includes a shuttle schedule that will take him to local events and shopping centers. The OT refers him to a community wellness program led by an OTA. Bill and his OT also work on developing a series of workshops that he will present at the local senior citizens center during tax season.

Note. OT = occupational therapy or occupational therapist, OTA = occupational therapy assistant.

Practitioner Education and Training

Occupational therapists and occupational therapy assistants complete nationally accredited educational programs that prepare them to address the psychological and social aspects of mental health of all their clients. The Accreditation Council for Occupational Therapy Education (ACOTE) standards for accreditation requirements of occupational therapy and occupational therapy assistants educational programs stipulate course work that will enable practitioners to demonstrate knowledge and understanding of (1) human behavior, including behavioral and social sciences; (2) support for the quality of life, well-being, and occupation of the individual, group, or population to promote physical and mental health; and (3) the ability to utilize the therapeutic use of self, which includes one's personality, insights, perceptions, and judgments as part of the therapeutic process (ACOTE, 2007a, 2007b). Coursework must include classes in psychology, abnormal psychology, sociology, or anthropology (ACOTE, 2007a, 2007b). In addition, many occupational therapy practitioners complete fieldwork training in areas where psychological and social factors are explicitly addressed. These settings include psychiatric units and hospitals, substance abuse facilities, prisons, juvenile detention centers, adult day care facilities, community practice, and the school system.

Outcomes

"The benefits of occupational therapy are multifaceted and may occur in all aspects of the domain of concern" (AOTA, 2008, p. 660). Improved occupational performance contributes to self-efficacy and hopefulness about the future. Clients subjective impressions related to performance goals may include improved outlook, confidence, hope, playfulness, self-efficacy, sustainability of valued occupations, resilience, or perceived well-being. These examples of subjective and observable outcomes contribute to improved occupational performance and support health and participation in life through engagement in occupation (AOTA, 2008).

Achievement of psychological and social aspects of mental health through adaptation to change by clients receiving occupational therapy services is a dynamic, nonlinear process that includes working through the initial responses of shock, anger, depression, hostility, and the intermediate coping strategy of denial. Positive mental health occurs when a client is able to acknowledge and positively adjust to their current situation. In cases where change in physical, mental, social, environmental, or health status are permanent, those individuals who can acknowledge and accept their new state, gain a new sense of self-concept, reappraise life value, and seek new meanings and goals will achieve the ultimate goal of adjustment. It is necessary for individuals to re-establish a positive sense of self-worth, realize the existence of remaining and newly discovered potentialities, actively pursue and implement social and vocational goals, and overcome obstacles while working toward those goals (Livneh & Antonak, 1997).

Summary and Conclusion

Supporting clients' engagement in meaningful occupations and routines involves understanding and harnessing individual psychological and social factors in order to promote mental and physical health and recovery and adaptation to their current life situation. An appreciation of the impact of psychological attributes and social capacities within the environment and contexts of the client is the foundation on which all occupational therapy evaluation, intervention, and outcomes are based. The efficacy of occupational therapy intervention is measured by these principles and beliefs in supporting health and participation in life regardless of the specific diagnosis or practice setting (Yerxa, 1967).

References

Accreditation Council for Occupational Therapy Education. (2007a). Accreditation standards for a master's-degree-level educational program for the occupational therapist. *American Journal of Occupational Therapy, 61,* 652–661.

Accreditation Council for Occupational Therapy Education. (2007b). Accreditation standards for educational program for the occupational therapy assistant. *American Journal of Occupational Therapy, 61,* 686–700.

American Occupational Therapy Association. (2006). Policy 1.44: Categories of occupational therapy personnel. In *Policy manual* (2007 ed., pp. 33–34). Bethesda, MD: Author.

American Occupational Therapy Association. (2008). Occupational therapy practice framework: Domain and process (2nd ed.). *American Journal of Occupational Therapy, 62,* 625–683.

American Occupational Therapy Association. (2009). Guidelines for supervision, roles, and responsibilities during the delivery of occupational therapy services. *American Journal of Occupational Therapy, 63,* 797–803.

Bandura, A. (1994). Self-efficacy. In V. S. Ramachaudran (Ed.), *Encyclopedia of human behavior* (Vol. 4, pp. 71–81). New York: Academic Press. (Reprinted in H. Friedman [Ed.], 1998, *Encyclopedia of mental health.* San Diego: Academic Press)

Baum, C. M., & Edwards, D. (2008). *Activity Card Sort* (2nd ed.). Bethesda, MD: AOTA Press.

Bonder, B. (1993). Issues in assessment of psychosocial components of function. *American Journal of Occupational Therapy, 47,* 211–216.

Bonder, B. (1997). Coping with psychological and emotional challenges. In C. Christiansen & C. Baum (Eds.), *Occupational therapy: Enabling function* (pp. 313–334). Thorofare, NJ: Slack.

Brodaty, H., Green, A., & Koschera, A. (2003). Meta-analysis of psychosocial interventions for caregivers of people with dementia. *Journal of the American Geriatrics Society, 51,* 657–664.

Drench, M., Noonan, A., Sharby, N., & Ventura, S. (2007). *Psychosocial aspects of health care* (2nd ed.). Upper Saddle River, NJ: Pearson.

Fidler, G. (1997). Position Paper—The psychosocial core of occupational therapy. *American Journal of Occupational Therapy, 51,* 868–869.

Graff, M., Vernooij-Dassen, M., Thijssen, M., Dekker, J., Hoefnagels, W., & Olde Rikkert, M. (2006). Community-based occupational therapy for patients with dementia and their care givers: Randomized controlled trial. *British Medical Journal, 333,* 1196–1202.

Jerusalem, M., & Schwarzer, R. (1992). Self-efficacy as a resources factor in stress appraisal processes. In R. Schwarzer (Ed.), *Self-efficacy: Thought control of action* (pp. 195–213). Washington, DC: Hemisphere.

Kielhofner, G. (Ed.). (1997). *Conceptual foundations of occupational therapy* (2nd ed.). Philadelphia: F. A. Davis.

Keyes, C. L. (2009). *Toward a science of mental health.* In C. R. Snyder & S. J. Lopez (Eds.), *Handbook of positive psychology* (2nd ed., pp. 89–96). New York: Oxford University Press.

Law, M., Baptiste, S., Carsweel, A., McColl, A., Polatajko, H., & Pollock, N. (2005). *Canadian Occupational Therapy Performance Measure* (4th ed.). Ottawa, Ontario: Canadian Occupational Therapy Association.

Livneh, H., & Antonak, R. (1997). *Psychosocial adaptation to chronic illness and disability.* New York: Aspen.

Meyer, A. (1922). The philosophy of occupational therapy. *Archives of Occupational Therapy, 1,* 1–10.

Mosey, A. (1996). *Psychosocial components of occupational therapy.* Philadelphia: Lippincott-Raven.

Schell, B. A., & Schell, J. W. (2008). *Clinical and professional reasoning in occupational therapy.* Baltimore: Lippincott Williams & Wilkins.

Slagle, E. C. (1924). A year's development of occupational therapy in New York state hospitals. *Modern Hospital, 11*(1), 98–1104.

Smith Roley, S., & DeLany, J. (2008). Improving the *Occupational Therapy Practice Framework: Domain and Process. OT Practice, 14*(2), 9–13.

Taylor, R. R. (2008). *The intentional relationship: Occupational therapy and use of self.* Philadelphia: F. A. Davis.

Wilcock, A., & Townsend, E. (2008). Occupational justice. In E. B. Crepeau, E. S. Cohn, & B. B. Schell (Eds.), *Willard and Spackman's occupational therapy* (11th ed., pp. 192–199). Baltimore: Lippincott Williams & Wilkins.

World Health Organization. (2001). *International classification of functioning, disability and health.* Geneva, Switzerland: Author.

World Health Organization. (2004). *Promoting mental health: Concepts, emerging evidence, practice* [Summary Report]. Geneva, Switzerland: Author.

Yerxa, E. (1967). Authentic occupational therapy [Eleanor Clarke Slagle Lecture]. *American Journal of Occupational Therapy, 21,* 1–9.

Further Reading

American Occupational Therapy Association. (2008). Occupational therapy services in the promotion of health and the prevention of disease and disability. *American Journal of Occupational Therapy, 62,* 694–703.

American Occupational Therapy Association. (2010). Specialized knowledge and skills in mental health promotion, prevention, and intervention in occupational therapy practice. *American Journal of Occupational Therapy, 64.*

Arntson, L., & Knudsen, C. (2004). *Psychosocial care and protection of children in emergencies: A field guide.* Westport, CT: Save the Children Foundation.

Bishop, M. (2005). Quality of life and psychosocial adaptation to chronic illness and acquired disability. *Journal of Rehabilitation, 71*(2), 5–13.

Brodaty, H., Green, A., & Koschera, A. (2003). Meta-analysis of psychosocial interventions for caregivers of people with dementia. *Journal of the American Geriatrics Society, 51,* 657–664.

Bruce, M., & Borg, B. (2002). *Psychosocial frames of reference for occupation-based practice* (3rd ed.). Thorofare, NJ: Slack.

Cara, E., & MacRae, A. (2004). *Psychosocial occupational therapy: A clinical practice* (2nd ed.). Albany, NY: Delmar.

Christiansen, C. H. (1999). Defining lives: Occupation as identity: An essay on competence, coherence, and the creation of meaning [Eleanor Clarke Slagle Lecture]. *American Journal of Occupational Therapy, 53,* 547–558.

Cole, M. (1998). *Group dynamics in occupational therapy* (2nd ed.). Thorofare, NJ: Slack.

Cottrell, R. (2000). *Proactive approaches in psychosocial occupational therapy.* Thorofare, NJ: Slack.

Creek, J. (Ed.). (1997). *Occupational therapy and mental health* (2nd ed.). New York: Churchill-Livingstone.

Fidler, G., & Velde, B. (1999). *Activities: Reality and symbol.* Thorofarc, NJ: Slack.

Given, B., Sherwood, P., & Given, C. (2008). What knowledge and skills do caregivers need? *Journal of Social Work Education, 44,* 115–123.

Graff, M., Adang, E., Vernoouj-Dassen, M., Dekker, J., Jomsson, L., Thijssen, M., et al. (2008). Community occupational therapy for older patients with dementia and their care givers: Cost effectiveness study. *British Medical Journal, 336,* 134–138.

Hellen, C. (1998). *Alzheimer's disease: Activity-focused care.* Boston: Butterworth-Heineman.

Hemphill-Pearson, B. (1999). *Assessments in occupational therapy mental health: An integrated approach.* Thorofare, NJ: Slack.

Lazarus, R. (2006). Emotions and interpersonal relationships: Toward a person-centered conceptualization of emotions and coping. *Journal of Personality 74*(1), 9–46.

Livneh, H. (2001). Psychosocial adaptation to chronic illness and disability: A conceptual framework. *Rehabilitation Counseling Bulletin, 44*(3), 151–160.

Livneh, H., & Antonak, R. (2005). Psychosocial adaptation to chronic illness and disability: A primer for counselors. *Journal of Counseling and Development, 83,* 12–20.

Livneh, H., Martz, E., & Bodner, T. (2006). Psychosocial adaptation to chronic illness and disability: A preliminary study of its factorial structure. *Journal of Clinical Psychology in Medical Settings, 13*(3), 251–261.

Mee, J., & Sumsion, T. (2001). Mental health clients confirm the motivating power of occupation. *British Journal of Occupational Therapy, 64*(3), 121–128.

Polkinghorne, D. E. (1996). Transformative narratives: From victimic to agentic life plots. *American Journal of Occupational Therapy, 50,* 299–305.

Ross, M., & Bachner, S (Eds.). (1998). *Adults with developmental disabilities: Current approaches in occupational therapy.* Bethesda, MD: AOTA Press.

Scott, A. (Ed.). (1998). *New frontiers in psychosocial occupational therapy.* New York: Haworth Press.

Additional Resources

American Occupational Therapy Association. (2008). *FAQ: School mental health.* Retrieved January 7, 2010, from http://www.aota.org/Practitioners/PracticeAreas/Pediatrics/Browse/MH/FAQSchool MH.aspx

American Occupational Therapy Association. (2009). *Fact Sheet: Occupational therapy and school mental health.* Retrieved January 7, 2010, from http://www.aota.org/Consumers/WhatisOT/CY/Fact-Sheets/School-MH.aspx

Authors
Kathleen Kannenberg, MA, OTR/L, CCM
Debbie Amini, EdD, OTR/L, CHT
Kimberly Hartmann, PhD, OTR/L, FAOTA

for

The Commission on Practice
Janet DeLany, DEd, OTR/L, FAOTA, *Chairperson*

Adopted by the Representative Assembly 2010CApr14

Physical Agent Modalities

The American Occupational Therapy Association (AOTA) asserts that physical agent modalities (PAMs) may be used by occupational therapists and occupational therapy assistants in preparation for or concurrently with purposeful and occupation-based activities or interventions that ultimately enhance engagement in occupation (AOTA, 2008a, 2008b). AOTA further stipulates that PAMs may be applied only by occupational therapists and occupational therapy assistants who have documented evidence of possessing the theoretical background and technical skills for safe and competent integration of the modality into an occupational therapy intervention plan (AOTA, 2008b). The purpose of this paper is to clarify the appropriate context for use of PAMs in occupational therapy. It is the professional and ethical responsibility of occupational therapy practitioners to be knowledgeable of and adhere to applicable state laws.

Physical agent modalities are those procedures and interventions that are systematically applied to modify specific client factors when neurological, musculoskeletal, or skin conditions are present that may be limiting occupational performance. PAMs use various forms of energy to modulate pain, modify tissue healing, increase tissue extensibility, modify skin and scar tissue, and decrease edema or inflammation. PAMs are used in preparation for or concurrently with purposeful and occupation-based activities (Bracciano, 2008).

Categories of physical agents include superficial thermal agents, deep thermal agents, and electrotherapeutic agents and mechanical devices.

- *Superficial thermal agents* include but are not limited to hydrotherapy/whirlpool, cryotherapy (cold packs, ice), Fluidotherapy™, hot packs, paraffin, water, infrared, and other commercially available superficial heating and cooling technologies.

- *Deep thermal agents* include but are not limited to therapeutic ultrasound, phonophoresis, short-wave diathermy, and other commercially available technologies.

- *Electrotherapeutic agents* use electricity and the electromagnetic spectrum to facilitate tissue healing, improve muscle strength and endurance, decrease edema, modulate pain, decrease the inflammatory process, and modify the healing process. Electrotherapeutic agents include but are not limited to neuromuscular electrical stimulation (NMES), functional electrical stimulation (FES), transcutaneous electrical nerve stimulation (TENS), high-voltage galvanic stimulation for tissue and wound repair (ESTR), high-voltage pulsed current (HVPC), direct current (DC), iontophoresis, and other commercially available technologies (Bracciano, 2008).

- *Mechanical devices* include but are not limited to vasopneumatic devices and continuous passive motion (CPM).

PAMs are categorized as preparatory methods (AOTA, 2008a) that also can be used concurrently with purposeful activity or during occupational engagement. Preparatory methods support and promote the acquisition of the performance skills necessary to enable an individual to resume or assume habits, routines, and roles for engagement in occupation.

The exclusive use of PAMs as a therapeutic intervention without direct application to occupational performance is not considered occupational therapy. When used, *PAMs are always integrated into a broader occupational therapy program* as a preparatory method for the therapeutic use of occupations or purposeful activities (AOTA, 2008a).

Occupational therapists and occupational therapy assistants must have demonstrated and verifiable competence in order to use PAMs in occupational therapy practice. The foundational knowledge necessary for proper use of these modalities requires appropriate, documented professional education, which includes continuing education courses, institutes at conferences, and accredited higher education courses or programs. Integration of PAMs in occupational therapy practice must include foundational education and training in biological and physical sciences. Modality-specific education consists of biophysiological, neurophysiological, and electrophysiological changes that occur as a result of the application of the selected modality. Education in the application of PAMs also must include indications, contraindications, and precautions; safe and efficacious administration of the modalities; and patient preparation, including the process and outcomes of treatment (i.e., risks and benefits). Education should include essential elements related to documentation, including parameters of intervention, subjective and objective criteria, efficacy, and the relationship between the physical agent and occupational performance.

Supervised use of the PAM should continue until service competency and professional judgment in selection, modification, and integration into an occupational therapy intervention plan is demonstrated and documented (AOTA, 2009).

The occupational therapist makes decisions and assumes responsibility for use of PAMs as part of the intervention plan. The occupational therapy assistant delivers occupational therapy services under the supervision of the occupational therapist. Services delivered by the occupational therapy assistant are selected and delegated by the occupational therapist (AOTA, 2009). When an occupational therapist delegates the use of a PAM to an occupational therapy assistant, both must comply with appropriate supervision and state regulatory requirements and ensure that preparation, application, and documentation are based on service competency and institutional rules. Only occupational therapists with service competency in this area may supervise the use of PAMs by occupational therapy assistants. Occupational therapy assistants may gain competency only in those modalities allowed by state and laws and regulations.

The *Occupational Therapy Code of Ethics and Ethics Standards (2010)* (AOTA, 2010) provides principles that guide safe and competent professional practice and that must be applied to the use of PAMs. The following principles from the *Code and Ethics Standards* are relevant to the use of PAMs:

Occupational therapy personnel shall:

- *Principle 1E:* provide occupational therapy services that are within each practitioner's level of competence and scope of practice (e.g., qualifications, experience, and the law).

- *Principle 1F:* use, to the extent possible, evaluation, planning, intervention techniques, and therapeutic equipment that are evidence-based and within the recognized scope of occupational therapy practice.

- *Principle 1G:* take responsible steps (e.g., continuing education, research, supervision, and training) and use careful judgment to ensure their own competence and weigh potential for client harm when generally recognized standards do not exist in emerging technology or areas of practice.

- *Principle 5:* take responsibility for maintaining high standards and continuing competence in practice, education, and research by participating in professional development and educational activities to improve and update knowledge and skills.

- *Principle 5G:* ensure that all duties assumed by or assigned to other occupational therapy personnel match credentials, qualifications, experience, and scope of practice.

- *Principle 5H:* provide appropriate supervision to individuals for whom they have supervisory responsibility in accordance with AOTA official documents and local, state, and federal or national laws, rules, regulations, policies, procedures, standards, and guidelines. (AOTA, 2010)

References

American Occupational Therapy Association. (2008a). Occupational therapy practice framework: Domain and process (2nd ed.). *American Journal of Occupational Therapy, 56*, 625–683.

American Occupational Therapy Association. (2008b). Physical agent modalities: A position paper. *American Journal of Occupational Therapy, 62*, 691–693.

American Occupational Therapy Association. (2009). Guidelines for supervision, roles, and responsibilities during the delivery of occupational therapy services. *American Journal of Occupational Therapy, 63*, 797–803.

American Occupational Therapy Association. (2010). Occupational therapy code of ethics and ethics standards (2010). *American Journal of Occupational Therapy, 64*, S17–S26.

Bracciano, A. G. (2008). *Physical agent modalities: Theory and application for the occupational therapist* (2nd ed.). Thorofare, NJ: Slack.

Authors

Alfred G. Bracciano, EdD, OTR, FAOTA
Scott D. McPhee, DrPH, OT, FAOTA
Barbara Winthrop Rose, MA, OTR, CVE, CHT, FAOTA

for

The Commission on Practice
Sara Jane Brayman, PhD, OTR/L, FAOTA, *Chairperson*
Adopted by the Representative Assembly 2003M37.
Edited by the Commission on Practice, 2007.

Revised by the Commission on Practice, 2012.
Debbie Amini, EdD, OTR/L, CHT, C/NDT, *Chairperson*
Adopted by the Representative Assembly Coordinating Council (RACC) for the Representative Assembly, 2012.

This revision replaces the 2008 document Physical Agent Modalities. Previously published and copyrighted 2008, by the American Occupational Therapy Association in the *American Journal of Occupational Therapy, 62*, 691–693.

The Role of Occupational Therapy in Wound Management

The American Occupational Therapy Association (AOTA) asserts that the prevention and amelioration of wounds and their impact on daily life occupations are within the scope of occupational therapy practice. Occupational therapists and occupational therapy assistants[1] routinely work with individuals and populations who are at risk for or have sustained wounds.

In the *Healthy People 2020* initiative, the U.S. Department of Health and Human Services (DHHS) called for a 10% reduction in pressure ulcer–related hospitalizations in persons age 65 or older by 2020 (DHHS, 2010), identifying this area as one of significant concern for individuals and society. This position paper serves to inform internal and external audiences, including employers and payer sources, about the role of occupational therapy related to prevention and amelioration of wounds to preserve and restore the ability of the individual to participate in meaningful, desired, and necessary daily life occupations.

Types, Incidence, and Prevalence of Wounds

Wounds, or impaired skin integrities, include abrasions, punctures, bites, surgical wounds, diabetic ulcers, pressure ulcers, traumatic wounds, venous stasis ulcers, and arterial ulcers. Certain populations either exhibit or are at risk for wounds and related complications. These populations include people with spinal cord injuries, cerebral palsy, hand injuries, diabetes, cancer, and burns and those with sensory or mobility impairments, including older adults. For example, the Centers for Disease Control and Prevention (CDC) has reported that in 2006, about 65,700 nontraumatic lower-limb amputations were performed in people with diabetes, representing approximately 60% of all nontraumatic lower-limb amputations (CDC, 2011).

Wounds and related conditions can affect a person's ability to participate fully in all daily life activities. Limitations can occur in performing self-care, work, educational activities, leisure activities, social participation, and rest and sleep. Wounds affect both the physical and the psychological well-being of individuals and can adversely affect quality of life. Pain, depression, social isolation, and anxiety can result from the existence of wounds, particularly those that are chronic in nature (Nogueira, Zanin, Miyazaki, & Godoy, 2009).

In addition, and depending on the location and severity of the wound, a person may also have difficulties with any of the following:

- Management of the wound site, including applying wound care treatments and products to promote healing as well as manage drainage or odor

- Management of clothing and footwear that may no longer fit correctly or that may worsen the wound condition

- Care, use, and application of pressure garments for scar management

---

[1]*Occupational therapists* are responsible for all aspects of occupational therapy service delivery and are accountable for the safety and effectiveness of the occupational therapy service delivery process. *Occupational therapy assistants* deliver occupational therapy services under the supervision of and in partnership with an occupational therapist (AOTA, 2009).

- Engaging in restful sleep due to the presence of pain

- Functional mobility related to the wound site or associated pain

- Engaging in physical activity necessary to prevent impairments in endurance, overall strength, cardio-vascular status, pulmonary status, and cognition

- Social participation, self-efficacy, and reported quality of life resulting from discoloration of the skin, visible scars, contracting or hypertrophic scars, and conspicuous use of compression garments

- Financial stability due to an inability to work

- Maintaining role identity in all aspects of life.

Occupational Therapy's Role in Wound Management

Occupational therapy's perspective on working in this area combines an understanding of the mechanism and progression of acute and chronic wound healing and management, related body functions and structures, positive mental health, and the benefits of participation in everyday activities. Occupational therapy interventions focus on supporting health and participation through engagement in daily life activities and occupations.

The profession of occupational therapy is grounded in the principle that participation in meaningful and relevant life activities leads to life satisfaction, longevity, health, and wellness (AOTA, 2008; Christiansen, 2011). The ability to actively pursue and participate in desired life tasks and activities can be altered temporarily or for sustained periods of time due to the presence of a significant or chronic wound. In addition, diminished engagement in activity and mobility are considered risk factors for pressure ulcer–type wounds, according to the Braden Scale wound risk assessment tool (Bergstrom, Braden, Kemp, Champagne, & Ruby, 1998).

Occupational therapy practitioners[2] understand and appreciate the transactional relationship between client factors, including body functions and structures, and performance skills and performance patterns that are fundamental to participation (AOTA, 2008). When a wound is sustained, such as a severe finger laceration, direct attention to the wound itself as part of the overall occupational therapy intervention may be required to prevent or reduce occupational dysfunction that may occur secondary to this breach in the integumentary system (AOTA, 2010b).

With established service competency, following a plan of care established by an occupational therapist and as allowed by federal and state regulations and third-party payer requirements, the occupational therapy practitioner can utilize preparatory techniques such as the following:

- Application of clean dressings using the principles of moist wound care with both exudating and non-exudating wounds

- Application of wound closure strips

- Removal of sutures and wound closure strips

- Monitoring of wound status

- Mechanical debridement using forceps, cotton-tipped applicators, and wet-to-dry dressings and pulsed lavage

---

[2]When the term *occupational therapy practitioner* is used in this document, it refers to both occupational therapists and occupational therapy assistants (AOTA, 2006).

- Sharp debridement using scalpel or scissors to remove denatured tissue

- Application of appropriate topical agents to facilitate wound healing and debridement

- Application of silver nitrate for reduction of hypertrophic granulation tissue

- Application of enzymatic agents (e.g., collagenase) for debridement

- Application of negative pressure wound therapy

- Application of physical agent modalities such as whirlpool, electrical stimulation, and ultrasound.

This care may be offered as part of a team approach to intervention or in collaboration with the referring physician. In addition, occupational therapy practitioners may provide accommodations while the wound is healing. For example, education and adaptive equipment can allow a client to assist with or perform dressing changes, basic activities of daily living (ADLs), instrumental activities of daily living (IADLs), and tasks within all other areas of occupation.

Occupational therapy practitioners also are skilled in the prevention of wounds for people with various acute and chronic conditions such as spinal cord injuries, burns, lymphedema, cancer, diabetes, hand injuries, and other sensory and mobility impairments. In these cases, individual attention is given to the client's health status, environmental and contextual status, patterns of activity, and lifestyle choices as part of an overall plan to maintain skin integrity. Some interventions focus on the client (persons, organizations, and populations), others address the way activities are performed, and still others seek to change the context or environment that surrounds the client and influences performance. Interventions may focus on treatment of the actual wound, treatment of the resulting dysfunction, or prevention of the wound from occurring.

The following are examples of types of interventions and intervention approaches used in the delivery of occupational therapy services:

- Position the body to alleviate points of pressure including positioning techniques to ensure postural alignment, distribution of weight, balance, and stability.

- Fabricate and provide splints and orthotic devices to protect healing structures, prevent deformity, and secure dressings.

- Recommend support surfaces such as specialized beds and customized wheelchairs, cushions, and seating systems.

- Educate client and caregivers in skin care techniques, including moisture control and dry skin prevention.

- Educate clients and caregivers in precautions and safety techniques for all areas of occupation.

- Modify and adapt the environment for safe functional performance.

- Educate in transfer techniques to minimize risk of skin tears.

- Work with clients to identify ways to incorporate recommended prevention measures into their ongoing daily routines. These measures include pressure-relief activities (techniques and frequency) and pressure reduction equipment such as tilt-in-space wheelchairs and seat cushions.

- Educate clients and caregivers in techniques for donning and doffing pressure garments to manage swelling.

- Utilize specialized techniques for the management of upper-extremity lymphedema.

In addition, occupation-based and purposeful activities are provided and designed to engage the client in tasks that are meaningful and relevant and that support the mind, body, and spirit. Skilled selection of appropriate activities will minimize the detrimental effects of physical inactivity; loss of habits, roles, and routines; and the social isolation that may result from the presence of wounds (AOTA, 2008).

Occupational therapy practitioners recognize that, in addition to neuromusculoskeletal concerns, clients experiencing wounds also may exhibit diminished sense of self and self-efficacy, anxiety, and depression that interfere with their ability to manage currently existing wounds or participate in relevant daily occupations. Individuals who currently do not present with a wound may be at risk due to various lifestyle choices or environmental situations. Occupational therapy practitioners engage the qualities of their personality; verbal and nonverbal communication; listening skills; and empathy to encourage, facilitate, and motivate clients as they seek and achieve personal health, wellness, and occupational participation (AOTA, 2008). Practitioners consider the contextual issues that affect availability and choice with regard to wound care methods and access to tools. Advocacy efforts are initiated by practitioners as appropriate to prevent and treat wounds when individuals are faced with these concerns.

Cultural issues are also considered in the course of occupational therapy intervention. The impact of beliefs and choices is considered and integrated as part of the holistic approach to treatment. For example, parents may prefer that only organic debridement agents be used on their child's wound. An occupational therapy practitioner who is aware of this decision may advocate for the family through a team conference in which a discussion about the use of autolytic debrident versus pharmaceutical agents can take place.

Education

Occupational therapy practitioners are knowledgeable in the areas of human biology and physiology and treatment methods and interventions used as part of wound management. According to the *Accreditation Council on Occupational Therapy Education Standards* (ACOTE, 2012), occupational therapists and occupational therapy assistants must demonstrate knowledge and understanding of the structure and function of the human body to include the biological and physical sciences (B.1.1). They select and provide interventions and procedures to enhance safety, health and wellness, and performance in all areas of occupation (i. e., ADLs, IADLs, work, play, leisure, social participation, education, rest and sleep; B.5.2). In addition, occupational therapy practitioners provide development, remediation, and compensation for physical, mental, cognitive, perceptual, sensory function, neuromuscular, and behavioral skills (B.5.6) and are able to design, fabricate, apply, fit, and train in assistive technologies and devices (e.g., electronic aids to daily living, seating and positioning systems) used to enhance occupational performance and foster participation (B.5.10). Occupational therapy practitioners are able to demonstrate safe and effective application of superficial thermal and mechanical modalities as a preparatory measure to manage pain and improve occupational performance (B.5.15).

Ethical Considerations

The *Occupational Therapy Code of Ethics and Ethics Standards (2010)* (AOTA, 2010a) provides principles that guide safe and competent professional practice in all areas, including wound management. Several principles from the Code and Ethics Standards are particularly relevant to the use of wound management interventions and state that occupational therapy personnel shall

- "Provide occupational therapy services that are within each practitioner's level of competence and scope of practice (e.g., qualifications, experience, the law)" (AOTA, 2010a, p. S19, Principle 1E).

- "Use, to the extent possible, evaluation, planning, intervention techniques, and therapeutic equipment that are evidence-based and within the recognized scope of occupational therapy practice" (AOTA, 2010a, p. S19, Principle 1F).

- "Take responsible steps (e.g., continuing education, research, supervision, training) and use careful judgment to ensure competence and weigh potential for client harm when generally recognized standards do not exist in emerging technology or areas of practice" (AOTA, 2010a, p. S19, Principle 1G).

- "Take responsibility for maintaining high standards and continuing competence in practice, education, and research by participating in professional development and educational activities to improve and update knowledge and skills" (AOTA, 2010a, p. S23, Principle 5F).

- "Ensure that all duties assumed by or assigned to other occupational therapy personnel match credentials, qualifications, experience, and scope of practice" (AOTA, 2010a, p. S23, Principle 5G).

- "Provide appropriate supervision to individuals for whom they have supervisory responsibility in accordance with AOTA official documents and local, state, and federal or national laws, rules, regulations, policies, procedures, standards, and guidelines" (AOTA, 2010a, p. S23, Principle 5H).

All state laws and regulations related to wound management have precedence over AOTA policies and positions.

Table 1 presents case examples of occupational therapy's role in wound management.

Table 1. Case Examples of Occupational Therapy's Role in Wound Management

CLIENT AND BACKGROUND	ASSESSMENT AND FINDINGS	INTERVENTIONS
Geneva, age 68, was referred to an occupational therapist specializing in hand rehabilitation following an extensive palmar fasciotomy resulting from progressive Dupuytren's contracture. A full-thickness skin graft harvested from her volar wrist/forearm was used to close a full-thickness wound on the volar surface of the small finger proximal phalanx and palm that sustained extensive loss of tissue due to long-standing MP and PIP contracture. At the time of the initial occupational therapy evaluation, about 4 days postsurgery, it was noted that the donor site (about 2 cm by 5 cm) was left to heal by secondary intention. Physician orders called for the initiation of a moist wound care regimen following removal of the postsurgical dressing.	Following a saline rinse, the occupational therapy practitioner visually inspected the wound site and measured it using a disposable tape measure. Possible undermining and tunneling were assessed using a sterile cotton swab; no undermining or tunneling were found. The depth of the wound (2 mm) was measured with a tongue depressor and tape measure overlay. Observation of wound color and exudate indicated a clean red wound with early granulation tissue. Exudate was minimal/moderate and clear, as would be expected for this type of donor site. No signs of infection were present. Circumferential measurements were taken of the arm just distal and proximal to the wound; when compared with the noninvolved side, no significant differences were noted. The measurements served as a baseline for levels of edema. An analog pain scale revealed that Geneva had very minimal pain, with a score of 2 on a scale of 1–10. The occupational profile included client-centered assessment tools and outlined areas of occupation of concern to Geneva.	The occupational therapy practitioner initiated moist wound care using hydrogel to maintain an appropriately moist environment for granulation tissue growth. She covered the wound and hydrogel with semipermeable film dressing to ensure adequate oxygenation and minimize the potential for anaerobic bacterial proliferation. A secondary dry gauze dressing was applied to protect the film dressing during splint wear and functional tasks. Geneva was instructed to keep the dressing in place until her next occupational therapy visit, at which time the wound was reassessed and re-dressed as appropriate. Geneva was instructed in modification and adaptation strategies to maintain involvement in areas of occupation such as cooking and gardening, from which she derived significant personal satisfaction. This wound care regimen was administered by the occupational therapy practitioner for 2 weeks until granulation tissue bed was established. Geneva was then instructed to continue with program at home. About 2 weeks later, moist wound care was discontinued, as the wound had epithelialized fully.

(Continued)

Table 1. Case Examples of Occupational Therapy's Role in Wound Management *(cont.)*

CLIENT AND BACKGROUND	ASSESSMENT AND FINDINGS	INTERVENTIONS
Mr. Adams, age 71, was referred to home health care services following a recent fall, resulting in a pelvic fracture; increased BP; and chronic Parkinson's disease. He was discharged home from the ER with no inpatient hospitalization. Upon admission to home care, a Stage II ischial tuberosity ulcer was discovered. According to Mr. Adams, he preferred to stay in a recliner during the day and occasionally sleeps there at night if he doesn't "feel strong." Mr. Adams lives with his daughter and son-in-law, both of whom work during the day. Mr. Adams reported decreased appetite and that family are available to help with bathing if needed. He prefers to wear adult diapers, as he occasionally "cannot get to the toilet in time."	During a visit to the home, the occupational therapist visually assessed the covered wound (a nurse provided documentation of measurements and granulation tissue, and occupational therapy documentation described the type of wound and dressing present). The nurse and occupational therapist collaborated to determine whether the wound dressing was appropriate for Mr. Adams to shower. A hydrocolloid dressing was recommended to the doctor to allow a moist healing environment but provide a waterproof seal to allow bathing and prevent contamination. Upon further visual assessment of skin integrity and evaluation of clinical factors (i.e., decreased mobility with prolonged sitting, occasional incontinence with moistness leading to potential maceration, and decreased nutrition due to poor meal planning), the occupational therapists noted 2 additional reddened areas over bony prominences on the coccyx. In addition, Mr. Adams presented with decreased pain awareness and fragile skin due to decreased weight, which contributed to pressure ulcer formation. The occupational therapist consulted with the nurse case manager to discuss a recommendation for a nutritionist consult, which the nurse followed up on and received from the doctor.	Although the home care nurse initially provided the direct application of the hydrocolloid dressing to the Stage II ulcer and monitored the wound status with photographs and diagrams, the occupational therapist was imperative in the wound care. As the wound began epithelialization, the dressing changes were reduced to every 4 days, and the nurse instructed the family in proper application, which the occupational therapist was able to reinforce during the performance of bathing. The therapist instructed Mr. Adams and his caregivers on the effects of prolonged pressure, shear forces, friction, and incontinence on the development of future ulcers and prevention of healing in the current ulcer. Bathing and toileting were addressed for thoroughness of drying skin as well as techniques for self-inspection. A toileting routine was established. Pressure relief was addressed (Mr. Adams and his caregivers were instructed on changing position every hour, and a chair cushion was introduced for the recliner). Adequate nutrition needs (to assist with healing) were met after meal preparation alternatives were addressed with Mr. Adams, his caregivers, and a nutritionist. The wound was considered healed after full epithelialization, and as the last health care professional involved, the occupational therapist completed proper Medicare documentation and staging of the healed wound.
Tanner, age 10, qualifies for special education services at school due to multiple impairments (e.g., orthopedic, cognitive, visual). As a result of a disability, Tanner is not able to independently change his position to relieve pressure points created by the gravitational pull on his body in any position. Tanner is supported with a customized wheelchair for mobility, adapted stander, and adaptive seating in the school setting to facilitate his highest level of participation in instructional activities. Tanner is recovering from a medical intervention to address a pressure area.	Occupational therapy services evaluated Tanner's participation at school using observation, parent and teacher interviews, and the School Function Assessment (Coster, Deeney, Haltiwanger, & Haley, 1998). From the evaluation process, it was identified that Tanner required alternative positioning options at school to facilitate his highest level of functional participation in the instructional activities presented in this setting. Additionally, the classroom personnel required training on the necessity to provide Tanner with a daily schedule for change in position to facilitate healing of the pressure area.	The occupational therapist provided training for the classroom personnel on how to transfer and position Tanner in the various positioning options provided in the classroom and the functional performance they should expect from Tanner in each option. The therapist also collaborated with the classroom teacher to develop a daily positioning schedule for Tanner while at school that not only facilitated function in the setting but also provided Tanner with a change in position at least every hour. The frequency of positional changes at school was determined in consultation with Tanner's orthopedic surgeon, who is medically managing the pressure area healing process.

(Continued)

Table 1. Case Examples of Occupational Therapy's Role in Wound Management *(cont.)*

CLIENT AND BACKGROUND	ASSESSMENT AND FINDINGS	INTERVENTIONS
Brian,[a] **age 36,** had a complete SCI at the T-8 level 2 years ago as a result of motor vehicle crash. He lives alone and uses a manual wheelchair for mobility. He drives a vehicle adapted with hand controls. He has been employed as a computer programmer and has had a history of pressure ulcers for the past year. Currently, he is admitted to the hospital for a UTI and a Stage 3 pressure ulcer on his left ischial tuberosity.	The rehabilitation team worked with the hospital urologist to determine the cause of Brian's recurrent UTIs. Brian uses intermittent catheterization and may not have always used the safest techniques. The team also reviewed Brian's pressure ulcer history. The pressure ulcer was cultured and treated according to the hospital's protocol, which may include dressings, whirlpool, vacuum-assisted closure, or surgery. Brian remains prone as much as possible while in the hospital. The occupational therapist evaluated Brian's ability to participate in bladder management and work. All equipment pertaining to seating (e.g., wheelchair, cushion) was evaluated for appropriateness, condition, and effectiveness. Pressure mapping may be necessary to find a wheelchair pressure reduction cushion that helps reduce the risk of pressure ulcers.	The occupational therapy practitioner reviewed with Brian strategies for reducing infection during intermittent catheterization. She discussed strategies for continued engagement in work and leisure tasks while he is hospitalized in the prone position. If necessary, Brian's wheelchair will be modified or replaced (if finances are available). Brian will participate in group and individual pressure ulcer prevention and management education sessions and will be provided with a home program to follow. Brian will be instructed on managing the ulcer (surgical site if he had surgery) with dressings and pressure redistribution (weight shifts if he is allowed to sit) during sitting or lying in bed, on nutrition, on transfers, and on sitting tolerance. Home and work site visits are recommended to help Brian identify situations that may be contributing to his recurrent pressure ulcers. He may be referred for home health services while the ulcer heals.

Note. BP = blood pressure; ER = emergency room; MP = metacarpophalangeal; PIP = proximal interphalangeal; SCI = spinal cord injury; UTI = urinary tract infection.

[a]The case study on Brian was contributed by Susan L. Garber, MA, OTR, FAOTA, FACRM.

References

Accreditation Council for Occupational Therapy Education. (2012). Accreditation Council for Occupational Therapy Education (ACOTE™) standards. *American Journal of Occupational Therapy, 66*(Suppl.), S6–S74. http://dx.doi.org/10.5014/ajot.2012.66S6

American Occupational Therapy Association. (2006). Policy 1.44: Categories of occupational therapy personnel. In *Policy manual* (2011 ed., pp. 33–34). Bethesda, MD: Author.

American Occupational Therapy Association. (2008). Occupational therapy practice framework: Domain and process (2nd ed.). *American Journal of Occupational Therapy, 62,* 525–683. http://dx.doi.org/10.5014/ajot.62.6.625

American Occupational Therapy Association. (2009). Guidelines for supervision, roles, and responsibilities during the delivery of occupational therapy services. *American Journal of Occupational Therapy, 63,* 797–803. http://dx.doi.org/10.5014/ajot.63.6.819

American Occupational Therapy Association. (2010a). Occupational therapy code of ethics and ethics standards (2010). *American Journal of Occupational Therapy, 64*(Suppl.), S17–S26. http://dx.doi.org/10.5014/ajot.2010.64S17

American Occupational Therapy Association. (2010b). Scope of practice. *American Journal of Occupational Therapy, 64*(Suppl.), S70–S77. http://dx.doi.org/10.5014/ajot.2010.64S70

Bergstrom, N., Braden, B. J., Kemp, M., Champagne, M., & Ruby, E. (1998). Reliability and validity of the Braden Scale: A multi-site study. *Nursing Research, 47,* 261–269.

Centers for Disease Control and Prevention. (2011). *National estimates and general information on diabetes and prediabetes in the United States, 2011* (National Diabetes Fact Sheet). Atlanta: Author.

Christiansen, C. (2011). The importance of participation in everyday activities. In C. H. Christiansen & K. M. Matuska (Eds.), *Ways of living: Intervention strategies to enable participation* (4th ed., pp. 1–26). Bethesda, MD: AOTA Press.

Coster, W. J., Deeney, T., Haltiwanger, J., & Haley, S. M. (1998). *School Function Assessment.* San Antonio, TX: Psychological Corporation.

Nogueira, G., Zanin, C., Miyazaki, M., & Godoy, J. (2009). Venous leg ulcers and emotional consequences. *International Journal of Lower Extremity Wounds, 8,* 194–196.

U.S. Department of Health and Human Services. (2010, December). OA-10. Reduce the rate of pressure ulcer–related hospitalizations among older adults. In *Healthy People 2020: Summary of objectives.* Retrieved December 29, 2011, from www.healthypeople.gov/2020/topicsobjectives2020/pdfs/OlderAdults.pdf

Additional Resources

Baker, T., Boyce, J., Gairy, P., & Mighty, G. (2011). Interprofessional management of a complex continuing care patient admitted with 18 pressure ulcers: A case report. *Ostomy Wound Management, 57*(2), 38–47.

Blanche, E. I., Fogelberg, D., Diaz, J., Carlson, M., & Clark, F. (2011). Manualization of occupational therapy interventions: Illustrations from the Pressure Ulcer Research Program. *American Journal of Occupational Therapy, 65,* 711–719. http://dx.doi.org/10.5014/ajot.2011.001172

Braden, B., & Bergstrom, N. (1988). *The Braden Scale.* Retrieved June 13, 2013, from http://www.in.gov/isdh/files/Braden_Scale.pdf

Author
Debbie Amini, EdD, OTR/L, CHT

for

The Commission on Practice
Debbie Amini, EdD, OTR/L, CHT, *Chairperson*

Adopted by the Representative Assembly 2012CO19

Note. This document replaces the 2009 Wound Management White Paper.

To be published and copyrighted in 2013 by the American Occupational Therapy Association in the
American Journal of Occupational Therapy, 67(Suppl.).

Scope of Practice

Statement of Purpose

The purpose of this document is to

A. Define the scope of practice in occupational therapy by

1. Delineating the domain of occupational therapy practice that directs the focus and actions of services provided by occupational therapists and occupational therapy assistants;

2. Delineating the dynamic process of occupational therapy evaluation and intervention services used to achieve outcomes that support the participation of clients in their everyday life activities (occupations);

3. Describing the education and certification requirements needed to practice as an occupational therapist and occupational therapy assistant;

B. Inform consumers, health care providers, educators, the community, funding agencies, payers, referral sources, and policymakers regarding the scope of occupational therapy.

Introduction

The occupational therapy scope of practice is based on the American Occupational Therapy Association (AOTA) document *Occupational Therapy Practice Framework: Domain and Process* (AOTA, 2008) and on the *Philosophical Base of Occupational Therapy*, which states that "the understanding and use of occupations shall be at the central core of occupational therapy practice, education, and research" (AOTA, 2006b, Policy 1.11). Occupational therapy is a dynamic and evolving profession that is responsive to consumer needs and to emerging knowledge and research.

This scope of practice document is designed to support and be used in conjunction with the *Definition of Occupational Therapy Practice for the Model Practice Act* (AOTA, 2004b). While this scope of practice document helps support state laws and regulations that govern the practice of occupational therapy, it does not supersede those existing laws and other regulatory requirements. Occupational therapists and occupational therapy assistants are required to abide by statutes and regulations when providing occupational therapy services. State laws and other regulatory requirements typically include statements about educational requirements to practice occupational therapy, procedures to practice occupational therapy legally within the defined area of jurisdiction, the definition and scope of occupational therapy practice, and supervision requirements.

It is the position of AOTA that a referral is not required for the provision of occupational therapy services and that "an occupational therapist accepts and responds to referrals in compliance with state laws or other regulatory requirements"(AOTA 2005a, Standard II.1, p. 664). State laws and other regulatory requirements should be viewed as minimum criteria to practice occupational therapy. Ethical guidelines that ensure safe and effective delivery of occupational therapy services to clients always influence occupational therapy practice (AOTA, 2005b). Policies of payers such as insurance companies also must be followed.

Occupational therapy services may be provided by two levels of practitioners—the occupational therapist and the occupational therapy assistant. Occupational therapists function as autonomous practitioners and are responsible for all aspects of occupational therapy service delivery and are accountable for the safety and effectiveness of the occupational therapy service delivery process.

The occupational therapy assistant delivers occupational therapy services under the supervision of and in partnership with the occupational therapist (AOTA, 2009). When the term *occupational therapy practitioner* is used in this document, it refers to both occupational therapists and occupational therapy assistants (AOTA, 2006a).

Definition of *Occupational Therapy*

AOTA's *Definition of Occupational Therapy for the Model Practice Act* defines *occupational therapy* as

> The therapeutic use of everyday life activities (occupations) with individuals or groups for the purpose of participation in roles and situations in home, school, workplace, community, and other settings. Occupational therapy services are provided for the purpose of promoting health and wellness and to those who have or are at risk for developing an illness, injury, disease, disorder, condition, impairment, disability, activity limitation, or participation restriction. Occupational therapy addresses the physical, cognitive, psychosocial, sensory, and other aspects of performance in a variety of contexts to support engagement in everyday life activities that affect health, well-being, and quality of life. (AOTA, 2004b)

Occupational Therapy Practice

Occupational therapists and occupational therapy assistants are experts at analyzing the performance skills and patterns necessary for people to engage in their everyday activities in the contexts and environments in which those activities and occupations occur. The practice of occupational therapy includes

A. Methods or strategies selected to direct the process of interventions, such as

 1. Establishment, remediation, or restoration of a skill or ability that has not yet developed or is impaired.

 2. Compensation, modification, or adaptation of activity or environment to enhance performance.

 3. Maintenance and enhancement of capabilities without which performance in everyday life activities would decline.

 4. Health promotion and wellness to enable or enhance performance in everyday life activities.

 5. Prevention of barriers to performance, including disability prevention.

B. Evaluation of factors affecting activities of daily living (ADLs), instrumental activities of daily living (IADLs), education, work, play, leisure, and social participation, including

 1. Client factors, including body functions (e.g., neuromuscular, sensory, visual, perceptual, cognitive) and body structures (e.g., cardiovascular, digestive, integumentary, genitourinary systems).

 2. Habits, routines, roles, and behavior patterns.

 3. Cultural, physical, environmental, social, and spiritual contexts and activity demands that affect performance.

 4. Performance skills, including motor, process, and communication/interaction skills.

C. Interventions and procedures to promote or enhance safety and performance in activities of daily living (ADLs), instrumental activities of daily living (IADLs), education, work, play, leisure, and social participation, including

1. Therapeutic use of occupations, exercises, and activities.

2. Training in self-care, self-management, home management, and community/work reintegration.

3. Development, remediation, or compensation of physical, cognitive, neuromuscular, sensory functions, and behavioral skills.

4. Therapeutic use of self, including one's personality, insights, perceptions, and judgments, as part of the therapeutic process.

5. Education and training of individuals, including family members, caregivers, and others.

6. Care coordination, case management, and transition services.

7. Consultative services to groups, programs, organizations, or communities.

8. Modification of environments (e.g., home, work, school, community) and adaptation of processes, including the application of ergonomic principles.

9. Assessment, design, fabrication, application, fitting, and training in assistive technology, adaptive devices, and orthotic devices, and training in the use of prosthetic devices.

10. Assessment, recommendation, and training in techniques to enhance functional mobility, including wheelchair management.

11. Driver rehabilitation and community mobility.

12. Management of feeding, eating, and swallowing to enable eating and feeding performance.

13. Application of physical agent modalities and use of a range of specific therapeutic procedures (e.g., wound care management; techniques to enhance sensory, perceptual, and cognitive processing; manual therapy techniques) to enhance performance skills (AOTA, 2004b).

Scope of Practice: Domain and Process

The scope of practice includes the domain (see Figure 1) and process (see Figure 2) of occupational therapy services. These two concepts are intertwined, with the *domain* defining the focus of occupational therapy and the *process* defining the delivery of occupational therapy (see Figure 3). The domain of occupational therapy is the everyday life activities (occupations) that people find meaningful and purposeful. Within this domain, occupational therapy services enable clients to engage (participate) in their everyday life activities in their desired roles, contexts and environments, and life situations. Clients may be individuals or persons, organizations or populations. The occupations in which clients engage occur throughout the life span and include

- ADLs (self-care activities);

- Education (activities to participate as a learner in a learning environment);

- IADLs (multistep activities to care for self and others, such as household management, financial management, and child care);

- Rest and sleep (activities relating to obtaining rest and sleep, including identifying need for rest and sleep, preparing for sleep, and participating in rest and sleep);

- Leisure (nonobligatory, discretionary, and intrinsically rewarding activities);

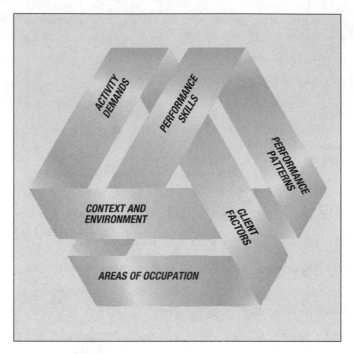

Figure 1. Occupational Therapy's Domain.
Supporting health and participation in life through engagement in
occupation (AOTA, 2008).

- Play (spontaneous and organized activities that promote pleasure, amusement, and diversion);

- Social participation (activities expected of individuals or individuals interacting with others); and

- Work (employment-related and volunteer activities).

Within their domain of practice, occupational therapists and occupational therapy assistants consider the repertoire of occupations in which the client engages the performance skills and patterns the client uses, the contexts and environments influencing engagement, the features and demands of the activity, and the client's body functions and structures. Occupational therapists and occupational therapy assistants use their knowledge and skills to help clients attain and resume daily life activities that support function and health throughout the lifespan. Participation in activities and occupations that are meaningful to the client involves emotional, psychosocial, cognitive, and physical aspects of performance. Participation in meaningful activities and occupations enhances health, well-being, and life satisfaction.

The domain of occupational therapy practice complements the World Health Organization's (WHO) conceptualization of participation and health articulated in the *International Classification of Functioning, Disability and Health (ICF;* WHO, 2001). Occupational therapy incorporates the basic constructs of *ICF*, including environment, participation, activities, and body structures and functions, when addressing the complexity and richness of occupations and occupational engagement.

The process of occupational therapy refers to the delivery of services and includes evaluating, intervening, and targeting outcomes. Occupation remains central to the occupational therapy process. It is client-centered, involving collaboration with the client throughout each aspect of service delivery. During the evaluation, the therapist develops an occupational profile; analyzes the client's ability to carry out everyday life activities; and determines the client's occupational needs, problems, and priorities for intervention.

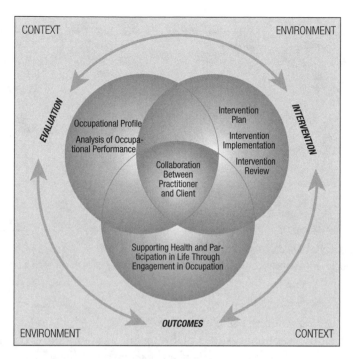

Figure 2. Occupational Therapy's Process.
Collaboration between the practitioner and the client is central to the interactive nature of service delivery (AOTA, 2008).

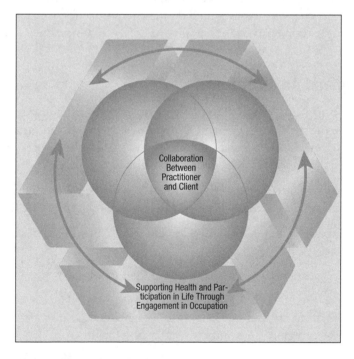

Figure 3. Occupational Therapy.
The domain and process are inextricably linked (AOTA, 2008).

Note: Mobius in figures 1 and 3 originally designed by Mark Dow. Used with permission.

AREAS OF OCCUPATION	CLIENT FACTORS	PERFORMANCE SKILLS	PERFORMANCE PATTERNS	CONTEXT AND ENVIRONMENT	ACTIVITY DEMANDS
Activities of Daily Living (ADL)* Instrumental Activities of Daily Living (IADL) Rest and Sleep Education Work Play Leisure Social Participation	Values, Beliefs, and Spirituality Body Functions Body Structures	Sensory Perceptual Skills Motor and Praxis Skills Emotional Regulation Skills Cognitive Skills Communication and Social Skills	Habits Routines Roles Rituals	Cultural Personal Physical Social Temporal Virtual	Objects Used and Their Properties Space Demands Social Demands Sequencing and Timing Required Actions Required Body Functions Required Body Structures
*Also referred to as *basic activities of daily living (BADL)* or *personal activities of daily living (PADL)*.					

Figure 4. Aspects of Occupational Therapy's Domain.
All aspects of the domain transact to support engagement, participation, and health. This figure does not imply a hierarchy (AOTA, 2008).

Evaluation and intervention may address one or more aspects of the domain (see Figure 4) that influence occupational performance. Intervention includes planning and implementing occupational therapy services and involves therapeutic use of self, activities, and occupations, as well as consultation, education, and advocacy. The occupational therapist and occupational therapy assistant utilize occupation-based theories, frames of reference, evidence, and clinical reasoning to guide the intervention (AOTA, 2008).

The outcome of occupational therapy intervention is directed toward "supporting health and participation in life through engagement in occupations" (AOTA, 2008, p. 660). Outcomes of the intervention determine future actions with the client. Outcomes include the client's occupational performance, adaptation, health and wellness, participation, prevention, quality of life, role competence, self-advocacy, and occupational justice initiatives (AOTA, 2008, pp. 662–663).

Sites of Intervention and Areas of Focus

Occupational therapy services are provided to persons, organizations, and populations. People served come from all age groups. Practitioners work with individuals one to one, in organizations, or at the population level to address occupational needs and issues in mental health, work and industry, rehabilitation, disability and participation, productive aging, and health and wellness.

Along the continuum of service, occupational therapy services may be provided to clients throughout the life span in a variety of settings. The settings may include, but are not limited to, the following:

- Institutional settings (inpatient) (e.g., acute rehabilitation, psychiatric hospital, community and specialty-focused hospitals, nursing facilities, prisons)

- Outpatient settings (e.g., hospitals, clinics, medical and therapy offices)

- Home and community settings (e.g., home care, group homes, assisted living, schools, early intervention centers, day care centers, industry and business, hospice, sheltered workshops, transitional-living facilities, wellness and fitness centers, community mental health facilities)

- Research facilities.

Education and Certification Requirements

To practice as an occupational therapist, an individual

- Must have graduated from an occupational therapy program accredited by the Accreditation Council for Occupational Therapy Education (ACOTE®) or predecessor organizations,[1] and

- Must have successfully completed a period of supervised fieldwork experience required by the recognized educational institution where the applicant met the academic requirements of an educational program for occupational therapists that is accredited by ACOTE® or predecessor organization.

- Must have successfully passed the national certification examination for occupational therapists and/or met state requirements for licensure/registration.

To practice as an occupational therapy assistant, an individual

- Must have graduated from an occupational therapy assistant program accredited by ACOTE® or predecessor organizations, and

- Must have successfully completed a period of supervised fieldwork experience required by the recognized educational institution where the applicant met the academic requirements of an educational program for occupational therapy assistants that is accredited by ACOTE® or predecessor organizations.

- Must have successfully passed the national certification examination for occupational therapy assistants and/or met state requirements for licensure/registration[2].

AOTA supports licensure of qualified occupational therapists and occupational therapy assistants (AOTA, 2004a, Policy 5.3). State and other legislative or regulatory agencies may impose additional requirements to practice as occupational therapists and occupational therapy assistants in their area of jurisdiction.

References

Accreditation Council for Occupational Therapy Education. (2007a). Accreditation standards for a doctoral-degree-level educational program for the occupational therapist. *American Journal of Occupational Therapy, 61,* 641–651.

Accreditation Council for Occupational Therapy Education. (2007b). Accreditation standards for a master's-degree-level educational program for the occupational therapist. *American Journal of Occupational Therapy, 61,* 652–661.

Accreditation Council for Occupational Therapy Education. (2007c). Accreditation standards for an educational program for the occupational therapy assistant. *American Journal of Occupational Therapy, 61,* 662–671.

American Occupational Therapy Association. (2004a). Policy 5.3: Licensure. *Policy manual* (2008 ed., p. 64). Bethesda, MD: Author.

American Occupational Therapy Association. (2004b). Definition of occupational therapy practice for the AOTA Model Practice Act. (Available from the State Affairs Group, American Occupational Therapy Association, PO Box 31220, Bethesda, MD 20824-1220. E-mail: stpd@aota.org)

---

[1] Foreign-educated graduates of occupational therapy programs approved by the World Federation of Occupational Therapy also may be eligible for certification/licensure as an occupational therapist provided that additional requirements are met.

[2] The majority of this information is taken from the *Accreditation Standards for a Doctoral-Degree-Level Educational Program for the Occupational Therapist* (ACOTE, 2007a), *Accreditation Standards for a Master's-Degree-Level Educational Program for the Occupational Therapist* (ACOTE, 2007b), and *Accreditation Standards for an Educational Program for the Occupational Therapy Assistant* (ACOTE, 2007c).

American Occupational Therapy Association. (2005a). Standards of practice for occupational therapy. *American Journal of Occupational Therapy, 59,* 663–665.

American Occupational Therapy Association. (2005b). Occupational therapy code of ethics (2005). *American Journal of Occupational Therapy, 54,* 614–616.

American Occupational Therapy Association. (2006a). Policy 1.44: Categories of occupational therapy personnel. In *Policy manual* (2008 ed., p. 10). Bethesda, MD: Author.

American Occupational Therapy Association. (2006b). Policy 1.11: The philosophical base of occupational therapy. In *Policy manual* (2008 ed., pp. 33–34). Bethesda, MD: Author.

American Occupational Therapy Association. (2008). Occupational therapy practice framework: Domain and process (2nd ed.). *American Journal of Occupational Therapy, 62,* 625–688.

American Occupational Therapy Association. (2009). Guidelines for supervision, roles, and responsibilities during the delivery of occupational therapy services. *American Journal of Occupational Therapy, 63.*

World Health Organization. (2001). *International classification of functioning, disability, and health (ICF).* Geneva, Switzerland: Author.

Additional Reading

Moyers, P., & Dale, L. (Eds.). (2007). *The guide to occupational therapy practice* (2nd ed.). Bethesda, MD: AOTA Press.

Authors
The Commission on Practice:
Sara Jane Brayman, PhD, OTR/L, FAOTA, *Chairperson, 2002–2005*
Gloria Frolek Clark, MS, OTR/L, FAOTA
Janet V. DeLany, DEd, OTR/L
Eileen R. Garza, PhD, OTR, ATP
Mary V. Radomski, MA, OTR/L, FAOTA
Ruth Ramsey, MS, OTR/L
Carol Siebert, MS, OTR/L
Kristi Voelkerding, BS, COTA/L
Patricia D. LaVesser, PhD, OTR/L, *SIS Liaison*
Lenna Aird, *ASD Liaison*
Deborah Lieberman, MHSA, OTR/L, FAOTA, *AOTA Headquarters Liaison*

for

The Commission on Practice
Sara Jane Brayman, PhD, OTR/L FAOTA, *Chairperson*

Adopted by the Representative Assembly 2004C23

Edited by the Commission on Practice 2005

Edited by the Commission on Practice 2009

Note: This replaces the 2004 document Scope of Practice (previously published and copyrighted in 2004 by the *American Journal of Occupational Therapy 58,* 673–677).

Telehealth

The purpose of this paper is to provide the current position of the American Occupational Therapy Association (AOTA) regarding the use of telehealth by occupational therapists and occupational therapy assistants[1] to provide occupational therapy services. This document describes the use of telehealth within occupational therapy practice areas, as described in the existing research. Additionally, occupational therapy practitioner[2] qualifications, ethics, and regulatory issues related to the use of telehealth as a service delivery model within occupational therapy are outlined. Occupational therapy practitioners are the intended audience for this document, although others involved in supervising, planning, delivering, regulating, and paying for occupational therapy services also may find it helpful.

Telecommunication and information technologies have prompted the development of an emerging model of health care delivery called *telehealth*, which involves health care services, health information, and health education. AOTA defines *telehealth* as the application of evaluative, consultative, preventative, and therapeutic services delivered through telecommunication and information technologies. Occupational therapy services provided by means of a telehealth service delivery model can be *synchronous*, that is, delivered through interactive technologies in real time, or *asynchronous*, using store-and-forward technologies. Occupational therapy practitioners can use telehealth as a mechanism to provide services at a location that is physically distant from the client, thereby allowing for services to occur where the client lives, works, and plays, if that is needed or desired (AOTA, 2010d). An overview of telehealth technologies is included in Appendix A. *Telerehabilitation* within the larger realm of telehealth is the application of telecommunication and information technologies for the delivery of rehabilitation services. Key terms related to telehealth and telehealth technologies are defined in Appendix B.

Use of Telehealth Within Occupational Therapy

Occupational therapy practitioners use telehealth as a service delivery model to help clients develop skills; incorporate assistive technology and adaptive techniques; modify work, home, or school environments; and create health-promoting habits and routines. Benefits of a telehealth service delivery model include increased accessibility of services to clients who live in remote or underserved areas, improved access to providers and specialists otherwise unavailable to clients, prevention of unnecessary delays in receiving care, and workforce enhancement through consultation and research among others (Cason, 2012a, 2012b). By removing barriers to accessing care, including social stigma, travel, and socioeconomic and cultural barriers, the use of telehealth as a service delivery model within occupational therapy leads to improved access to care and ameliorates the impact of personnel shortages in underserved areas. Occupational therapy outcomes aligned with telehealth include the facilitation of occupational performance, adaptation, health and wellness, prevention, and quality of life.

---

[1]The *occupational therapist* is responsible for all aspects of occupational therapy service delivery and is accountable for the safety and effectiveness of the occupational therapy service delivery process. The *occupational therapy assistant* delivers occupational therapy services under the supervision of and in partnership with the occupational therapist (AOTA, 2009).

[2]When the term *occupational therapy practitioner* is used in this document, it refers to both occupational therapists and occupational therapy assistants (AOTA, 2006).

Telehealth has potential as a service delivery model in each major practice area within occupational therapy. Note that given the variability of client factors, activity demands, performance skills, performance patterns, and contexts and environments, the candidacy and appropriateness of a telehealth service delivery model "should be determined on a case-by-case basis with selections firmly based on clinical judgment, client's informed choice, and professional standards of care" (Brennan et al., 2010, p. 33). See Appendix C for applications and evidence supporting the use of telehealth within occupational therapy practice areas.

Evaluation Using Telehealth Technologies: Tele-Evaluation

The traditional telephone system continues to be a low-cost alternative for effectively conducting interview assessments by various health care professionals (Cooper et al., 2002; Dreyer, Dreyer, Shaw, & Wittman, 2001; Winters, 2002), and advanced communication technologies have broadened the possibilities for conducting evaluations. Studies have described the use of telehealth in areas that are of concern to occupational therapy, such as evaluation and consultative services for wheelchair prescription (Barlow, Liu, & Sekulic, 2009; Schein, Schmeler, Brienza, Saptono, & Parmanto, 2008; Schein, Schmeler, Holm, Saptono, & Brienza, 2010; Schein et al., 2011), neurological assessment (Savard, Borstad, Tkachuck, Lauderdale, & Conroy, 2003), adaptive equipment prescription and home modification (Sanford et al., 2007), and ergonomic assessment (Baker & Jacobs, 2013).

Clinical reasoning guides the selection and application of appropriate telehealth technologies necessary to evaluate client needs and environmental factors. Therapists should consider the reliability and validity of specific assessment tools when administered remotely. Researchers have investigated the reliability of assessments such as the Functional Reach Test and European Stroke Scale (Palsbo, Dawson, Savard, Goldstein, & Heuser, 2007); the Kohlman Evaluation of Living Skills and the Canadian Occupational Performance Measure (Dreyer et al., 2001); and the FIM™, the Jamar Dynamometer, the Preston Pinch Gauge, the Nine-Hole Peg Test, and the Unified Parkinson's Disease Rating Scale (Hoffman, Russell, Thompson, Vincent, & Nelson, 2008) and found these tools to be reliable when administered remotely through telehealth technologies. In some cases, an in-person assistant, such as a paraprofessional or other support person, may be used to relay assessment tool measurements or other measures (e.g., environmental, wheelchair and seating) to the remote therapist during the evaluation process.

When choosing a telehealth model for conducting an evaluation, occupational therapists need to consider the client's diagnosis, client's preference, access to technology, and ability to measure outcomes when using that model. The occupational therapist may determine that an in-person evaluation is required for some clients. Because of the evolving knowledge and technology related to telehealth, occupational therapists should review the latest research to remain current about the appropriate use of telehealth technologies for conducting evaluations.

Intervention Using Telehealth Technologies: Teleintervention and Telerehabilitation

A telehealth model of service delivery may be used for providing interventions that are preventative, habilitative, or rehabilitative in nature. When planning and providing interventions delivered with telehealth technologies, Scheideman-Miller et al. (2003) reported that the appropriateness and maintenance of the technology and the sustainability of participation by the client are important factors to consider. As related to occupational therapy interventions, some factors to consider include technology availability and options for the occupational therapy practitioner and the client; the safety, effectiveness, sustainability, and quality of interventions provided exclusively through telehealth or in combination with in-person interventions; the client's choice about receiving interventions by means of telehealth technologies; the client's outcomes, including the client's perception of services provided; reimbursement; and compliance with federal and state laws, regulation, and policy, including licensure requirements (Cason & Brannon, 2011).

Consultation Using Telehealth Technologies: Teleconsultation

Teleconsultation is a virtual consultation that includes the

- Expert provider and client,

- Expert provider and local provider with the client present, or

- Expert provider and local provider without the client present.

Teleconsultation uses telecommunication and information technologies for the purpose of obtaining health and medical information or advice.

Teleconsultation has been used to overcome the shortage of various rehabilitation professionals across the United States. For example, an occupational therapist or prosthetist can remotely evaluate and adjust a client's prosthetic device using computer software with videoconferencing capability and remote access to a local clinician's computer screen despite the physical distance between the expert and client (Whelan & Wagner, 2011). Similarly, Schein et al. (2008) demonstrated positive outcomes associated with teleconsultation between a remote seating specialist and a local therapist for evaluating wheelchair prescriptions. The Veterans Health Administration is using teleconsultation for veterans with traumatic brain injuries in a process that involves interactive videoconferencing technology and Web-based management systems (Girard, 2007). In the practice area of pediatrics, Wakeford (2002) used videoconferencing technologies to consult on play performance in children with special needs.

Practitioners should contact state professional licensure boards in their state as well as in the state where the client is located for further clarification on policies related to teleconsultation before rendering services. Some states do have consultation and licensure exemption provisions, although application of the consultation and licensure exemption provisions to facilitate temporary (i.e., consultative) interstate occupational therapy practice using telehealth technologies has not been established (Cason & Brannon, 2011).

Monitoring Using Telehealth Technologies: Telemonitoring

Occupational therapy practitioners can use telehealth technologies to monitor a client's adherence to an intervention program, assist a client in progressing toward achieving desired outcomes, and track and respond to follow-up issues and concerns within a client's natural environments. For example, the Gator Tech Smart House (Mann & Milton, 2005) developed at the University of Florida provides an array of *self-monitoring analysis and reporting technology* (SMART) technologies that monitor and cue clients remotely. Examples include the SmartShoe (Naditz, 2009), which determines fall risk by analyzing walking behavior patterns in a client's own environment and sends the information to a remote site. Similarly, home exercise programs can be monitored remotely using a *haptic* (touch-sensitive) control interface to track a client's hand position while providing resistive forces remotely (Popescu, Burdea, Bouzit, & Hentz, 2000).

Tang and Venables (2000) used smartphones to deliver rehabilitation interventions remotely by using wireless Internet or Intranet access and by providing frequent prompts and cues regarding when and how to complete daily living occupations. Wireless technologies such as these are expanding opportunities for occupational therapy practitioners to implement interventions using telehealth technologies where clients live, work, and play and to provide services throughout the day rather than only within the occupational therapy clinic.

Appendix D provides case examples of how occupational therapy practitioners use telehealth technologies to support health and participation in occupations.

Practitioner Qualifications and Ethical Considerations

AOTA asserts that the same ethical and professional standards that apply to in-person delivery of occupational therapy services also apply to the delivery of services by means of telehealth technologies. Occupational therapy practitioners should refer to the *Occupational Therapy Code of Ethics and Ethics Standards (2010)* (AOTA, 2010a). As stated in this document, occupational therapy practitioners are responsible for ensuring their individual competence in the areas in which they provide services. In addition, Principle 1B of the *Code and Ethics Standards* states that "occupational therapy personnel shall provide appropriate evaluation and a plan of intervention for all recipients of occupational therapy services specific to their needs" (AOTA, 2010a, p. S19). This requirement reinforces the importance of careful consideration about whether evaluation or intervention through a telehealth service delivery model will best meet the client's needs and is the most appropriate method of providing services given the client's situation.

Clinical and ethical reasoning guides the selection and application of appropriate telehealth technology necessary to evaluate and meet client needs. Occupational therapy practitioners should consider whether the use of technology and service provision through telehealth will ensure the safe, effective, appropriate delivery of services. To determine whether providing occupational therapy by means of telehealth is in the best interest of the client, the occupational therapist must consider the following:

- Complexity of the client's condition

- Knowledge, skill, and competence of the occupational therapy practitioner

- Nature and complexity of the intervention

- Requirements of the practice setting

- Client's context and environment.

Additionally, the American Telemedicine Association's "A Blueprint for Telerehabilitation Guidelines" outlines important administrative, clinical, technical, and ethical principles associated with the use of telehealth (Brennan et al., 2010). Occupational therapy practitioners may use various educational approaches to gain competency in using telehealth technologies. They may gain an understanding about basic telehealth service delivery model and telehealth technologies as a part of entry-level education (Standard B.1.8; Accreditation Council for Occupational Therapy Education, 2012) or may participate in continuing education opportunities as clinicians to acquire expertise in this area (Theodorus & Russell, 2008). Examples of ethical considerations related to telehealth are outlined in Table 1.

The *Specialized Knowledge and Skills in Technology and Environmental Interventions for Occupational Therapy Practice* document (AOTA, 2010b) describes the knowledge and skills necessary for entry- and advanced-level practice in technology. Practitioners should have a working knowledge of the hardware, software, and other elements of the technology they are using and have technical support personnel available should problems arise (Schopp, Hales, Brown, & Quetsch, 2003). They should use evidence, mentoring, and continuing education to maintain and enhance their competency related to the use of a telehealth service delivery model within occupational therapy.

Supervision Using Telehealth Technologies

State licensure laws, institution-specific guidelines regarding supervision of occupational therapy students and personnel, the AOTA *Guidelines for Supervision, Roles, and Responsibilities During the Delivery of Occupational Therapy Services* (AOTA, 2009), and the *Occupational Therapy Code of Ethics and Ethics Standards (2010)* (AOTA, 2010a) must be followed, regardless of the method of supervision. Telehealth technologies may be used within those guidelines to the extent that they take into account the unique characteristics of telehealth supervision, to support students and practitioners working in isolated or rural areas (Miller, Miller,

Table 1. Ethical Considerations and Strategies for Practice Using Telehealth Technologies

ETHICAL CONSIDERATIONS	STRATEGIES FOR ETHICAL PRACTICE
Fully inform the client regarding the implications of a telehealth service delivery model versus an in-person service delivery model.	Occupational therapy personnel shall . . .
	"Establish a collaborative relationship with recipients of service including families, significant others, and caregivers in setting goals and priorities throughout the intervention process. This includes full disclosure of the benefits, risks, and potential outcomes of any intervention; the personnel who will be providing the intervention(s); and/or any reasonable alternatives to the proposed intervention." (Principle 3A)
	"Obtain consent before administering any occupational therapy service, including evaluation, and ensure that recipients of service (or their legal representatives) are kept informed of the progress in meeting goals specified in the plan of intervention/care." (Principle 3B)
Abide by laws and scope of practice related to licensure and provision of occupational therapy services using telehealth technologies.	"Occupational therapy personnel shall comply with institutional rules, local, state, federal, and international laws and AOTA documents applicable to the profession of occupational therapy." (Principle 5)
Adhere to professional standards.	Occupational therapy personnel shall . . .
	"Provide occupational therapy services that are within each practitioner's level of competence and scope of practice (e.g., qualification, experience, the law)." (Principle 1E)
	"Take responsible steps (e.g., continuing education, research, supervision, training) and use careful judgment to ensure their own competence and weigh potential for client harm when generally recognized standards do not exist in emerging technology or areas of practice." (Principle 1G)
	"Take responsibility for maintaining high standards and continuing competence in practice, education, and research by participating in professional development and educational activities to improve and update knowledge and skills." (Principle 5F)
	"Occupational therapy personnel shall comply with institutional rules, local, state, federal, and international laws and AOTA documents applicable to the profession of occupational therapy." (Principle 5)
Understand and abide by approaches that ensure that privacy, security, and confidentiality are not compromised as a result of using telehealth technologies.	Occupational therapy personnel shall . . .
	"Ensure that confidentiality and the right to privacy are respected and maintained regarding all information obtained about recipients of service, students, research participants, colleagues, or employees. The only exceptions are when a practitioner or staff member believes that an individual is in serious foreseeable or imminent harm. Laws and regulations may require disclosure to appropriate authorities without consent." (Principle 3G)
	"Maintain the confidentiality of all verbal, written, electronic, augmentative, and nonverbal communications, including compliance with HIPAA regulations." (Principle 3H)
Understand and adhere to procedures if there is any compromise of security related to health information.	Report any breach of security to an appropriate health privacy officer, or seek guidance of an independent legal counsel.

(Continued)

Table 1. Ethical Considerations and Strategies for Practice Using Telehealth Technologies *(Cont.)*

ETHICAL CONSIDERATIONS	STRATEGIES FOR ETHICAL PRACTICE
Assess the effectiveness of interventions provided through telehealth technologies by consulting current research and conducting ongoing monitoring of client response.	Occupational therapy personnel shall . . . "Refer to other health care specialists solely on the basis of the needs of the client." (Principle 1I) "Reevaluate and reassess recipients of service in a timely manner to determine if goals are being achieved and whether intervention plans should be revised." (Principle 1C) "Use, to the extent possible, evaluation, planning, intervention techniques, and therapeutic equipment that are evidence-based and within the recognized scope of occupational therapy practice." (Principle 1F)
Recognize the need to be culturally competent in the provision of services via telehealth, including language, ethnicity, socioeconomic and educational background that could affect the quality and outcomes of services provided.	Occupational therapy personnel shall . . . "Provide services that reflect an understanding of how occupational therapy service delivery can be affected by factors such as economic status, age, ethnicity, race, geography, disability, marital status, sexual orientation, gender, gender identity, religion, culture, and political affiliation." (Principle 4F) "Make every effort to facilitate open and collaborative dialogue with clients and/or responsible parties to facilitate comprehension of services and their potential risks/benefits." (Principle 3J)

Note. HIPAA = Health Insurance Portability and Accountability Act of 1996 (Pub. L. 104–191). Ethical principles are from AOTA's (2010a) *Occupational Therapy Code of Ethics and Ethics Standards (2010).*

Burton, Sprang, & Adams, 2003; Hubbard, 2000). However, practitioners engaged in telehealth supervision should be cautious when relying on legal or other standards that were not necessarily established with telehealth supervision in mind. Factors that may affect the model of supervision and frequency of supervision include the complexity of client needs, number and diversity of clients, skills of the occupational therapist and the occupational therapy assistant, type of practice setting, requirements of the practice setting, and other regulatory requirements (AOTA, 2009). Supervision must comply with applicable state and federal practice regulations, state and federal insurance programs, relevant workplace policies, and the *Occupational Therapy Code of Ethics and Ethics Standards (2010)* (AOTA, 2010a).

Legal and Regulatory Considerations

Occupational therapy practitioners are to abide by state licensure laws and related occupational therapy regulations regarding the use of a telehealth service delivery model within occupational therapy (Cwiek, Rafiq, Qamar, Tobey, & Merrell, 2007). Given the inconsistent adoption and nonuniformity of language regarding the use of telehealth within occupational therapy, it is incumbent upon the practitioner to check a state's statutes, regulations, and policies before beginning to practice using a telehealth service delivery model. Typically, information may be found on state licensure boards' Web sites. The absence of statutes, regulations, or policies that guide the practice of occupational therapy by means of telehealth delivery should not be viewed as authorization to do so. State regulatory boards should be contacted directly in the absence of written guidance to determine the appropriateness of using telehealth technologies for the delivery of occupational therapy services within their jurisdictions. In addition, the policies and guidelines of payers should be consulted. At this time, occupational therapy practitioners are to comply with the licensure and regulatory requirements in the state where they are located and the state where the client is located (Cason & Brannon, 2011).

Occupational therapy practitioners are to abide by Health Insurance Portability and Accountability Act (HIPAA, 1996; Pub. L. 104–191) regulations to maintain security, privacy, and confidentiality of all records and interactions. Additional safeguards inherent in the use of technology to deliver occupational therapy services must be considered to ensure privacy and security of confidential information (Watzlaf, Moeini, & Firouzan, 2010; Watzlaf, Moeini, Matusow, & Firouzan, 2011). Occupational therapy practitioners are to consult with their practice setting's privacy officer or legal counsel or to consult with independent legal counsel if they are in independent or other practice outside of an institutional setting to ensure that the services they provide through telehealth are consistent with protocol and HIPAA regulations.

Funding and Reimbursement

It is the position of AOTA that occupational therapy services provided with telehealth technologies should be valued, recognized, and reimbursed the same as occupational therapy services provided in person. At this writing, Medicare does not list occupational therapy practitioners as eligible providers of services delivered through telehealth technologies. However, AOTA supports the inclusion of occupational therapy practitioners on Medicare's approved list of telehealth providers. The U.S. Department of Defense and Veteran's Health Administration use occupational therapy practitioners for select telehealth programming.

Opportunities for reimbursement exist through some state Medicaid programs; insurance companies; and private pay with individuals, school districts, agencies, and organizations. Medicaid reimbursement is available at the discretion of each state, because it is subject to specific requirements or restrictions within a state. It is recommended that occupational therapy practitioners contact their state Medicaid or other third-party payers to determine the guidelines for reimbursement of services provided through telehealth technologies.

When billing occupational therapy services provided by means of telehealth technologies, practitioners must distinguish the service delivery model, often designated with a *modifier* (Cason & Brannon, 2011). However, regardless of whether the services are reimbursed or the practitioner is responsible for completing paperwork related to billing, the nature of the service delivery as being performed through telehealth should be thoroughly documented.

Summary

Telehealth is a service delivery model that uses telecommunication technologies to deliver health-related services at a distance. Occupational therapy practitioners are using synchronous or asynchronous telehealth technologies to provide evaluative, consultative, preventative, and therapeutic services to clients who are physically distant from the practitioner. Occupational therapy practitioners using telehealth as a service delivery model must adhere to the *Occupational Therapy Code of Ethics and Ethics Standards (2010)* (AOTA, 2010a), maintain the *Standards of Practice for Occupational Therapy* (AOTA, 2010c), and comply with federal and state regulations to ensure their competencies as practitioners and the well-being of their clients.

Occupational therapy practitioners must give careful consideration as to whether evaluation or intervention through a telehealth service delivery model will best meet the client's needs and provide the most appropriate method of providing services given the individual's situation. Clinical and ethical reasoning guides the selection and application of appropriate telehealth technology necessary to evaluate and meet client needs.

References

Accreditation Council for Occupational Therapy Education. (2012). 2011 Accreditation Council for Occupational Therapy Education (ACOTE®) standards. *American Journal of Occupational Therapy, 66*(6, Suppl.), S6–S74. http://dx.doi.org/10.5014/ajot.2012.66S6

American Medical Association. (2011). *CPT 2012.* Chicago: Author.

American Occupational Therapy Association. (2006). Policy 1.44: Categories of occupational therapy personnel. In *Policy manual* (2009 ed., pp. 33–34). Bethesda, MD: Author.

American Occupational Therapy Association. (2009). Guidelines for supervision, roles, and responsibilities during the delivery of occupational therapy services. *American Journal of Occupational Therapy, 63,* 797–803. http://dx.doi.org/10.5014/ajot.63.6.797

American Occupational Therapy Association. (2010a). Occupational therapy code of ethics and ethics standards (2010). *American Journal of Occupational Therapy, 64,* S17–S26. http://dx.doi.org/10.5014/ajot.2010.64S17

American Occupational Therapy Association. (2010b). Specialized knowledge and skills in technology and environmental interventions for occupational therapy practice. *American Journal of Occupational Therapy, 64,* S44–S56. http://dx.doi.org/10.5014/ajot.2010.64S44

American Occupational Therapy Association. (2010c). Standards of practice for occupational therapy. *American Journal of Occupational Therapy, 64,* S106–S111. http://dx.doi.org/10.5014/ajot.2010.64S106

American Occupational Therapy Association. (2010d). Telerehabilitation. *American Journal of Occupational Therapy, 64*(Suppl.), S92–S102. http://dx.doi.org/10.5014/ajot.2010.64S92

Backman, C. L., Village, J., & Lacaille, D. (2008). The Ergonomic Assessment Tool for arthritis: Development and pilot testing. *Arthritis and Rheumatism, 59,* 1495–1503. http://dx.doi.org/10.1002/art.24116

Baker, N., & Jacobs, K. (2010). Tele-ergonomics: A novel approach to computer workstation ergonomic assessment and modification. In *Proceedings of the Human Factors and Ergonomics Society 54th Annual Meeting (2010)* (p. 36). Santa Monica, CA: Human Factors and Ergonomics Society.

Baker, N., & Jacobs, K. (2013). Tele-ergonomics. In S. Kumar & E. Cohn (Eds.), *Telerehabilitation* (pp. 163–174). London: Springer.

Barlow, I. G., Liu, L., & Sekulic, A. (2009). Wheelchair seating assessment and intervention: A comparison between telerehabilitation and face-to-face service. *International Journal of Telerehabilitation, 1,* 17–28. http://dx.doi.org/10.5195/ijt.2009.868

Bendixen, R., Horn, K., & Levy, C. (2007). Using telerehabilitation to support elders with chronic illness in their homes. *Topics in Geriatric Rehabilitation, 23,* 47–51.

Bendixen, R., Levy, C., Lutz, B. J., Horn, K. R., Chronister, K., & Mann, W. C. (2008). A telerehabilitation model for victims of polytrauma. *Rehabilitation Nursing, 33,* 215–220. http://dx.doi.org/10.1002/j.2048-7940.2008.tb00230.x

Bendixen, R., Levy, C., Olive, E., Kobb, R., & Mann, W. (2009). Cost-effectiveness of a telerehabilitation program to support chronically ill and disabled elders in their homes. *Telemedicine and e-Health, 15,* 31–38. http://dx.doi.org/10.1089/tmj.2008.0046

Brennan, D., Tindall, L., Theodoros, D., Brown, J., Campbell, M., Christiana, D., . . . Lee, A. (2010). A blueprint for telerehabilitation guidelines. *International Journal of Telerehabilitation, 2,* 31–34. http://dx.doi.org/10.5195/ijt.2010.6063

Brewer, B. R., Fagan, M., Klatzky, R. L., & Matsuoka, Y. (2005). Perceptual limits for a robotic rehabilitation environment using visual feedback distortion. *IEEE Transactions on Neural Systems and Rehabilitation Engineering, 13,* 1–11. http://dx.doi.org/10.1109/TNSRE.2005.843443

Bruce, C., & Sanford, J. A. (2006). Development of an evidence-based conceptual framework for workplace assessment. *Work, 27,* 381–389.

Cason, J. (2009). A pilot telerehabilitation program: Delivering early intervention services to rural families. *International Journal of Telerehabilitation, 1,* 29–38. http://dx.doi.org/10.5195/ijt.2009.6007

Cason, J. (2011). Telerehabilitation: An adjunct service delivery model for early intervention services. *International Journal of Telerehabilitation, 3,* 19–28. http://dx.doi.org/10.5195/ijt.2011.6071

Cason, J. (2012a). An introduction to telehealth as a service delivery model within occupational therapy. *OT Practice, 17*(7), CE1–CE8.

Cason, J. (2012b). Telehealth opportunities in occupational therapy through the Affordable Care Act. *American Journal of Occupational Therapy, 66,* 131–136. http://dx.doi.org/10.5014/ajot.2012.662001

Cason, J., & Brannon, J. A. (2011). Telehealth regulatory and legal considerations: Frequently asked questions. *International Journal of Telerehabilitation, 3,* 15–18. http://dx.doi.org/10.5195/ijt.2011.6077

Chumbler, N., Quigley, P., Sanford, J., Griffiths, P., Rose, D., Morey, M., . . . Hoenig, H. (2010). Implementing telerehabilitation research for stroke rehabilitation with community dwelling veterans: Lessons learned. *International Journal of Telerehabilitation, 2,* 15–21. http://dx.doi.org/10.5195/ijt.2010.6047

Cooper, R., Fitzgerald, S., Boninger, M. L., Cooper, R. A., Shapcott, N., & Cohen, L. (2002). Using telerehabilitation to aid in selecting a wheelchair. In R. Simpson (Ed.), *RESNA 2002 annual conference proceedings* (pp. 245–247). Minneapolis, MN: RESNA Press.

Cwiek, M. A., Rafiq, A., Qamar, A., Tobey, C., & Merrell, R. C. (2007). Telemedicine licensure in the United States: The need for a cooperative regional approach. *Telemedicine and e-Health, 13,* 141–147. http://dx.doi.org/10.1089/tmj.2006.0029

Darkins, A., Ryan, P., Kobb, R., Forster, L., Edmonson, E., Wakefield, B., & Lancaster, A. E. (2008). Care coordination/home telehealth: The systematic implementation of health informatics, home telehealth, and disease management to support the care of veteran patients with chronic conditions. *Telemedicine and e-Health, 14,* 1118–1126. http://dx.doi.org/10.1089/tmj.2008.0021

Diamond, B. J., Shreve, G. M., Bonilla, J. M., Johnston, M. V., Morodan, J., & Branneck, R. (2003). Telerehabilitation, cognition and user accessibility. *NeuroRehabilitation, 18,* 171–177.

Dreyer, N. C., Dreyer, K. A., Shaw, D. K., & Wittman, P. P. (2001). Efficacy of telemedicine in occupational therapy: A pilot study. *Journal of Allied Health, 30,* 39–42.

Federal Communications Commission. (2010). *Voice-over-Internet protocol.* Retrieved from www.fcc.gov/voip/

Forducey, P. G., Ruwe, W. D., Dawson, S. J., Scheideman-Miller, C., McDonald, N. B., & Hantla, M. R. (2003). Using telerehabilitation to promote TBI recovery and transfer of knowledge. *NeuroRehabilitation, 18,* 103–111.

Gallagher, T. E. (2004). Augmentation of special-needs services and information to students and teachers "ASSIST"—A telehealth innovation providing school-based medical interventions. *Hawaii Medical Journal, 63,* 300–309.

Germain, V., Marchand, A., Bouchard, S., Drouin, M. S., & Guay, S. (2009). Effectiveness of cognitive behavioural therapy administered by videoconference for posttraumatic stress disorder. *Cognitive Behaviour Therapy, 38,* 42–53. http://dx.doi.org/10.1080/16506070802473494

Girard, P. (2007). Military and VA telemedicine systems for patients with traumatic brain injury. *Journal of Rehabilitation Research and Development, 44,* 1017–1026. http://dx.doi.org/10.1682/JRRD.2006.12.0174

Gros, D. F., Yoder, M., Tuerk, P. W., Lozano, B. E., & Acierno, R. (2011). Exposure therapy for PTSD delivered to veterans via telehealth: Predictors of treatment completion and outcome and comparison to treatment delivered in person. *Behavior Therapy, 42,* 276–283. http://dx.doi.org/10.1016/j.beth.2010.07.005

Harada, N. D., Dhanani, S., Elrod, M., Hahn, T., Kleinman, L., & Fang, M. (2010). Feasibility study of home telerehabilitation for physically inactive veterans. *Journal of Rehabilitation Research and Development, 47*, 465–475. http://dx.doi.org/10.1682/JRRD.2009.09.0149

Harrison, A., Derwent, G., Enticknap, A., Rose, F. D., & Attree, E. A. (2002). The role of virtual reality technology in the assessment and training of inexperienced powered wheelchair users. *Disability and Rehabilitation, 24*, 599–606. http://dx.doi.org/10.1080/09638280110111360

Health Insurance Portability and Accountability Act, Pub. L. 104–191, 101 Stat. 1936 (1996).

Hegel, M. T., Lyons, K. D., Hull, J. G., Kaufman, P., Urguhart, L., Li, Z., & Ahles, T. A. (2011). Feasibility study of a randomized controlled trial of a telephone-delivered problem solving occupational therapy intervention to reduce participation restrictions in rural breast cancer survivors undergoing chemotherapy. *Psycho-Oncology, 20*, 1092–1101. http://dx.doi.org/10.1002/pon.1830

Heimerl, S., & Rasch, N. (2009). Delivering developmental occupational therapy consultation services through telehealth. *Developmental Disabilities Special Interest Section Quarterly, 32*(3), 1–4.

Hermann, V. H., Herzog, M., Jordan, R., Hofherr, M., Levine, P., & Page, S. J. (2010). Telerehabilitation and electrical stimulation: An occupation-based, client-centered stroke intervention. *American Journal of Occupational Therapy, 64*, 73–81. http://dx.doi.org/10.5014/ajot.64.1.73

Hoffman, H. G., Patterson, D. R., & Carrougher, G. J. (2000). Use of virtual reality for adjunctive treatment of adult burn pain during physical therapy: A controlled study. *Clinical Journal of Pain, 16*, 244–250. http://dx.doi.org/10.1097/00002508-200009000-00010

Hoffmann, T., Russell, T., Thompson, L., Vincent, A., & Nelson, M. (2008). Using the Internet to assess activities of daily living and hand function in people with Parkinson's disease. *NeuroRehabilitation, 23*, 253–261.

Hori, M., Kubota, M., Kihara, T., Takahashi, R., & Kinoshita, A. (2009). The effect of videophone communication (with Skype and webcam) for elderly patients with dementia and their caregivers. *Gan To Kagaku Ryoho, 36S*, 36–38. Retrieved from www.ncbi.nlm.nih.gov/pubmed/20443395

Hubbard, S. (2000, December 4 & 18). A case example of remote supervision. *OT Practice, 5*, 16–18.

Individuals With Disabilities Education Act Amendments of 1997, Pub. L. 105–117, 20 U.S.C. § 1400 *et seq.*

Kairy, D., Lehoux, P., Vincent, C., & Visintin, M. (2009). A systematic review of clinical outcomes, clinical process, healthcare utilization and costs associated with telerehabilitation. *Disability and Rehabilitation, 31*, 427–47. http://dx.doi.org/10.1080/09638280802062553

Kelso, G., Fiechtl, B., Olsen, S., & Rule, S. (2009). The feasibility of virtual home visits to provide early intervention: A pilot study. *Infants and Young Children, 22*, 332–340. http://dx.doi.org/10.1097/IYC.0b013e3181b9873c

Kim, J. B., & Brienza, D. M. (2006). Development of a remote accessibility assessment system through three-dimensional reconstruction technology. *Journal of Rehabilitation Research and Development, 43*, 257–272. http://dx.doi.org/10.1682/JRRD.2004.12.0163

Kim, J. B., Brienza, D. M., Lynch, R. D., Cooper, R. A., & Boninger, M. L. (2008). Effectiveness evaluation of a remote accessibility assessment system for wheelchair users using virtualized reality. *Archives of Physical Medicine and Rehabilitation, 89*, 470–479. http://dx.doi.org/10.1016/j.apmr.2007.08.158

Lewis, J. A., Boian, R. F., Burdea, G., & Deutsch, J. E. (2005). Remote console for virtual telerehabilitation. *Studies in Health Technology and Informatics, 111*, 294–300.

Lewis, J. A., Deutsch, J. E., & Burdea, G. (2006). Usability of the remote console for virtual reality telerehabilitation: Formative evaluation. *Cyberpsychology and Behavior, 9*, 142–147. http://dx.doi.org/10.1089/cpb.2006.9.142

450

Mann, W. C., & Milton, B. R. (2005). Home automation and SMART homes to support independence. In W. C. Mann (Ed.), *Smart technology for aging, disability, and independence* (pp. 33–66). Hoboken, NJ: Wiley.

Merians, A. S., Jack, D., Boian, R., Tremaine, M., Burdea, G. C., Adamovich, S. V., . . . Poizner, H. (2002). Virtual reality–augmented rehabilitation for patients following stroke. *Physical Therapy, 82,* 898–915.

Miller, T. W., Miller, J. M., Burton, D., Sprang, R., & Adams, J. (2003). Telehealth: A model for clinical supervision in allied health. *Internet Journal of Allied Health Sciences and Practice, 1*(2), 1–8.

Naditz, A. (2009). Still standing: Telemedicine devices and fall prevention. *Telemedicine and e-Health, 15,* 137–141. http://dx.doi.org/10.1089/tmj.2009.9989

Neubeck, L., Redfern, J., Fernandez, R., Briffad, T., Bauman, A., & Freedman, S. B. (2009). Telehealth interventions for the secondary prevention of coronary heart disease: A systematic review. *European Journal of Preventive Cardiology, 16,* 281–289. http://dx.doi.org/0.1097/HJR.0b013e32832a4e7a

Palsbo, S. E., Dawson, S. J., Savard, L., Goldstein, M., & Heuser, A. (2007). Televideo assessment using Functional Reach Test and European Stroke Scale. *Journal of Rehabilitation Research and Development, 44,* 659–664. http://dx.doi.org/10.1682/JRRD.2006.11.0144

Popescu, V. G., Burdea, G. C., Bouzit, M., & Hentz, V. R. (2000). A virtual-reality-based telerehabilitation system with force feedback. *IEEE Transactions on Information Technology in Biomedicine, 4,* 45–51. http://dx.doi.org/10.1109/4233.826858

Rand, D., Katz, N., & Weiss, P. L. (2009). Intervention using the VMall for improving motor and functional ability of the upper extremity in poststroke participants. *European Journal of Physical and Rehabilitation Medicine, 45,* 113–121.

Rand, D., Kizony, R., & Weiss, P. T. (2008). The Sony PlayStation II EyeToy: Low-cost virtual reality for use in rehabilitation. *Journal of Neurologic Physical Therapy, 32,* 155–163. http://dx.doi.org/10.1097/NPT.0b013e31818ee779

Rand, D., Weiss, P. L., & Katz, N. (2009). Training multitasking in a virtual supermarket: A novel intervention after stroke. *American Journal of Occupational Therapy, 63,* 535–542. http://dx.doi.org/10.5014/ajot.63.5.535

Sanford, J., Hoenig, H., Griffiths, P., Butterfield, T., Richardson, P., & Hargraves, K. (2007). A comparison of televideo and traditional in-home rehabilitation in mobility impaired older adults. *Physical and Occupational Therapy in Geriatrics, 25,* 1–18. http://dx.doi.org/10.1080/J148v25n03_01

Savard, L., Borstad, A., Tkachuck, J., Lauderdale, D., & Conroy, B. (2003). Telerehabilitation consultations for clients with neurologic diagnoses: Cases from rural Minnesota and American Samoa. *NeuroRehabilitation, 18,* 93–102.

Scheideman-Miller, C., Clark, P. G., Moorad, A., Post, M. L., Hodge, B. G., & Smeltzer, S. (2003, January). Efficacy and sustainability of a telerehabilitation program. In *Proceedings of the 36th Annual Hawaii International Conference on System Sciences* (pp. 11–21). Washington, DC: IEEE Computer Society.

Schein, R. M., Schmeler, M. R., Brienza, D., Saptono, A., & Parmanto, B. (2008). Development of a service delivery protocol used for remote wheelchair consultation via telerehabilitation. *Telemedicine and e-Health, 14,* 932–938.

Schein, R. M., Schmeler, M. R., Holm, M. B., Pramuka, M., Saptono, A., & Brienza, D. M. (2011). Telerehabilitation assessment using the Functioning Everyday with a Wheelchair-Capacity instrument. *Journal of Rehabilitation Research and Development, 48,* 115–124. http://dx.doi.org/10.1682/JRRD.2010.03.0039

Schein, R. M., Schmeler, M. R., Holm, M. B., Saptono, A., & Brienza, D. M. (2010). Telerehabilitation wheeled mobility and seating assessments compared with in person. *Archives of Physical Medicine and Rehabilitation, 91,* 874–878. http://dx.doi.org/10.1016/j.apmr.2010.01.017

Schopp, L. H., Hales, J. W., Brown, G. D., & Quetsch, J. L. (2003). A rationale and training agenda for rehabilitation informatics: Roadmap for an emerging discipline. *NeuroRehabilitation, 18,* 159–170.

Sheridan, T. B. (1992). Musings on telepresence and virtual presence. *Presence, 1,* 120–125.

Steel, K., Cox, D., & Garry, H. (2011). Therapeutic videoconferencing interventions for the treatment of long-term conditions. *Journal of Telemedicine and Telecare, 17,* 109–117. http://dx.doi.org/10.1258/jtt.2010.100318

Tang, P., & Venables, T. (2000). "Smart" homes and telecare for independent living. *Journal of Telemedicine and Telecare, 6,* 8–14. http://dx.doi.org/10.1258/1357633001933871

Theodorus, D., & Russell, T. (2008). Telerehabilitation: Current perspectives. *Current Principles and Practices of Telemedicine and e-Health, 131,* 191–209.

Verburg, G., Borthwick, B., Bennett, B., & Rumney, P. (2003). Online support to facilitate the reintegration of students with brain injury: Trials and errors. *NeuroRehabilitation, 18,* 113–123.

Wakeford, L. (2002, November 25). Telehealth technology for children with special needs. *OT Practice, 7,* 12–16.

Watzlaf, V., Moeini, S., & Firouzan, P. (2010). VoIP for telerehabilitation: A risk analysis for privacy, security, and HIPAA compliance, Part I. *International Journal of Telerehabilitation, 2,* 3–14. http://dx.doi.org/10.5195/ijt.2010.6056

Watzlaf, V., Moeini, S., Matusow, L., & Firouzan, P. (2011). VoIP for telerehabilitation: A risk analysis for privacy, security, and HIPAA compliance, Part II. *International Journal of Telerehabilitation, 3,* 3–10. http://dx.doi.org/10.5195/ijt.2011.6070

Weiss, P. L., & Jessel, A. S. (1998). Virtual reality applications to work. *Work, 11,* 277–293.

Whelan, L., & Wagner, N. (2011). Technology that touches lives: Teleconsultation to benefit persons with upper limb loss. *International Journal of Telerehabilitation, 3,* 19–22. http://dx.doi.org/10.5195/ijt.2011.6080

Winters, J. M. (2002). Telerehabilitation research: Emerging opportunities. *Annual Review of Biomedical Engineering, 4,* 287–320. http://dx.doi.org/10.1146/annurev.bioeng.4.112801.121923

Additional Resources

American Telemedicine Association's Telerehabilitation Special Interest Group/Resources, www.americantelemed.org/i4a/pages/index.cfm?pageid=3328

Center for Telehealth and e-Health Law (CTel), http://ctel.org/

International Journal of Telerehabilitation, http://telerehab.pitt.edu/ojs/index.php/telerehab

Journal of Telemedicine and Telecare, http://jtt.rsmjournals.com/

Rehabilitation Engineering Research Center for Telerehabilitation, www.rerctr.pitt.edu

Telehealth Resource Centers, http://www.telehealthresourcecenter.org/

Telemedicine and e-Health, www.liebertpub.com/TMJ

Authors
Jana Cason, DHS, OTR/L, FAOTA
Kim Hartmann, PhD, OTR/L, FAOTA
Karen Jacobs, EdD, CPE, OTR/L, FAOTA
Tammy Richmond, MS, OTR/L, FAOTA

for

The Commission on Practice
Debbie Amini, EdD, OTR/L, CHT, *Chairperson*

The COP would like to acknowledge the contributions of the authors of the 2010 Telerehabilitation
Position Paper:
Mark R. Schmeler, PhD, OTR/L, ATP
Richard M. Schein, PhD
Andrea Fairman, MOT, OTR/L, CPRP
Amanda Brickner, MOT, OTR/L
William C. Mann, PhD, OTR

Adopted by the Representative Assembly Coordinating Council (RACC) for the Representative Assembly, 2012.

Revised by the Commission on Practice 2012.

Note. This revision replaces the 2010 document *Telerehabilitation Position Paper,* previously published and copyrighted
2010 by the American Occupational Therapy Association in the *American Journal of Occupational Therapy, 64,* S92–S102.
http://dx.doi.org/10.5014/ajot.2010.64S92

To be published and copyrighted in 2013 by the American Occupational Therapy Association in the *American Journal
of Occupational Therapy, 67*(Suppl.).

Appendix A. Overview of Telehealth Technologies

Synchronous Technologies: Videoconferencing

Synchronous technologies enable the exchange of health information in *real time* (i.e., live) by interactive audio and video between the patient or client and a health care provider located at a distant site. Several options for videoconferencing are available; they include voice over the Internet protocol (VoIP) services, mobile videoconferencing systems, "plain old telephone service" (POTS), videoconferencing, and high-definition television (HDTV) technologies (see Table A1).

VoIP services use a computer, special VoIP phone, or traditional phone with adapter to convert voice into a digital signal that travels over the Internet (Federal Communications Commission, 2010). Integrated with video software, VoIP provides a mechanism for Internet-based videoconferencing. Similarly, mobile videoconferencing uses a mobile device (e.g., smartphone, electronic tablet) with videoconferencing capabilities to transmit audio and video over a wireless or cellular network. POTS videoconferencing primarily uses an analog telephone line or landline to support audio and video transmission through a videophone or specialized equipment connected to a television. HDTV videoconferencing requires an HD television, console, HD camera, remote control, and high-speed broadband connection at both locations. Unlike the technologies described above and marketed for consumer use, telehealth networks use high-end videoconferencing technologies (e.g., Polycom, Tandberg) and fiber-optic telephone lines (e.g., T1 lines) or high-speed Internet to connect sites.

Advantages of VoIP, mobile, POTS, and consumer HDTV technologies include service provision within the context where occupations naturally occur (e.g., home, work, community), minimal infrastructure requirements, and lower costs for equipment and connectivity (e.g., residential service plan, data plan). Disadvantages may include privacy, security, and confidentiality risks; lack of infrastructure (e.g., limited access to high-speed Internet/broadband; inadequate bandwidth for connectivity); recurring expense (e.g., residential service plan, data plan); diminished sound or image quality; and technological challenges associated with end-user experience and expertise with videoconferencing technology (Cason, 2011; see Table A1).

Asynchronous Technologies

Telehealth applications that are asynchronous, commonly referred to as "store-and-forward" data transmission, may include video clips, digital photographs, virtual technologies, and other forms of electronic communications. With *asynchronous technologies*, the provider and client are not connected at the same time. Potential applications for asynchronous telehealth technologies within occupational therapy include home assessments and recommendations for home modifications that are based on recorded data of the home environment; recommendations for inclusion of ergonomic principles and workstation modifications that are based on recorded data of the work environment; and secure viewing of video segments for evaluation and intervention purposes.

Technologies That May Be Synchronous or Asynchronous

Telemonitoring Technologies

Occupational therapy practitioners providing services through telehealth technologies can take advantage of self-monitoring analysis and reporting technology (SMART) to monitor a client's occupational performance within the home and community. SMART technologies that are wireless allow the occupational therapy practitioner to provide services within varied environments without restricting the client's movements within those environments. These technologies provide information that allows an offsite occupational therapy practitioner to assess performance and modify services and the environment and also enable occupational therapy practitioners to understand the real-life occupations and performance challenges of the client and to plan appropriate interventions. As a result, occupational therapy practitioners can tailor environmental accommodations for clients with physical limitations or can develop individualized technology-based cueing systems for clients with cognitive disabilities so that they can live more independently.

Virtual Reality Technologies

Virtual reality (VR) typically refers to the use of interactive simulations created with computer hardware and software to present users with opportunities to engage in environments that appear and feel similar to real-world objects and events (Sheridan, 1992; Weiss & Jessel, 1998). Although typical use of VR technologies does not constitute a telehealth service delivery model, live data (synchronous) streamed to a remote occupational therapy practitioner or recorded data (asynchronous) used by an occupational therapy practitioner to monitor and adjust a client's course of treatment would constitute the use of VR technologies within a telehealth service delivery model. Occupational therapy practitioners can use a telehealth service delivery model with VR technologies when conducting evaluations and providing interventions. A remote console telerehabilitation system (ReCon, Rutgers University, New Brunswick, NJ) incorporating VR technology provides occupational therapy practitioners with three-dimensional representations of the client's movements, VR-based exercise progress, and motor performance updates (Lewis, Boian, Burdea, & Deutsch, 2005; Lewis, Deutsch, & Burdea, 2006). Telehealth combined with VR has been used to provide feedback and information remotely as part of occupational therapy intervention (Merians et al., 2002), to distract people from physical pain, and to improve their adherence to therapeutic exercises (Hoffman, Patterson, & Carrougher, 2000).

Further, VR provided through telehealth technologies is effective in enabling people to compare the difference between their desired level of occupational engagement and their current functional status after a stroke (Brewer, Fagan, Klatzky, & Matsuoka, 2005; Merians et al., 2002; Rand, Katz, & Weiss, 2009; Rand, Weiss, & Katz, 2009), using virtual environments as part of the assessment and training of users of power wheelchairs (Harrison, Derwent, Enticknap, Rose, & Attree, 2002), and evaluating and determining home accessibility using three-dimensional construction of the architectural features of the environment (Kim & Brienza, 2006; Kim, Brienza, Lynch, Cooper, & Boninger, 2008).

Low-cost video capture gaming systems (e.g., Nintendo Wii, Sony Playstation's EyeToy and MOVE, XBOX-360 Kinect) were not developed specifically for rehabilitation, but they offer an easy-to-set-up, fun, and less expensive alternative to the expensive VR systems (Rand, Kizony, & Weiss, 2008). Although typical use of gaming systems does not constitute telehealth, live data (synchronous) streamed to a remote occupational therapy practitioner or recorded data (asynchronous) used by an occupational therapy practitioner to monitor and adjust a client's course of treatment would constitute a telehealth application of the devices.

Table A1. Telehealth Technologies

TECHNOLOGY TYPE	EXAMPLES	CONSIDERATIONS
Synchronous	• Voice over Internet protocol software • Mobile videoconferencing • Consumer high-definition television videoconferencing • "Plain old telephone service" • Videoconferencing • Telehealth network with commercial videoconferencing system • Virtual reality (VR) technologies (with live-streaming data to remote practitioner)	• Confidentiality (security, privacy) • Integrity (information protected from changes by unauthorized users) • Availability (information, services) • Cost–benefit ratio • Socioeconomic considerations • Leveraging existing infrastructure (equipment and personnel) • Technology connection requirements (e.g., broadband, T1 line) • Sound and image quality
Asynchronous	• Video recording devices • Cameras (photographs) • Devices enabling electronic communication • VR technologies (with store-and-forward data to remote practitioner)	• Equipment accessibility • Provider and end-user comfort, experience, and expertise with technology
Synchronous (interactive) or asynchronous (store-and-forward data)	• Telemonitoring technologies – Home monitoring systems/devices – Wireless sensors • VR technologies – Remote use of VR systems/devices	

Note. From "Telerehabilitation: An Adjunct Service Delivery Model for Early Intervention Services," by J. Cason, 2011, *International Journal of Telerehabilitation, 3*(1), p. 24. http://dx.doi.org/10.5195/ijt.2011.6071 Copyright © 2011 by Jana Cason. Adapted with permission.

Appendix B. Glossary

asynchronous—A method of exchanging health information whereby the provider and patient or client are not connected at the same time; commonly referred to as "store-and-forward" data transmission and may include video clips, digital photographs, virtual technologies, and other forms of electronic communications.

eHealth—A broad term encompassing health-related information and educational resources (e.g., health literacy Web sites and repositories, videos, blogs), commercial "products" (e.g., apps), and direct services delivered electronically (often through the Internet) by professionals, nonprofessionals, businesses, or consumers. May also be written as *e-Health* or *E-Health;* sometimes used interchangeably with *health informatics.*

haptic technology A tactile feedback technology that takes advantage of a user's sense of touch by applying forces, vibrations, or motions upon the user.

health informatics—Use of information technologies for health care data collection, storage, and analysis to enhance health care decisions and improve quality and efficiency of health care services.

mHealth—The delivery of health-related information and services using mobile communication technology (e.g., smartphone, electronic tablet, or other mobile devices).

modifier—A modifier used in conjunction with a *Current Procedural Terminology* (American Medical Association, 2011) code to identify the type of technology used within a telehealth service delivery model. GT is the most common modifier; it indicates use of interactive audio and video telecommunications technology. The GQ modifier designates the use of asynchronous technologies; reimbursement for this modifier is limited.

privacy officer A position or office that responds to concerns over the use of personal information, including medical data and financial information. It ensures adherence to regulations but is not limited to legislation concerning the protection of patient medical records (e.g., Health Insurance Portability and Accountability Act of 1996, Pub. L. 104–191).

protocol A written document specifying standard operating policies and procedures for application of telehealth technologies in delivering services.

synchronous A method of exchanging health information in real time (i.e., live) between the patient or client and a health care provider located at a distant site.

telehealth The application of evaluative, consultative, preventative, and therapeutic services delivered through telecommunication and information technologies.

telehealth technologies The hardware and software used in delivering services remotely by means of a telehealth service delivery model.

telemedicine—Medical services delivered through communication and information technologies.

telerehabilitation The application of telecommunication and information technologies for the delivery of rehabilitation services.

virtual reality—A computer-simulated environment of the real world; can be coupled with telehealth technologies as part of a telehealth service delivery model.

Appendix C. Applications of Telehealth Within Occupational Therapy Practice Areas

Children and Youth

Evidence supports the use of a telehealth service delivery model to deliver appropriate early intervention (EI) and school-based services effectively and efficiently. EI services, mandated by Part C of the Individuals With Disabilities Education Act Amendments of 1997 (IDEA; Pub. L. 105–117), are designed to promote development of skills and enhance the quality of life of infants and toddlers who have been identified as having a disability or developmental delay (Cason, 2011). Telehealth technology supports delivery of EI services (Cason, 2009, 2011; Heimerl & Rasch, 2009; Kelso, Fiechtl, Olsen, & Rule, 2009).

Similarly, evidence supports the use of telehealth for the delivery of occupational therapy services within the school setting for evaluation and intervention (Gallagher, 2004) as well as for reintegration of students with traumatic injury following acute rehabilitation (Verburg, Borthwick, Bennett, & Rumney, 2003). Telehealth may be used within school-based interprofessional team models for wellness programming, including efforts to combat the obesity epidemic among children and for programming targeting prevention of violence among youth (Cason, 2012b). School-based occupational therapy services focus on helping children with disabilities participate in and, thus, benefit from the instructional program.

In addition to what has been stated, telehealth technology may provide another avenue for the occupational therapy practitioner to observe the child's level of participation in a school setting without risk of altering the setting by being physically present. This unobtrusive observation strategy can allow the occupational therapy practitioner to consult with the teacher and offer strategies to alter the child's level of participation (e.g., strategies to facilitate a child's use of self-regulation skills, encourage appropriate interaction with peers, or facilitate the child's physical participation in an instructional activity).

The potential benefit of this observation strategy is to ensure the maintenance of the day-to-day integrity of the classroom while providing the practitioner with an understanding of the specific sensory, cognitive, physical, and emotional demands placed on the child in the setting. This technology may also provide the ability to record observations that contribute to the therapist's data collection during evaluation; this information can then be used as a baseline from which to support Individualized Education Program teams in developing goals and objectives and measuring progress in the child's level of participation in the setting. In rural or large urban school districts, this technology can assist the occupational therapy practitioner with more efficiently supporting multiple campuses that may be located across large distances, thereby facilitating the interprofessional team process as well as reducing costs incurred to allow a practitioner the time and transportation resources to support multiple campuses.

Productive Aging

The growing number of older adults in the United States creates opportunities for occupational therapy practitioners to use telehealth to promote health and wellness, prevention, and productive aging while reducing health care costs. The use of telerehabilitation to remotely monitor and provide self-management strategies to older adults who are chronically ill and living in their homes has been found to decrease hospitalizations and nursing home stays (Bendixen, Levy, Olive, Kobb, & Mann, 2009). Interactive videoconferencing technologies promote health and aging in place among older adults (Bendixen, Horn, & Levy, 2007; Harada et al., 2010; Hori, Kubota, Kihara, Takahashi, & Kinoshita, 2009). The use of home monitoring devices such as *self-m*onitoring *a*nalysis and *r*eporting *t*echnology (SMART) enable occupational therapy practitioners to remotely monitor clients' occupational performance and provide recommendations for environmental modifications and interventions to support occupational performance (Mann & Milton, 2005).

Health and Wellness

Telehealth also supports health and wellness and prevention programming through assessment and management of obesity (Neubeck et al., 2009) and chronic diseases such as diabetes mellitus, congestive heart failure, and hypertension (Darkins et al., 2008; Steel, Cox, & Garry, 2011).

Mental Health

Opportunities exist for occupational therapy practitioners to use telehealth to promote participation and psychological and social functioning for clients within the home, at work, and in the community through engagement in meaningful occupations. Research demonstrates efficacy of telehealth as a delivery model for psychological and behavioral interventions among individuals with posttraumatic stress disorder (PTSD) and other mental health issues (Germain, Marchand, Bouchard, Drouin, & Guay, 2009; Gros, Yoder, Tuerk, Lozano, & Acierno, 2011).

Rehabilitation, Disability, and Participation

In the practice area of rehabilitation, disability, and participation, the use of a telehealth service delivery model promotes occupational performance, adaptation, participation, and quality of life for clients with polytrauma, neurological, and orthopedic conditions. Telehealth provides remote access to occupational therapy services through assessment of physical function and goal setting, integration of individualized exercise interventions, training in adaptive strategies such as environmental modifications and energy conservation, and consultation on durable medical and adaptive equipment (Chumbler et al., 2010; Sanford et al., 2007).

Published studies support the use of telehealth in improving functional outcomes with individuals with stroke (Chumbler et al., 2010; Hermann et al., 2010), survivors of breast cancer (Hegel et al., 2011), veterans with polytrauma (Bendixen et al., 2008), and individuals with traumatic brain injury (Diamond et al., 2003; Forducey et al., 2003; Girard, 2007; Verburg et al., 2003). Additional studies have used a telehealth service delivery model to evaluate activities of daily living and hand function in individuals with Parkinson's disease (Hoffman, Russell, Thompson, Vincent, & Nelson, 2008) and other neurological impairments (Savard, Borstad, Tkachuck, Lauderdale, & Conroy, 2003). Seating experts used telehealth to provide remote wheelchair prescription and consultation to individuals with neurological and orthopedic conditions (Barlow, Liu, & Sekulic, 2009; Schein, Schmeler, Holm, Saptono, & Brienza, 2010; Schein et al., 2011). In addition to positive clinical outcomes, evidence indicates a high level of practitioner and client satisfaction associated with a telehealth service delivery model (Kairy, Lehoux, Vincent, & Visintin, 2009; Steel et al., 2011).

Work and Industry

Schmeler, Schein, McCue, and Betz (2009) detailed the use of assistive technology via a telehealth service delivery model for clinical and vocational applications. Telehealth is also being used to support work through remote assessment and analysis of work spaces. Bruce and Sanford (2006) described using teleconferencing to complete remote assessments and discussed the need for a highly structured and comprehensive assessment tool to be able to complete remote assessments.

Backman, Village, and Lacaille (2008) developed the Ergonomic Assessment Tool for Arthritis (EATA) to evaluate the workplace for people with arthritis. The EATA was designed so that the worker could gather the data for the assessment without an expert visiting the workplace. Pilot testing of the method indicated that workers could successfully gather the necessary information for appropriate intervention identification (Baker & Jacobs, 2013). Baker and Jacobs (2010) developed a systematic two-step program, the Telere-habilitation Computer Ergonomics System *(tele-CES)*. This systematic program will allow ergonomically trained health professionals to (1) remotely assess the computer workstation and (2) on basis of the assess-ment, generate explicit, participant-specific workstation modification recommendations. The recommen-dations will be easily implemented; reduce pain, discomfort, and fatigue; and eliminate barriers to productivity.

Appendix D. Telehealth Case Examples

CASE DESCRIPTION	USE OF TELEHEALTH	OUTCOME
Lisa is a 70-year-old woman who has difficulty performing her daily occupations because of a stroke resulting in right-sided weakness. Although she had learned compensatory techniques for completing activities of daily living (ADLs), instrumental ADLs, and work, she still wants to increase the use of her right hand, particularly for tasks related to managing her farm. Lisa learned of a program in a nearby community using new technology that might be beneficial for people with hemiparesis; however, the clinic is 2 hours from her home.	Lisa meets with her occupational therapist in a clinic for the initial evaluation. During the evaluation, Lisa learns additional strategies for incorporating the use of her right hand to perform her farm work. She is fitted for a functional electrical stimulation orthosis that she can use at home once it is programmed in the clinic. Twice each week, Lisa meets with her occupational therapist by computer, using a Web camera and online video software. As Lisa continues to make progress, the occupational therapist instructs her in how to more effectively use her right hand for completion of ADLs and farm chores.	Lisa is able to make functional gains in using her right hand for everyday occupations. She reports that she is able to rely less on compensatory strategies and use her right hand more easily, especially while completing ADLs. Lisa achieved these outcomes with only two trips to the clinic and without therapist travel.
José is a 35-year-old administrative assistant working at an urban university. He has been employed in this position for 5 years. Recently, he began experiencing discomfort in his neck, shoulder, and back areas. He reported this discomfort, which he associated with computer work, to his immediate supervisor.	Josh scheduled an appointment with an occupational therapist who had expertise in ergonomic workstation evaluation. During his initial contact with the occupational therapist, he requested that because of his busy schedule, he would prefer to have his evaluation conducted through telehealth technology. The occupational therapist asked Josh to have photographs taken of him while working at his office computer workstation. The occupational therapist requested that the photographs be from multiple angles and then e-mailed to a secure platform, where the therapist would be able to review them. In addition, Josh was asked to keep a time log for a week into which he would input information on his activities along with when he experienced discomfort. A telephone consultation was arranged, during which the occupational therapist reviewed findings from the photographs along with the time log. Josh reported on the time log that he sat at his computer workstation 100% of the time during the work day. During this time, he multitasked by using a hand-held telephone while keying. It was observed from the photographs that Josh was using a notebook computer, which placed him in an awkward posture for computing.	Explicit workstation modification recommendations were provided by the occupational therapist by means of a telephone consultation with Josh. The recommendations included raising the notebook computer so that his head was not positioned in flexion or extension and that the monitor was about arm's length away (closed fist) and using a keyboard and mouse as input devices. An adjustable keyboard tray was recommended for the keyboard and mouse. On the basis of data from the time log, the occupational therapist encouraged Josh to change his work behaviors by taking regular stretch breaks every 20 minutes. A second telephone consultation occurred within 2 weeks. Josh reported that his supervisor ordered the external notebook computer accessories and that this new workstation arrangement had reduced his discomfort.

(Continued)

Appendix D. Telehealth Case Examples *(Cont.)*

CASE DESCRIPTION	USE OF TELEHEALTH	OUTCOME
Angela is a 10-year-old girl with a complicated medical history that includes spina bifida. She is significantly limited in her ability to be mobile in the home and community. Although she uses a basic power wheelchair to drive around town and attend her family activities, it is in poor condition and too small for her. Angela cannot adequately reposition herself or properly perform a weight shift because of decreased upper-extremity strength and range of motion.	Angela has trouble traveling and sitting for long distances. She and her mother meet with an occupational therapy generalist in person at a nearby clinic. Concurrently, an occupational therapist who has expertise in wheeled mobility participates in an occupational therapy session remotely using a videoconferencing system. The remote occupational therapist provides consultation to the local occupational therapist, Angela, and her mother about seating system frames, bases, and accessories; policy implications and funding mechanisms; and wheeled mobility and seating options.	After interviewing Angela and her mother and observing Angela navigate in her current chair, the remote occupational therapist recommends the appropriate power wheelchair and power seat functions. Upon approval from the insurance company, the remote occupational therapist uses the videoconferencing system to monitor the delivery, evaluate the fitting, and provide feedback and advice to Angela about use of the wheelchair within the community and home. Angela has benefited from services without the need to travel a long distance. The local practitioner gained additional knowledge about wheeled mobility and seating options.
Ethan is a 55-year-old self-employed entrepreneur who has severe depression, anxiety, and isolation after head and neck cancer resection surgery. The surgery left one side of his face disfigured. He plans to have reconstructive surgery in the future. Meanwhile, Ethan has difficulties with eating, fatigue, facial–body image, depression, and pain. He lives alone and over 50 minutes away from the hospital/outpatient therapy clinic. Ethan was seen by an occupational therapist in the hospital and prescribed outpatient occupational therapy for his physical and mental impairments. Due to travel distance to the outpatient therapy clinic and anxiety associated with being seen in public, Ethan is interested in the option to continue his therapy at home through secure videoconferencing technology.	Ethan completed a telehealth participation screening and initial occupational therapy evaluation during his hospital stay. It was determined that he would continue with occupational therapy twice a week via telehealth using secure videoconferencing software and a Web camera within his home environment. During the biweekly occupational therapy sessions delivered via telehealth technologies, focus is on establishing a therapeutic wellness plan and implementing compensatory eating techniques, pain management and relaxation techniques, stress management, and engagement in progressive physical activities. Ethan completes a home program and a daily journal sent to him by his occupational therapist through electronic communications technology.	Ethan is able to manage his physical and mental impairments and is able to leave his house to purchase groceries and complete other errands in his community. His pain is tolerable, and breathing and stamina have improved to allow 20–30 minutes of physical activity after 6 weeks of occupational therapy delivered through telehealth technologies. Ethan continues his daily journaling. The occupational therapist will follow up with Ethan via telehealth technologies weekly until reconstruction surgery and again after surgery to make sure Ethan continues his wellness plan.

SECTION I.H.
Standards

Standards for Continuing Competence

Continuing competence is a process involving the examination of current competence and the development of capacity for the future. It is a component of ongoing professional development and lifelong learning. Continuing competence is a dynamic and multidimensional process in which the occupational therapist and occupational therapy assistant develop and maintain the knowledge, performance skills, interpersonal abilities, critical reasoning, and ethical reasoning skills necessary to perform current and future roles and responsibilities within the profession. Continuing competence is maintained through self-assessment of the practitioner's capacities in the core of occupational therapy, which reflects the knowledge of the domain of the profession and the process used in service delivery.

Occupational therapists and occupational therapy assistants use these standards to assess, maintain, and document continuing competence. Basic to these standards is the belief that all occupational therapists and occupational therapy assistants share core values and knowledge, guiding actions within their roles and responsibilities. The core of occupational therapy involves an understanding of occupation and purposeful activities and their influence on human performance. The unique "contribution of occupational therapy is the application of core values, knowledge, and skills to assist clients (people, organizations, and populations) to engage in everyday activities or occupations that they want and need to do in a manner that supports health and participation" (American Occupational Therapy Association [AOTA], 2008, p. 626).

Standard 1. Knowledge

Occupational therapists and occupational therapy assistants shall demonstrate understanding and comprehension of the information required for the multiple roles and responsibilities they assume. The individual must demonstrate

- Mastery of the core of occupational therapy as it is applied in the multiple responsibilities assumed;

- Expertise associated with primary responsibilities;

- Integration of relevant evidence, literature, and epidemiological data related to primary responsibilities and to the consumer population(s) served;

- Integration of current AOTA documents and legislative, legal, and regulatory issues into practice; and

- The ability to anticipate how new knowledge is necessary to meet client needs.

Standard 2. Critical Reasoning

Occupational therapists and occupational therapy assistants shall use reasoning processes to make sound judgments and decisions. The individual must demonstrate

- Deductive and inductive reasoning in making decisions specific to roles and responsibilities;

- Problem-solving skills necessary to carry out responsibilities;

465

- The ability to analyze occupational performance as influenced by environmental factors;
- The ability to reflect on one's own practice;
- Management and synthesis of information from a variety of sources in support of making decisions;
- Application of evidence, research findings, and outcome data in making decisions; and
- The ability to assess previous assumptions against new evidence and revise decision-making process.

Standard 3. Interpersonal Skills

Occupational therapists and occupational therapy assistants shall develop and maintain their professional relationships with others within the context of their roles and responsibilities. The individual must demonstrate

- Use of effective communication methods that match the abilities, personal factors, learning styles, and therapeutic needs of consumers and others;
- Effective interaction with people from diverse backgrounds;
- Use of feedback from clients, supervisors, and colleagues to modify one's professional behavior;
- Collaboration with clients and professionals to attain optimal consumer outcomes; and
- The ability to develop, sustain, and refine team relationships to meet identified outcomes.

Standard 4. Performance Skills

Occupational therapists and occupational therapy assistants shall demonstrate the expertise, aptitudes, proficiencies, and abilities to competently fulfill their roles and responsibilities. The individual must demonstrate expertise in

- Practice grounded in the core of occupational therapy;
- The therapeutic use of self, the therapeutic use of occupations and activities, the consultation process, and the education process to bring about change;
- Integrating current practice techniques and technologies;
- Updating performance based on current evidence-based literature with consideration given to client desires and practitioner judgment; and
- Quality improvement processes that prevent practice error and optimize client outcomes.

Standard 5. Ethical Practice

Occupational therapists and occupational therapy assistants shall identify, analyze, and clarify ethical issues or dilemmas to make responsible decisions within the changing context of their roles and responsibilities. The individual must demonstrate in practice

- Understanding and adherence to the profession's *Code of Ethics and Ethics Standards (2010)* (AOTA, 2010), other relevant codes of ethics, and applicable laws and regulations;
- The use of ethical principles and the profession's core values to understand complex situations;
- The integrity to make and defend decisions based on ethical reasoning; and
- Integration of varying perspectives in the ethics of clinical practice.

References

American Occupational Therapy Association. (2008). Occupational therapy practice framework: Domain and process (2nd ed.). *American Journal of Occupational Therapy, 62*(6), 625–683.

American Occupational Therapy Association. (2010). Occupational therapy code of ethics and ethics standards (2010). *American Journal of Occupational Therapy, 64.*

Authors

The Commission on Continuing Competence and Professional Development:
Barbara A. Schell, PhD, OT, FAOTA, *Chairperson*
Ron Cevero, PhD
Mary Kay Currie, OT, BCPR
Jan Davis, MS, OTR/L
Pamela Roberts, PhD, OTR/L, SCFES, CPHQ, FAOTA
Winifred Schultz-Krohn, PhD, OTR/L, BCP, FAOTA
Christine Urish, PhD, BCMH, FAOTA
Maria Elena E. Louch, OT, *AOTA Staff Liaison*

for

The Commission on Continuing Competence and Professional Development
Barbara A. Schell, PhD, OT, FAOTA, *Chairperson*

Adopted by the Representative Assembly 1999
Revisions adopted 2005C243
Edited 2006
Revisions adopted 2010CApr12

Note: This document replaces the 2005 document *Standards for Continuing Competence (American Journal of Occupational Therapy, 59,* 661–662).

Standards of Practice for Occupational Therapy

This document defines minimum standards for the practice of occupational therapy. The practice of occupational therapy means the therapeutic use of everyday life activities (occupations) with individuals, groups, organizations, and populations for the purpose of participation in roles and situations in the home, school, workplace, community, or other settings. Occupational therapy services are provided for the purpose of promoting health and wellness and to those who have or are at risk for developing an illness, injury, disease, disorder, condition, impairment, disability, activity limitation, or participation restriction. Occupational therapy addresses physical, cognitive, psychosocial, sensory, communication, and other areas of performance in various contexts and environments in everyday life activities that affect health, well-being, and quality of life (American Occupational Therapy Association [AOTA], 2004). The overarching goal of occupational therapy is "to support [people's] health and participation in life through engagement in occupations" (AOTAa, 2008, p. 626).

The *Standards of Practice for Occupational Therapy* are requirements for occupational therapists and occupational therapy assistants for the delivery of occupational therapy services. *The Reference Manual of Official Documents of the American Occupational Therapy Association, Inc.* (current version as of press time, AOTA, 2010) contains documents that clarify and support occupational therapy practice, as do various issues of the *American Journal of Occupational Therapy.* These documents are reviewed and updated on an ongoing basis for their applicability.

Education, Examination, and Licensure Requirements

All occupational therapists and occupational therapy assistants must practice under federal and state law.

To practice as an occupational therapist, the individual trained in the United States

- Has graduated from an occupational therapy program accredited by the Accreditation Council for Occupational Therapy Education (ACOTE®) or predecessor organizations;

- Has successfully completed a period of supervised fieldwork experience required by the recognized educational institution where the applicant met the academic requirements of an educational program for occupational therapists that is accredited by ACOTE or predecessor organizations;

- Has passed a nationally recognized entry-level examination for occupational therapists; and

- Fulfills state requirements for licensure, certification, or registration.

To practice as an occupational therapy assistant, the individual trained in the United States

- Has graduated from an occupational therapy assistant program accredited by ACOTE or predecessor organizations;

- Has successfully completed a period of supervised fieldwork experience required by the recognized educational institution where the applicant met the academic requirements of an educational program for occupational therapy assistants that is accredited by ACOTE or predecessor organizations;

- Has passed a nationally recognized entry-level examination for occupational therapy assistants; and

- Fulfills state requirements for licensure, certification, or registration.

Definitions

The following definitions are used in this document:

- *Activity (Activities):* A class of human behaviors that are goal directed.

- *Assessment:* Specific tools or instruments that are used during the evaluation process.

- *Client:* The entity that receives occupational therapy services. Clients may include (1) individuals and other persons relevant to the individual's life, such as family, caregivers, teachers, employers, and others who also may help or be served indirectly; (2) organizations such as business, industry, or agencies; and (3) populations within a community (Moyers & Dale, 2007).

- *Evaluation:* The process of obtaining and interpreting data necessary for intervention. This includes planning for and documenting the evaluation process and results.

- *Intervention:* The process and skilled actions taken by occupational therapy practitioners in collaboration with the client to facilitate engagement in occupation related to health and participation. The intervention process includes the plan, implementation, and review.

- *Occupation:* "Goal-directed pursuits that typically extend over time, have meaning to their performance, and involve multiple tasks" (Christiansen, Baum, & Bass-Haugen, 2005, p. 548); "all the things that people want, need, or have to do, whether of a physical, mental, social, sexual, political, spiritual, or any other nature, including sleep and rest activities." (Wilcock & Townsend, 2009, p. 193); "activities of everyday life named, organized, and given meaning by individuals and a culture" (Law, Polatajko, Baptiste, & Townsend, 1997, p. 32).

- *Outcomes:* What occupational therapy actually achieves for the client. Changes desired by the client that can focus on any area of the client's occupational performance.

- *Re-evaluation:* The process of critical analysis of client response to intervention. This analysis enables the therapist to make any necessary changes to intervention plan in collaboration with the client.

- *Screening:* Obtaining and reviewing data relevant to a potential client to determine the need for further evaluation and intervention.

- *Transitions:* "Actions coordinated to prepare for or facilitate a change, such as from one functional level to another, from one life [change] to another, from one program to another, or from one environment to another" (AOTA, 1998, p. 866).

Standard I. Professional Standing and Responsibility

1. An occupational therapy practitioner (occupational therapist or occupational therapy assistant) delivers occupational therapy services that reflect the philosophical base of occupational therapy and are consistent with the established principles and concepts of theory and practice.

2. An occupational therapy practitioner is knowledgeable about and delivers occupational therapy services in accordance with AOTA standards, policies, and guidelines and state, federal, and other regulatory and payer requirements relevant to practice and service delivery.

3. An occupational therapy practitioner maintains current licensure, registration, or certification as required by law or regulation.

4. An occupational therapy practitioner abides by the *Occupational Therapy Code of Ethics* (AOTA, 2005a).

5. An occupational therapy practitioner abides by the *Standards for Continuing Competence* (AOTA, 2005b) by establishing, maintaining, and updating professional performance, knowledge, and skills.

6. An occupational therapist is responsible for all aspects of occupational therapy service delivery and is accountable for the safety and effectiveness of the occupational therapy service delivery process (AOTA, 2009).

7. An occupational therapy assistant is responsible for providing safe and effective occupational therapy services under the supervision of and in partnership with the occupational therapist and in accordance with laws or regulations and AOTA documents (AOTA, 2009).

8. An occupational therapy practitioner maintains current knowledge of legislative, political, social, cultural, societal, and reimbursement issues that affect clients and the practice of occupational therapy.

9. An occupational therapy practitioner is knowledgeable about evidence-based research and applies it ethically and appropriately to provide occupational therapy services consistent with best practice approaches.

10. An occupational therapy practitioner respects the client's sociocultural background and provides client-centered and family-centered occupational therapy services.

Standard II. Screening, Evaluation, and Re-evaluation

1. An occupational therapist is responsible for all aspects of the screening, evaluation, and re-evaluation process.

2. An occupational therapist accepts and responds to referrals in compliance with state or federal laws, other regulatory and payer requirements, and AOTA documents.

3. An occupational therapist, in collaboration with the client, evaluates the client's ability to participate in daily life by considering the client's history, goals, capacities, and needs; the activities and occupations the client wants and needs to perform; and the environments and context in which these activities and occupations occur.

4. An occupational therapist initiates and directs the screening, evaluation, and re-evaluation process and analyzes and interprets the data in accordance with federal and state law, other regulatory and payer requirements, and AOTA documents.

5. An occupational therapy assistant contributes to the screening, evaluation, and re-evaluation process by implementing delegated assessments and by providing verbal and written reports of observations and client capacities to the occupational therapist in accordance with federal and state laws, other regulatory and payer requirements, and AOTA documents.

6. An occupational therapy practitioner uses current assessments and assessment procedures and follows defined protocols of standardized assessments during the screening, evaluation, and re-evaluation process.

7. An occupational therapist completes and documents occupational therapy evaluation results. An occupational therapy assistant contributes to the documentation of evaluation results. An occupational therapy practitioner abides by the time frames, formats, and standards established by practice settings, federal and state law, other regulatory and payer requirements, external accreditation programs, and AOTA documents.

8. An occupational therapy practitioner communicates screening, evaluation, and re-evaluation results within the boundaries of client confidentiality and privacy regulations to the appropriate person, group, organization, or population.

9. An occupational therapist recommends additional consultations or refers clients to appropriate resources when the needs of the client can best be served by the expertise of other professionals or services.

10. An occupational therapy practitioner educates current and potential referral sources about the scope of occupational therapy services and the process of initiating occupational therapy services.

Standard III: Intervention

1. An occupational therapist has overall responsibility for the development, documentation, and implementation of the occupational therapy intervention based on the evaluation, client goals, best available evidence, and professional and clinical reasoning.

2. An occupational therapist ensures that the intervention plan is documented within the time frames, formats, and standards established by the practice settings, agencies, external accreditation programs, state and federal law, and other regulatory and payer requirements.

3. An occupational therapy practitioner collaborates with the client to develop and implement the intervention plan, on the basis of the client's needs and priorities, safety issues, and relative benefits and risks of the interventions.

4. An occupational therapy practitioner coordinates the development and implementation of the occupational therapy intervention with the intervention provided by other professionals, when appropriate.

5. An occupational therapy practitioner uses professional and clinical reasoning to select the most appropriate types of interventions, including therapeutic use of self, therapeutic use of occupations and activities, consultation, education, and advocacy.

6. An occupational therapy assistant selects, implements, and makes modifications to therapeutic interventions that are consistent with the occupational therapy assistant's demonstrated competency and delegated responsibilities, the intervention plan, and requirements of the practice setting.

7. An occupational therapist modifies the intervention plan throughout the intervention process and documents changes in the client's needs, goals, and performance.

8. An occupational therapy assistant contributes to the modification of the intervention plan by exchanging information with and providing documentation to the occupational therapist about the client's responses to and communications throughout the intervention.

9. An occupational therapy practitioner documents the occupational therapy services provided within the time frames, formats, and standards established by the practice settings, agencies, external accreditation programs, federal and state laws, other regulatory and payer requirements, and AOTA documents.

Standard IV. Outcomes

1. An occupational therapist is responsible for selecting, measuring, documenting, and interpreting expected or achieved outcomes that are related to the client's ability to engage in occupations.

2. An occupational therapist is responsible for documenting changes in the client's performance and capacities and for transitioning the client to other types or intensity of service or discontinuing services when the client has achieved identified goals, reached maximum benefit, or does not desire to continue services.

3. An occupational therapist prepares and implements a transition or discontinuation plan based on the client's needs, goals, performance, and appropriate follow-up resources.

4. An occupational therapy assistant contributes to the transition or discontinuation plan by providing information and documentation to the supervising occupational therapist related to the client's needs, goals, performance, and appropriate follow-up resources.

5. An occupational therapy practitioner facilitates the transition or discharge process in collaboration with the client, family members, significant others, other professionals (e.g., medical, educational, or social services), and community resources, when appropriate.

6. An occupational therapist is responsible for evaluating the safety and effectiveness of the occupational therapy processes and interventions within the practice setting.

7. An occupational therapy assistant contributes to evaluating the safety and effectiveness of the occupational therapy processes and interventions within the practice setting.

References

American Occupational Therapy Association. (1998). Standards of practice. *American Journal of Occupational Therapy, 52,* 866–869.

American Occupational Therapy Association. (2004). Policy 5.3.1: Definition of occupational therapy practice for state regulation. *American Journal of Occupational Therapy, 58,* 694–695.

American Occupational Therapy Association. (2005a). Occupational therapy code of ethics (2005). *American Journal of Occupational Therapy, 59,* 639–642.

American Occupational Therapy Association. (2005b). Standards for continuing competence. *American Journal of Occupational Therapy, 59,* 661–662.

American Occupational Therapy Association. (2008). Occupational therapy practice framework: Domain and process (2nd ed.). *American Journal of Occupational Therapy, 62,* 625–683.

American Occupational Therapy Association. (2009). Guidelines for supervision, roles, and responsibilities during the delivery of occupational therapy services. *American Journal of Occupational Therapy, 63,* 173–179.

American Occupational Therapy Association. (2010). *The reference manual of the official documents of the American Occupational Therapy Association, Inc.* (15th ed.). Bethesda, MD: AOTA Press.

Christiansen, C., Baum, M. C., & Bass-Haugen, J. (Eds.). (2005). *Occupational therapy: Performance, participation, and well-being.* Thorofare, NJ: Slack.

Law, M., Polatajko, H., Baptiste, W., & Towsend, E. (1997). Core concepts of occupational therapy. In E. Towsend (Ed.), *Enabling occupation: An occupational therapy perspective* (pp. 29–56). Ottawa, ON: Canadian Association of Occupational Therapists.

Moyers, P. A., & Dale, L. M. (2007). *The guide to occupational therapy practice* (2nd ed.). Bethesda, MD: AOTA Press.

Wilcock, A. A., & Townsend, E. A. (2009). Occupational justice. In E. Crepeau, E. Cohn, & B. Schell (Eds.), *Willard and Spackman's occupational therapy* (11th ed., pp. 192– 215). Philadelphia: Lippincott Williams & Wilkins.

Authors

The Commission on Practice

Janet V. DeLany, DEd, OTR/L, FAOTA, *Chairperson*

Debbie Amini, MEd, OTR/L, CHT

Ellen Cohn, ScD, OTR/L, FAOTA

Jennifer Cruz, MAT, MOTS, *ASD Liaison*

Kimberly Hartmann, PhD, OTR/L, FAOTA, *SISC Liaison*

Jeanette Justice, COTA/L

Kathleen Kannenberg, MA, OTR/L, CCM

Cherylin Lew, OTD, OTR/L

James Marc-Aurele, MBA, OTR/L

Mary Jane Youngstrom, MS, OTR, FAOTA

Deborah Lieberman, MHSA, OTR/L, FAOTA, *AOTA Headquarters Liaison*

for

The Commission on Practice

Janet V. DeLany, DEd, OTR/L, FAOTA, *Chairperson*

The COP wishes to acknowledge the authors of the 2005 edition of this document: Sara Jane Brayman, PhD, OTR/L, FAOTA, *Chairperson;* Susanne Smith Roley, MS, OTR/L, FAOTA, *Chairperson-Elect;* Gloria Frolek Clark, MS, OTR/L, FAOTA; Janet V. DeLany, DEd, MSA, OTR/L, FAOTA; Eileen R. Garza, PhD, OTR, ATP; Mary V. Radomski, MA, OTR/L, FAOTA; Ruth Ramsey, MS, OTR/L; Carol Siebert, MS, OTR/L; Kristi Voelkerding, BS, COTA/L; Lenna Aird, COTA/L, *ASD Liaison;* Patricia D. LaVesser, PhD, OTR/L, *SIS Liaison;* and Deborah Lieberman, MHSA, OTR/L, FAOTA, *AOTA Headquarters Liaison.*

Adopted by the Representative Assembly Coordinating Council (RACC) for the Representative Assembly

Revised by the Commission on Practice 2010

Note: This revision replaces the 2005 document *Standards of Practice for Occupational Therapy* (previously published and copyrighted in 2005 by the American Occupational Therapy Association in the *American Journal of Occupational Therapy, 59,* 663–665).

Note. These standards are intended as recommended guidelines to assist occupational therapy practitioners in the provision of occupational therapy services. These standards serve as a minimum standard for occupational therapy practice and are applicable to all individual populations and the programs in which these individuals are served.

Statements

Academic Terminal Degree

Although there are doctoral-degree programs in occupational therapy and occupational science, currently it is customary for occupational therapy faculty to have a doctorate in related areas of science or social science, including but not limited to education, neuroscience, public health, psychology, policy, law, or sociology. Thus, a degree in any of these areas would be considered a terminal degree for occupational therapists in academia.

Prepared by

René Padilla, PhD, OTR/L, FAOTA

for

The Commission on Education
René Padilla, PhD, OTR/L, FAOTA, *Chairperson*

Note: This replaces the 2003 document "Academic Terminal Degree" (*American Journal of Occupational Therapy, 58*, 648).

Adopted by the Representative Assembly 2008C4

Cognition, Cognitive Rehabilitation, and Occupational Performance

The American Occupational Therapy Association (AOTA) asserts that occupational therapists and occupational therapy assistants, through the use of occupations and activities, facilitate individuals' cognitive functioning to enhance occupational performance, self-efficacy, participation, and perceived quality of life. Cognition is integral to effective performance across the broad range of daily occupations such as work, educational pursuits, home management, and play and leisure. Cognition also plays an integral role in human development and in the ability to learn, retain, and use new information in response to changes in everyday life.

The purpose of this statement is to clarify the role of occupational therapy in evaluating and addressing cognitive functioning and the provision of cognitive rehabilitation to maintain and improve occupational performance. The intended primary audience for this statement is practitioners within the profession of occupational therapy. The statement also may be used to inform recipients of occupational therapy services, practitioners in other disciplines, and the wider community regarding occupational therapy theory and methods and to articulate the expertise of occupational therapy practitioners in addressing cognition and cognitive dysfunction.

Occupational therapy theory and research support the principle that cognition is essential to the performance of everyday tasks (Toglia & Kirk, 2000). Occupational therapy practitioners'[1] educational preparation and focus on occupational performance are grounded in an understanding of the relationship between cognitive processes and performance of daily life occupations. This understanding is in keeping with the disciplinary perspective of occupational therapy that emphasizes engagement in the client's desired occupations as a means of promoting cognitive functioning and occupational performance (Baum & Katz, 2010; Giles, 2010). Occupation is understood as both the means and the end of occupational therapy intervention. Participation in occupations enhances client functioning in areas such as cognition, the improvement in which leads to enhanced participation in desired daily activities.

Occupational therapy practitioners administer assessments and interventions that focus on cognition as it relates to participation and occupational performance. Furthermore, occupational therapy practitioners believe that cognitive functioning can only be understood and facilitated fully within the context of occupational performance. This understanding of the relationship among the client, his or her roles, daily occupations, and context make occupational therapy a profession that is uniquely qualified to address cognitive deficits that negatively affect the daily life experience of the individual.

Occupational therapy practitioners may choose from a range of interventions that use engagement in the client's desired occupations and activities with a focus on function-based outcomes. Considerable progress has been made over the past decade in advancing the knowledge of cognition and in identifying effective rehabilitative strategies.

---

[1]When the term *occupational therapy practitioner* is used in this document, it refers to both occupational therapists and occupational therapy assistants (AOTA, 2006). *Occupational therapists* are responsible for all aspects of occupational therapy service delivery and are accountable for the safety and effectiveness of the occupational therapy service delivery process. *Occupational therapy assistants* deliver occupational therapy services under the supervision of and in partnership with an occupational therapist (AOTA, 2009).

Definitions

In this document, *cognition* refers to information-processing functions carried out by the brain (Diller & Weinberg, 1993) that include attention, memory, executive functions (i.e., planning, problem solving, self-monitoring, self-awareness), comprehension and formation of speech (Sohlberg & Mateer, 1989), calculation ability (Roux, Boetto, Sacko, Chollet, & Trémoulet, 2003), visual perception (Warren, 1993), and praxis skills (Donkervoort, Dekker, Stehmann-Saris, & Deelman, 2001). Cognitive processes can be conscious or unconscious (Eysenck & Keane, 1990) and often are divided into basic level skills (e.g., attention and memory processes) and executive functions (Schutz & Wanlass, 2009).

Cognitive dysfunction (or cognitive impairment) can be defined as functioning below expected normative levels or loss of ability in any area of cognitive functioning. The term *cognitive rehabilitation* has been widely discussed and used in a variety of contexts. However, there is no singular, consensus-based definition. In general, it refers to a broad category of "therapeutic interventions designed to improve cognitive functioning and participation in activities that may be affected by difficulties in one or more cognitive domains" (Brain Injury Association of America, 2011, p. 1). When occupational therapy practitioners provide intervention to improve cognitive functioning (i.e., cognitive rehabilitation), the therapeutic goal is always to enhance some aspect of occupational performance.

Occupations refer to "everyday activities" that are important to the individual and that help define the individual to himself or herself and others and that serve an individual's life roles (AOTA, 2008; Baum & Christiansen, 2005). Occupations help structure everyday life and contribute to health and well-being. Engagement in occupation as the focus of occupational therapy intervention involves addressing both the neurologically mediated occupational performance deficits and the individual's psychological responses to those deficits.

Cognitive Dysfunction

Cognitive dysfunction may occur across the lifespan and may be associated with a wide range of clinical conditions. Cognitive dysfunction can be transient or permanent, progressive or static, general or specific, and of different levels of severity affecting individuals in different domains of their lives. Even subtle cognitive impairments consistently influence social participation, subjective well-being, academics, employment, and functional performance across different ages and populations (Foster et al., 2011; Frittelli et al., 2009; Wadley, Okonkwo, Crowe, & Ross-Meadows, 2008). Most often, cognitive impairments are categorized by severity (mild or major neurocognitive disorder; American Psychiatric Association, 2000) or clinical condition that causes the dysfunction (i.e., by diagnostic group).

Cognitive rehabilitation interventions for persons with stroke, traumatic brain injury (TBI), and dementias have the most robust empirical support (Cicerone et al., 2011; Golisz, 2009; Rohling, Faust, Beverley, & Demakis, 2009), and persons with these conditions are among the most frequently seen by occupational therapy practitioners. Additionally, occupational therapy practitioners address cognitive barriers to functioning resulting from developmental disorders, environmental factors, or disease. Specifically, these populations include those experiencing cognitive dysfunction related to

- Human genetics and/or development (e.g., environmental deprivation, fetal alcohol syndrome, learning disabilities, pervasive developmental disorders);

- Neurologic disease, events, injuries, and disorders (e.g., stroke, TBI, Parkinson's and Huntington's diseases, HIV/AIDS, Alzheimer's disease and related dementias, rheumatoid arthritis, diabetes, lupus, Lyme disease, multiple sclerosis, chronic fatigue syndrome, chronic obstructive pulmonary disease, cardiac and circulatory conditions);

- Mental illness (e.g., schizophrenia, major depressive disorder, bipolar disorder, substance use disorders); or

- Transient or continuing life stresses or changes (e.g., stress-related disorders, pain syndromes, anxiety disorders, grief and loss).

In addition to rehabilitative approaches, occupational therapy practitioners recognize that there are many circumstances in which interventions to support cognitive functions can optimize occupational performance and quality of life. Habilitative approaches to cognitive functioning can be appropriate for populations with normative neurological development (e.g., interventions to enhance executive functions in the school-age population; see Case 1 in Appendix C) and the well elderly (in an attempt to prevent cognitive disability and occupational performance problems). Occupational therapy practitioners are in the forefront of using novel approaches to assess and enhance function among these diverse populations (Rand, Basha-Abu Rukan, Weiss, & Katz, 2009).

Occupational Therapy Service Delivery

The occupational therapy service delivery process is broadly composed of evaluation and intervention leading to the outcome of participation in areas of occupation. Occupational therapists are often a valuable part of an interdisciplinary team in which practitioner knowledge of cognition, participation, and context complements the interventions of other clinicians on the team, including, but not limited to, neuropsychologists and speech–language pathologists.

Evaluation of Occupational Performance

Occupational therapy evaluation focuses on determining what the client most needs and wants to be able to do and identifying the factors that either support or hinder the desired performance (AOTA, 2008). The *Occupational Therapy Practice Framework: Domain and Process* (2nd ed., AOTA, 2008) identifies the underlying factors and areas of occupation that occupational therapy practitioners consider during the evaluation and intervention process (i.e., client factors, performance skills, performance patterns, context and environment, activity demands). The interaction between a person's cognitive functioning and each factor is transactional in nature and, as such, cognitive functioning is always embedded in occupational performance and cannot be accurately understood in isolation.

In addition, the relationship of cognitive dysfunction to occupational performance is complex. Therefore, a thorough understanding of the contributions of various client factors and the current level of client participation must be sought (Giles, 2011; Lowenstein & Acevedo, 2010).

Occupational therapists examine cognition and performance from multiple perspectives and use multiple methods during the evaluation process, including interviewing the client and others (e.g., parent, teacher, caregiver), cognitive screening, performance-based assessments, environmental assessment, and specific cognitive measures.

The Cognitive Functional Evaluation (CFE) process is an example of a multifaceted approach used by occupational therapists for individuals with suspected cognitive disabilities (Baum & Katz, 2010; Hartman-Maeir, Katz, & Baum, 2009). The CFE process is intended to be customized to each person's needs and can include up to six types of assessments, as outlined in Appendix A.

Models for Intervention and Cognitive Rehabilitation

Occupational therapy scholars have developed several theoretical models that explain and guide intervention. These models, and the specific approaches and methods that they espouse, are used by occupational therapy practitioners to address cognition and to provide evidence-based cognitive rehabilitation as it affects occupational performance. These models include, but are not limited to, the

- Dynamic Interactional Model (Toglia, 2011),
- Cognitive Rehabilitation Model (Averbach & Katz, 2011),

- Cognitive Disabilities Model (Allen, Earhart, & Blue, 1992),

- Cognitive Orientation to Daily Occupational Performance model (CO–OP; Polatajko, Mandich, & McEwen, 2011), and the

- Neurofunctional Approach (NFA; Giles, 2010, 2011; Giles & Clark-Wilson, 1993; Parish & Oddy, 2007; Vanderploeg et al., 2008).

The development of occupational therapy theoretical models is ongoing, as is the refinement of their applicability to particular client populations, severity of deficits, and environmental contexts. Additional information about these theoretical models is included in Appendix B.

Key Features of Interventions

Many occupational therapy intervention models are multimodal and include a range of strategies adapted to an individual client's needs. Occupational therapists may select different approaches to address different types of occupational performance deficits in the same client. The following key features are found within various models and can assist practitioners in choosing an approach or approaches that are best suited to the client.

Global Strategy Learning and Awareness Approaches

Global strategy learning focuses on improving awareness of cognitive processes and assisting clients to develop higher order compensatory approaches (e.g., internal problem-solving and reasoning strategies) versus attempting to remediate basic cognitive deficits. This type of intervention relies on the holistic analysis skills of the occupational therapist in understanding the whole person and helping the client deconstruct his or her own performance. This approach enables clients to be able to generalize the application of these compensatory strategies to novel circumstances (Dawson et al., 2009; Polatajko et al., 2011). Case studies illustrating these approaches can be found in Appendix C (see Cases 1, 2, and 3).

Domain-Specific Strategy Training

Domain-specific strategy training focuses on teaching clients particular strategies to manage specific perceptual or cognitive deficits versus being taught the task itself. For example, the client may learn an internal routine to scan the whole environment to assist with left-sided neglect, may learn a social skills strategy to manage interpersonal interactions, or may learn to use a mental checklist to identify things to be recorded in a personal digital assistant. Case studies illustrating these approaches can be found in Appendix C (see Cases 3 and 4).

Cognitive Retraining Embedded in Functional Activity

In cognitive retraining, cognitive processes are addressed within the context of the activity (e.g., attention retraining during driving reeducation); the retraining is "context specific." The transfer appropriate processing hypothesis of Park, Moscovitch, and Robertson (1999) suggests that performance on a particular task after training will improve to the extent that processing operations required to carry out that task overlap with the processes engaged during training. For example, problem-solving strategies developed in the context of a simple front-closing shirt-donning activity will carry over to a front-closing jacket-donning activity when that process is engaged.

Specific-Task Training

Specific-task training assists clients to perform a specific functional behavior (Mastos, Miller, Eliasson, & Imms, 2007; Parish & Oddy, 2007). In specific-task training, the therapist attempts to circumvent the cognitive deficit that hampers performance by teaching an actual functional task. The intervention is designed to help the individual achieve the occupational performance goal by learning a routine so that the cognitive deficits no longer interfere with occupational performance (Giles, 2010; Giles & Clark-Wilson, 1993).

"Errorless" learning is often used in preference to trial-and-error learning. By addressing basic-skills training, clients may be able to improve self-awareness, mental efficiency, and organization, resulting in continued cognitive improvements (Parish & Oddy, 2007). Case studies illustrating these approaches can be found in Appendix C (see Cases 3–6).

Environmental Modifications and Use of Assistive Technology

Environmental modifications and simplifications are a component of most of the approaches described. Part of the process of occupational therapy intervention involves addressing the complexity of activity demands and altering environmental contexts to enhance the match between the client's abilities and the environmental demands (Evans et al., 2000; Wilson, Baddeley, Evans, & Shiel, 1994). Several technology-based cognitive prosthetics have been developed as a scheduling assistant (to assist with memory impairment) and for task initiation and task guidance (to cue persons with cognitive impairment to undertake and complete functional routines; Bergman, 2003; Gorman, Dayle, Hood, & Rumrell, 2003; Wilson, Scott, Evans, & Emslie, 2003).

The cueing systems may be used as an ongoing prosthetic or as a way to "extend" therapy and to become second nature as the client internalizes the routine. When occupational therapists think about the environment, they do not limit themselves to consideration of the physical environment (Giles, Wager, Fong, & Waraich, 2005). In addition to physical objects, Barris, Kielhofner, Levine, and Neville (1985) conceptualized other aspects of the environment that influence behavior, including the structure and sequence of tasks, the content of the social network, and values and beliefs embedded in culture (Giles, 2011). Case studies illustrating these approaches can be found in Appendix C (see Cases 2, 6, and 7).

Contributions to the Interdisciplinary Team

Occupational therapy practitioners are important members of interdisciplinary rehabilitation teams. As part of these teams, practitioners bring a unique focus on occupational performance as both an intervention and an outcome (AOTA, 2008; Baum & Katz, 2010; Giles, 2010). Interdisciplinary programs that address cognition are variously described as *comprehensive outpatient programs, postacute rehabilitation,* and *holistic neurologic rehabilitation* (Geurtsen, van Heugten, Martina, & Geurts, 2010; Turner-Stokes, 2008; Turner-Stokes, Nair, Sedki, Disler, & Wade, 2005) and often emphasize the integration of cognitive, interpersonal, and functional interventions within a therapeutic milieu.

Occupational therapy practitioners bring an understanding of the interrelatedness of the mind, body, and spirit and the transactional relationship of client factors, the environment, and occupational performance to the rehabilitation team (AOTA, 2008). Clients in these programs have been found to show increased self-awareness, increased self-efficacy for symptom management, increased perceived quality of life, and increased community integration (Cicerone et al., 2008, 2011).

Advancing Future Research

Considerable progress has been made over the past decade in advancing knowledge and rehabilitative strategies that improve the clients' occupational performance, self-efficacy, and perceived quality of life. Occupational therapy practitioners use existing and emerging evidence as summarized in systematic reviews (such as Cicerone et al., 2000, 2005, 2011) and the *Occupational Therapy Practice Guidelines for Adults With Traumatic Brain Injury* (Golisz, 2009) to guide their approach to evaluation and intervention. All of the occupational therapy approaches described in this statement have (at minimum) case-series and proof-of-concept designs showing effectiveness, and some have been found effective in large-scale, multi-center, randomized controlled trials (Giles, 2010; Vanderploeg et al., 2008).

There is now a general consensus among several payers (including insurance companies and Medicare contractor policy statements) that sufficient information is available to support evidence-based protocols and implement empirically supported treatments for disability caused by cognitive impairment after TBI and stroke (Rohling et al., 2009). However, although there is some support from systematic reviews of cognitive interventions for persons with Alzheimer's disease, multiple sclerosis, and schizophrenia, no consensus as yet exists for these and other diagnostic groupings in regard to cognitive rehabilitation (McGurk, Twamley, Sitzer, McHugo, & Mueser, 2007; Sitzer, Twamley, & Jeste, 2006; Wykes, Huddy, Cellard, McGurk, & Czobor, 2011; Zarit & Femia, 2008). Occupational therapy practitioners continue to work to advance the evidence base in these areas.

Qualifications of Occupational Therapy Practitioners

Occupational therapy practitioners are well qualified to assess and address cognitive performance issues affecting daily activity performance because of their education and training in cognitive functioning, task analysis, learning, diagnostic conditions, and a holistic understanding of the wide range of factors and contexts that affect performance (Accreditation Council for Occupational Therapy Education [ACOTE], 2012). The occupational therapist is responsible for the overall evaluation process, interpretation of the results, development, and management of the intervention plan. The occupational therapy assistant can perform those portions of the assessment as delegated by the occupational therapist, in which service competency has been established and in keeping with state laws and other regulations. All occupational therapy practitioners assume ethical responsibility for maintaining competence and determining whether they are qualified for independent or supervised practice (ACOTE, 2012).

AOTA asserts the importance of cognition to human performance and to the superordinate goals of occupational therapy. On the basis of theoretical models and evidence-supported methods and approaches, occupational therapy practitioners assess and address cognition so that clients may optimally perform the roles and activities that advance their productivity, wellness, and life satisfaction.

References

Accreditation Council for Occupational Therapy Education. (2012). 2011 Accreditation Council for Occupational Therapy Education (ACOTE®) standards. *American Journal of Occupational Therapy, 66*(6, Suppl.), S6–S74. http://dx.doi.org/10.5014/ajot.2012.66S6

Allen, C. K., Earhart, C., & Blue, T. (1992). *Occupational therapy treatment goals for the physically and cognitively disabled.* Rockville, MD: American Occupational Therapy Association.

American Occupational Therapy Association. (2006). Policy 1.44: Categories of occupational therapy personnel. In *Policy manual* (2011 ed., pp. 33–34). Bethesda, MD: Author.

American Occupational Therapy Association. (2008). Occupational therapy practice framework: Domain and process (2nd ed.). *American Journal of Occupational Therapy, 62,* 625–683. http://dx.doi.org/10.5014/ajot.62.6.625

American Occupational Therapy Association. (2009). Guidelines for supervision, roles, and responsibilities during the delivery of occupational therapy services. *American Journal of Occupational Therapy, 63,* 797–803. http://dx.doi.org/10.5014/ajot.63.6.797

American Psychiatric Association. (2000). *Diagnostic and statistical manual of mental disorders* (4th ed., text rev.). Washington, DC: Author.

Amundson, S. J. (1995). *Evaluation Tool of Children's Handwriting.* Homer, AK: OT Kids.

Arnadottir, G. (1990). *Brain and behavior: Assessing cortical dysfunction through activities of daily living (ADL).* St. Louis, MO: Mosby.

Arnadottir, G. (2011). Impact of neurobehavioral deficits on activities of daily living. In G. Gillen (Ed.), *Stroke rehabilitation: A function-based approach* (3rd ed., pp. 456–500). St. Louis, MO: Elsevier/Mosby.

Averbach, S., & Katz, N. (2011). Cognitive rehabilitation: A retraining model for clients with neurological disabilities. In N. Katz (Ed.), *Cognition, occupation, and participation across the life span: Neuroscience, neurorehabilitation, and models of intervention in occupational therapy* (3rd ed., pp. 277–298). Bethesda, MD: AOTA Press.

Barris, R., Kielhofner, G., Levine, R. E., & Neville, A. (1985). Occupation as interaction with the environment. In G. Kielhofner (Ed.), *A model for human occupation* (pp. 42–62). Baltimore: Williams & Wilkins.

Baum, C. M., & Christiansen, C. H. (2005). Person–environment–occupation–performance: An occupation-based framework for practice. In C. Christiansen, C. M. Baum, & J. Bass-Haugen (Eds.), *Occupational therapy: Performance, participation, and well-being* (pp. 242–267). Thorofare, NJ: Slack.

Baum, C. M., Connor, L. T., Morrison, T., Hahn, M., Dromerick, A. W., & Edwards, D. F. (2008). Reliability, validity, and clinical utility of the Executive Function Performance Test: A measure of executive function in a sample of people with stroke. *American Journal of Occupational Therapy, 62,* 446–455. http://dx.doi.org/10.5014/ajot.62.4.446

Baum, C. M., & Edwards, D. (2008). *Activity Card Sort* (2nd ed.). Bethesda, MD: AOTA Press.

Baum, C. M., & Katz, N. (2010). Occupational therapy approach to assessing the relationship between cognition and function. In T. D. Marcotte & I. Grant (Eds.), *Neuropsychology of everyday functioning* (pp. 63–90). New York: Guilford Press.

Baum, C. M., Morrison, T., Hahn, M., & Edwards, D. F. (2003). *Executive Function Performance Test: Test protocol booklet.* St. Louis, MO: Washington University School of Medicine, Program in Occupational Therapy.

Bergman, M. M. (2003). The essential steps cognitive orthotic. *NeuroRehabilitation, 18,* 31–46.

Brain Injury Association of America. (2011). *Cognitive rehabilitation evidence.* Retrieved July 5, 2011, from www.BIAUSA.org

Brown, C. E., & Dunn, W. (2002). *Adolescent/Adult Sensory Profile: User's manual.* San Antonio, TX: Psychological Corporation.

Brown, L., & Alexander, J. (1991). *Self-Esteem Index.* Austin, TX: Pro-Ed.

Burns, T. (1991). *Cognitive Performance Test: A measure of cognitive capacity for the performance of routine tasks.* Minneapolis: Minneapolis Veterans Administration Medical Center, GRECC Center.

Cermak, S. A., & Maeir, A. (2011). Cognitive rehabilitation of children and adults with attention-deficit/hyperactivity disorder. In N. Katz (Ed.), *Cognition, occupation, and participation across the life span: Neuroscience, neurorehabilitation, and models of intervention in occupational therapy* (3rd ed., pp. 249–276). Bethesda, MD: AOTA Press.

Chui, T., Oliver, R., Ascott, P., Choo, L. C., Davis, T., Gaya, A., . . . Letts, L. (2006). *Safety Assessment of Function and the Environment for Rehabilitation–Health Outcome Measurement and Evaluation (SAFER–Home), Version 3 manual.* Toronto: COTA Health.

Cicerone, K. D., Dahlberg, C., Kalmar, K., Langenbahn, D. M., Malec, J. F., Bergquist, T. F., . . . Morse, P. A. (2000). Evidence-based cognitive rehabilitation: Recommendations for clinical practice. *Archives of Physical Medicine and Rehabilitation, 81,* 1596–1615. http://dx.doi.org/10.1053/apmr.2000.19240

Cicerone, K. D., Dahlberg, C., Malec, J. F., Langenbahn, D. M., Felicetti, T., Kneipp, S., . . . Catanese, J. (2005). Evidence-based cognitive rehabilitation: Updated review of the literature from 1998 through 2002. *Archives of Physical Medicine and Rehabilitation, 86,* 1681–1692. http://dx.doi.org/10.1016/j.apmr.2005.03.024

Cicerone, K. D., Langenbahn, D. M., Braden, C., Malec, J. F., Kalmar, K., Fraas, M., . . . Ashman, T. (2011). Evidence-based cognitive rehabilitation: Updated review of the literature from 2003 through 2008. *Archives of Physical Medicine and Rehabilitation, 92,* 519–530. http://dx.doi.org/10.1016/j.apmr.2010.11.015

Cicerone, K. D., Mott, T., Azulay, J., Sharlow-Galella, M. A., Ellmo, W. J., Paradise, S., & Friel, J. C. (2008). A randomized controlled trial of holistic neuropsychologic rehabilitation after traumatic brain injury. *Archives of Physical Medicine and Rehabilitation, 89,* 2239–2249. http://dx.doi.org/10.1016/j.apmr.2008.06.017

Corcoran, M. (Ed.). (2006). *Neurorehabilitation for dementia-related diseases* (AOTA Self-Paced Clinical Course). Bethesda, MD: American Occupational Therapy Association.

Dawson, D. R., Gaya, A., Hunt, A., Levine, B., Lemsky, C., & Polatajko, H. J. (2009). Using the Cognitive Orientation to Occupational Performance (CO–OP) with adults with executive dysfunction following traumatic brain injury. *Canadian Journal of Occupational Therapy, 76,* 115–127. http://dx.doi.org/10.1177/000841740907600209

Diller, L., & Weinberg, J. (1993). Response styles in perceptual retraining. In W. A. Gordon (Ed.), *Advances in stroke rehabilitation* (pp. 162–182). Boston: Andover Medical.

Donkervoort, M., Dekker, J., Stehmann-Saris, F. C., & Deelman, B. G. (2001). Efficacy of strategy training in left-hemisphere stroke patients with apraxia: A randomized clinical trial. *Neuropsychological Rehabilitation, 11,* 549–566. http://dx.doi.org/10.1080/09602010143000093

Evans, J. J., Wilson, B. A., Schuri, U., Andrade, J., Baddeley, A., Bruna, O., . . . Taussik, I. (2000). A comparison of "errorless" and "trial-and-error" learning methods for teaching individuals with acquired memory deficits. *Neuropsychological Rehabilitation, 10,* 67–101. http://dx.doi.org/10.1080/096020100389309

Eysenck, M. W., & Keane, M. T. (1990). *Cognitive psychology: A student's handbook.* East Sussex, England: Erlbaum.

Fisher, A. G., & Bray Jones, K. (2010a). *Assessment of Motor and Process Skills: Vol. 1. Development, standardization, and administration manual* (7th ed.). Fort Collins, CO: Three Star Press.

Fisher, A. G., & Bray Jones, K. (2010b). *Assessment of Motor and Process Skills: Vol. 2. User manual* (7th ed.). Fort Collins, CO: Three Star Press.

Folstein, M. F., Folstein, S. E., & McHugh, P. R. (1975). "Mini-Mental State." A practical method for grading the cognitive state of patients for the clinician. *Journal of Psychiatric Research, 12,* 189–198. http://dx.doi.org/10.1016/0022-3956(75)90026-6

Foster, E. R., Cunnane, K. B., Edwards, D. F., Morrison, M. T., Ewald, G. A., Geltman, E. M., & Zazulia, A. R. (2011). Executive dysfunction and depressive symptoms associated with reduced participation of people with severe congestive heart failure. *American Journal of Occupational Therapy, 65,* 306–313. http://dx.doi.org/10.5014/ajot.2011.000588

Frittelli, C., Borghetti, D., Iudice, G., Bonanni, E., Maestri, M., Tognoni, G., . . . Iudice, A. (2009). Effects of Alzheimer's disease and mild cognitive impairment on driving ability: A controlled clinical study by simulated driving test. *International Journal of Geriatric Psychiatry, 24,* 232–238. http://dx.doi.org/10.1002/gps.2095

Gentry, T., Wallace, J., Kvarfordt, C., & Lynch, K. B. (2008). Personal digital assistants as cognitive aids for individuals with severe traumatic brain injury: A community-based trial. *Brain Injury, 22,* 19–24. http://dx.doi.org/10.1080/02699050701810688

Geurtsen, G. J., van Heugten, C. M., Martina, J. D., & Geurts, A. C. H. (2010). Comprehensive rehabilitation programmes in the chronic phase after severe brain injury: A systematic review. *Journal of Rehabilitation Medicine, 42,* 97–110. http://dx.doi.org/10.2340/16501977-0508

Giles, G. M. (2010). Cognitive versus functional approaches to rehabilitation after traumatic brain injury: Commentary on a randomized controlled trial. *American Journal of Occupational Therapy, 64,* 182–185. http://dx.doi.org/10.5014/ajot.64.1.182

Giles, G. M. (2011). A neurofunctional approach to rehabilitation after brain injury. In N. Katz (Ed.), *Cognition, occupation, and participation across the life span: Neuroscience, neurorehabilitation, and models of intervention in occupational therapy* (3rd ed., pp. 351–381). Bethesda, MD: AOTA Press.

Giles, G. M., & Clark-Wilson, J. (Eds.). (1993). *Brain injury rehabilitation: A neurofunctional approach.* San Diego, CA: Singular.

Giles, G. M., Wager, J., Fong, L., & Waraich, B. S. (2005). Twenty-month effectiveness of a non-aversive, long-term, low-cost programme for persons with persisting neurobehavioural disability. *Brain Injury, 19,* 753–764. http://dx.doi.org/10.1080/02699050500110108

Gillen, G. (2009). *Cognitive and perceptual rehabilitation: Optimizing function.* St. Louis, MO: Mosby.

Gillespie, L. D., Robertson, M. C., Gillespie, W. J., Lamb, S. E., Gates, S., Cumming, R. G., & Rowe, B. H. (2009). Interventions for preventing falls in older people living in the community. *Cochrane Database of Systematic Reviews, 2012*(9), Art. No. CD007146. http://dx.doi.org/10.1002/14651858.CD007146.pub2

Gioia, G. A., Isquith, P. K., Guy, S. C., & Kenworthy, L. (2000). *Behavior Rating Inventory of Executive Function.* Lutz, FL: Psychological Assessment Resources.

Gitlin, L. N. (2003). Conducting research on home environments: Lessons learned and new directions. *Gerontologist, 43,* 628–637. http://dx.doi.org/10.1093/geront/43.5.628

Gitlin, L. N., & Corcoran, M. (Eds.). (2005). *An occupational therapy guide to helping caregivers of persons with dementia: The Home Environment Skill-Building Program.* Bethesda, MD: AOTA Press.

Gitlin, L. N., Schinfeld, S., Winter, L., Corcoran, M., Boyce, A. A., & Hauck, W. W. (2002). Evaluating home environments of persons with dementia: Interrater reliability and validity of the Home Environmental Assessment Protocol (HEAP). *Disability and Rehabilitation, 24,* 59–71. http://dx.doi.org/10.1080/09638280110066325

Goldenberg, G., Daumuller, M., & Hagmann, S. (2001). Assessment and therapy of complex activities of daily living in apraxia. *Neuropsychological Rehabilitation, 11,* 549–566. http://dx.doi.org/10.1080/09602010042000204

Goldenberg, G., & Hagman, S. (1998). Therapy of activities of daily living in patients with apraxia. *Neuropsychological Rehabilitation, 8,* 123–141. http://dx.doi.org/10.1080/713755559

Golisz, K. (2009). *Occupational therapy practice guidelines for adults with traumatic brain injury.* Bethesda, MD: AOTA Press.

Gorman, P., Dayle, R., Hood, C.-A., & Rumrell, L. (2003). Effectiveness of the ISAAC cognitive prosthetic system for improving rehabilitation outcomes with neurofunctional impairment. *NeuroRehabilitation, 18,* 57–67.

Guy, S. C., Isquith, P. K., & Gioia, G. A. (2004). *Behavior Rating Inventory of Executive Function—Self-Report Version.* Lutz, FL: Psychological Assessment Resources.

Hartman-Maeir, A., Katz, N., & Baum, C. M. (2009). Cognitive Functional Evaluation (CFE) process for individuals with suspected cognitive disabilities. *Occupational Therapy in Health Care, 23,* 1–23.

Izal, M., Montorio, I., Márquez, M., & Losada, A. (2005). Caregivers' expectations and care receivers' competence: Lawton's ecological model of adaptation and aging revisited. *Archives of Gerontology and Geriatrics, 41,* 129–140. http://dx.doi.org/10.1016/j.archger.2005.01.001

Josman, N. (2011). The Dynamic Interactional Model in schizophrenia. In N. Katz (Ed.), *Cognition, occupation, and participation across the lifespan: Neuroscience, neurorehabilitation, and models of intervention in occupational therapy* (3rd ed., pp. 203–221). Bethesda, MD: AOTA Press.

Katz, N. (2006). *Routine Task Inventory–Expanded manual.* Retrieved from www.allen-cognitive-network.org

Katz, N., Itzkovich, M., Averbuch, S., & Elazar, B. (1989). Loewenstein Occupational Therapy Cognitive Assessment (LOTCA) battery for brain-injured patients: Reliability and validity. *American Journal of Occupational Therapy, 43,* 184–192. http://dx.doi.org/10.5014/ajot.43.3.184

Katzman, R., Brown, T., Fuld, P., Peck, A., Schechter, R., & Schimmel, H. (1983). Validation of a short Orientation–Memory–Concentration Test of cognitive impairment. *American Journal of Psychiatry, 140,* 734–739.

Kielhofner, G. (2009). *Conceptual foundations of occupational therapy* (3rd ed.). Philadelphia: F. A. Davis.

Law, M., Baptiste, S., Carswell, A., McColl, M. A., Polatajko, H., & Pollock, N. (1998). *Canadian Occupational Performance Measure* (2nd rev. ed.). Ottawa, ON: CAOT Publications.

Law, M., Baptiste, S., Carswell, A., McColl, M. A., Polatajko, H., & Pollock, N. (2005). *Canadian Occupational Performance Measure* (4th ed.). Ottawa, ON: CAOT Publications.

Law, M., Cooper, B., Strong, S., Stewart, D., Rigby, P., & Letts, L. (1996). The Person–Environment–Occupation Model: A transactive approach to occupational performance. *Canadian Journal of Occupational Therapy, 63,* 10–23.

Lawton, M. P., & Nahemow, L. (1973). Ecology and the aging process. In C. Eisdorfer & M. P. Lawton (Eds.), *Psychology of adult development and aging* (pp. 619–674). Washington, DC: American Psychological Association.

Lowenstein, D., & Acevedo, A. (2010). The relationship between activities of daily living and neuropsychological performance. In T. D. Marcotte & I. Grant (Eds.), *Neuropsychology of everyday functioning* (pp. 93–112). New York: Guilford Press.

Mastos, M., Miller, K., Eliasson, A. C., & Imms, C. (2007). Goal-directed training: Linking theories of treatment to clinical practice for improved functional activities in daily life. *Clinical Rehabilitation, 21,* 47–55. http://dx.doi.org/10.1177/0269215506073494

McGurk, S. R., Twamley, E. W., Sitzer, D. I., McHugo, G. J., & Mueser, K. T. (2007). A meta-analysis of cognitive remediation in schizophrenia. *American Journal of Psychiatry, 164,* 1791–1802. http://dx.doi.org/10.1176/appi.ajp.2007.07060906

Nasreddine, Z. S., Phillips, N. A., Bédirian, V., Charbonneau, S., Whitehead, V., Collin, I., . . . Chertkow, H. (2005). The Montreal Cognitive Assessment, MoCA: A brief screening tool for mild cognitive impairment. *Journal of the American Geriatrics Society, 53,* 695–699. http://dx.doi.org/10.1111/j.1532-5415.2005.53221.x

Neistadt, M. E. (1992). The Rabideau Kitchen Evaluation–Revised: An assessment of meal preparation skill. *OTJR: Occupation, Participation and Health, 12,* 242–253.

Parish, L., & Oddy, M. (2007). Efficacy of rehabilitation for functional skills more than 10 years after extremely severe brain injury. *Neuropsychological Rehabilitation, 17,* 230–243. http://dx.doi.org/10.1080/09602010600750675

Park, N. W., Moscovitch, M., & Robertson, I. H. (1999). Divided attention impairments after traumatic brain injury. *Neuropsychologia, 37,* 1119–1133. http://dx.doi.org/10.1016/S0028-3932(99)00034-2

Polatajko, H. J., & Mandich, A. (2004). *Enabling occupation in children: The Cognitive Orientation to Daily Occupational Performance.* Ottawa, ON: CAOT Publications.

Polatajko, H. J., Mandich, A., & McEwen, S. E. (2011). Cognitive Orientation to Daily Occupational Performance (CO–OP): A cognitive-based intervention for children and adults. In N. Katz (Ed.), *Cognition, occupation, and participation across the life span: Neuroscience, neurorehabilitation, and models of intervention in occupational therapy* (3rd ed., pp. 299–321). Bethesda, MD: AOTA Press.

Rand, D., Basha-Abu Rukan, S., Weiss, P. L., & Katz, N. (2009). Validation of the Virtual MET as an assessment tool for executive functions. *Neuropsychological Rehabilitation, 19,* 583–602. http://dx.doi.org/10.1080/09602010802469074

Riska-Williams, L., Allen, C. A., Austin, S., David, S., Earhart, C., & McCraith, D. B. (2007). *Manual for the ACLS–5 and LACLS–5.* Camarillo, CA: ACLS & LACLS Committee.

Robertson, I. H., Ward, T., Ridgeway, V., & Nimmo-Smith, I. (1994). *The Test of Everyday Attention.* Bury St. Edmunds, England: Thames Valley Test Company.

Rocke, K., Hays, P., Edwards, D., & Berg, C. (2008). Development of a performance assessment of executive function: The Children's Kitchen Task Assessment. *American Journal of Occupational Therapy, 62,* 528–537. http://dx.doi.org/10.5014/ajot.62.5.528

Rohling, M. L., Faust, M. E., Beverly, B., & Demakis, G. (2009). Effectiveness of cognitive rehabilitation following acquired brain injury: A meta-analytic re-examination of Cicerone et al.'s (2000, 2005) systematic reviews. *Neuropsychology, 23,* 20–39. http://dx.doi.org/10.1037/a0013659

Roux, F. E., Boetto, S., Sacko, O., Chollet, F., & Trémoulet, M. (2003). Writing, calculating, and finger recognition in the region of the angular gyrus: A cortical stimulation study of Gerstmann syndrome. *Journal of Neurosurgery, 99,* 716–727. http://dx.doi.org/10.3171/jns.2003.99.4.0716

Schutz, L. E., & Wanlass, R. L. (2009). Interdisciplinary assessment strategies for capturing the elusive executive. *American Journal of Physical Medicine and Rehabilitation, 88,* 419–422. http://dx.doi.org/10.1097/PHM.0b013e3181a0e2d3

Shallice, T., & Burgess, P. W. (1991). Deficits in strategy application following frontal lobe damage in man. *Brain, 114,* 727–741. http://dx.doi.org/10.1093/brain/114.2.727

Sheikh, J. L., & Yesavage, J. A. (1986). Geriatric Depression Scale (GDS): Recent evidence and development of a shorter version. *Clinical Gerontologist, 5,* 165–173.

Sitzer, D. I., Twamley, E. W., & Jeste, D. V. (2006). Cognitive training in Alzheimer's disease: A meta-analysis of the literature. *Acta Psychiatrica Scandinavica, 114,* 75–90. http://dx.doi.org/10.1111/j.1600-0447.2006.00789.x

Sohlberg, M. M., & Mateer, C. A. (1989). *Introduction to cognitive rehabilitation.* New York: Guilford Press.

Tariq, S. H, Tumosa, N., Chibnall, J. T., Perry, M. H., III, & Morley, J. E. (2006). Comparison of the Saint Louis University Mental Status Examination and the Mini-Mental State Examination for detecting dementia and mild neurocognitive disorder: A pilot study. *American Journal of Geriatric Psychiatry, 14,* 900–910. http://dx.doi.org/10.1097/01.JGP.0000221510.33817.86

Toglia, J. P. (1993). *The Contextual Memory Test.* Tucson, AZ: Therapy Skill Builders.

Toglia, J. P. (2011). The Dynamic Interactional Model of Cognition in cognitive rehabilitation. In N. Katz (Ed.), *Cognition, occupation, and participation across the life span: Neuroscience, neurorehabilitation, and models of intervention in occupational therapy* (3rd ed., pp. 161–201). Bethesda, MD: AOTA Press.

Toglia, J. P., Johnston, M. V., Goverover, Y., & Dain, B. (2010). A multicontext approach to promoting transfer of strategy use and self regulation after brain injury: An exploratory study. *Brain Injury, 24,* 664–677. http://dx.doi.org/10.3109/02699051003610474

Toglia, J. P., & Kirk, U. (2000). Understanding awareness deficits following brain injury. *NeuroRehabilitation, 15,* 57–70.

Turner-Stokes, L. (2008). Evidence for the effectiveness of multi-disciplinary rehabilitation following acquired brain injury: A synthesis of two systematic approaches. *Journal of Rehabilitation Medicine, 40,* 691–701. http://dx.doi.org/10.2340/16501977-0265

Turner-Stokes, L., Nair, A., Sedki, I., Disler, P. B., & Wade, D. (2005). Multi-disciplinary rehabilitation for acquired brain injury in adults of working age. *Cochrane Database of Systematic Reviews, 2005*(3), Art. No. CD004170. http://dx.doi.org/10.1002/14651858.CD004170.pub2

Vanderploeg, R. D., Schwab, K., Walker, W. C., Fraser, J. A., Sigford, B. J., Date, E. S., . . . Warden, D. L. (2008). Rehabilitation of traumatic brain injury in active duty military personnel and veterans: Defense and Veterans Brain Injury Center randomized controlled trial of two rehabilitation approaches. *Archives of Physical Medicine and Rehabilitation, 89,* 2227–2238. http://dx.doi.org/10.1016/j.apmr.2008.06.015

van Heugten, C. M., Dekker, J., Deelman, B. G., Stehmann-Saris, J. C., & Kinebanian, A. (1999). Assessment of disabilities in stroke patients with apraxia: Internal consistency and inter-observer reliability. *OTJR: Occupation, Participation and Health, 19,* 55–73.

van Heugten, C. M., Dekker, J., Deelman, B. G., van Dijk, A., Stehmann Saris, J. C., & Kinebanian, A. (2000). Measuring disabilities in stroke patients with apraxia: A validation of an observational method. *Neuropsychological Rehabilitation, 10,* 401–414. http://dx.doi.org/10.1080/096020100411989

Wadley, V. G., Okonkwo, O., Crowe, M., & Ross-Meadows, L. A. (2008). Mild cognitive impairment and everyday function: Evidence of reduced speed in performing instrumental activities of daily living. *American Journal of Geriatric Psychiatry, 16,* 416–424. http://dx.doi.org/10.1097/01.JGP.0000310780.04465.13

Warren, M. (1993). A hierarchical model for evaluation and treatment of visual perceptual dysfunction in adult acquired brain injury, Part 1. *American Journal of Occupational Therapy, 47,* 42–54. http://dx.doi.org/10.5014/ajot.47.1.42

Wilson, B. A., Alderman, N., Burgess, A. W., Emslie, H., & Evans, J. J. (1996). *Behavioral assessment of the dysexecutive syndrome.* Bury St. Edmunds, England: Thames Valley Test Company.

Wilson, B. A., Baddeley, A., Evans, J. J., & Shiel, A. (1994). Errorless learning in the rehabilitation of memory impaired people. *Neuropsychological Rehabilitation, 4,* 307–326. http://dx.doi.org/10.1080/09602019408401463

Wilson, B. A., Clare, E., Baddeley, A. D., Cockburn, J., Watson, P., & Tate, R. (1999). *The Rivermead Behavioural Memory Test–Extended Version*. London: Pearson Assessment.

Wilson, B. A., Cockburn, J., & Baddeley, A. (1991). *The Rivermead Behavioral Memory Test*. Bury St. Edmunds, England: Thames Valley Test Company.

Wilson, B. A., Cockburn, J., & Baddeley, A. D. (2003). *The Rivermead Behavioural Memory Test* (2nd ed.). London: Pearson Assessment.

Wilson, B. A., Scott, H., Evans, J., & Emslie, H. (2003). Preliminary report of a NeuroPage service within a health care system. *NeuroRehabilitation, 18,* 3–8.

Wykes, T., Huddy, V., Cellard, C., McGurk, S. R., & Czobor, P. (2011). A meta-analysis of cognitive remediation for schizophrenia: Methodology and effect sizes. *American Journal of Psychiatry, 168,* 472–485. http://dx.doi.org/10.1176/appi.ajp.2010.10060855

Zarit, S. H., & Femia, E. E. (2008). A future for family care and dementia intervention research? Challenges and strategies. *Aging and Mental Health, 12,* 5–13. http://dx.doi.org/10.1080/13607860701616317

Related Readings

Gitlin, L. N., Winter, L., Dennis, M. P., Corcoran, M., Schinfeld, S., & Hauck, W. W. (2002). Strategies used by families to simplify tasks for individuals with Alzheimer's disease and related disorders: Psychometric analysis of the Task Management Strategy Index (TMSI). *Gerontologist, 42,* 61–69. http://dx.doi.org/10.1093/geront/42.1.61 PubMed

Katz, N. (Ed.). (2011). *Cognition, occupation, and participation across the life span: Neuroscience, neurorehabilitation, and models of intervention in occupational therapy* (3rd ed.). Bethesda, MD: AOTA Press.

Authors
Gordon Muir Giles, PhD, OTR/L, FAOTA
Mary Vining Radomski, PhD, OTR/L, FAOTA
Tina Champagne, OTD, OTR/L
Mary A. Corcoran, PhD, OT/L, FAOTA
Glen Gillen, EdD, OTR/L, FAOTA
Heather Miller Kuhaneck, PhD, OTR/L, FAOTA
M. Tracy Morrison, OTD, OTR/L
Barbara Nadeau, MA, OTR/L
Izel Obermeyer, MS, OTR/L
Joan Toglia, PhD, OTR/L
Timothy J. Wolf, OTD, MSCI, OTR/L

for

The Commission on Practice
Debbie Amini, EdD, OTR/L, CHT, *Chairperson*

Adopted by the Representative Assembly 2012OctCO21

To be published and copyrighted in 2013 by the American Occupational Therapy Association in the *American Journal of Occupational Therapy, 67*(Suppl.).

Appendix A. Types of Cognitive Evaluations in Occupational Therapy Based on Cognitive Functional Evaluation Process

EVALUATION TYPE	DESCRIPTION	EXAMPLES
Interview	Provides the occupational therapist with background information from the client or significant others and delineates the client's occupational profile (occupational history, current status, and occupational goals) as well as the client's views regarding the nature of any deficits he or she might have.	• Activity Card Sort (Baum & Edwards, 2008) • Canadian Occupational Performance Measure (Law et al., 1998)
Cognitive screening tools	Used to create a preliminary overview of the client's strengths and weaknesses using standardized assessments.	• Mini-Mental State Examination (Folstein, Folstein, & McHugh, 1975) • Short Blessed Memory Test (Katzman et al., 1983) • Montreal Cognitive Assessment (Nasreddine et al., 2005) • Allen Cognitive Level Screen–5 (Riska-Williams et al., 2007) • Loewenstein Occupational Therapy Cognitive Assessment (Katz, Itzkovich, Averbuch, & Elazar, 1989) • St. Louis University Mental Status Examination (Tariq, Tumosa, Chibnall, Perry, & Morley, 2006)
Performance-based assessments that may be used to assess cognitive- and executive function–based performance deficits once those have been established	Used to identify the occupational performance concerns to address in occupational therapy intervention. These measures themselves may or may not implicate specific cognitive or executive function deficits, and this relationship is established on the basis of the skilled observation of the occupational therapist.	• Routine Task Inventory (Katz, 2006) • Rabideau Kitchen Task Assessment–Revised (Neistadt, 1992) • Assessment of Motor and Process Skills (AMPS; Fisher & Bray Jones, 2010a, 2010b) • Executive Function Performance Test (EFPT; Baum, Morrison, Hahn, & Edwards, 2003) • Multiple Errands Test (Shallice & Burgess, 1991) • Árnadóttir OT-ADL Neurobehavioral Evaluation (Arnadottir, 1990) • Children's Kitchen Task Assessment (Rocke, Hays, Edwards, & Berg, 2008)
Measures of specific cognitive functions and client factors (e.g., memory, attention), preferably those with established ecological validity	Used to develop a detailed understanding of the client's occupational performance deficits or to inform in the design of interventions to help clients overcome occupational performance deficits.	• Contextual Memory Test (Toglia, 1993) • Rivermead Behavioral Memory Test (Wilson et al., 1999; Wilson, Cockburn, & Baddeley, 1991, 2003) • Test of Everyday Attention (Robertson, Ward, Ridgeway, & Nimmo-Smith, 1994) • Behavioral Assessment of the Dysexecutive Syndrome (Wilson, Alderman, Burgess, Emslie, & Evans, 1996)
Specific measures of cognitive performance in the context of specific occupations	Used to determine how specific cognitive deficits manifest themselves in occupational performance.	• ADL checklist for neglect • EFPT (Baum et al., 2008) • AMPS (Fisher & Bray Jones, 2010a, 2010b)
Environmental assessment	Provides the therapist with information about the environment and context in which the client needs to function in his or her daily life.	• Safety Assessment of Function and the Environment for Evaluation (Chui et al., 2006) • Home Environmental Assessment Protocol (Gitlin et al., 2002)

Appendix B. Theoretical Models Guiding Occupational Therapy Cognitive Rehabilitation

Occupational therapy scholars have developed several theoretical models that explain and guide the intervention approaches used by occupational therapy practitioners to address the impact of cognition on occupational performance.

Toglia's Dynamic Interactional Model (Toglia, 2011) was developed for persons with stroke or traumatic brain injury (TBI) but is relevant to many people with cognitive dysfunction, including children with attention deficit hyperactivity disorder and adolescents (Cermak & Maeir, 2011; Josman, 2011). The Dynamic Interactional Model utilizes multiple activities in a variety of contexts to help individuals understand performance problems and develop strategies to enhance occupational performance. The overall goal of multicontextual intervention is to help the client gain more control over symptoms by efficiently and independently using strategies for information processing (Toglia, Johnston, Goverover, & Dain, 2010).

The **Cognitive Rehabilitation Model of Katz and Averbach** (Averbach & Katz, 2011) provides a comprehensive approach to clients with neurological impairment of differing severities. The approach focuses on enhancing retained cognitive abilities, the development of self-awareness, and the use of remedial cognitive-training strategies (targeting specific areas of cognitive function such as visual perception, visual–motor organization, and thinking operations), learning strategies (interventions designed to help the client develop learning strategies), and remedial strategies (to develop basic activities of daily living [ADLs]).

Allen's Cognitive Disabilities Model (Allen, Earhart, & Blue, 1992) has been applied to persons with dementia, TBI, and severe mental health disorders. The cognitive disabilities model provides a way to describe deficits arising from damage in the physical or chemical structures of the brain and producing observable limitations in "routine task behavior." The Allen battery of assessments provides tools that are used to predict what a person will be able to do (level, mode, patterns) across multiple domains of functioning; identifies the assistance that he or she will require, including safety considerations; and guides appropriate communication and teaching methods when appropriate (Allen et al., 1992; Kielhofner, 2009).

The **Cognitive Orientation to Daily Occupational Performance (CO–OP)** model was developed for children with developmental coordination disorder but has been used widely with neurological and adult populations and across different types of dysfunction (Polatajko, Mandich, & McEwen, 2011). CO–OP is a client-centered problem-solving and performance-based intervention that facilitates performance acquisition through a process of guided discovery of strategies that enable learning of skills. Strategies may be global and provide a general method of approaching any problem (i.e., goal, plan, do, check) or domain-specific (i.e., relating to one area of dysfunction only).

The **Neurofunctional Approach** was developed for persons with independent living goals after TBI but has also been applied to persons after stroke and other acquired neurological impairment (Giles, 2010, 2011; Giles & Clark-Wilson, 1993; Parish & Oddy, 2007; Vanderploeg et al., 2008). The client and therapist collaboratively select specific performance goals. A task analysis is developed, and a "constraint" model is used to establish the client's specific strengths and limitations and construct specific interventions to allow learning to take place (e.g., "cue experimentation" to determine the types of cues the client needs to be successful). Automatic behavioral routines are viewed as the foundation of effective functional and behavioral competencies for all individuals. Interventions are specifically tailored to the client's abilities and are experiential. Evidence from social psychology, learning theory, errorless learning, self-generation, and overlearning literature is used in the design of task-specific skill-retraining programs.

Several occupational therapy models focus on the influence of the environment and the modification of task demands on cognition and function. The **Cognitive Disabilities Model** is an important occupational therapy model that assists in the development of an understanding of a client's needs for environmental support (Kielhofner, 2009). Many other occupational therapy models (Baum & Christiansen, 2005; Gitlin, 2003; Law et al., 1996) trace their roots to the **Press-Competence Model** (Izal, Montorio, Márquez, & Losada, 2005; Lawton & Nahemow, 1973), which was developed to explain the transactional relationship between an individual's capacity and attributes of the environment (e.g., natural, physical, social). Gitlin and Corcoran's (2005) **Environmental Skill-Building Program** is designed to help family caregivers of persons with dementia learn specific strategies to modify their living space and develop a more supportive environment so that the person with dementia will exhibit fewer disruptive behaviors and experience a slower rate of decline and dependence in instrumental and basic ADLs.

Appendix C. Cognition Case Examples

Case 1. Students in a 5th-Grade Classroom: Improving cognitive performance using the Multicontext Approach

CLIENT DESCRIPTION	EVALUATION AND GOAL-SETTING	OCCUPATIONAL THERAPY INTERVENTION AND OUTCOME
The teachers and principal expressed concerns about the organizational skills of **5th graders,** who, in this district, are required for the first time to manage lockers and switch classes. The class included 35 students (7 with special needs) with an average age of 10 years and had 3 teacher's aides.	*Occupational Profile:* The occupational therapist interviewed the principal and teachers. The teachers indicated that more than half of the students had difficulty keeping track of class materials and homework and often lost or misplaced required materials. *Analysis of Occupational Performance:* The therapist observed the classroom and analyzed the classroom and locker routines and the school demands placed on the students' organizational skills. *Goal Setting:* Analysis of interviews and classroom observations indicated that disorganization of lockers, desks, and folders appeared to contribute to students' difficulties. The teachers agreed with this analysis. Goals were for students to be able to 1. Identify at least 2 strategies for improving locker or desk organization; 2. Recognize situations in which they need to use organizational strategies; and 3. Apply self-generated organizational strategies to other school and home activities.	*Intervention Approach:* The occupational therapist collaborated with the teacher to design a 12-session pilot program to address the identified goals and assess initial feasibility, student engagement, and response. The therapist led each weekly 42-minute session. The teacher reinforced the information between sessions. The program was based on the Multicontext Approach (Toglia, Johnston, Goverover, & Dain, 2010), which provides a framework to promote strategy use and metacognitive skills across different situations. Activities are systematically varied to help persons make connections across activities. The approach emphasizes anticipation of challenges and self-monitoring skills. During the intervention sessions, students discussed identifying "roadblocks" and challenges to staying organized in school and daily life (e.g., locker, desk, folders, backpack). Once students identified these, they generated strategies. For example, to address locker management, students were asked to develop or draw a personalized locker plan and checklist, carry it out, and then assess whether it worked for them. During the week, students made daily ratings of their locker organization. Next session they identified factors that influenced their performance and revised or generated new strategies. Students were encouraged to use organizational strategies in different activities (e.g., homework, backpack, binder, folder, or desk organization; organizing information on a page or worksheet). Every session focused on making connections to previous sessions. *Outcome:* The lead teacher indicated that 80% of the students came to class prepared, with the correct materials. The majority of students rated their lockers as more organized and reported high satisfaction with the program. Students indicated that although their lockers could still become disorganized, they knew when to stop, reorganize, or make a new plan.

Case 2. Client With Asperger's Syndrome: Addressing cognition to optimize occupational performance at school using a CO–OP and Environmental Adaptation Approach

Cody, age 12 and in 6th grade, was diagnosed with Asperger's syndrome at age 8. Cody currently lives with his mother, father, and 2 siblings. He received occupational therapy through his school system and from an occupational therapist in private practice beginning in kindergarten and	*Occupational Profile:* Cody stated that he dislikes writing by hand, cannot read his own notes, and often wastes time in school so he can do schoolwork at home on the computer. He reported having trouble concentrating and being distracted by noise and classroom activity. He described him-	*Intervention Approach:* The occupational therapy practitioner used the CO–OP approach (Polatajko & Mandich, 2004) to develop the intervention plan. In the CO–OP approach, children develop their own goals and are guided in developing and applying cognitive strategies.

(Continued)

Appendix C. Cognition Case Examples *(cont.)*

CLIENT DESCRIPTION	EVALUATION AND GOAL-SETTING	OCCUPATIONAL THERAPY INTERVENTION AND OUTCOME
continuing through 3rd grade. Following 3rd grade, his occupational therapy services were discontinued, but he continued to use assistive technology to reduce the writing demands of schoolwork. Cody's mother requested renewed occupational therapy services for him at an outpatient facility because of her concerns with his coordination and self-image and his reported concerns regarding relationships with his peers.	self as bad at sports because he doesn't have good reflexes. His interests are primarily sedentary and digital. Cody's mother reported that he needs structure and routine and becomes upset when routines are altered. A phone interview with his teacher suggested that Cody is disorganized with his work, has trouble initiating appropriate activity, does not seek assistance, and often loses track of time. *Analysis of Occupational Performance:* While completing the Evaluation Tool of Children's Handwriting (ETCH; Amundson, 1995), Cody exhibited problems with both legibility and speed. Cody's scores on the Self-Esteem Index (Brown & Alexander, 1991) indicated that he is most comfortable with himself and his family relationships and least comfortable with himself in relation to his peers. His scores on the Sensory Profile (Brown & Dunn, 2002) indicated difficulties with sensory seeking and sensitivity. Cody's score on the Behavior Rating Inventory of Executive Function (BRIEF; Gioia, Isquith, Guy, & Kenworthy, 2000) and the BRIEF Self-Report (Guy, Isquith, & Gioia, 2004) suggested problems with inhibition, behavioral shift, emotional control, planning and organizing, and task completion. Cody reported feeling comfortable and secure in his family and discussed his difficulties easily. He reported being motivated to play sports and games with his peers. *Goal Setting:* Cody, his mother, and the occupational therapist collaborated to set therapy goals. After 6 months, Cody will 1. Independently manage the homework process (knowing what homework is required and due dates, initiating its completion, and turning it in on time); 2. Complete homework while seated at the kitchen table; 3. Write legibly during note taking and homework; 4. Sit at a desk and attend during class time; and 5. Select at least 1 peer sport to try.	For the first month, Cody attended twice-weekly occupational therapy sessions. Cody was then seen monthly and provided with home practice and phone consultation for strategy implementation and modification. Therapy focused on the use of cognitive strategies to improve performance as well as environmental and task adaptations. Cognitive–behavioral interventions were taught to assist Cody with the specific social situations he identified as difficult; role-playing was completed in occupational therapy. The skills were then practiced with a peer. These included the problem-solving steps of 1. Stopping and thinking before acting, 2. Identifying the problem, 3. Thinking about 2 or 3 possible solutions, 4. Considering the consequences of each action, and 5. Deciding on and implementing a strategy. Cody was also taught skills of task analysis so he could begin to develop his own adaptations. By gaining control over his own behaviors, he hoped to improve his ability to engage with peers. *Outcome:* After 6 months, Cody participated in a reevaluation. Improvements were noted in all goal areas. Cody had begun playing soccer with neighborhood friends. His handwriting was more legible. The combination of improved legibility and the use of technology allowed him to take notes, read them, complete his written class work, and document to his teacher what he was learning. He was better able to attend to his classroom activities using the strategies he had implemented at school. He also found that by keeping data on his performance, with his mother's help, he was able to see how much better he was doing and that motivated him to continue and practice. Cody reported that his self-esteem is better now that he believes he can learn the things he wants to learn.

Case 3. Client With Mild Stroke: Addressing cognition to advance occupational performance using a combined Problem-Solving and Task-Specific Approachand Environmental Adaptation Approach

Until a month ago, **Martha, age 65,** was living independently in the community with her husband. Martha had worked as a circuit judge for the previous 10 years. She has 3 children and 3 grandchildren younger than age 5. Martha had cared for her grandchildren every Saturday while her daughter worked. Martha frequently trav-	*Occupational Profile:* The occupational therapist conducted an informal interview with Martha and her husband and concluded that Martha was aware of her deficits. Martha revealed she found situations that are out of her control to be the most difficult: "I don't like not knowing what is going to happen. I lose my cool,	*Intervention Approach:* A goal-setting/problem-solving approach aims to empower the client so that the client uses a specific problem-solving framework to develop (with the occupational therapist's guidance) his or her own self-training program, which when successful acts as reinforcement for the whole process.

(Continued)

496

Appendix C. Cognition Case Examples *(cont.)*

CLIENT DESCRIPTION	EVALUATION AND GOAL-SETTING	OCCUPATIONAL THERAPY INTERVENTION AND OUTCOME

eled for work and pleasure. One month ago, Martha fell down a flight of stairs in her home.

Symptom/Complaints: Since the fall, Martha has felt dizzy and fatigued and reported several functional changes. For example, it takes more effort for her to smile and make facial expressions. She reports difficulty picking up items, such as her hairbrush, and holding on to them during functional tasks. Prior to her fall she enjoyed spending time with her grandchildren, but now she feels impatient and intolerant with them. During a recent work trip, Martha lost track of time while having a meal at the airport and missed her flight.

Medical Evaluation and Referral to Occupational Therapy: Martha's physician referred her to an imaging center for a MRI scan. The physician informed Martha that she had had a stroke. Martha was referred to a neurologist, who told her she had had a mild stroke, due to a clot in her right anterior cerebral artery, damaging the middle region of her right frontal lobe. The neurologist noted that Martha had mild facial weakness and dysarthria and mild weakness in her left hand. The neurologist recommended that Martha take a couple of weeks to rest before returning to work. He also referred her to outpatient occupational therapy.

and that is when I make mistakes." According to Martha and her family, these errors are new and appear to be a consequence of her stroke.

The Canadian Occupational Performance Measure (COPM; Law et al., 2005) was used to identify Martha's priorities for treatment. The Activity Card Sort (Baum & Edwards, 2008) revealed that Martha retained only 80% of her usual activities since her stroke. Among the activities she had given up were eating in restaurants, playing golf, dancing, going to parties and picnics, and doing laundry and yard work.

Analysis of Occupational Performance: The occupational therapist used informal observation methods as Martha worked on complex everyday tasks, such as child care, to assess Martha's ability to deal with unforeseen frustrations and challenges.

The Executive Function Performance Test (EFPT) helped determine the underlying factors that limited Martha's occupational performance (Baum, Morrison, Hahn, & Edwards, 2003; Baum et al., 2008). The EFPT results suggested that Martha required some support in planning and organizing complex tasks (e.g., paying bills). Additionally, results from the EFPT suggested Martha could use support in terms of her judgment during high-stress times. During the EFPT assessment, the occupational therapist noted Martha would get off task if she felt challenged on test items (e.g., bill paying).

Martha accurately predicts the environmental factors that result in her performance errors. Problematic situations for Martha are dynamic and novel, such as going to a conference or going out to lunch. Additionally, Martha has motor weakness that affects her speech, facial expressions, and ability to grasp objects.

On the basis of Martha's occupational therapy evaluation, the following long-term (1-month) goals were established:

1. Resume caring for her grandchildren with support from her husband 1 day a week.
2. Schedule all weekly meetings independently using an organizing system.
3. Complete desired functional activities using her upper extremity as an active assist.
4. Continue with desired leisure activities through planning and engaging in trips to novel restaurants with her husband.

Appropriate steps for problem-solving training include problem orientation, definition, and formulation; generation of alternatives; decision making; and solution verification. Task-specific training requires task analysis and a graded approach as the client accomplishes sequential tasks. Using both training methods, Martha accomplished her goal to improve child care skills by identifying specific aspects of child care that resulted in her feeling stressed and frustrated. Martha was encouraged to define the problem (e.g., "When the children yell, I feel anxious and frustrated"). She was then encouraged to formulate alternatives to reacting in a negative manner.

With practice Martha improved at self-monitoring and needed her husband's assistance less and less. With the encouragement and guidance of the occupational therapy practitioner, Martha identified her organizational problems and identified the use of a day planner as a preferred solution. Martha also developed methods that worked for her in entering and checking for information. Martha developed a program to work on her upper extremity and used her day planner to arrange a novel restaurant trip for her and her husband once per week.

Outcome: After 1 month of twice-weekly occupational therapy sessions, the COPM was readministered, and Martha reported significant improvements in both her performance and satisfaction with performance associated with tasks of importance to her. She was taking care of her grandchildren (with her husband) and routinely using a planner to organize her day and to plan restaurant trips. In addition to upper-extremity exercises, Martha continued to set and meet daily goals involving use of her left upper extremity to perform routine tasks.

Martha and the occupational therapist discussed whether the therapist could be of assistance in problem solving about return to work. Martha reported that she had not yet determined if she was going to transition back to work at a reduced schedule or retire, but she felt confident that she would be able to make the right decision.

(Continued)

Appendix C. Cognition Case Examples *(cont.)*

Case 4. Client With Severe Stroke: Addressing cognition to advance occupational performance using a Task-Specific, Strategy-Training Approach

CLIENT DESCRIPTION	EVALUATION AND GOAL-SETTING	OCCUPATIONAL THERAPY INTERVENTION AND OUTCOME
Jamie, age 55, was healthy and living independently in the community with her husband Carl prior to a left middle cerebral artery occlusion and subsequent fall. Following 6 days at the acute hospital, the acute care team documented her ADL/mobility status as maximum assist and determined that Jamie was a candidate for inpatient rehabilitation.	*Occupational Profile:* On admission, Jamie presented with global aphasia, so an interview with Carl served to develop Jamie's occupational profile. Carl reported that Jamie enjoyed long walks, trying new recipes, and was planning her daughter's wedding. Carl reported that Jamie "takes pride in her appearance" and "always has a positive outlook on life." Carl saw himself as Jamie's primary support. He reported that Jamie becomes tearful when he has to assist her in feeding.	*Intervention Approach:* Following goal identification, a task-specific strategy-training approach was chosen (Donkervoort, Dekker, Stehmann-Saris, & Deelman, 2001), because it is focused on improving occupational performance and has been shown to promote generalization (Gillen, 2009). The intervention is aimed at improving the performance of those with apraxia by teaching them internal (e.g., verbalizing steps during task performance) or external (e.g., referring to a sequence of pictures) compensatory strategies that enable more independent functioning despite the persisting apraxia. Strategy training occurred in the context of ADLs. A task-specific errorless-completion approach (Goldenberg, Daumuller, & Hagmann, 2001; Goldenberg & Hagman, 1998) was used during mealtimes for achieving errorless completion of feeding.
	Analysis of Occupational Performance: The occupational therapist administered the A–ONE (Arnadottir, 1990, 2011) instrument, which helped determine the underlying factors that limited occupational performance. Jamie required maximum assistance for self-care and mobility due to the presence of ideational apraxia (e.g., using a comb as a toothbrush, putting her sock on her hand), motor apraxia (e.g., inability to plan left-sided movements to propel her wheelchair, unable to generate motor plans for tooth brushing resulting in clumsy and awkward movements), impaired organization and sequencing (attempting to don socks after donning her shoes, attempting to get out of bed prior to removing the blanket), and impaired motor function (i.e., a flaccid right upper extremity preventing Jamie from washing her left arm or right axilla, weak right lower extremity making transfers unsafe).	*Outcome:* Jamie spent 18 days in inpatient rehabilitation. Jamie met her grooming goal, surpassed her toileting goal, and met her feeding goal (Goals 1, 2, and 4, respectively). Although improvement was noted, Jamie did not meet her meal preparation goal (Goal 3) by discharge, as her performance still fluctuated between minimal and moderate assistance.

The team and Carl decided that Jamie would be discharged home with a home health aide and occupational, speech, and physical therapy. |
| | The Assessment of Disabilities in Stroke Patients With Apraxia (van Heugten et al., 1999, 2000) revealed that Jamie required physical assistance to initiate task performance, to execute the correct sequence of action, and to correct her errors. | |
| | *Goal Setting:* On the basis of the evaluation, the following long-term (1-month) goals were established:

1. Jamie will complete grooming tasks with supervision and 3 demonstration cues for object use;
2. Jamie will transfer to the toilet with minimal assist for sequencing;
3. Jamie will prepare a simple sandwich with minimal assist; and
4. Jamie will eat a sandwich with supervision. | |

Case 5. Client With Severe Traumatic Brain Injury: Addressing cognition to advance occupational performance using Specific-Skill Training and an Environmental Modification Approach

Chloe, age 19, had sustained a traumatic brain injury 2 years ago when she collided with a tree while skiing. At the scene she had a Glasgow Coma Scale of 8 and was intubated. Injuries included a right basilar skull fracture, bilateral subarachnoid hemorrhage, a mandibular fracture, and a fractured right wrist. Chloe was transported via	*Occupational Profile:* The occupational therapist met with Chloe and her mother to develop the occupational profile. Chloe's daily activities consist primarily of watching TV and occasionally completing simple household chores assigned by her mother. Chloe uses her smartphone to text message her mother more than 30 times a day,	*Intervention Approach:* Occupational therapy was provided as a weekly consultative service and was a collaboration among the therapist, Chloe, and her support staff. A compensatory approach using an electronic memory aid (Gentry, Wallace, Kvarfordt, & Lynch, 2008) was chosen, as Chloe was already comfortable with the use of

(Continued)

Appendix C. Cognition Case Examples *(cont.)*

CLIENT DESCRIPTION	EVALUATION AND GOAL-SETTING	OCCUPATIONAL THERAPY INTERVENTION AND OUTCOME
medical helicopter to a Level 1 trauma center. Six weeks later, Chloe was transferred to a subacute rehabilitation hospital where she received occupational therapy, physical therapy, and speech and language therapy for 1 month before being discharged home. Two years post injury, Chloe has been unable to hold a job and lives at home with her mother. Chloe's most recent neuropsychological evaluation indicated significant impairments in visual and verbal memory and processing speed as well as in verbal comprehension. Deficits also were noted in executive functioning, including problem solving and planning and organization. Chloe recently was approved to receive services through her state's Brain Injury Medicaid Waiver program. This program provides support staff for individuals who meet specified financial and functional criteria so that individuals who have sustained a severe brain injury can remain in the community rather than be institutionalized. Chloe was approved to have support staff 8 hours per day while her mother was at work. An occupational therapy consult was ordered to provide input to the program.	asking repetitive questions and for reassurance. Chloe states that she feels anxious and does not know what to do. Chloe states that the memory book that she was asked to use "made her look stupid"; however, she verbalizes that she "can't remember anything." Prior to her injury, Chloe was very active and was on the softball and volleyball teams at school. She also liked to cook but no longer does so because she "burns stuff." Chloe stated that she loves animals and wants to be a veterinarian. *Analysis of Occupational Performance:* The occupational therapist administered several measures of functional cognition and observed Chloe plan, shop for, and prepare a simple meal. Chloe required moderate cueing when making the grocery list and at the grocery store to proceed to the next step of the task. She required reorientation to the task twice because she stated she could not remember what she was doing. She was able to use the list, locate needed items, and pay for items appropriately, although she reported being anxious throughout the shopping trip and rechecked the list multiple times. She was able to make the sandwich without cueing but required a verbal cue to turn off the stove. *Goal Setting:* Chloe and her mother agreed that developing strategies to manage Chloe's memory deficits would have the largest impact on her functional status. A list of goals was established: 1. Chloe will refer to her smartphone to determine the next activity in her day with minimal cues from staff. 2. Chloe will refer to her smartphone to determine the next step of IADL tasks with minimal cues from staff. 3. Chloe will refer to her smartphone to determine the next steps in each task in a volunteer position at local animal shelter with minimal cues from staff.	her smartphone and regarded this device as socially acceptable. Chloe's staff were instructed to enter her daily schedule into the calendar of the smartphone each morning. Chloe was then cued at the completion of each task to check her calendar and determine what activity she should do next. When Chloe was comfortable with using the calendar function, a task management application was added to the phone. The occupational therapist worked with staff to enter step-by-step instructions for IADLs that initially required moderate verbal cueing from staff. Staff then cued Chloe to check the next step in the phone rather than helping her with tasks. When Chloe was comfortable with using the smartphone for familiar tasks, the therapist worked with her and her staff to program steps for tasks undertaken as part of a volunteer job at a local animal shelter. *Outcome:* After 6 months the Brain Injury Medicaid Waiver program hours were decreased from 8 hours per day to 4 hours per day because Chloe was now using the smartphone to guide her through IADLs. However, through the frequent repetition of task performance the same way each day, Chloe is relying less on the phone with no increase in errors. Text messages to her mother have decreased from 30 messages per day to 3 per day. Chloe volunteers 15 hours per week at the local animal shelter and rarely reports feeling anxious. Any new tasks need to be programmed into the smartphone and monitored for the first few weeks. Chloe has learned that for any new tasks she must rely on her smartphone.

Case 6. Client With Alzheimer's Disease: Addressing cognition to advance occupational performance using an Task/Environmental Modification Approach

Raymond, age 79, lives with his wife Dorothy in a small central Pennsylvania town. Raymond and Dorothy have lived in the same house for 42 years, where they have raised 5 children. Very few upgrades have been made to the home, so all the bedrooms and the only full bath are on the second floor (clawfoot tub only). The event that first led to medical evaluation occurred 1 year ago, when Raymond became lost when driving to a neighboring town and ended up 150 miles beyond his intended destination. A state trooper	*Occupational Profile:* Dorothy responds to most of the questions at the initial interview, with Raymond responding only if specifically asked. Dorothy reports that Raymond is requiring assistance for most self-care tasks, with the exception of feeding and toileting, in which he is independent. Raymond owned his own furniture repair business before retiring and until about 3 months ago was able to make very simple repairs around the house or in his workshop. Dorothy does not feel it is currently safe for him to work unsupervised.	*Intervention Approach:* The intervention approach was based on the Person–Environment–Occupation–Performance model and involved teaching Dorothy and Raymond to use environmental and verbal cuing, plus task simplification during self-care, leisure, and work activities and to provide a calming atmosphere. The occupational therapist proposed 6 visits per month (twice weekly for 2 weeks; once weekly for 2 weeks) followed by a reevaluation. In collaboration with Dorothy, the therapist worked with Raymond to

(Continued)

Appendix C. Cognition Case Examples *(cont.)*

CLIENT DESCRIPTION	EVALUATION AND GOAL-SETTING	OCCUPATIONAL THERAPY INTERVENTION AND OUTCOME

CLIENT DESCRIPTION

helped him when his car ran out of gas, and Raymond was returned home to a worried Dorothy. Subsequently, Raymond was diagnosed with Alzheimer's disease, and over the following year his symptoms have progressed, triggering a referral to occupational therapy by Raymond's internist.

EVALUATION AND GOAL-SETTING

Raymond no longer drives or does home chores and is angry about these losses. Dorothy says he is easily angered and bored. She is concerned that he will "sit around the house all day and do nothing."

Dorothy wants to help her husband and has given up activities she enjoys to do so. The occupational therapist is concerned about role overload for Dorothy.

Analysis of Occupational Performance: Direct observation of Raymond in his workshop and the Cognitive Performance Test (Burns, 1991) provided findings for symptoms consistent with the moderate stage of Alzheimer's disease and difficulties completing detailed tasks. This score was consistent with Dorothy's report of Raymond's need for assistance with most IADLs and supervision and setup for ADLs. The occupational therapist also administered the following assessments:

1. *Geriatric Depression Scale* (Sheikh & Yesavage, 1986). Raymond's score on this measure indicated that he should visit his physician for diagnostic testing for possible major depressive disorder. Dorothy's score was within the normal range.
2. *Safety Assessment of Function and the Environment for Rehabilitation–Health Outcome Measurement and Evaluation* (SAFER–Home), Version 3 (Chui et al., 2006). Using this tool, the therapist determined that overall safety issues were moderate and were primarily isolated to lighting and bathroom issues.
3. *Task Management Strategy Index* (TMSI; Gitlin et al., 2002). This tool was administered to Dorothy to assess her use of task simplification and objects modification. Scores suggested that training was needed in environmental and verbal cueing and guidance.

Goal Setting: On the basis of Raymond's occupational profile, the analysis of occupational performance, and consultation with Dorothy, the following long-term (1-month) goals were established:

1. Through use of environmental and verbal cueing, Raymond will
   • Dress and bathe independently on 5 of 7 days,
   • Complete simple home chores with distant supervision, and
   • Assemble simple wooden kits with distant supervision.
2. Engage in desired activities, with agitated outbursts reduced to no more than 1 per week.

OCCUPATIONAL THERAPY INTERVENTION AND OUTCOME

determine the types of cueing that work best to support his occupational performance. The overall approach was to support his retained procedural memory with cues (e.g., lists or other types of instructions, placement of objects, verbal instruction).

Interventions with empirical evidence were implemented (Corcoran, 2006; Gillespie et al., 2009; Gitlin & Corcoran, 2005) and included the folllowing approaches:

1. *Environmental Cueing*—Modifying objects so their use is unambiguous (may require use of labels), eliminating power tools or other items that could cause injury, reducing the number of items available (clutter), and improved lighting for safety. In addition, suggestions were made regarding specific adaptive equipment for bathing and a monitoring system to provide distant supervision. Raymond's favorite music was used to create a calming atmosphere.
2. *Verbal Cueing*—To avoid conflict, Dorothy was taught to use implicit guiding by setting up the environment and making appropriate activity choices. When explicit guidance is needed, Dorothy was taught to provide instructions one step at a time in a neutral voice. Dorothy also decided to make or purchase audio or video recordings with explicit instructions for wooden assembly kits. Dorothy was shown how to provide tactile guidance.
3. *Task Simplification*—Dorothy and Raymond learned to choose simple activities or to modify existing activities so they involve few steps and reduced opportunities for errors.

Outcome: At the 4-week reevaluation visit, the occupational therapist observed Raymond during a leisure activity in the workshop, interviewed the couple, and readministered the SAFER–HOME and the TMSI. Scores improved on the standardized tests, and the couple reported that all goals were met. The therapist developed a discharge plan that included identification of behaviors that should trigger a request for additional occupational therapy (e.g., reduced performance in ADLs or leisure activities, daily agitation, increased risk of or actual falls or injury).

(Continued)

Appendix C. Cognition Case Examples *(cont.)*

Case 7. Client With Schizophrenia: Addressing cognition to optimize occupational performance based on the Cognitive Disabilities Model

CLIENT DESCRIPTION	EVALUATION AND GOAL-SETTING	OCCUPATIONAL THERAPY INTERVENTION AND OUTCOME
George, age 62, resides in a group home that has 24-hour staff supervision. George was diagnosed with schizophrenia, paranoid type, at age 21. He works at a local furniture workshop but is having difficulty with attendance, staying on task, and some aspects of job satisfaction. George was referred to occupational therapy to evaluate his abilities, goals, and employment expectations and also the job site.	*Occupational Profile:* George described two key areas of challenge at work: (1) work performance limitations and (2) strained interactions with his supervisor. George could explain most of the steps of his upholstery job, but he had difficulties with memory and sequencing when demonstrating the tasks. Additionally he reported problems with task transitions and indicated that he is frequently expected to shift to a new task before achieving mastery of the prior task. George reported that he likes his job but that his boss is often angry with him and he does not know why. George's boss appeared equally frustrated and confused. For example, the boss appeared puzzled by George's daily questions about familiar tasks. In private, George's boss admitted that he thought George was lazy. *Analysis of Occupational Performance:* Using clinical observations within the work setting, an analysis of cognitive performance actions with the Allen level and mode correlations (Allen, Earhart, & Blue, 1992) was completed for 3 of George's job activities (e.g., measuring, cutting, and gluing fabric) on 3 different days. George's scores on the Allen Cognitive Level Battery ranged between 4.4 and 4.6, suggesting that "scaffolding" would help George optimize his work performance. At this cognitive level and mode range, assistance for setup and organization, sequencing, and cues as needed is recommended. *Goal Setting:* The following long-term (3-month) goals were established: 1. George will demonstrate an increase of 25% in his productivity, with assistance for setup, the use of pictures outlining the steps of each task, and one full demonstration of each task and object use prior to the supervisor leaving George to complete the task. 2. George will increase attendance from 50% to 90% of the time. 3. George will check in at the end of each shift on a daily basis to discuss with his supervisor what works and what might be more helpful in order for George to meet his vocational goals. 4. George will report a 75% increase in job satisfaction by the end of 3 months.	*Intervention Approach:* The occupational therapist met with George's supervisor to provide education about schizophrenia to help him better understand George's experiences and needs. The supervisor was very appreciative of this information, which heightened his receptiveness to the therapist's recommendations. The therapist also met jointly with George and his boss to explain the results of the evaluation process, review George's work-related goals, and discuss recommended types and amount of assistance. Together they decided to create weekly schedule in which George spends each day doing one specific task in the upholstery department rather than multiple tasks in the same day. The occupational therapist developed pictorial sequencing booklets for each task that George was to complete. The supervisor agreed to provide the organizational setup for the day's tasks and one full demonstration of the directions at the start of each shift. He would then observe George fully complete what was demonstrated and provide any needed additional verbal cues. These external cues (e.g., setup, demonstration, referring to a sequence of pictures) provided the compensatory strategies necessary to enable George to function more independently and productively at work. *Outcome:* • *Goal 1:* George demonstrated an increase of 40% in his productivity rate. • *Goal 2:* George demonstrated an increase of 95% in his attendance at work. • *Goal 3:* George and his supervisor met at the end of each workday 100% of the time and identified and addressed all issues that came up within their sessions. • *Goal 4:* George reported an increase in his job satisfaction by 80%.

Note. ADLs = activities of daily living; CO–OP = Cognitive Orientation to Daily Occupational Performance; IADLs = instrumental activities of daily living; MRI = magnetic resonance imaging.

Driving and Community Mobility

The purpose of this paper is to describe the role of occupational therapy in the area of driving and community mobility. The intended audience for this paper includes occupational therapists, occupational therapy assistants, and stakeholders outside of the occupational therapy profession.

Community mobility, an instrumental activity of daily living (IADL), is defined as "moving around in the community and using public or private transportation, such as driving, walking, bicycling, or accessing and riding in buses, taxi cabs, or other transportation systems" (American Occupational Therapy Association [AOTA], 2008, p. 631). Community mobility or transportation is essential for independence and access to engagement in other everyday life activities (occupations). Community mobility, specifically driving, contributes to health and quality of life (U.S. Department of Transportation, 2003) by supporting independence, a sense of identity, social participation, and access to health services and the community (Oxley & Whelan, 2008). Loss of the fundamental privilege of driving and community mobility in adult life is exemplified by the feelings of loneliness, isolation, and depressive symptoms that often arise when one suddenly loses the ability to drive (Marottoli et al., 1997).

Driving and community mobility are included within the domain of occupational therapy (AOTA, 2008) and in the profession's *Scope of Practice* (AOTA, 2010). Appendix A illustrates some of the aspects of driving and community mobility within the domain of occupational therapy practice and describes the complexity and influence of this critical IADL.

Service Provision Across the Lifespan and Modes of Transportation

Occupational therapists and occupational therapy assistants address driving and other aspects of community mobility in a variety of practice settings with individual clients of all ages, organizations, and populations. When addressing community mobility and driving, occupational therapy practitioners[1] assess the client's sensory, cognitive, and motor performance skills; performance patterns; safety concerns; the contextual and environment supports or barriers; and the influence of community mobility and driving on the client's ability to participate in daily life. Occupational therapy practitioners also address mental health issues that may arise when community mobility is compromised. This comprehensive set of skills deems occupational therapy a critical and essential health care discipline to meet the complex demands of driving and community mobility concerns.

These occupational therapy practitioners share the common goals of supporting participation in the community; optimizing independence in community mobility; and reducing crashes, injuries, and fatalities. The extent of that therapeutic attention is provided along a continuum of specialization, with some specialty practitioners offering a very focused approach in which driving or community mobility is the pri-

---

[1]When the term *occupational therapy practitioner* is used in this document, it refers to both occupational therapists and occupational therapy assistants (AOTA, 2006). *Occupational therapists* are responsible for all aspects of occupational therapy service delivery and are accountable for the safety and effectiveness of the occupational therapy service delivery process. *Occupational therapy assistants* deliver occupational therapy services under the supervision of and in partnership with an occupational therapist (AOTA, 2009b).

mary goal, while other generalist practitioners address driving and community mobility as part of a larger agenda to optimize occupational engagement in their clients. Clients may be persons, organizations, or populations. Appendix B outlines the clients served, their respective community mobility concerns, and the examples of possible occupational therapy services.

Knowledge and Skill of Occupational Therapy Practitioners in Driving and Community Mobility

Occupational therapists and occupational therapy assistants possess the foundational education and training necessary to address driving and community mobility as an IADL as identified in the *Occupational Therapy Practice Framework: Domain and Process, 2nd Edition* (AOTA, 2008). Throughout the evaluation and intervention process, occupational therapy practitioners recognize the influence of disability and aging on client factors and can translate those influences into implications of risk in driving and community mobility. Through the use of clinical reasoning skills, occupational therapy practitioners use information about the client's performance skills, performance patterns, contextual and environmental factors, and client factors to deduce strengths and potential weaknesses with occupational performance in driving and community mobility.

Some occupational therapy practitioners specialize in *driving rehabilitation* by entirely focusing their practice on the occupation of driving. Occupational therapy specialists in driving rehabilitation have advanced education and expertise that enable them to present varying challenges and complexities during the in vivo observation and assessment of performance evaluation process to replicate actual driving experiences for a valid judgment of performance and safety. Those who are occupational therapists administer comprehensive driving evaluations; recommend continued, modified, or cessation of driving; and suggest appropriate vehicle modifications, adaptive equipment for driving, and driver retraining or specialized driver education. Those who are occupational therapy assistants contribute to this process. Many states require that occupational therapy practitioners who specialize in driving also become licensed as certified driver instructors to be able to perform on-road assessments and provide training to novice drivers or persons whose driver's license has expired.

AOTA asserts that occupational therapists and occupational therapy assistants require advanced education prior to working directly in specialized driving rehabilitation services. In addition, occupational therapy practitioners also can benefit from specialized certification in driving and community mobility. The available certification programs are further explained in Appendix C. These specialist occupational therapy practitioners administer evidence-based assessments specific to the requirements involved in driving, including clinical assessments of motor and praxis skills, sensory–perceptual skills, emotional regulation skills, cognitive skills, and communication and social skills, in addition to reaction time, knowledge of traffic rules, and on-road assessment of driving skills. The primary purpose of conducting or contributing to these comprehensive driving evaluations is to determine the client's occupational performance and safety to engage in driving. Specialist occupational therapy practitioners also provide intervention services to individuals for whom safe driving is a possibility or will require intervention to transition from driver to passenger. Interventions for the client with potential to drive may include remediation of performance skills, education in adaptive strategies, and training in the use of adaptive equipment to optimize performance and safety while operating or traveling in a motor vehicle.

Occupational therapists addressing community mobility assess clients as well as their communities to determine the client's ability to access transportation choices and utilize available resources and equipment. Individual assessments may include clinical testing similar to those in the area of driving evaluation. In vivo assessments are conducted using the mode of transportation desired or required by the client and may include buses, taxis, trains, airplanes, bicycles, or pedestrian means of travel. The focus of the evaluation for individual clients is to determine the client's ability to access and utilize transportation resources to enable engagement in community occupations. Intervention implemented with individuals using community mobility may include travel training, recommendation and training in the use of adaptive equipment, route planning, and advocacy.

Clients also may be organizations that provide transportation services. In these situations, an assessment of the community context may involve analysis of the various modes of transportation; professional skills of transit agency employees; effectiveness of para-transit eligibility tools and protocols; accessibility of sidewalks, intersection, bus stops, and transit vehicles; safety checks on equipment; community resources available; location of supplemental agencies; and policy review. Interventions implemented with transportation organizations may include employee training programs, development or revision of para-transit eligibility protocols, development of a travel training program, recommendations for adaptive equipment or vehicle modifications, and accessibility modifications to ingress/egress locations such as bus stops and train stations.

The roles of the occupational therapist and the occupational therapy assistant in providing community mobility services are different from each other per the AOTA supervision guidelines (AOTA, 2009b). Consistent with these guidelines, the occupational therapist carries the overall responsibility for the evaluation and intervention process. The occupational therapist oversees the evaluation process and may delegate specific assessments to the occupational therapy assistant if the occupational therapy assistant has demonstrated competency in administration of the individual assessment. Examples include clinic-based tests of vision, cognition, and motor performance or the on-road assessment. The occupational therapist is responsible for interpreting the results of any assessments and incorporating the results into the analysis of the entire evaluation. The occupational therapist also may delegate the responsibility of implementing the intervention to the occupational therapy assistant in accordance with the occupational therapist's plan and the client's intervention goals (AOTA, 2009b). The *Guidelines for Supervision, Roles, and Responsibilities During the Delivery of Occupational Therapy Services* (AOTA, 2009b) recommends that the occupational therapist and the occupational therapy assistant develop a collaborative plan for supervision to guide the evaluation and the intervention process. The supervision must follow state and federal regulations, as well as the policies of the workplace and the *Occupational Therapy Code of Ethics* (AOTA, 2005).

Both federal and state laws, as well as the activities of key professional organizations, influence delivery of and payment for occupational therapy services related to driving and community mobility. Reimbursement for driving and community mobility services is highly variable in the United States. There are mechanisms for reimbursement for these professional services as well as vehicle modifications including the Veterans Administration system, Medicaid in some states, state vocational rehabilitation departments, worker's compensation carriers, legal settlements, and self-pay. Community mobility services are paid for by several different funding sources, including paratransit budgets, transit agencies, state departments of vocational rehabilitation, office on aging, school systems, and grant funding through a variety of sources such as the United We Ride and Safe Routes to School (see Appendix C for a summary of external influences on service delivery).

Summary

Driving and community mobility is a growing area of importance due to the implications of safe transportation and mobility across the life span. The association between transportation and occupational engagement is increasingly relevant to clients, the community, and other organizational entities (see Appendix C). The skills, knowledge base, and scope of practice of occupational therapy enhanced by advanced education in driving and community mobility place the profession of occupational therapy in the forefront of driving and community mobility services. The focus on injury prevention, engagement in occupation, and the intervention strategies used in driving rehabilitation and community mobility services are consistent with *The Philosophical Base of Occupational Therapy* (AOTA, 1995) and, therefore, warrant attention in all areas of occupational therapy practice. Occupational therapy practitioners provide a critical and essential combination of skills and abilities to support people's driving and community mobility and thus to expand or maintain their engagement in community activities and their quality of life.

References

American Academy of Pediatrics. (1994). School bus transportation of children with special needs. *Pediatrics, 93*, 129–130.

American Association of Motor Vehicle Administrators, & National Highway Traffic Safety Administration. (2009). *Driver fitness medical guidelines* (No. DOT HS 811 210). Washington, DC: National Highway Traffic Safety Administration.

American Automobile Association, AARP, & American Occupational Therapy Association. (2008). *CarFit technician manual.* Washington, DC: American Automobile Association.

American Medical Association, Council on Ethical and Judicial Affairs. (1999). *Impaired drivers and their physicians* (No. 1-I-99). Chicago: Author.

American Occupational Therapy Association. (1995). The philosophical base of occupational therapy. *American Journal of Occupational Therapy, 49*, 1026.

American Occupational Therapy Association. (2005). Occupational therapy code of ethics (2005). *American Journal of Occupational Therapy, 59*, 639–642.

American Occupational Therapy Association. (2006). Policy 1.44: Categories of occupational therapy personnel. In *Policy manual* (2009 ed., pp. 33–34). Bethesda, MD: Author.

American Occupational Therapy Association. (2008). Occupational therapy practice framework: Domain and process (2nd ed.). *American Journal of Occupational Therapy, 62*, 625–683.

American Occupational Therapy Association. (2009a). *About AOTA.* Retrieved October 26, 2009, from http://www.aota.org/general/about.asp

American Occupational Therapy Association. (2009b). Guidelines for supervision, roles, and responsibilities during the delivery of occupational therapy services. *American Journal of Occupational Therapy, 63*, 797–803.

American Occupational Therapy Association. (2010). Scope of practice. *American Journal of Occupational Therapy, 64*.

Association for Driver Rehabilitation Specialists. (2004). *Association for driver rehabilitation specialists.* Retrieved January 29, 2004, from http://www.aded.net

Association for Driver Rehabilitation Specialists. (2009). *Best practice guidelines for delivery of driver rehabilitation services.* Hickory, NC: Author.

Barlow, J. H., Cullen, L. A., Foster, N. E., Harrison, K., & Wade, M. (1999). Does arthritis influence perceived ability to fulfill a parenting role? Perceptions of mothers, fathers, and grandparents. *Patient Education and Counseling, 37*, 141–151.

Best, K. L., Kirby, R. L., Smith, C., & MacLeod, D. A. (2005). Wheelchair skills training for community-based manual wheelchair users: A randomized controlled trial. *Archives of Physical Medicine and Rehabilitation, 86*, 2316–2323.

Bicycle Safety Resource Center. (2009). *Federal Highway Administration.* Retrieved February 23, 2010, from http://www.bicyclinginfo.org/education/resource/fhwa.html?/ee/fhwa.html

Boulias, C., Meikle, B., Pauley, T., & Devlin, M. (2006). Return to driving after lower-extremity amputation. *Archives of Physical Medicine and Rehabilitation, 87*, 1183–1188.

Brown, C. (2009). Functional assessment and intervention in occupational therapy. *Psychiatric Rehabilitation Journal, 32,* 162–170.

Bull, M. J., Stroup, K. B., Stout, J., Doll, J. P., Jones, J., & Feller, N. (1990). Establishing special needs car seat loan program. *Pediatrics, 85,* 540–547.

Classen, S., Levy, C., McCarthy, D., Mann, W. C., Lanford, D., & Waid-Ebbs, J. K. (2009). Traumatic brain injury and driving assessment: An evidence-based literature review. *American Journal of Occupational Therapy, 64,* 580–591.

Falkmer, T. (n.d.). *Visual–perceptual abilities in children and adults with autism spectrum disorders.* Jönköping University, School of Health Sciences, Sweden. Retrieved February 23, 2010, from http://www.hhj.hj.se/upload_dir/95ee696d1a523135b7fd9845444fb3fd.pdf

Federal Highway Administration. (2001). *Highway design handbook: For older drivers and pedestrians* (No. FHWA-RD-01-103). McLean, VA: U.S. Department of Transportation.

Federal Highway Administration. (2010). *Safe routes to school.* Retrieved March 8, 2010, from http://safety.fhwa.dot.gov/saferoutes/

Koffman, D., & Salstrom, R. (2001). *How to best serve seniors on existing transit services* (MTI Report 01-04). San Jose, CA: San Jose State University, College of Business, Mineta Transportation Institute.

Lillie, S. (2006). Transportation, community mobility, and driving assessment. In H. M. Pendleton & W. Schultz-Krohn (Eds.), *Predretti's occupational therapy practice skills for physical dysfunction* (6th ed., pp. 224–247). St. Louis, MO: Mosby.

Marottoli, R. A., Mendes de Leon, C. F., Glass, T. A., Williams, C. S., Cooney, L. M., Jr., Berkman, L. F., et al. (1997). Driving cessation and increased depressive symptoms: Prospective evidence from the New Haven EPESE. Established populations for epidemiologic studies of the elderly. *Journal of the American Geriatrics Society, 5,* 202–206.

National Highway Traffic Safety Administration. (1999). *Safe mobility for older people notebook* (DOT HS 808 853). Springfield, VA: Author.

National Highway Traffic Safety Administration. (2009a). *Driving transitions education: Tools, scripts, and practice exercises* (No. DOT HS 811 152). Washington, DC: Author.

National Highway Traffic Safety Administration. (2009b). *NHTSA's core values and commitment to serving customers.* Retrieved October 26, 2009, from http://www.nhtsa.dot.gov/portal/site/nhtsa/menuitem.30351f8e7e40c1cbf62a63101891ef9a/

National Highway Traffic Safety Administration, & American Society on Aging. (2007). *DriveWell: Promoting older driver safety and mobility in your community.* Washington, DC: National Highway Traffic Safety Administration.

Oxley, J., & Whelan, M. (2008). It cannot be all about safety: The benefits of prolonged mobility. *Traffic Injury Prevention, 9,* 367–378.

Perkinson, M. A., Berg-Weger, M. L., Carr, D. B., Meuser, T. M., Palmer, J. L., Buckles, V. D, et al. (2005). Driving and dementia of the Alzheimer type: Beliefs and cessation strategies among stakeholders. *The Gerontologist, 45,* 676–685.

Stav, W. B., Hunt, L. A., & Arbesman, M. (2006). *Occupational therapy practice guidelines for driving and community mobility for older adults.* Bethesda, MD: AOTA Press.

Stav, W. B., & Lieberman, D. (2008). From the desk of the editor. *American Journal of Occupational Therapy, 62*(2), 127–129.

Stern, E. (2007). *Driving safely at home after combat driving.* Military OneSource. Retrieved February 23, 2010, from http://www.militaryonesource.com/portals/0/aspx/material_getpdf.ashx?MaterialID =15086

Stout, J. D., Bull, M. J., & Stroup, K. B. (1989a). Safe transportation for infants and preschoolers with special needs. *Infants and Young Children: An Interdisciplinary Journal of Special Care Practices, 2,* 67–73.

Stout, J. D., Bull, M. J., & Stroup, K. B. (1989b). Safe transportation for children with disabilities. *American Journal of Occupational Therapy, 43,* 31–36.

U.S. Department of Transportation. (2003). *Safe mobility for a maturing society: Challenges and opportunities.* Washington, DC: Author.

Wang, C. C., Kosinski, C. J., Schwartzberg, J. G., & Shanklin, A. V. (2003). *Physician's guide to assessing and counseling older drivers.* Washington, DC: National Highway Traffic Safety Administration.

Authors
Wendy B. Stav, PhD, OTR/L, SCDCM, FAOTA
Susan Pierce, OTR/L, SCDCM, CDRS

for

The Commission on Practice
Janet DeLany, DEd, OTR/L, FAOTA, *Chairperson*

The COP wishes to acknowledge the authors of the 2005 edition of this document: Carol J. Wheatley, OTR/L, CDRS and Elin Schold Davis, OTR/L, CDRS

Adopted by the Representative Assembly Coordinating Council (RACC) for the Representative Assembly

Revised by the Commission on Practice 2010

Note: This revision replaces the 2005 document *Driving and Community Mobility Statement* (previously published and copyrighted in 2005 by the American Occupational Therapy Association in the *American Journal of Occupational Therapy, 59,* 666–670).

Appendix A. Domain of Occupational Therapy Specific to Driving and Community Mobility

Aspects of the Domain (American Occupational Therapy Association [AOTA], 2008)	Examples
Areas of Occupation − Instrumental Activity of Daily Living (IADL) − Community Mobility	"Moving around in the community and using public or private transportation, such as driving, walking, bicycling, or accessing and riding in buses, taxi cabs, or other transportation systems" (AOTA, 2008, p. 631). In addition to being an IADL, community mobility is an occupation enabler, as it allows for engagement in several other areas of occupation including education, work, leisure, social participation, and other IADLs (Stav & Lieberman, 2008).
Performance Skills (Sensory–Perceptual Skills, Motor and Praxis Skills, Emotional Regulation Skills, Cognitive Skills, Communication and Social Skills)	Driving and community mobility require one to possess and execute adequate performance skills. • Engagement in driving and community mobility requires one to have intact sensation and ability to perceive sensory input accurately. • Individuals must use motor and praxis skills to physically move in a planned, coordinated, sequenced manner to operate a motor vehicle, travel using transit services, or exert bodily control while walking or bicycling. • Emotional regulation is used while engaging in driving and community mobility to perform appropriately on shared roadways and pathways with other users. • Driving and community mobility require cognitive skills to exercise sufficient attention, judgment, organization, memory, and multitasking while moving through the dynamic, unpredictable environment of the community. • Communication and social skills are used as individuals exchange information, relate, and physically communicate to move through a community in which other individuals are also mobile.
Performance Patterns (Habits, Routines, and Roles)	Driving and community mobility involve performance patterns using habits to operate equipment and routines to travel on an established route. Individuals fulfill the duties and responsibilities of life roles by engaging in community mobility.
Contexts (Cultural, Personal, Temporal, Virtual, Physical, and Social)	The context in which driving and community mobility take place is critical in understanding who, what, where, when, how, and why individuals move through the community. • The cultural context may dictate which driver in family with 5 licensed individuals operates an automobile during an outing. • An individual's personal context indicates whether travel will be performed as a passenger or operator on the basis of age or socioeconomic status. • Temporal context affects community mobility on the basis of the stage of life, time of day, season of year, and duration of driving. • Recent technologies permit virtual engagement in community mobility through the use of computers and simulators. • The physical context relates to travel in urban or rural settings; on different types of roadways; over a street, sidewalk, or path; or using underground, waterway, air, or land travel. • The social context may influence independent vs. group travel.
Activity Demands	Driving and community mobility have many activity demands consisting of the objects and properties of tools and vehicles used, space and social demands, sequence and timing, required actions and performance skills, required body functions, and required body structures.
Client Factors	Individuals use their body functions—neuromusculoskeletal and movement-related functions; cardiovascular; voice and speech functions; and metabolic and endocrine system function—as well as related body structures, to effectively and safely move about in the community.

Appendix B. Case Examples of Driving and Community Mobility Services

Service Recipients	Community Mobility Concerns	Occupational Therapy Services
Persons		
Traveling in a car with a 3-year-old with cerebral palsy	• Secure safe seating for the child safely • Adherence to state child passenger safety laws	• Assistance in selection of appropriate child safety seat for the child's size/weight/age • Parent education for seat installation • Parent education for managing extensor tone and fastening the child • Development of a child safety seat loan closet for short term client needs (Bull et al., 1990; Stout, Bull, & Stroup, 1989a, 1989b)
Fastening a child into a safety seat by a parent with rheumatoid arthritis	• Secure, safe seating for the child • Adherence to state child passenger safety laws • Joint protection for the parent • Energy conservation for the parent	• Assistance in the identification of the appropriate seat for child's size/weight/age • Assistance in the identification of child safety seats for ease of use • Parent education for seat installation • Identification of child safety seat installation stations • Client education in joint protection and energy conservation seat installation and child fastening • Training in the use of adaptive equipment to aide in fastening (Barlow, Cullen, Foster, Harrison, & Wade, 1999)

Bicycling with an 8-year-old with muscular dystrophy	• Strength and coordination to operate a bicycle
	• Balance to remain upright on the bicycle
	• Awareness of risks and rules of the road
		• Evaluation to determine potential for independent bicycling
		• Therapeutic exercise for
		  o Strength
		  o Coordination
		  o Balance
		• Client education on environmental awareness and rules of the road
		(Bicycle Safety Resource Center, 2009)

Learning to drive for a 16-year-old with Asperger's syndrome	• Interpersonal relations with other road users using non-verbal communication • Coordination to operate a motor vehicle • Awareness of the driving environment and risks • Awareness of rules of the road	• Referral to an occupational therapist specialist in driving for an individualized structured driver education • Evaluation to determine potential for driving • Client education for environmental awareness consistent with client's cognitive capacities and learning needs • Assistance with applying for a driver license (Falkmer, n.d.)
Traveling in a community as a 19-year-old pedestrian with a spinal cord injury	• Negotiation of intersections • Navigation across uneven terrain	• Client education of curb cuts, safety awareness • Route planning for accessible paths • Training in advocacy strategies for promotion of accessible communities (Best, Kirby, Smith, & MacLeod, 2005)

Appendix B. Case Examples of Driving and Community Mobility Services *(cont.)*

Service Recipients	Community Mobility Concerns	Occupational Therapy Services
Persons *(cont.)*		

Return to driving for a 45-year-old following a traumatic brain injury	• Operation of the vehicle controls with impaired motor skills and abnormal muscle tone
	• Full and accurate visual access to the driving environment
	• Safe maneuvering in the driving environment using
	  o Attention
	  o Memory
	  o Judgment
	  o Planning
	  o Organization
	  o Impulse control
	• Transfer in and out of the vehicle
	• Storage of mobility aids
		• Determination of readiness for driving rehabilitation services
		• Evaluation to identify client-centered transportation option and potential to return to driving*
		• Client and family education related to delayed return to driving
		• Assessment to determine capability of learning how to use adaptive equipment and traffic safety rules*
		• Therapeutic exercises and activities to maximize
		  o Sensory–perceptual skills
		  o Motor and praxis skills
		  o Emotional regulation skills
		  o Cognitive skills
		  o Communication and social skills
		• Behind-the-wheel training*
		• Recommendation and training in the use of adaptive equipment*
		• Assistance in the selection of an automobile capable of accommodating adaptive equipment*
		• Assistance with applying for a modified driver license
		• Guidance for applying to vehicle manufacturer for an adaptive equipment rebate
		(Classen et al., 2009; Lillie, 2006)

Return to driving for a 20-year-old wounded veteran with a traumatic right lower-extremity amputation and posttraumatic stress disorder (PTSD) related to combat driving	• Operation of the vehicle foot pedals with a prosthetic limb or left-foot gas pedal
	• Continuation of dangerous combat driving post deployment
	  o Maneuvering around traffic
	  o Avoidance of roadside debris
	  o Proceeding through traffic lights and stop signs
	• Panic attacks when driving under bridges
	• Safety related to return to driving
		• Evaluation to determine potential for safe return to driving*
		• Assessment to determine capability to learn how to use adaptive equipment*
		• Referral for psychological counseling to address PTSD concerns
		• Behind-the-wheel training*
		• Recommendation and training in the use of adaptive equipment*
		• Assistance in the selection of an automobile capable of accommodating adaptive equipment*
		• Assistance with applying for a modified driver license
		• Guidance in applying to veteran's benefits for a vehicle stipend and vehicle manufacturer for an adaptive equipment rebate
		(Boulias, Meikle, Pauley, & Devlin, 2006; Stern, 2007)

(Continued)

Appendix B. Case Examples of Driving and Community Mobility Services *(cont.)*

Service Recipients	Community Mobility Concerns	Occupational Therapy Services
Persons *(cont.)*		

Driving for a 64-year-old woman with dementia	• Safe operation an automobile in a variety of driving environments, particularly unfamiliar roads or routes due to impaired
	  o Memory
	  o Judgment
	  o Cognitive processing speed
	  o Recognition of errors
	• Potential for wandering and getting lost
		• Comprehensive driving evaluation to determine potential for continued driving*
		• Identification of plan for driving restrictions and/or re-evaluation
		• Analysis of a person's historical and current daily occupational patterns as part of an occupational profile to identify community mobility needs. Assistance in the transition to driving cessation, including
		  o Identification of transportation alternatives and service delivery resources in the client's area
		  o Training in supervised travel on existing transit systems, assistance with the application for paratransit and family education
		  o Referral to counseling or support services to address feelings of loss related to driving cessation
		  o Provision of support for family members
		  o Provision of cessation strategies to counter persistent determination to drive
		(Perkinson et al., 2005)

Traveling by transit systems for an adult with schizophrenia	• Safe and timely negotiation of routes and transfers
	• Management of fare or bus pass
	• Potential for victimization
		• Travel training in the use of the local transit system
		• Therapeutic activities for
		  o Money management
		  o Time management
		  o Trip planning
		  o Community reintegration
		• Assistance in the application for prepaid bus passes
		• Training in strategies to protect one's person and possessions
		(Brown, 2009)

Organizations		

Transit company seeking to increase ridership among disabled passengers and reduce costly paratransit services	• Availability and accessibility of
	  o Vehicles
	  o Bus stops
	  o Shelters
	• Leniency of paratransit eligibility
	• Disability awareness
	• Ability of drivers to operate lift, wheelchair tie-downs, and manage behavioral issues
	• Ability of schedulers to meet the needs of riders with cognitive impairments
		• Accessibility evaluations and recommendations for vehicles, bus stops, and shelters to elevate to Americans with Disabilities Act compliance
		• Modification of paratransit eligibility evaluation
		• Equipment training for drivers
		• Sensitivity training of drivers and schedulers
		(Koffman & Salstrom, 2001)

Appendix B. Case Examples of Driving and Community Mobility Services *(cont.)*

Service Recipients	Community Mobility Concerns	Occupational Therapy Services
Organizations *(cont.)*		
School system looking to increase the safety of transport of students with special needs	• Availability, appropriateness, and currency of child safety seats • Proper fastening techniques for children with special needs • Management of students with behavioral issues while operating the vehicle	• Assessment of child safety seats in use and system-wide needs • Training drivers and bus aides in child passenger safety • Training bus aides in behavior management strategies to alleviate duty from driver (American Academy of Pediatrics, 1994)
Populations		

Populations that need to safely engage in mobility within the community	• Roadway design to support older drivers
	• Bike lanes, pedestrian paths, and sidewalks to support multiple modes of transportation
	• Signage visible to road users of varying literacy and visual levels
	• Access to common areas
		• Collaboration with municipal planning organizations to promote
		  o Multi-user roadway design
		  o Inclusion of bicycle and pedestrian paths
		  o Centralized common areas of equidistant travel from all residences
		  o Separation of locations with high-risk drivers (e.g., high school and senior center should not be across the street from each other)
		  o Legible signage with large fonts and symbols
		(Federal Highway Administration, 2001)
		• Participation in multidisciplinary programming, such as Safe Routes to School (Federal Highway Administration, 2010)

Population of older drivers at risk for injuries and fatalities during crashes	• Increased frailty/fragility of the aging body, which is less able to sustain energy forces of a crash
	• Knowledge about operation and use of safety features that emerged in the past several decades
	• Poor driver–vehicle fit among older drivers
		• Provide education to stakeholder groups (National Highway Traffic Safety Administration & American Society on Aging, 2007)
		• Participation in CarFit events to
		  o Measure driver–vehicle fit
		  o Identify areas of concern
		  o Make suggestions related to adjustment of vehicle safety features (e.g., air bag, seat belt, head restraint) and positioning of driver's body in the vehicle
		  o Educate about commonly used assistive devices (American Automobile Association, AARP, & American Occupational Therapy Association, 2008)

(Continued)

Appendix B. Case Examples of Driving and Community Mobility Services *(cont.)*

Service Recipients	Community Mobility Concerns	Occupational Therapy Services
Populations *(cont.)*		

Population of medically at risk drivers placing all road users at risk with undefined medical reporting guidelines	• Drivers with medical impairments at increased risk for crashes
	• Subsequent increased risk of injury and fatality for all road users
	• Narrow or non-existent medical reporting guidelines
	• Confidentiality of reporting
	• Legal immunity for reporting parties
	• Evidence-based guidelines supporting licensing decisions
		• Conduct an evidence-based literature review of diagnostic groups and report to state licensing agency (American Association of Motor Vehicle Administrators & National Highway Traffic Safety Administration, 2009)
		• Advocate for the development of new and more comprehensive medical reporting laws inclusive of
		  o Recognition of occupational therapy as a discipline capable of reporting
		  o Confidentiality of reporting
		  o Legal immunity for reporters
		• Serve as a member of state Medical Review Board or state constituency group

*Services performed by an occupational therapy practitioner who specializes in driving rehabilitation.

Appendix C. External Influence on Occupational Therapy Practice Related to Driving and Community Mobility

Governmental Influences

Federal Government: National Highway Traffic Safety Administration (NHTSA)

NHTSA's mission is to "save lives, prevent injuries, and reduce economic costs due to road traffic crashes, through education, research, safety standards, and enforcement activity" (2009b, para. 1). NHTSA focuses attention and programs on occupant protection specific to safety belt use, air bags, child passenger safety, graduated licensing, new drivers, vehicle modifications, and impaired driving due to alcohol or illegal drug use. The recent activity on older driver safety has generated educational materials such as the *Drive Well Toolkit: Promoting Older Driver Safety and Mobility in Your Community* (NHTSA & American Society on Aging, 2007) and *Driving Transitions Education: Tools, Scripts, and Practice Exercises* (NHTSA, 2009a). Concerns related to driving with specific medical conditions prompted the development of 11 educational brochures about driving with specific diagnoses, including Alzheimer's disease, Parkinson's disease, diabetes, stroke, arthritis, and glaucoma. Similar resources and educational materials have been developed on child passenger safety, bicycle and pedestrian safety, occupant protection, and school buses that guide occupational therapy practice by outlining safety standards, laws, and best practices.

State Government: State Licensure Laws

Laws related to driving and community mobility vary by state and jurisdiction with regard to vision standards, medical reporting, legal immunity, licensure laws, licensing restrictions, and credentials required for practitioners. Therefore, occupational therapists and occupational therapy assistants must become knowledgeable of the statutes and guidelines specific to the state or jurisdiction of practice.

Professional Organizations

American Association of Motor Vehicle Administrators (AAMVA)

In response to concerns from motor vehicle agencies nationwide about making driver licensing decisions for individuals with medical conditions, AAMVA coordinated an evidence-based literature review and subsequent development of the *Driver Fitness Medical Guidelines* (AAMVA & NHTSA, 2009) to aid state agencies in making licensing decisions.

American Medical Association (AMA)

- The AMA believes that older driver safety is a public health issue and that physicians play an important role in ensuring the safety of older drivers (Wang, Kosinski, Schwartzberg, & Shanklin, 2003). The AMA has dedicated efforts to a safe driver initiative resulting in a physician training program and several publications.
- The AMA collaborated with aging, driving rehabilitation, and transportation experts nationwide to write guidelines for physician practice related to older drivers (Wang et al., 2003). The book advises several alternatives that physicians might pursue, such as referring older drivers to driver rehabilitation specialists.
- On December 7, 1999, the AMA's Council on Ethical and Judicial Affairs adopted a report outlining physicians' ethical obligation to address driving issues with their clients (AMA, 1999). The report included 7 recommendations for physicians to recognize impairments and act on that knowledge when a patient's driving posed a strong threat to public safety.

Association for Driver Rehabilitation Specialists (ADED)

ADED (2004) is a multidisciplinary group comprised of occupational therapy practitioners, driver educators, vehicle modification manufacturers and dealers, rehabilitation engineers, physical therapists, kinesiotherapists, and rehabilitation specialists. ADED provides certification for driver rehabilitation specialists (CDRS) by means of a portfolio review and standardized exam. ADED (2009) passed a revised *Best Practice Guidelines for Delivery of Driver Rehabilitation Services*.

American Occupational Therapy Association (AOTA)

AOTA "advances the quality, availability, use, and support of occupational therapy through standard-setting, advocacy, education, and research on behalf of its members and the public" (AOTA, 2009a, para. 5). Specific to driving and community mobility, AOTA has created an Older Driver Initiative to coordinate multiple projects related to awareness and professional training, which has grown beyond older drivers to community mobility across the lifespan. Projects include

- Collaborative activities and awareness-building activities within the profession, to the growing community of providers, and stakeholder agencies and associations (e.g., American Automobile Association, American Society on Aging, AARP, ADED, National Mobility Equipment Dealers Association, Transportation Research Board) concerned with safe mobility across the lifespan.
- Interagency strategic planning initiatives in support of transportation and community mobility with organizations such as Easter Seals/National Center on Senior Transportation and the U.S. Department of Defense.
- Completion and dissemination of an evidence-based literature review specific to driving and community mobility; publication of practice guidelines on driving and community mobility (Stav, Hunt, & Arbesman, 2006).
- Older Driver Microsite (www.aota.org/olderdriver) offering resources and links for professionals and consumers, including a resource toolkit for the development of driving and community mobility programs. Annual Older Driver Week launched in 2009, during the first week in December.
- Specialty Certification in Driving and Community Mobility by means of a reflective portfolio demonstrating competencies in the practice area organized around AOTA's Standards of Continuing Competence.
- Fact sheets on older drivers, community mobility across the lifespan, collaborating with judges.
- Online and CD-based continuing education materials about older drivers, driving rehabilitation for new drivers with cognitive and social limitations, and community mobility for adolescents.

Occupational Therapy Fieldwork Education: Value and Purpose

The purpose of fieldwork education is to propel each generation of occupational therapy practitioners from the role of student to that of practitioner. Through the fieldwork experience, future practitioners achieve competence in applying the occupational therapy process and using evidence-based interventions to meet the occupational needs of a diverse client population. Fieldwork assignments may occur in a variety of practice settings, including medical, educational, and community-based programs. Moreover, fieldwork placements also present the opportunity to introduce occupational therapy services to new and emerging practice environments.

Fieldwork assignments constitute an integral part of the occupational therapy and occupational therapy assistant education curricula. Through fieldwork, students learn to apply theoretical and scientific principles learned from their academic programs to address actual client needs within the context of authentic practice environments. While on fieldwork, each student develops competency to ascertain client occupational performance needs to identify supports or barriers affecting health and participation and document interventions provided. Fieldwork also provides opportunities for the student to develop advocacy, leadership, and managerial skills in a variety of practice settings. Finally, the student develops a professional identity as an occupational therapy practitioner, aligning his or her professional judgments and decisions with the American Occupational Therapy Association (AOTA) *Standards of Practice* (AOTA, 2005b) and the *Occupational Therapy Code of Ethics* (AOTA, 2005a).

As students proceed through their fieldwork assignments, performance expectations become progressively more challenging. *Level I fieldwork* experiences occur concurrently with academic coursework and are "designed to enrich didactic coursework through directed observation and participation in selected aspects of the occupational therapy process" (Accreditation Council for Occupational Therapy Education [ACOTE], 2007a, 2007b, 2007c). *Level II fieldwork* experiences occur at or near the conclusion of the didactic phase of occupational therapy curricula and are designed to develop competent, entry-level, generalist practitioners (ACOTE, 2007a, 2007b, 2007c). Level II fieldwork assignments feature in-depth experience(s) in delivering occupational therapy services to clients, focusing on the application of purposeful and meaningful occupation and evidence-based practice through exposure to a "variety of clients across the life span and to a variety of settings" (ACOTE, 2007a, 2007b, 2007c).

The value of fieldwork transcends the obvious benefits directed toward the student. Supervising students enhances fieldwork educators' own professional development by providing exposure to current practice trends, evidence-based practice, and research. Moreover, the experience of fieldwork supervision is recognized by the National Board for Certification in Occupational Therapy (NBCOT) and many state regulatory boards as a legitimate venue for achieving continuing competency requirements for occupational therapy practitioners.

Another benefit to the fieldwork site for sponsoring a fieldwork education program is with the recruitment of qualified occupational therapy personnel. Through the responsibilities expected during Level II fieldwork, occupational therapy staff and administration are given opportunity for an in-depth view of a student's potential as a future employee. In turn, an active fieldwork program allows the student, as a potential employee, to view first-hand the agency's commitment to the professional growth of its occupational therapy personnel and to determine the "fit" of his or her professional goals with agency goals. The fieldwork program also creates a progressive, state-of-the-art image to the professional community, consumers, and other external audiences through its partnership with the academic programs.

In summary, fieldwork education is an essential bridge between academic education and authentic occupational therapy practice. Through the collaboration between academic faculty and fieldwork educators, students are given the opportunity to achieve the competencies necessary to meet the present and future occupational needs of individuals, groups, and indeed, society as a whole.

References

Accreditation Council for Occupational Therapy Education. (2007a). Accreditation standards for a doctoral-degree level educational program for the occupational therapist. *American Journal of Occupational Therapy, 61*, 641–651.

Accreditation Council for Occupational Therapy Education (2007b) Accreditation standards for a master's-degree level educational program for the occupational therapist. *American Journal of Occupational Therapy, 61*, 662–671.

Accreditation Council for Occupational Therapy Education. (2007c) Accreditation standards for an educational program for the occupational therapy assistant. *American Journal of Occupational Therapy, 61*, 652–661.

American Occupational Therapy Association. (2005a). Occupational therapy code of ethics (2005). *American Journal of Occupational Therapy, 59*, 639–642.

American Occupational Therapy Association. (2005b). Standards of practice for occupational therapy. *American Journal of Occupational Therapy, 59*, 663–665.

The Commission on Education
René Padilla, PhD, OTR/L, FAOTA, *Chairperson*
Andrea Bilics, PhD, OTR/L
Judith C. Blum, MS, OTR/L
Paula C. Bohr, PhD, OTR/L, FAOTA
Jennifer C. Coyne, COTA/L
Jyothi Gupta, PhD, OTR/L
Linda Musselman, PhD, OTR, FAOTA
Linda Orr, MPA, OTR/L
Abbey Sipp, *ASD Liaison*
Patricia Stutz-Tanenbaum, MS, OTR
Neil Harvison, PhD, OTR/L, *AOTA Staff Liaison*

Adopted by the Representative Assembly 2009FebCS115

Note: This document replaces the document *The Purpose and Value of Occupational Therapy Fieldwork Education* 2003M41.

Occupational Therapy in the Promotion of Health and the Prevention of Disease and Disability

Introduction

The purpose of this paper is to describe occupational therapy's contribution in the areas of health promotion and prevention and is intended for internal and external audiences. The American Occupational Therapy Association (AOTA) supports and promotes involvement of occupational therapists and occupational therapy assistants in the development and provision of health promotion and disease or disability prevention programs and services.

It is important to frame the discussion of occupational therapy's role in health promotion and disease or disability prevention by defining these terms as they are used in this paper. The World Health Organization (WHO) provides the following definition in the Ottawa Charter for Health Promotion:

> *Health promotion* is the process of enabling people to increase control over, and to improve, their health. To reach a state of complete physical, mental, and social well-being, an individual or group must be able to identify and realize aspirations, to satisfy needs, and to change or cope with the environment. Health is, therefore, seen as a resource for everyday life, not the objective of living. Health is a positive concept emphasizing social and personal resources, as well as physical capacities. Therefore, health promotion is not just the responsibility of the health sector, but goes beyond healthy lifestyles to well-being. (WHO, 1986, italics added)

Trentham and Cockburn (2005) expand on this definition by stating that

> Health promotion is equally and essentially concerned with creating the conditions necessary for health at individual, structural, social, and environmental levels through an understanding of the determinants of health: peace, shelter, education, food, income, a stable ecosystem, sustainable resources, *social justice,*[1] and equity. (p. 441, italics added)

For the past two decades, the U.S. Department of Health and Human Services (DHHS) has used health promotion and disease prevention objectives to improve the health of the American people. The primary goal of *Healthy People 2010* (DHHS, 1998), the national prevention initiative, is to increase the quality as well as the number of years of healthy life. It emphasizes health status and not just longevity. From an individual perspective, healthy life means a full range of functional capacities across the life span, allowing one to enter into satisfying relationships with others, to work, and to play. From a national perspective, healthy life means a vital, creative, and productive citizenry contributing to thriving communities and a thriving nation.

The second goal of *Healthy People 2010* is to eliminate health disparities (DHHS, 2000). The Health Resources and Services Administration (HRSA) defines health disparities as "population-specific differences in the presence of disease, health outcomes, or access to health care" (HRSA, 2000). Addressing health disparities is consistent with the occupational therapy profession's official document on nondiscrimination and inclusion, which states "inclusion requires that we ensure not only that everyone is treated fairly and equitably but also that all individuals have the same opportunities to participate in the naturally occurring activities of society" (AOTA, 2004b, p. 668). Population health focuses on *aggregates,* or communities of

---

[1]Some italicized terms in this statement are defined in the glossary.

people, and the many factors that influence their health. A population health approach strives to identify and reduce health disparities as well as enhance the overall health and well-being of a population (Finlayson & Edwards, 1997).

Health promotion programs and services may target individuals, organizations, communities and populations, and policymakers. The focus of these programs is to

- Prevent or reduce the incidence of illness or disease, accidents, injuries, and disabilities in the population;

- Reduce health disparities among racial and ethnic minorities and other underserved populations;

- Enhance mental health, resiliency, and quality of life;

- Prevent secondary conditions and improve the overall health and well-being of people with chronic conditions or disabilities and their caregivers; and

- Promote healthy living practices, social participation, *occupational justice,* and healthy communities, with respect for cross-cultural issues and concerns.

A key purpose of health promotion is the prevention of disease and disability in individuals and populations. Prevention is generally categorized into three levels: primary, secondary, and tertiary. *Primary prevention* is defined as education or health promotion strategies designed to help people avoid the onset and reduce the incidence of unhealthy conditions, diseases, or injuries. Primary prevention attempts to identify and eliminate risk factors for disease, injury, and disability. *Secondary prevention* includes early detection and intervention after disease has occurred and is designed to prevent or disrupt the disabling process. *Tertiary prevention* refers to treatment and services designed to arrest the progression of a condition, prevent further disability, and promote social opportunity (Patrick, Richardson, Starks, Rose, & Kinne, 1997).

Occupational Therapy and Health Promotion

Healthy People 2010 and the Ottawa Chapter of Health Promotion parallel occupational therapy's belief that engagement in meaningful occupations supports health and leads to a productive and satisfying life. Wilcock (2006) states that

> Following an occupation-focused health promotion approach to well-being embraces a belief that the potential range of what people can do, be, and strive to become is the primary concern and that health is a by-product. A varied and full occupational lifestyle will coincidentally maintain and improve health and well-being if it enables people to be creative and adventurous physically, mentally, and socially. (p. 315)

According to Christiansen (1999), "Health enables people to pursue the tasks of everyday living that provide them with the life meaning necessary for their well-being" (p. 547).

The Guide to Occupational Therapy Practice (Moyers & Dale, 2006) affirms the profession's participation in disability prevention and health promotion at both the individual and population levels. Occupational therapy services are provided to clients of all age groups, infants through older adults, from a variety of socioeconomic, cultural, and ethnic backgrounds, who possess or who are at risk for impairments, activity limitations, or participation restrictions. According to the *Occupational Therapy Practice Framework* (AOTA, 2002), occupational therapy practitioners[2] recognize that health is supported when individuals are able to engage in occupations and activities that allow them to achieve the desired outcome of participation in their chosen environments. This focus on the outcome of "engagement in occupation to support participation" (p. 611) is interwoven through the delivery of service, beginning with the evaluation and continuing through the intervention phase. Health management and maintenance are included within the domain of occupational therapy as an instrumental activity of daily living; health promotion and preven-

---

[2]When the term *occupational therapy practitioner* is used in this document, it refers to both occupational therapists and occupational therapy assistants (AOTA, 2006).

tion are listed as occupational therapy intervention approaches; and health, wellness, and quality of life are potential outcomes of occupational therapy services (AOTA, 2002).

Occupations are purposeful and meaningful daily activities that fill a person's time and are typically categorized as self-care, work, play or leisure, and rest (AOTA, 1995; Meyer, 1922). *Occupational health and wellness* includes the elements of choice, meaning, balance, satisfaction, opportunity, and self-actualization (Wilcock, 1998). A natural, balanced pattern of occupations is believed to be health enhancing and fulfills both the needs of the individual and the demands of the environment (Kielhofner, 2004; Meyer, 1922). This belief has been supported in studies with well elderly individuals (Clark et al., 1997).

Occupational imbalance, deprivation, and *alienation* are risk factors for health problems in and of themselves. They also may result from or lead to the development of other risk factors, which in turn can result in larger health and social problems. Causes are varied (e.g., unanticipated caregiving responsibilities, losses in employment or housing) and can lead to occupational imbalance, deprivation, and alienation, which can then lead to individual health problems (e.g., stress, sleep disturbance, depression). People who experience these health problems may be at greater risk for suicide; elder, spousal, and child abuse; substance use disorders; and so forth (Wilcock, 1998). Belle et al. (2006) demonstrated that caregivers of people with dementia experienced significant improvement in quality of life and a decrease in depression after intervention that included stress management; strategies for engaging in pleasant events; and teaching of healthy behaviors, communication skills, and problem-solving skills regarding behavior management of care recipients' difficult behaviors. Occupational therapy practitioners are in a prime position to recognize these occupational health problems and offer interventions to alleviate them through task analysis and modification.

Role of Occupational Therapy

There are three critical roles for occupational therapy practitioners in health promotion and disease or disability prevention: to promote healthy lifestyles; to emphasize occupation as an essential element of health promotion strategies; and to provide interventions, not only with individuals but also with populations. It is important that occupational therapy practitioners promote a healthy lifestyle for all individuals and their families, including people with physical, mental, or cognitive impairments. An occupation-focused approach to prevention of illness and disability is defined by Wilcock (2006) as

> The application of medical, behavioral, social, and *occupational science* to prevent physiological, psychological, social, and occupational illness; accidents; and disability; and to prolong quality of life for all people through advocacy and mediation and through occupation-focused programs aimed at enabling people to do, be, and become according to their natural health needs. (p. 282, italics added)

The following are some examples of occupation-based primary prevention intervention that target individuals:

- Musculoskeletal injury prevention and management programs;

- Anger management and conflict resolution training for parents, teachers, and school-aged youth to reduce the incidence of violence;

- Parenting skills training for adolescent mothers;

- Fall prevention programs for community-dwelling seniors.

Examples of secondary prevention carried out by occupational therapy practitioners may include

- Education and training regarding eating habits, activity levels, and prevention of secondary disability subsequent to obesity;

- Education and training on stress management and adaptive coping strategies for people with mood disorders and post traumatic stress disorder;

521

- Osteoporosis prevention and management classes for individuals recently diagnosed or at high risk for this condition.

Examples of occupation-based tertiary prevention intervention may include

- Transitional or independent-living skills training for people who have mental illness and those with cognitive impairments;

- Groups for older adults with dementia to prevent depression, enhance socialization, and improve quality of life;

- A program of leisure and educational activities for a drop-in center for adults with severe mental illness;

- Stroke support groups.

Occupational therapy practitioners have an opportunity to complement existing health promotion efforts by adding the contribution of occupation to programs developed by experts in health education, nutrition, exercise, and so forth. For example, when working with a person with a lower-extremity amputation due to diabetes, the occupational therapy practitioner may focus on the occupation of meal preparation using foods and preparation methods recommended in the nutritionist's health promotion program. This enables achievement of the occupational therapy goal of functional independence in the kitchen and reinforces the importance of proper nutrition for the prevention of further disability (Scaffa, 2001).

To be effective, health promotion efforts cannot focus only on intervention at the individual level. Because of the inextricable and reciprocal links between people and their environments, larger groups, organizations, communities, populations, and government policymakers must also be considered for intervention (Law, 1991; Wilcock, 2006). The function of occupational therapy at these levels uses the knowledge and perspective of occupational science in a variety of roles and settings (Baum & Law, 1997; Brownson, 1998).

Organizational-level interventions may include

- Providing consultation to businesses to promote emotional well-being through identification of problems and solutions for balance among work, leisure, and family life;

- Consulting to schools regarding implementation of Americans With Disabilities Act (ADA) requirements;

- Providing education for day care staff regarding normal growth and development, handling behavior problems, and identifying children at risk for developmental delays; and

- Promoting ergonomically correct work stations in schools and offices.

Community or population-level interventions may include

- Consulting on accessible public transportation;

- Consulting with contractors, architects, and city planners regarding accessibility and universal design;

- Implementing a community-wide screening program for depression at nursing homes, assisted-living facilities, and senior centers for the purpose of developing group and individual prevention and intervention programs addressing depression;

- Conducting needs assessments and implementing intervention strategies to reduce health disparities in communities with high rates of disease or injury; intervention strategies may include lifestyle management programs addressing issues such as hypertension, diabetes, and obesity;

- Addressing the health and occupation needs of the homeless population by eliminating barriers and enhancing opportunities for occupational engagement; and

- Training volunteers to function effectively in special needs shelters during disasters.

Governmental or policy-level interventions may include

- Promoting policies that offer affordable, accessible health care to everyone, including people with disabilities;

- Promoting policies that support economic self-sufficiency for all people;

- Supporting full inclusion of children with disabilities in schools and day care programs;

- Lobbying for public funds to support research and program development in areas related to improvement in quality of life for people at risk and those with disabilities; and

- Promoting policies that establish opportunities for rehabilitation in the community for people discharged from inpatient psychiatric programs.

Occupational Therapy's Contributions

Occupational therapy has an important role in health promotion and disease or disability prevention due to its focus on the health effects of purposeful, productive, and meaningful occupation. It is the profession's focus and associated knowledge base that is occupational therapy's contribution to the health and well-being of Americans. Occupational therapy practitioners can

- Evaluate occupational capabilities, values, and performance;

- Provide education regarding occupational role performance and balance;

- Reduce risk factors and symptoms through engagement in occupation;

- Provide skill development training in the context of everyday occupations;

- Provide self-management training to prevent illness and manage health;

- Modify environments for healthy and safe occupational performance;

- Consult and collaborate with health care professionals, organizations, communities, and policymakers regarding the occupational perspective of health promotion and disease or disability prevention;

- Promote the development and maintenance of mental functioning abilities through engagement in productive and meaningful activities and relationships (adapted from DHHS, 1999, p. 4); and

- Provide training in adaptation to change and in coping with adversity to promote mental health (adapted from DHHS, 1999, p. 4).

While recognizing the role of occupational therapy in health promotion and disease and disability prevention, it is important to acknowledge and respect the contributions of other health care professions in this important arena. Occupational therapy practitioners should operate within their scope of practice and training and partner with other health promotion disciplines with specialized expertise such as in the areas of public health, health education, nutrition, and exercise physiology. The roles of the occupational therapist and the occupational therapy assistant in evaluation and intervention in health promotion practice are based on the *Guidelines for Supervision, Roles, and Responsibilities During the Delivery of Occupational Therapy Services* (AOTA, 2004a). Occupational therapists and occupational therapy assistants possess the basic knowledge to carry out health promotion and interventions to prevent disability and disease. However, this is a very broad area of practice, and practitioners need to continually expand their knowledge in health promotion to be effective and competent members of the team.

As in all other areas of practice, health promotion services should be evidence based. Law, Steinwender, and LeClair (1998) conducted an extensive review of the literature on the relationship between occupation and health. The longitudinal studies that were reviewed found that activity participation had a significant effect on perceived health. Maintenance of everyday activities, social interactions, and community mobility influenced self-reported quality of life. A long-term benefit attributable to preventive occupational therapy was demonstrated by Clark et al. (2001) when they re-evaluated participants from the Well Elderly Study and found that 90% of therapeutic gain observed following intervention was retained at the 6-month follow-up.

Funding for health promotion programs can come from governmental agencies, foundations, nonprofit organizations, insurance companies, and large corporations, among others. In addition, fee for service is an option. Typically, health promotion and prevention programs do not rely on a single source of funding (Brownson, 1998; Scaffa, 2001).

The following case studies provide examples of the role of occupational therapy in health promotion and prevention of disease and disability.

Case Study: Primary Prevention—Individual Level

A retired husband and wife consult an occupational therapist regarding a home safety assessment for the purpose of remaining in their home as they age.

Assessment: The occupational therapist uses a semi-structured interview format to gather information about the clients' health, occupational performance, and satisfaction level within the various performance areas, as well as social connectedness and overall life satisfaction. Both the husband and wife are healthy and able to perform daily tasks with a high level of satisfaction. They have a strong social support network and report being very satisfied with their life. The occupational therapist also explores the health history of their parents and learns of a history of Alzheimer's disease and diabetes. The environment (i.e., home, yard, neighborhood) is assessed regarding accessibility and safety.

The occupational therapist notes that the living area is on three levels (several steps have no railings); rooms and hallways are generally poorly lit; and too much furniture is in each room, leaving narrow or obstructed passageways. The yard has uneven and poorly defined walkways. The couple lives in a residential neighborhood with a distance of 3 miles to shopping. No public transportation is available (even for people with mobility impairments).

Intervention: For immediate consideration, the occupational therapist recommends that the couple install railings by all steps, increase the level of lighting, and decrease the amount of furniture. She works with them to find the best configuration of furniture placement to maximize safety when walking in a room. She recommends that they consider changing the landscape to include clearly defined and level walkways that also will accommodate wheeled mobility, should that ever be needed.

A second set of recommendations includes how to retrofit the house if mobility impairments preclude climbing stairs in the future. Optimal placement of an elevator from the first to the second floor is described. There is not an easy placement of an elevator from the basement to the first floor, so the occupational therapist describes how the occupations now performed in the basement (exercise, laundry, and computer use) may be transferred to the other two floors. The occupational therapist works with the couple on problem solving around transportation, should driving become difficult.

Case Study: Primary Prevention—Organizational Level

A commercial bakery contacts an occupational therapist to assess the various work stations in the bakery and make recommendations for improvements. Management goals are to increase productivity and to decrease sick days and worker compensation claims.

Assessment: The occupational therapist observes the work performed at the various work stations and interviews the workers. She notes body mechanics, repetitive motions, machine design, layout of work stations with travel distances, weights lifted and number of lifts per time unit, work speed and load, noise, temperature, air quality, clothing comfort, and length and frequency of rest breaks. Worker-to-worker interaction and interaction among workers, supervisors, and management also are noted. In general, the supervisors and management seem approachable and open to suggestions from the workers.

The occupational therapist finds much lifting and repetitive motion done by the workers. Work stations require much static standing, which contributes to many musculoskeletal problems. Travel distances are long, work speed is rapid, noise level is high in certain parts of the factory, and the temperature is uncomfortably warm.

Intervention: The occupational therapist recommends ergonomically designed work stations with decreased amount of static work, time standing, travel, or lifting and improved working positions. Because some jobs involve repetitive motions that may not be avoided, the occupational therapist instructs the managers in the benefits of rest breaks and instructs the workers in stretching exercises. Each worker also is instructed in proper body mechanics at his or her work station. The occupational therapist works with the management on designing a daily schedule that allows for an even workflow to decrease times of high stress. The occupational therapist is asked to return every 6 months to reassess and instruct new employees.

Case Study: Primary Prevention—Community/Population Level

An elementary school is planning a new playground, which must be accessible to every child in the school. An occupational therapist is consulted for input on design features that will make the playground aesthetically pleasing, fun, and challenging to use for children of all abilities.

Assessment: The occupational therapist surveys the area where the school is planning to locate the playground. He uses the guidelines for play areas developed by the U.S. Access Board (2005) to make sure the minimum requirements are met. He then researches commercially available playground equipment to find equipment that will be fun and challenging to use for all populations in the school as well as encourage interactions among the children.

Intervention: The occupational therapist provides the school with a report detailing his recommendations for important features in the playground equipment and the layout of the playground. He is careful to identify all the safety issues and suggests ways to make the playground as safe as possible. The report also includes recommendations for landscaping so that children using wheeled mobility can easily navigate around the playground. The occupational therapist remains on the design team for consultation until the playground is completed.

Case Study: Primary Prevention—Governmental/Policy Level

An occupational therapist working in home health has noticed that her elderly clients who no longer drive have no other means of transportation to go grocery shopping, run errands, and visit friends. The occupational therapist contacts the Occupational Science Department at the local university to collaborate on a grant proposal asking for start-up money to research the need for and develop a system of transportation for non-drivers in the community.

Case Study: Tertiary Prevention—Individual Level

A rehabilitation unit in a hospital decides to offer health promotion classes to former patients with chronic conditions. An occupational therapy assistant is chosen to lead a class for patients with chronic obstructive pulmonary disease.

Assessment: The occupational therapy assistant researches information on the disease, existing programs, and their content and outcomes. She researches optimal group size, length of each session frequency, and number of sessions.

Intervention: Using the assessment information, the supervising occupational therapist works with the occupational therapy assistant to develop the health promotion class, including number of participants, length of session, and topics offered. It is decided that a maximum of 15 participants will meet monthly for 1.5 hours for a total of 12 sessions. Topics include self-management, assertive communication, information seeking, and problem-solving skills. The group also will function as a support group.

Appendix: Glossary

Occupational alienation: "Sense of isolation, powerlessness, frustration, loss of control, and estrangement from society or self as a result of engagement in occupation that does not satisfy inner needs" (Wilcock, 2006, p. 343).

Occupational deprivation: "Deprivation of occupational choice and diversity because of circumstances beyond the control of individuals or communities" (Wilcock, 2006, p. 343).

Occupational imbalance: "A lack of balance or disproportion of occupation resulting in decreased well-being" (Wilcock, 2006, p. 343).

Occupational justice: To experience meaning and enrichment in one's occupations; to participate in a range of occupations for health and social inclusion; to make choices and share decision-making power in daily life; and to receive equal privileges for diverse participation in occupations (Townsend & Wilcock, 2004).

Occupational science: "An interdisciplinary academic discipline in the social and behavioral sciences dedicated to the study of the form, the function, and the meaning of human occupations" (Zemke & Clark, 1996, p. vii).

Social justice: "The promotion of social and economic change to increase individual, community, and political awareness, resources, and opportunity for health and well-being" (Wilcock, 2006, p. 344).

References

American Occupational Therapy Association. (1995). Occupation: A position paper. *American Journal of Occupational Therapy, 49,* 1015–1018.

American Occupational Therapy Association. (2002). Occupational therapy practice framework: Domain and process. *American Journal of Occupational Therapy, 56,* 609–639.

American Occupational Therapy Association. (2004a). Guidelines for supervision, roles, and responsibilities during the delivery of occupational therapy services. *American Journal of Occupational Therapy, 58,* 663–667.

American Occupational Therapy Association. (2004b). Occupational therapy's commitment to nondiscrimination and inclusion. *American Journal of Occupational Therapy, 58,* 668.

American Occupational Therapy Association (2006). Policy 1.44: Categories of occupational therapy personnel. *American Journal of Occupational Therapy, 60,* 683–684.

Baum, C. M., & Law, M. (1997). Occupational therapy practice: Focusing on occupational performance. *American Journal of Occupational Therapy, 51,* 277–287.

Belle, S. H., Burgio, L., Burns, R., Coon, D., Czaja, S. J., Gallagher-Thompson, D., et al. (2006). Enhancing the quality of life of dementia caregivers from different ethnic or racial groups. *Annals of Internal Medicine, 145,* 727–738.

Brownson, C. A. (1998). Funding community practice: Stage 1. *American Journal of Occupational Therapy, 52,* 60–64.

Christiansen, C. H. (1999). Defining lives: Occupation as identity: An essay on competence, coherence, and the creation of meaning. *American Journal of Occupational Therapy, 53,* 547–558.

Clark, F., Azen, S. P., Zemke, R., Jackson, J., Carlson, M., Mandel, D., et al. (1997). Occupational therapy for independent-living older adults: A randomized controlled trial. *Journal of the American Medical Association, 278,* 1321–1326.

Clark, F., Azen, S. P., Carlson, M., Mandel, D., LaBree, L., Hay, J., et al. (2001). Embedding health-promoting changes into the daily lives of independent-living older adults: Long-term follow-up of occupational therapy intervention. *Journal of Gerontology: Psychological Sciences, 56,* 60–63.

Finlayson, M., & Edwards, J. (1997). Evolving health environments and occupational therapy: Definitions, descriptions, and opportunities. *British Journal of Occupational Therapy, 60,* 456–460.

Health Resources and Services Administration. (2000). *Eliminating health disparities in the United States.* Retrieved June 12, 2006, from http://newsroom.hrsa.gov/NewsBriefs/2001/eliminatingdisparities.htm

Kielhofner, G. (2004). *Conceptual foundation of occupational therapy* (3rd ed.). Philadelphia: F. A. Davis.

Law, M. (1991). The environment: A focus for occupational therapy [Murial Driver Memorial Lecture]. *Canadian Journal of Occupational Therapy, 58,* 171–179.

Law, M., Steinwender, S., & LeClair, L. (1998). Occupation, health, and well-being. *Canadian Journal of Occupational Therapy, 65,* 81–91.

Meyer, A. (1922). The philosophy of occupation therapy. *Archives of Occupational Therapy, 1,* 1–10.

Moyers, P., & Dale, L. (2006). *The guide to occupational therapy practice* (2nd ed.). Bethesda, MD: AOTA Press.

Patrick, D. L., Richardson, M., Starks, H. E., Rose, M. A., & Kinne, S. (1997). Rethinking prevention for people with disabilities part II: A framework for designing interventions. *American Journal of Health Promotion, 11,* 261–263.

Scaffa, M. E. (2001). *Occupational therapy in community-based practice settings.* Philadelphia: F. A. Davis.

Townsend, E., & Wilcock, A. A. (2004). Occupational justice and client-centered practice: A dialogue in progress. *Canadian Journal of Occupational Therapy, 71,* 75–87.

Trentham, B., & Cockburn, L. (2005). Participatory action research: Creating new knowledge and opportunities for occupational engagement. In F. Kronenberg, S. Simó Algado, & N. Pollard (Eds.), *Occupational therapy without borders: Learning from the spirit of survivors* (pp. 440–453). Philadelphia: Elsevier/Churchill Livingstone.

U.S. Access Board. (2005). *Accessible play areas: A summary of accessibility guidelines for play areas.* Retrieved August 8, 2007, from http://www.access-board.gov/play/guide/guide.pdf

U.S. Department of Health and Human Services. (1998). *Healthy People 2010 objectives: Draft for public comment.* Washington, DC: Author.

U.S. Department of Health and Human Services. (1999). *Mental health: A report of the Surgeon General.* Rockville, MD: Author.

U.S. Department of Health and Human Services. (2000). *Healthy People 2010: Understanding and improving health* (2nd ed.). Washington, DC: U.S. Government Printing Office.

Wilcock, A. A. (1998). *An occupational perspective of health.* Thorofare, NJ: Slack.

Wilcock, A. A. (2006). *An occupational perspective of health* (2nd ed.). Thorofare, NJ: Slack.

World Health Organization. (1986). The Ottawa charter for health promotion. *Health Promotion, 1,* iii–v.

Zemke, R., & Clark, F. (1996). *Occupational science: The evolving discipline.* Philadelphia: F. A. Davis.

Authors

Marjorie E. Scaffa, PhD, OTR, FAOTA
Nancy Van Slyke, EdD, OTR, FAOTA
Carol A. Brownson, MSPH

for

The Commission on Practice
Susanne Smith Roley, MS, OTR/L, FAOTA, *Chairperson*

Adopted by the Representative Assembly 2007CO146

Note: This document replaces the 2000 Statement *Occupational Therapy in the Promotion of Health and the Prevention of Disease and Disability.*

Occupational Therapy Services for Individuals Who Have Experienced Domestic Violence

The primary purpose of this statement is to define the role of occupational therapy and the scope of services available for survivors and families who have experienced domestic violence. The American Occupational Therapy Association (AOTA) supports and promotes the use of this document by occupational therapists, occupational therapy assistants, and individuals interested in this topic as it relates to the profession of occupational therapy.

Domestic Violence

Prevalence

Domestic violence is a societal problem in the United States and internationally that affects not only the survivor of the violence but also the children witnessing it, the family and friends of the survivor, and the communities in which it occurs. In 2008, there were approximately 552,000 reported cases of nonfatal domestic violence against females and approximately 101,000 reported cases against males (U.S. Department of Justice [USDOJ], 2011). These are the reported cases; it is estimated that the numbers are much higher because many cases of abuse are unreported (National Coalition Against Domestic Violence [NCADV], 2007; Centers for the Disease Control and Prevention [CDC], 2010).

Definitions

The term *victim* is sometimes used to describe individuals who are or have been in an abusive relationship. The term *survivor* is used to describe individuals who are currently in the abusive relationship or who have overcome the abuse. We choose to use the term survivor because it is more empowering and denotes the strength and courage needed to endure as well as leave the abusive relationship.

There are numerous definitions of domestic violence depending on the state and organization. This document defines *domestic violence* as a pattern of "coercive behavior designed to exert power and control over a person in an intimate relationship through the use of intimidating, threatening, harmful, or harassing behavior" (Office for Victims of Crime [OVC], 2002). The emphasis is on a *pattern* of abuse and violence that becomes part of their lives, leaving lasting effects on the survivor and children. *Domestic violence* often is used more globally to account for the broad impact it has on the family, whereas the term *intimate partner violence (IPV)* specifically refers to the violence between a former or current partner or spouse (National Institute of Justice [NIJ], 2007).

For the purposes of this paper, the term *domestic violence* is used because of its broader connotation. Although women are abused in 85% to 95% of the reported domestic violence cases (Fisher & Shelton, 2006), men also are abused and face an additional stigma of gender roles, which often prevents them from coming forward (OVC, 2002). Therefore, it is important to view domestic violence as an issue of obtaining power and control over a partner without assuming that the partner is female.

Survivor Characteristics

Domestic violence occurs in both heterosexual and homosexual relationships at nearly the same rate (National Coalition of Anti-Violence Programs, 1998). In a national study, Tjaden and Thoennes (2000a) indicated that 11% of lesbians reported violence by their female partner and 15% of gay men who had lived with a male partner reported being victimized by that partner. Survivors of domestic violence in a homosexual relationship may have more difficulty accessing services and may face further stigma and marginalization due to their sexual orientation.

Domestic violence knows no boundaries; it crosses into all socioeconomic classes, races, societies, and ages, regardless of the sexual orientation that defines the relationships. The key issue in domestic violence is the use of a pattern of abusive behavior by the abuser to establish fear, power, and control over an intimate or formerly intimate partner.

Women with disabilities who are abused may face additional barriers that make it more difficult to leave the abusive relationship and access services. Although there are inconsistent findings regarding the incidence of abuse of women with disabilities, several sources indicate that women with disabilities are assaulted, raped, and abused at a rate twice that of women without disabilities (Brownridge, 2006; Helfrich, Lafata, MacDonald, Aviles, & Collins, 2001; Milberger et al., 2002; NIJ, 2000; Nosek, Hughes, Taylor, & Taylor, 2006). Analysis of data from the 2007 National Crime Victimization Survey indicated that the rates of violence against women with disabilities was highest among women with cognitive disabilities (Rand & Harrell, 2009).

Women with disabilities may be dependent on their partners for financial, physical, and/or medical support and thus may stay in abusive relationships for longer periods of time (Helfrich et al., 2001; NIJ, 2000). Their abusers may withhold necessary equipment such as wheelchairs, braces, medications, and transportation as a means to control them (NIJ, 2000).

Domestic violence also affects older adults. Domestic violence in older adults has unique considerations due to the chronic exposure to abuse over a lifetime (Jacobson, Pabst, Regan, & Fisher, 2006; Zink, Regan, Jacobson, & Pabst, 2003). The couple may experience feelings of guilt mixed with responsibility, particularly when the abuser is also the caregiver or when the caregiver needs to care for the abuser. As the couple gets older and experiences changes in their health, the violence may be masked by conditions such as Alzheimer's disease, or it may be heightened by the added stress that caregiving brings to the relationship (National Coalition Against Domestic Violence, n.d.; Zink et al., 2003).

Causes and Contributing Factors

Factors that cause or contribute to domestic violence have been discussed and contested by social scientists for decades, with little agreement about the commonalities (Jewkes, 2005). The exception is poverty, which is the only factor that consistently has been found to be a key contributor to domestic violence (Davies, 2008; Jewkes, 2005; Josephson, 2005; Lyon, 2000, 2002; Sokoloff & Dupont, 2005). The most recent USDOJ (2007) statistics from an analysis of reported and unreported family violence indicate that persons in households with annual incomes less than $7,500 (below the U.S. poverty threshold) have higher rates of assault than do persons in households with higher income levels. Furthermore, the data also indicate that social class appears to be inversely related to the severity of the violence; more severe domestic violence occurs against women within the lowest socioeconomic group (Bograd, 2005; Browne & Bassuk, 1997; Davies, 2008; Lyon, 2000, 2002; Rank, 2004; Rice, 2001).

Limited education and being a victim of child maltreatment, especially sexual abuse, also have been found to be strong links to subsequent victimization (Browne & Bassuk, 1997; Tjaden & Thoennes, 2000b). Being verbally abused has been found to be a highly predictive variable for abuse by an intimate partner (Tjaden & Thoennes, 2000b).

Being economically poor also has serious implications in terms of whether a woman stays in an abusive relationship. Studies of female survivors of domestic violence have consistently indicated that a survivor's ability to earn an independent source of income that allows her to successfully sustain her family is the most significant indicator that she will be able to permanently leave the abusive relationship (Economic Stability Working Group, 2002; Waldner, 2003). It makes sense, then, that the lack of a sustainable income is a significant reason why, on average, survivors return to abusive relationships 5–7 times (Adair, 2003; Brush, 2003; Harris, 2003).

Childhood Exposure

Between 7 and 14 million children and youth are exposed to adult domestic violence each year (Edleson et al., 2007). In addition to witnessing the violence between their parents or a parent and partner, it is estimated that child abuse occurs in 30% to 60% of domestic violence cases (Appel & Holden, 1998; McKibben, DeVos, & Newberger, 1998). Children who grow up in a domestic violence household often have low self-esteem, psychosomatic complaints, nightmares, impaired social skills, and poor academic performance. As a result, they may be aggressive, withdrawn, anxious, depressed, and even suicidal (Israel & Stover, 2009; OVC, 2002). In families where there is domestic violence, young boys may model their father's behavior, while girls may model their mother's behavior and show more signs of withdrawal and isolation (Cummings, Peplar, & Moore, 1999; Holt, Buckley, &Whelan, 2008; Huth-Beck, Levendosky, & Semel, 2001; Stiles, 2002).

Some children may have difficulty expressing their feelings and stress and may exhibit aggressive behaviors as a way to try to communicate with their mother. Studies of children exposed to domestic violence indicate that they also may have difficulty with self-calming, sleeping, and eating activities; may demonstrate developmental delays or maladaptive behaviors; and may have poor verbal and social skills that negatively affect their academic performance. They may have higher rates of somatic complaints and interpersonal problems (Cummings et al., 1999; Huth-Beck et al., 2001; Norwood, Swank, Stephens, Ware, & Buzy, 2001; Sternberg et al., 1993; Stiles, 2002).

Types of Violence

Abuse in domestic violence comes in many forms; it may be physical, psychological, sexual, or economic. *Physical violence* may include such behaviors as hitting, slapping, punching, or stabbing. *Psychological violence* may take the form of verbal abuse, harassment, possessiveness, destruction of personal property, cruelty to pets, and isolation (OVC, 2002; USDOJ, n.d.). The abuser often isolates the victim from family and friends, thus limiting access to support systems. *Sexual abuse* can occur between two intimate partners when the abuser forces or coerces the victim into a sexual act. Survivors also may experience *economic abuse* in which the abuser controls the finances, leaving the victim with no money or a limited allowance.

Challenges With Occupation or Activities

Research indicates that women who are survivors of domestic violence may struggle when performing several of their daily life occupations or activities, particularly work performance, educational participation, home management, parenting, and leisure participation (Gorde, Helfrich, & Finlayson, 2004; Helfrich & Rivera, 2006; Javaherian, Krabacher, Andriacco, & German, 2007). They may experience problems with money management, task initiation, self-confidence, coping skills, stress management, and interpersonal relationships (Carlson, 1997; D'Ardenne & Balakrishna, 2001; Helfrich, Aviles, Badiani, Walens, & Sabol, 2006; Levendosky & Graham-Bermann, 2001; Monahan & O'Leary, 1999). They may have difficulty with higher level mental functions, including decision making, judgment, problem solving, and direction following.

Survivors of domestic violence often face challenges sustaining employment (Josephson, 2005; Riger & Staggs, 2004; Tolman & Raphael, 2000). One common reason is that abuse, including stalking and excessive phone calls or other forms of contact, often happens at the workplace (Corporate Alliance to End Partner Violence, 2002–2008). Survivors' inconsistent work histories can cause difficulties with finding a job once they have left the abusive relationship.

In addition, leaving an abusive relationship and becoming a single parent can increase the risk of being unemployed or among the working poor in the United States. The jobless rate for unmarried mothers is almost 3 times that of married mothers, 8.5% as compared to 3.1% (U.S. Department of Labor, 2010).

Occupational Therapy and Domestic Violence

In its broadest sense, the domain of occupational therapy is the facilitation of people's ability to engage in meaningful, daily life activities, or occupations in a manner that supports their full participation in various contexts and positively affects health, well-being, and life satisfaction (AOTA, 2008). Occupational therapists and occupational therapy assistants view occupations as central to a person's identity and competence, influencing how a person spends time and makes decisions (AOTA, 2008). Domestic violence negatively affects the ability of the survivors and their families to engage in their daily life occupations in a competent, healthy, and satisfying manner. Consequently, in the spirit of social and occupational justice, occupational therapy practitioners[1] focus on developing or restoring these abilities. Specifically, occupational therapy practitioners focus on enhancing the ability of the survivors and their families to participate in activities of daily living (ADLs), instrumental activities of daily living (IADLs), rest and sleep, education, work, leisure, play, and social participation for the purpose of gaining skills and abilities needed to take control of their lives, find purpose, and develop a healthy independent lifestyle.

Occupational therapy practitioners work directly and indirectly with survivors of domestic violence and their families in a variety of settings such as hospitals, rehabilitation centers, skilled nursing facilities, outpatient therapy clinics, mental health facilities, school systems, shelters, home health care, and other community programs. Occupational therapy practitioners may work with survivors and family members who have

- Sustained injuries or disabilities as a result of domestic violence,

- Chosen to remain in and rebuild a relationship in which abuse has occurred, or

- Decided to leave the abusive relationship and reconstruct their lives.

In the course of their practice, occupational therapy practitioners also may work with individuals whom they suspect or discover are victims or survivors of domestic violence but who have not reported the domestic violence. In such cases, occupational therapy practitioners have a professional and ethical responsibility to take action that promotes the health and safety of these individuals. As health care professionals, occupational therapy practitioners are mandated to report suspected child abuse. Some states also mandate that they report suspected abuse in adults, particularly in older adults or adults who have intellectual disabilities.

Occupational therapy practitioners need to consult their state regulations and facility guidelines regarding procedures to follow when they suspect or know that domestic violence has occurred. Actions that practitioners may take include

---

[1]When the term *occupational therapy practitioner* is used in this document, it refers to both occupational therapists and occupational therapy assistants (AOTA, 2006). *Occupational therapists* are responsible for all aspects of occupational therapy service delivery and are accountable for the safety and effectiveness of the occupational therapy service delivery process. *Occupational therapy assistants* deliver occupational therapy services under the supervision of and in partnership with an occupational therapist (AOTA, 2009).

- Filing a report to the local law enforcement agency or children's protective services;

- Interviewing, evaluating, and providing interventions without the abuser present to allow the client the opportunity to discuss the situation in relative safety;

- Identifying and assessing injuries and their potential cause;

- Talking to the client about healthy relationships and addressing areas of occupation and performance patterns and skills that may have been affected by the abusive relationship, such as leisure, IADLs, work, and ADLs;

- Respecting the client's perception of the relative danger of the situation to his or her life and the well-being of other family members and remaining empathetic and nonjudgmental about the client's decision to remain in or leave the abusive situation;

- Providing the client with contact information for the local domestic violence hotline; and

- Following safety precautions to determine if it is appropriate to conduct home visits.

Occupational Therapy Evaluation and Intervention

The occupational therapy service delivery process occurs in collaboration with the survivors of domestic violence, their family members, and other service providers. Throughout the occupational therapy evaluation, intervention, and assessment of outcomes, occupational therapy practitioners value and consider the desires, choices, needs, personal and spiritual values, and sociocultural backgrounds of the survivors and their family members. Practitioners also consider the service delivery context. Important outcomes of occupational therapy service provision include, but are not limited to, facilitating the ability of the survivors and their family members to consistently engage in and perform their daily activities, achieving personal satisfaction and role competence, developing healthy performance patterns, and improving their quality of life.

The occupational therapy evaluation is focused on determining what the survivors and their family members want and need to do and identifying the factors that act as supports or barriers to performance of the desired occupations (AOTA, 2008). Occupational performance; routines, roles, and habits; activity demands; sociocultural beliefs/expectations; spirituality; and physical, cognitive, and psychosocial factors are addressed during the evaluation process. Evaluations and assessments that are client-centered and occupation-based are effective for this population.

Occupational therapy service delivery is based on findings from the evaluation and the survivors' and the family members' stated priorities. Interventions with adults who are survivors of domestic violence focus on empowerment and active participation in healthy occupations or daily life activities. Findings from several studies of survivors have indicated that during the early period after leaving the abusive situation, survivors continue to devote themselves to the care of others, especially their children, while often not taking care of themselves (Giles & Curreen, 2007; Underwood, 2009; Wuest & Merritt-Gray, 1999).

Occupational therapy interventions with adult women survivors may include working on the development of a realistic budget; facilitating the use of effective decision-making skills regarding employment opportunities; learning parenting skills and calming techniques to use with their children; encouraging and supporting efforts to attain further education; learning assertiveness skills; and teaching stress management and relaxation techniques to improve sleep patterns (Gorde et al., 2004; Helfrich et al., 2006; Helfrich & Rivera, 2006; Javaherian et al., 2010). Therapy sessions focused on performance patterns may be helpful, because findings from several studies have indicated that survivors are constantly juggling family, work, and possibly school responsibilities without a significant other to assist them with their obligations (Butler & Deprez, 2002; Jones-DeWeever & Gault, 2006; Underwood, 2009).

Interventions with children who have witnessed domestic violence may include facilitation of developmentally appropriate play skills, social skills training, the use of techniques for improving concentration and attention span during school activities, and assistance with the organization of study habits and school materials. Adolescents may benefit from interventions addressing relationship skills, life skills, stress management, and coping strategies (Javaherian-Dysinger et al., 2011).

Occupational therapy practitioners focus on outcomes throughout the occupational therapy service delivery process. Assessing outcome results assists occupational therapy practitioners with making decisions about future directions of interventions at the individual as well as at the organizational or population level (AOTA, 2008). At the individual level, the selection of outcomes is based on the survivors' priorities and may be modified based on changing needs, contexts, and performance abilities (AOTA, 2008). For example, an occupational therapy practitioner may work with a woman who is a survivor of domestic violence on her goal of obtaining housing. After the woman moves into the new living situation, the practitioner may help the woman work on her goal of maintaining a healthy home environment for herself and her children.

At the organizational or population level, data about targeted outcomes can be aggregated and reported to boards of directors of community agencies, state and federal regulators, and funding agencies. An example of this type of outcome assessment would be the reporting of the number of children who demonstrated difficulty participating in their daily life activities at home, at school, and in their communities because of exposure to domestic violence and the progress they have made during the occupational therapy intervention to increase their level of healthy participation.

Occupational therapy practitioners also may work with the abusers in collaboration with other professionals such as psychologists, social workers, and pastoral counselors. Sometimes the judicial system issues a court order for the abuser to participate in a formal program to address the violent behaviors. These programs are generally based on six principles: (1) the abuser is responsible for the behavior; (2) provocation does not justify violence; (3) violent behavior is a choice; (4) there are nonviolent alternatives; (5) violence is a learned behavior; and (6) domestic violence affects the entire family, whether it is directly or indirectly witnessed (OVC, 2002). Occupational therapy interventions with the abuser may include training in social skills, assertiveness, anger management, stress management, parenting, and spiritual exploration as related to daily occupations.

Education, Training, and Competencies

Occupational therapists and occupational therapy assistants are educationally prepared to address the various occupation-related concerns of survivors of domestic violence. The Accreditation Council for Occupational Therapy Education (ACOTE) standards for educational programs require content related to daily life occupations, human development, human behavior, sociocultural issues, diversity factors, medical conditions, theory, models of practice, evaluation, and techniques for the development and implementation of intervention plans under the scope of occupational therapy (ACOTE, 2010). Occupational therapy practitioners are competent to address life skills, lifestyle management, adaptive coping strategies, adaptation, time management, and values clarification that affect the ability of survivors of domestic violence to participate in their ADLs, IADLs, education, work, play, leisure, and social participation activities. In addition, occupational therapy practitioners have the expertise to work with individuals, organizations, and populations.

Occupational therapists and occupational therapy assistants who are supervised by an occupational therapist are competent in the following areas:

- Establishing and maintaining therapeutic relationships;

- Conducting interviews;

- Administering functional assessments to determine occupational performance needs and to develop an intervention plan;

- Utilizing interpersonal communication skills;

- Designing and facilitating therapeutic groups;

- Developing individualized teaching and learning processes with clients, family, and significant others;

- Coordinating program interventions in collaboration with clients, caregivers, families, and communities grounded in evidence-based practice;

- Developing therapeutic programs;

- Promoting health and wellness through engagement in meaningful occupations; and

- Understanding the effects of health, disability, and social conditions on the individual within the context of family and society (ACOTE, 2010).

Participating in continuing education initiatives advances occupational therapy practitioners' understanding of and capacity to provide interventions that address domestic violence.

Supervision of Other Personnel

When provided as part of an occupational therapy program, the occupational therapist is responsible for all aspects of the service delivery and is accountable for the safety and effectiveness of the service delivery process. The occupational therapy assistant delivers occupational therapy services under the supervision of and in partnership with the occupational therapist (AOTA, 2009). The education and knowledge of occupational therapy practitioners also prepare them for employment in arenas other than those related to traditional delivery of occupational therapy. In these circumstances, the occupational therapy practitioner should determine whether the services they provide are related to the delivery of occupational therapy by referring to their state practice acts, regulatory agency standards and rules, domain of occupational therapy practice, and written or verbal agreement with the agency or payer about the services provided (AOTA, 2009). Occupational therapy practitioners should obtain and use credentials and a job title commensurate with their roles in the specific arena. In such arenas, non–occupational therapy professionals may provide the supervision of occupational therapy assistants.

Case Studies

The following case studies provide examples of the role of occupational therapy in domestic violence.

Adult Case Study: Maria

An occupational therapist working in a shelter for survivors of domestic violence was asked to assess Maria, a 28-year-old mother of two children.

Evaluation

Using the Canadian Occupational Performance Measure (Law et al., 2005), Maria identifies the occupational performance areas are the most important to her. She would like to feel competent in her ability to take care of a house, parent her children, and keep them safe. She also wants to work with the occupational therapist on finding and maintaining a job, budgeting, and completing her GED. Maria rates her performance as 1— *unable to do it* and her satisfaction levels as 1—*not satisfied at all* for these performance areas.

When budgeting is discussed, Maria states that she had never been responsible for money management. She went straight from her parent's home into her marriage at age 17, and her husband would not allow her to have anything to do with the money. He constantly told her that she was "too stupid" to take care of money. She was not allowed to work outside the home, so she was dependent on her husband for money.

Intervention

The occupational therapist helps Maria procure and complete job applications and practice job interviewing skills. After Maria finds a steady job, she and her children move into the shelter's transitional living program. To stay in this program, Maria needs to put a certain amount of money into a savings account on a monthly basis to secure a home for her and her children. Following her first paycheck, the occupational therapist meets with Maria to project a budget for her expenses and savings. Maria asks the occupational therapist to develop her budget for her because she "isn't smart enough to do it herself." She states that math was her worst subject in school. The occupational therapist grades the complexity of the task to enable Maria to develop problem-solving skills and reasoning abilities for budgeting.

The occupational therapist then models for Maria how to contact community agencies to obtain information about GED programs. They determine a daily schedule and identify support networks so that Maria can work, complete her studies, and care for her children.

Older Adult Case Study: Mr. Lee

An occupational therapist in an outpatient clinic receives a referral to provide occupational therapy services to Mr. Lee, a 72-year-old man with a right distal radius fracture and a boxer's fracture. Mr. Lee has chronic obstructive pulmonary disease (COPD) and uses a wheelchair for mobility. He has been living with his current partner for the past 10 years.

Evaluation

During the evaluation the occupational therapist asks Mr. Lee to explain how the injury occurred. He is vague in his responses and simply states that he became weak and fell out of his wheelchair. Over the next few sessions, while providing interventions to address Mr. Lee's hand injuries and COPD, the occupational therapist notices additional bruises on his arms and suspects that he is involved in an abusive relationship.

Intervention

Because the occupational therapist lives in a state that mandates reporting of abuse in adults, she files a report to the appropriate law enforcement agency. She lets Mr. Lee know that law requires such action. The therapist then initiates conversation about domestic violence. Research (Bacchus, 2003; McCauley, 1998) has shown that victims of domestic violence want their health care provider to ask them about domestic violence, thereby creating a venue for them to open up as they feel able.

While continuing to provide interventions related to hand function and energy management, the occupational therapist also reassesses Mr. Lee's areas of occupation, performance skills, and performance patterns to identify additional home and community supports he may need because of the domestic violence. She provides Mr. Lee with resources on domestic violence and the local crisis center's contact information. She includes interventions to focus on building self-esteem and empowerment.

Adolescent Case Study: Heang

Heang is a 16-year-old girl in 10th grade. For the past 2 months she has dated a popular young man who is in the 11th grade. Heang initially thought that his frequent phone calls and text messages throughout the day were very romantic. He started telling her that he did not want her to go out with her friends and got into several fights with Heang's male classmates. After dating for about 1 month, he began to slap and punch her. The next day he would bring her flowers. Rather than tell anyone, Heang withdrew from her friends and after-school activities; she did not socialize with other boys at school or work.

A representative from the local women's shelter spoke to Heang's 10th-grade class about teen dating violence. Realizing that she was a victim of this violence, Heang spoke to her guidance counselor. The counselor referred her to a teen dating violence group run by the school occupational therapist.

Evaluation

The occupational therapist conducts an initial evaluation to assess Heang's occupational needs, problems, and concerns. The therapist analyzes Heang's occupational performance skills, performance patterns, context, and activity demands (AOTA, 2008). After reviewing the results of the evaluation, the therapist develops collaborative goals with Heang related to her school and after-school activities, social participation, leisure activities, and job.

Intervention

Using a cognitive–behavioral approach, the occupational therapist helps Heang explore the impact that the dating violence has had on her school and work performance, social participation, and sense of identity. She encourages Heang to identify the importance of social participation in the development of self-esteem, friendships, health, and identity. Together they develop a plan for Heang to participate again in familiar leisure occupations as well as in new ones.

Infant Case Study: Jonella and Kia

Jonella brought her 4-month-old daughter Kia to an occupational therapist as part of an early intervention service for infants and toddlers. Jonella tells the occupational therapist that she is concerned about Kia, who sleeps only 30 minutes at a time and consistently wakes up screaming. Jonella explains that she and Kia have just left an abusive relationship and now live with friends. Since infancy, Kia has been awakened many times because of the shouting and physical violence. In addition, Jonella could not establish a daily nap and sleep routine for Kia because she frequently had to rush Kia out of the house to keep her safe.

Evaluation

The occupational therapist administers the Test of Sensory Functions in Infants (DeGangi & Greenspan, 1989) and the Transdisciplinary Play-Based Assessment (Linder, 2008) to Kia to assess for sensory issues focusing on self-regulation and for potential developmental complications.

Intervention

The occupational therapist and Jonella collaborate to identify strategies for establishing a consistent nap and sleep routine for Kia. The occupational therapist models strategies that Jonella can use to help calm Kia and modulate the amount of sensory input she receives. They also identify strategies for modifying the environment in the room where Kia sleeps and for helping Jonella relax with Kia before putting her to bed.

Child Case Study: Daniel

A school system occupational therapist is asked to assess Daniel, a 5-year-old student who has an individual education program (IEP), to address learning challenges. His teacher states that Daniel is having extreme problems with manipulating crayons and performing gross motor activities. The teacher informs the therapist that his mother has just left an abusive situation. His mother has stated that Daniel's father would not let her place Daniel in a preschool or in a Mother's Morning Out program. She was not allowed to take Daniel outside to play. In addition, when his father was home, Daniel was expected to sit quietly and not play with toys. In spite of these restrictions, Daniel's mother did her best to expose her son to books and songs and teach him ways to play with household materials.

Evaluation

The occupational therapist performs the Quick Neurological Screening Test II (QNST–II; Mutti, Sterling, Spalding, & Spalding, 1998) and sends the Sensory Profile (Dunn, 1999) home with Daniel for his mother to complete. Daniel scores within the "Definite Difference" range on the following factors on the Sensory Profile: Emotionally Reactive, Oral Sensory Sensitivity, Inattention/Distractibility, Auditory Processing, Vestibular Processing, and Multisensory Processing. As measured by the QNST–II, Daniel also has difficulty with gross motor skills, balance, tactile processing, visual tracking, motor planning, impulsivity, and anxiety.

Intervention

The occupational therapist observes Daniel in the classroom and makes recommendations for strategies that the teacher can use to decrease Daniel's distractibility and to increase his attention and participation at school. The occupational therapy assistant works with Daniel for 45 minutes twice a week, with time divided between intervention in the classroom to address cutting and drawing activities and outside the classroom to increase motor control, sensory awareness, and problem-solving skills.

Family Case Study: Herminie's Family

An occupational therapist is part of a treatment team for individuals who have diabetes. The physician wants the therapist to assess and provide services to Herminie, a 34-year-old woman who is not routinely checking her glucose levels or taking her insulin. Because Herminie speaks limited English, her sister accompanies her to the session and translates for her.

Evaluation

During the interview, Herminie shares that her 13-year-old daughter has taken on the responsibility for prompting Herminie to perform the techniques necessary to keep the diabetes under control. The 13-year-old daughter also takes care of her 7-year-old brother while Herminie works. Herminie left home with her children a year ago because her husband was physically and emotionally abusive to her. According to Herminie's sister, as a result of witnessing the abuse, the daughter is continually afraid that something is going to happen to her mother and brother. She is afraid to leave the house, except to go to school, and does not socialize with friends.

Intervention

With the aid of Herminie's sister, who provides verbal and written translation, the occupational therapist develops a daily checklist that Herminie can use to prompt herself to independently check her glucose levels and take her insulin. She discusses with Herminie how important it is for her, rather than her daughter, to be responsible for managing her diabetes. The occupational therapist meets with Herminie and her daughter weekly for several weeks to reinforce and monitor the progress that Herminie is making and to assist the daughter with reducing her anxiety. With Herminie's and her daughter's permission, the therapist called the daughter's school guidance counselor to discuss the situation and request help with decreasing the daughter's anxiety while facilitating increased socialization. In addition, the occupational therapist recommends that Herminie participate in a domestic violence counseling program.

References

Accreditation Council for Occupational Therapy Education. (2010). *ACOTE standards and interpretive guidelines.* Available online at http://www.aota.org/Educate/Accredit/StandardsReview/guide/42369.aspx?FT=.pdf

Adair, V. (2003). Fulfilling the promise of higher education. In V. Adair & S. Dahlberg (Eds.), *Reclaiming class: Women, poverty, and the promise of higher education in America* (pp. 240–265). Philadelphia: Temple University.

American Occupational Therapy Association. (2006). Policy 1.44: Categories of occupational therapy personnel. In *Policy manual* (2009 ed.). Bethesda, MD: Author.

American Occupational Therapy Association. (2008). Occupational therapy practice framework: Domain and process (2nd ed.). *American Journal of Occupational Therapy, 62*(6), 625–683.

American Occupational Therapy Association. (2009). Guidelines for supervision, roles, and responsibilities during the delivery of occupational therapy services. *American Journal of Occupational Therapy, 63*(6), 796–803.

Appel, A., & Holden, G. (1998). The co-occurrence of spouse and physical child abuse: A review and appraisal. *Journal of Family Psychology, 12,* 578–599.

Bacchus, L. (2003). Experiences of seeking help from health professionals in a sample of women who experienced domestic violence. *Health and Social Care in the Community, 11,* 10–18.

Bograd, M. (2005). Strengthening domestic violence theories: Intersections of race, class, sexual orientation, and gender. In N. J. Sokoloff (Ed.), *Domestic violence at the margins: Readings on race, class, gender, and culture* (pp. 25–38). New Brunswick, NJ: Rutgers University.

Browne, A., & Bassuk, S. (1997). Intimate violence in the lives of homeless and poor housed women: Prevalence and patterns in an ethnically diverse sample. *American Journal of Orthopsychiatry, 6*(2), 261–278.

Brownridge, D. A. (2006). Partner violence against women with disabilities: Prevalence, risk, and explanations. *Violence Against Women, 12,* 805–822. doi:10.1177/1077801206292681

Brush, L. (2003). "That's why I'm on Prozac": Battered women, traumatic stress, and education in the context of welfare reform. In V. Adair & S. Dahlberg (Eds.), *Reclaiming class: Women, poverty, and the promise of higher education in America* (pp. 215–239). Philadelphia: Temple University.

Butler, S., & Deprez, L. (2002). Something worth fighting for: Higher education for women on welfare. *Afflia, 17*(1), 30–54.

Carlson, B. (1997). A stress and coping approach to intervention with abused women. *Family Relations, 46,* 291–298.

Centers for Disease Control and Prevention. (2010). *Intimate partner violence: Consequences.* Retrieved from http://www.cdc.gov/violenceprevention/intimatepartnerviolence/consequences.html.

Corporate Alliance to End Partner Violence. (2002–2008). *Workplace statistics.* Available online at http://www.caepv.org/getinfo/facts_stats.php?

Cummings, J., Peplar, D., & Moore, T. (1999). Behavior problems in children exposed to wife abuse: Gender differences. *Journal of Family Violence, 14,* 133–156.

D'Ardenne, P., & Balakrishna, J. (2001). Domestic violence and intimacy: What the relationship therapist needs to know. *Sexual and Relationship Therapy, 16,* 229–246.

Davies, J. (2008). *Building comprehensive solutions to domestic violence Publication 20: Policy blueprint on domestic violence and poverty: When battered women stay: Advocacy beyond leaving.* Retrieved February 24, 2011, from National Resource Center on Domestic Violence at http://new.vawnet.org/Assoc_Files_VAWnet/BCS20_Staying.pdf

DeGangi, G. A., & Greenspan, S. I. (1989). *Test of Sensory Function in Infants: Manual.* Los Angeles: Western Psychological Services.

Dunn, W. (1999). *Sensory Profile: User's manual.* San Antonio, TX: Psychological Corporation.

Economic Stability Working Group of the Transition Subcommittee of the Governors' Commission on Domestic Violence. (2002, October). *Voices of survival: The economic impacts of domestic violence, A blueprint for action.* Available online at http://www.harborcov.org/pages/publications/voices_of_survival.pdf

Edleson, J. L., Ellerton, A. L., Seagren, E. A., Kirchberg, S. L., Schmidt, S. O., & Ambrose, A. T. (2007). Assessing child exposure to adult domestic violence. *Children and Youth Services Review, 29*(7), 961–971. doi:10.1016/j.childyouth.2006.12.009

Fisher, J., & Shelton, A. (2006). Survivors of domestic violence: Demographics and disparities in visitors to an interdisciplinary specialty clinic. *Community Health, 29,* 118–130.

Giles, J., & Curreen, H. (2007). Phases of growth for abused New Zealand women: A Comparison with other studies. *Afflia, 22*(4), 371–384.

Gorde, M. W., Helfrich, C. A., & Finlayson, M. L. (2004). Trauma symptoms and life skills needs of domestic violence victims. *Journal of Interpersonal Violence, 19*, 691–708.

Harris, A. (2003). Choosing the lesser evil: The violence of the welfare stereotype. In V. Adair & S. Dahlberg (Eds.), *Reclaiming class: Women, poverty, and the promise of higher education* (pp. 131–138). Philadelphia: Temple University.

Helfrich, C. A., Aviles, A. M., Badiani, C., Walens, D., & Sabol, P. (2006). Life skill interventions with homeless youth, domestic violence victims, and adults with mental illness. *Occupational Therapy in Health Care, 20*(3/4), 189–207.

Helfrich, C. A., Lafata, M. J., MacDonald, S. L., Aviles, A., & Collins, L. (2001). Domestic abuse across the lifespan: Definitions, identification, and risk factors for occupational therapists. In C. A. Helfrich (Ed.), *Domestic violence across the lifespan. The role of occupational therapy* (pp. 5–34). Binghamton, NY: Haworth Press.

Helfrich, C. A., & Rivera, Y. (2006). Employment skills and domestic violence survivors: A shelter-based intervention. *Occupational Therapy in Mental Health, 22*(1), 33–48. doi:10.1300/J004v22n01_03

Holt, S., Buckley, H., & Whelan, S. (2008). The impact of exposure to domestic violence on children and young people: A review of the literature. *Child Abuse and Neglect, 32*(8), 797–810. doi:10.1016/j.chiabu.2008.02.004

Huth-Beck, A., Levendosky, A., & Semel, M. (2001). The direct and indirect effects of domestic violence on young children's intellectual functioning. *Journal of Family Violence, 16*, 269–290.

Israel, E., & Stover, C. (2009). Intimate partner violence: The role of the relationship between perpetrators and children who witness violence. *Journal of Interpersonal Violence, 24*(10), 1755–1764. doi:10.1177/0886260509334044

Jacobson, C. J., Pabst, S., Regan, S., & Fisher, B. (2006). A lifetime of intimate partner violence: Coping strategies of older women. *Journal of Interpersonal Violence, 21*(5), 634–651. doi:10.1177/0886260506286878

Javaherian, H., DeBrun, J., Moesser, A., Murphy, R., Salvati, B., & Shaffer, T. (2010). *The Mothering experiences of survivors of domestic violence: An in-depth analysis.* Loma Linda, CA: Loma Linda University, Department of Occupational Therapy.

Javaherian, H., Krabacher, V., Andriacco, K., & German, D. (2007). Surviving domestic violence: Rebuilding one's life. *Occupational Therapy in Health Care, 21*(3), 35–59.

Javaherian-Dysinger, H., Cameron, K., Harding, K., Hedgecock, A., Lopez, A., & Unterseher, R. (2011). *Occupational experiences of youth exposed to domestic violence.* Loma Linda, CA: Loma Linda University, Department of Occupational Therapy.

Jewkes, R. (2005). Domestic violence has many causes. In H. Cothran (Series Ed.) & D. Haugen (Vol. Ed.), *Opposing Viewpoints Series: Domestic violence* (pp. 104–114). Farmington Hills, MI: Thomson Gale.

Jones-DeWeever, A. A., & Gault, B. (2006). *Resilient and reaching for more: Challenges and benefits of higher education for welfare participants and their children.* Available online from Institute for Women's Policy Research at www.iwpr.org/publications

Josephson, J. (2005). The intersectionality of domestic violence and welfare in the lives of poor women. In N. Sokoloff (Ed.), *Domestic violence at the margins: Readings on race, class, gender, and culture* (pp. 83–100). New Brunswick, NJ: Rutgers University.

Law, M., Baptiste, S., Carswell, A., McColl, M. A., Polatajko, H., & Pollock, N. (2005). *Canadian Occupational Performance Measure.* Ottawa, ON: CAOT Publications ACE.

Levendosky, A., & Graham-Bermann, S. (2001). Parenting in battered women: The effects of domestic violence on women and their children. *Journal of Family Violence, 16*, 171–192.

Linder, T. (2008). *Transdisciplinary Play-Based Assessment* (2nd ed.). Baltimore: Paul H. Brookes.

Lyon, E. (2000, October). *Welfare, poverty, and abused women: New research and its implications* (Pub. No. 10). Available online at http://new.vawnet.org?Assoc_Files_VAWnet?BCS10_POV.pdf

Lyon, E. (2002, August). *Welfare and domestic violence against women: Lessons from research.* Retrieved February 24, 2010, from National Resource Center on Violence Against Women at http://new.vawnet.org/category/Main_Doc.php?docid=317

McCauley, J. (1998). Abused women's experiences with clinicians and health services. *Journal of General Internal Medicine, 13,* 549–555.

McKibben, L., DeVos, E., & Newberger, E. (1998). Victimization of mothers of abused children: A controlled study. *Pediatrics, 84,* 531–535.

Milberger, S., LeRoy, B., Martin, A., Israel, N., Potter, L., & Patchak-Schuster, P. (2002). *Michigan study on women with physical disabilities* (Final Report, National Institute of Justice Grant 2000-WT-VX-0018). Available online at http://www.ncjrs.gov/pdffiles1/nij/grants/193769.pdf

Monahan, K., & O'Leary, K. D. (1999). Health injury and battered women: An initial inquiry. *Health and Social Work, 24,* 269–279.

Mutti, M., Sterling, H., Spalding, M., & Spalding, N. (1998). *Quick Neurological Screening Test II (QNST–II).* Los Angeles: Western Psychological Assessment.

National Coalition Against Domestic Violence. (2007). *Domestic violence facts.* Available online at http://www.ncadv.org/files/DomesticViolenceFactSheet(National).pdf

National Coalition Against Domestic Violence. (n.d.). *The problem: What is battering?* Available online at http://www.ncadv.org/learn/TheProblem.php

National Coalition of Anti-Violence Programs. (1998). *Annual report on lesbian, gay, bisexual, transgender domestic violence.* Available online at http://www.mincava.umn.edu/documents/glbtdv/glbtdv.html

National Institute of Justice. (2000). *Extent, nature, and consequences of intimate partner violence.* Washington, DC: U.S. Department of Justice.

National Institute of Justice. (2007). *Intimate partner violence.* Available online at http://www.ojp.usdoj.gov/nij/topics/crime/intimate-partner-violence/welcome.htm

Norwood, W., Swank, P., Stephens, N., Ware, H., & Buzy, W. (2001). Reducing conduct problems among children of battered women. *Journal of Counseling and Clinical Psychology, 69,* 774–785.

Nosek, M., Hughes, R. B., Taylor, H., & Taylor, P. (2006). Disability, psychosocial, and demographic characteristics of abused women with physical disabilities. *Violence Against Women, 129,* 823–837. doi:10.1177/1077801206292671

Office for Victims of Crime. (2002). *National Victim Assistance Academy: Foundations in victimology and victims' rights and services* (Ch. 9. Domestic Violence). Retrieved February 25, 2011, from http://www.valor-national.org/ovc/chapter9.html.

Rand, M., & Harrell, E . (2009, October). *National Crimes Victimization Survey: Crime against people with disabilities, 2007.* Available online at http://bjs.ojp.usdoj.gov/content/pub/pdf/capd07.pdf

Rank, M. (2004). *One nation underprivileged: Why American poverty affects us all.* New York: Oxford University.

Rice, J. (2001). Poverty, welfare, and patriarchy: How macro-level changes in social policy can help low income women. *Journal of Social Issues, 57*(2), 355–374.

Riger, S., & Staggs, S. (2004). Welfare reform, domestic violence, and employment: What do we know and what do we need to know? *Violence Against Women, 10,* 961–990.

Sokoloff, N., & Dupont, I. (2005). Domestic violence: Examining the intersections of race, class, and gender—An introduction. In N. Sokoloff (Ed.), *Domestic violence at the margins: Readings on race, class, gender, and culture* (pp. 1–13). Piscataway, NJ: Rutgers University.

Sternberg, K., Lamb, M., Greenbaum, C., Cicchetti, D., Dawud, S., Cortes, R., et al. (1993). Effects of domestic violence on children's behavior problems and depression. *Developmental Psychology, 29,* 44–52.

Stiles, M. (2002). Witnessing domestic violence: The effect on children. *American Family Physician, 66,* 2052–2058.

Tjaden, P., & Thoennes, N. (2000a, July). *Extent, nature and consequences of intimate partner violence: Findings from the National Violence Against Women Survey* (NCJ 181867). Available online at http://www.ncjrs.gov/pdffiles1/nij/181867.pdf

Tjaden, P., & Thoennes, N. (2000b, November). *Full report of the Prevalence, Incidence, and Consequences of Violence Against Women: Findings From the National Violence Against Women Survey* (NCJ 183781). Available online at http://www.ojp.usdoj.gov/nij/pubs-sum/183781.htm

Tolman, R. M., & Raphael, J. (2000). A review of research on welfare and domestic violence. *Journal of Social Issues, 56,* 644–682.

Underwood, R. (2009). *Care of self: Construction of subjectivities of low-income, female survivors of domestic violence as they pursue postsecondary education.* Unpublished doctoral dissertation, University of Georgia, Athens.

U.S. Department of Justice, Office of Justice Programs, Bureau of Justice Statistics. (2007, December 19). *Intimate partner violence in the U.S.* Available online at http://www.ojp.usdoj.gov/nij/topics/crime/intimate-partner-violence/welcome.htm

U.S. Department of Justice, Office of Justice Programs, Bureau of Justice Statistics. (2011). *Intimate partner violence.* Retrieved from http://bjs.ojp.usdoj.gov/index.cfm?ty=tp&tid=971#summary.

U.S. Department of Justice. (n.d.). *About domestic violence.* Available online at http://www.ovw.usdoj.gov/domviolence.htm

U.S. Department of Labor. (2010). *Employment characteristics of families summary.* Retrieved February 25, 2011, from http://www.bls.gov/news.release/famee.nr0.htm

Waldner, L. (2003). If you want me to pull myself up, give me bootstraps. In V. Adair & S. Dahlberg (Eds.), *Reclaiming class: Women, poverty, and promise of higher education in America* (pp. 97–110). Philadelphia: Temple University.

Wuest, J., & Merritt-Gray, M. (1999). Not going back: Sustaining the separation in the process of leaving abusive relationships. *Violence Against Women, 5*(2), 110–134.

Zink, T., Regan, S., Jacobson, C. J., & Pabst, S. (2003). Cohort, period, and aging effects: A qualitative study of older women's reasons for remaining in abusive relationships. *Violence Against Women, 9*(12), 1429–1441. doi:10.1177/1077801203259231

Authors

Heather Javaherian-Dysinger, OTD, OTR/L
Robin Underwood, PhD, OTR/L

for

The Commission on Practice
Janet V. DeLany, DEd, MSA, OTR/L, FAOTA, *Chairperson*

Adopted by the Representative Assembly Coordinating Council (RACC) for the Representative Assembly. Revised by the Commission on Practice 2011.

This revision replaces the 2006 document *Occupational Therapy Services for Individuals Who Have Experienced Domestic Violence* (previously published and copyrighted in 2007 by the American Occupational Therapy Association in the *American Journal of Occupational Therapy, 61,* 704–709).

Occupational Therapy Services in Early Childhood and School-Based Settings

The primary purpose of this document is to describe how occupational therapy supports children's and youth's learning and development in early childhood and school-based settings. This document is intended for occupational therapists and occupational therapy assistants in practice, academia, research, advocacy, and administrative positions. Other audiences for this statement include regulatory and policymaking bodies, provider groups, accreditation agencies, other professionals, and the general public who may be seeking clarification about occupational therapy's scope of practice and domain of concern related to this topic. The American Occupational Therapy Association (AOTA) provides information and resources to support occupational therapists and occupational therapy assistants in the delivery of effective services for children and youth in a variety of settings, including school-based and early intervention programs, child care, Head Start and Early Head Start, preschool and pre-kindergarten programs, and at home.

Occupational therapists and occupational therapy assistants[1] work with children and youth, parents, caregivers, educators, and other team members to facilitate children's and youth's ability to participate in everyday activities, or *occupations*. Occupations are "activities…of everyday life, named, organized, and given value and meaning by individuals and a culture" (Law, Polatajko, Baptiste, & Townsend, 1997, p. 34). Occupations are meaningful for the child and are based on social or cultural expectations or peer performance. In early childhood (birth–8 years of age) and school-based settings, occupational therapy practitioners[2] use their unique expertise to help children and youth with and without challenges prepare for and perform important learning and developmental activities within their natural environment. Occupational therapy services support a child's participation in activities of daily living (ADLs), instrumental activities of daily living (IADLs), education, work, play, leisure, rest and sleep, and social participation.

Occupational therapists have knowledge and skills in the biological, physical, social, and behavioral sciences to evaluate and intervene with individuals across the life course. Occupational therapy practitioners apply evidence-based research ethically and appropriately to the evaluation and intervention process following professional *Standards of Practice* (AOTA, 2010b) and the *Occupational Therapy Code of Ethics and Ethics Standards* (AOTA, 2010a).

Legislative Influences on Service Delivery

Occupational therapy practice in schools and early childhood settings is affected by many federal and state laws and regulations, as well as local policies and procedures. Table 1 summarizes some of the policies that directly affect the provision of occupational therapy for children and youth. Additional

---

[1]*Occupational therapists* are responsible for all aspects of occupational therapy service delivery and are accountable for the safety and effectiveness of the occupational therapy service delivery process. *Occupational therapy assistants* deliver occupational therapy services under the supervision of and in partnership with an occupational therapist (AOTA, 2009).

[2]When the term *occupational therapy practitioner* is used in this document, it refers to both occupational therapists and occupational therapy assistants (AOTA, 2006).

Table 1. Federal Laws and Their Influence on Occupational Therapy Services

Law	Influence on Occupational Therapy Services
Individuals with Disabilities Education Improvement Act (IDEA), P.L. 108-446	Federal legislation that specifically includes occupational therapy as a related service for eligible students with disabilities, ages 3–21 years, to benefit from special education (Part B) or as a primary service for infants and toddlers who are experiencing developmental delays (Part C). IDEA may be reauthorized and amended in 2011.
Elementary and Secondary Education Act (ESEA) Amendments, No Child Left Behind Act (NCLB), P.L. 107-110	Federal legislation that requires public schools to raise the educational achievement of all students, particularly those from disadvantaged backgrounds, students with disabilities, and those with limited English proficiency, and that states establish high standards for teaching and student learning. While not specifically mentioned in the statute, occupational therapy is generally considered to be a pupil service under ESEA. ESEA may be reauthorized and amended in 2011.
Section 504 of the Rehabilitation Act of 1973, as amended, 29 U.S.C. 794; Americans with Disabilities Act (ADA, as amended); Americans with Disabilities Act Amendments Act of 2008 (ADAAA), P.L. 110-325	Civil rights statutes that prohibit discrimination on the basis of disability by programs receiving federal funds (Section 504) and by services and activities of state and local government (ADA and ADAAA). Disability here is defined more broadly than in IDEA. Children and youth who are not eligible for IDEA may be eligible for services under Section 504 or the ADA, such as for environmental adaptations and other reasonable accommodations, to help them access and succeed in the learning environment. Each state or local education agency determines eligibility procedures for children and youth served under Section 504 or the ADA.
Title XIX of the Social Security Act of 1965, as amended; Medicaid, P.L. 89-97	Federal–state match program that provides medical and health services for low-income children and adults. Occupational therapy is an optional service under the state plan but mandatory for children and youth under the Early Periodic Screening, Diagnosis and Treatment (EPSDT) services mandate. Occupational therapy services provided in early intervention programs are frequently covered by Medicaid. School-based services also may be covered by Medicaid but also must meet applicable medical necessary requirements as well as be educationally relevant.
Improving Head Start for School Readiness Act of 2007, P.L. 110-134	Federal program that provides comprehensive child development services to economically disadvantaged children (ages birth–5 years) and their families, including children with disabilities. Early Head Start serves children up to 3 years of age. Occupational therapy may be provided in these settings under the Head Start requirements or under IDEA.
Assistive Technology Act of 2004, P.L. 108-364, as amended	Federal program that promotes access to assistive technology for persons with disabilities so that they can more fully participate in education, employment, and daily activities.
U.S. Department of Agriculture Food and Nutrition Service (USDA, 2001)	National School Breakfast and Lunch Programs are required to provide food substitutions and modifications of school meals for students whose disabilities restrict their diets, as determined by a doctor.

information about these laws is provided in *Occupational Therapy Services for Children and Youth Under IDEA* (Jackson, 2007).

AOTA believes that occupational therapy practitioners working in early childhood and school settings should have working knowledge of the federal and state requirements to ensure that their program policies are in compliance. Occupational therapy practitioners also should be familiar with their state's occupational therapy practice act and related rules and regulations to ensure that occupational therapy services are provided accordingly.

Occupational Therapy Domain and Process

Occupational therapy supports client health and participation in life through engagement in occupations (AOTA, 2008). Occupational therapy focuses on the following occupations: ADLs, IADLs, education, leisure, play, social participation, work, and rest and sleep.

Occupational therapy practitioners provide services that enable children and youth to organize, manage, and perform their daily life occupations and activities. For example, a middle-school-age child with physical limitations may have difficulty completing written work. The occupational therapy practitioner collaborates with the student, parents, and educators to identify the skills of the student, the demands of the environment, and appropriate solutions for interventions. Another example is the family of a newborn baby with poor feeding skills. The occupational therapist may provide training and support for the family to enhance the baby's ability to drink from a bottle.

In early childhood and school-based practice, occupational therapy clients include individuals (e.g., child, family, caregivers, teachers), organizations (e.g., school districts, community preschools, Head Start), and populations within a community (e.g., homeless children, children at risk for social–emotional difficulties). Occupational therapy services are directed toward facilitating the client's participation in meaningful occupations that are desired and important in the school, family, and community contexts.

Occupational therapy services include evaluation, intervention, and documenting outcomes. During the evaluation, the occupational therapist gains an understanding of the client's priorities and his or her problems when engaging in occupations and activities. Evaluation and intervention address factors that influence occupational performance, including

- Performance skills (e.g., motor and praxis skills, sensory–perceptual skills, emotional regulation skills, cognitive skills, communication and social skills);

- Performance patterns (e.g., as habits, routines, rituals, roles);

- Contexts and environments (e.g., physical, social, cultural, virtual, personal, temporal);

- Activity demands (e.g., required actions, body functions); and

- Client factors (e.g., values and beliefs; mental, neuromuscular, sensory, visual, perceptual, digestive, cardiovascular, and integumentary functions and structures).

Desired outcomes are identified to guide future actions with the client. They also are a means for evaluating the effectiveness of occupational therapy services.

Occupational Therapy Service Provision

Occupational therapy practitioners provide early childhood services in children's homes, child care centers, preschools, Early and Head Start programs, early intervention programs, and clinical settings. Occupational therapy practitioners provide school-based services in both public and private facilities. Funding sources for occupational therapy services vary and may include federal and state funding (e.g., funding through state agencies, Medicaid), insurance, and self-pay.

Children and adolescents may be served under the Individuals with Disabilities Education Act (IDEA) Part C, if they are ages 3 years or younger, or Part B, if they are between the ages of 3 and 21 years. Some states are extending their Part C program to include preschool-age children.

Early Intervention (IDEA Part C; Birth Through Age 2 Years)

Early intervention occupational therapy services are provided to infants and toddlers with developmental delays, with diagnosed physical or mental conditions, or who are at risk for having a developmental delay in order to enhance the family's ability to care for their child with a disability. To be eligible for early intervention services under Part C, a child must have a delay in one or more of five developmental areas: (1) physical (including vision and hearing), (2) cognitive, (3) communication, (4) social–emotional, and (5) adaptive. When evaluating infants or toddlers, the occupational therapist considers aspects of the child's performance that are strengths or barriers to participation within the natural environment and daily routines. The occupational therapist's knowledge of brain development, assessment, and intervention across developmental domains, early literacy, and feeding/eating skills enables them to work with children with disabilities and their families. Infants and toddlers with significant medical or developmental concerns (e.g, feeding, neurological) should receive services from trained professionals, as they are vulnerable and require ongoing evaluation.

IDEA requires that child and family outcomes and services be developed in collaboration with the child's caregivers, other members of the team, and community agencies. These services become part of the individualized family service plan (IFSP). Some examples of occupational therapy services for the five developmental domains are listed in Table 2.

In Part C programs, occupational therapy is a primary service. The occupational therapist may be the sole service provider but most often is part of a collaborative team that works to enhance the family's capacity to care for the child's health and development within daily routines and natural environments. An occupational therapist may serve as the service coordinator to monitor the implementation of the IFSP and coordinate services with other team members and agencies. When the child is turning 3 years of age, the occupational therapist works collaboratively with the IFSP team to transition children to appropriate community-based programs or to preschool special education services, as applicable.

School Age (IDEA Part B; Ages 3–21 Years)

The local school district is responsible for determining whether school-age children and youth with disabilities, including preschool children from ages 3 to 5 years, qualify for special education and related services under IDEA Part B (§602(3)(A)(ii)). A full and individual evaluation is conducted, and an individualized education program (IEP) is developed if the student is eligible for services. Students with disabilities may be eligible for IDEA if they meet one or more of 10 disability categories:

1. Mental retardation;

2. Hearing impairments, including deafness;

3. Speech or language impairments;

4. Visual impairments, including blindness;

5. Serious emotional disturbance;

6. Orthopedic impairment;

7. Autism;

8. Traumatic brain injury;

9. Other health impairment; or

10. Specific learning disabilities (see §602(3)(A)).

Occupational therapy is one of the related services that may be provided to IDEA-eligible students who are receiving special education in schools; homes; hospitals; and other settings, including juvenile justice and alternative education settings. Related services are "transportation, and such developmental, corrective, and other supportive services (including…occupational therapy)…as may be required to assist a child with a disability to benefit from special education, and includes early identification and assessment of disabling conditions in children" (see §602(26)(A)). As such, occupational therapy is a support service for students and teachers.

When an occupational therapy evaluation is required, data collection is focused on identifying the academic, developmental, and functional needs of the student (see §614(d)(3)(A)(iv)). Information is sought regarding the student's strengths and factors that may be interfering with his or her learning and participation in the context of the educational activities, routines, and environments. Observations are made

Table 2. Occupational Therapy's Role in Early Intervention Developmental Areas

Developmental Area	Occupational Therapy's Role
Adaptive	Promote independence in self-care, such as eating and drinking, dressing, and grooming; collaborate with parents about safe positioning and modification of food textures to enhance eating
Cognitive	Promote ability to notice and attend to objects and people in the environment; promote ability to sort and classify objects and to generalize learning to new daily living tasks; promote ability to sequence steps to complete daily living occupations
Communication	Facilitate language development through social interactions, assistive communication devices, switches, toys
Physical	Promote movement for exploration of the environment, facilitate use of arms and hands to handle and manipulate objects, educate caregivers in handling and positioning techniques
Social–emotional	Foster self-regulation, social participation, and play through interactions with peers and adults

where and when difficulties occur at school (i.e., at the times and in the location in which the student normally engages in the activities and is demonstrating behaviors that are of concern). These locations include the classroom, hallways, cafeteria, restrooms, gym, and playground. The student's work, participation, and behaviors are compared with other students in the same environments and situations. Curricular demands and existing task and environmental modifications are reviewed.

Interviews with instructional personnel, the student, and family members are conducted to gather information about the student's participation and performance. Cultural differences that may exist between home and school are explored. Existing special education supports and services, including strategies utilized to improve performance, are reviewed. Practices consistent with universal design for learning (UDL) guidelines (CAST, 2008) and the availability of assistive technologies to support school performance are assessed. Standardized testing may be conducted when needed to gather additional data.

Occupational therapy evaluation results then are shared with the parents and the multidisciplinary IEP team. According to Nolet and McLaughlin (2005), decisions about an IEP are individualized but "start from the expectation that the student is to learn the general education curriculum, and special education's role is to help the student learn and progress in that curriculum" (p. 14). Annual goals for special education instruction are determined by the IEP team, as well as the accommodations and services and supports required to help the student access and progress in the general curriculum. Occupational therapy practitioners collaborate with the IEP team regarding the educational need for occupational therapy services.

On the basis of current occupational therapy evaluation data; the occupational therapist's professional judgment; and other available information about the student's skills, abilities, goals, and objectives to be achieved, the IEP team decides whether occupational therapy services are needed. The development of the IEP is a collaborative process with participation from all team members. The team determines when the student goals need the expertise of an occupational therapy practitioner, as well as the amount of time, frequency, duration, and location of those services. The team meets regularly (at least annually) to assess whether the student is making progress toward achieving his or her goals and whether special education and/or related services (including occupational therapy) need to be continued, modified, or discontinued.

Intervention can be directed toward individuals (including teachers and other adults working with the child), groups, environmental factors, and programmatic needs (see Table 3). According to Brannen et al. (2002), effective implementation includes consultation, collaboration, and teamwork. Throughout the intervention process, the occupational therapy practitioner works collaboratively with the client and other team members such as family members, instructional personnel, school administrators, and

Table 3. Occupational Therapy Services and Supports for Students 3–21 Years Under IDEA Part B

IDEA Part B Performance Areas	Occupational Therapy Services and Supports
Academic	Provide consultation with curriculum planners to support academic achievement by identifying needed curriculum accommodations and modifications for standardized testing; suggest adaptations to curriculum materials, methods, processes, and production; identify and provide needed transition supports and services targeting post-secondary goals
Developmental	Foster development of pre-academic skills, including prewriting and pre-scissor skills, toileting skills, eating and drinking skills, dressing and grooming tasks, communication skills, management of sensory needs, social skills
Functional	Facilitate use and management of school-related materials; daily routines/schedule; written school work: task/activity completion; transitions among activities and persons; adherence to rules; self-regulation; interactions with peers and adults; participation in leisure and recreational occupations at home, school, and the community; use of adaptive and assistive technology to support participation and performance
	Assist school in locating driver education training for students with disabilities. Collaborate with family and school staff in the development and implementation of transition programs, including preschool and high school transition. Collaborate with school personnel in the design and implementation of positive mental health programs and positive behavioral support systems

private practitioners who may serve the student. Interventions are respectful of the customs, beliefs, activity patterns, behavior standards, and expectations accepted by the society of which the client is a member. Along with the provision of strategies and techniques that assist the child with making progress, education and training of other team members also is an important service that occupational therapy practitioners provide. Interventions are provided in natural school environments (e.g., classroom, playground, cafeteria), occurring in the time and place that is most beneficial for the student. As noted in Hanft and Shepherd (2008), the primary setting for occupational therapy services incorporates daily routine and contexts important to the student.

Outcomes are measured by student achievement of the IEP goals and other educational objectives such as curriculum expectations. Outcome measurement for instruction may include participation on national, state, and/or district-wide assessments that are supported by services provided by the occupational therapy practitioner. Outcome measurement for occupations such as self-care, play, leisure, social participation, and work transition that typically are addressed by occupational therapy practitioners in the school setting is accomplished by monitoring progress on IEP goals focused on these areas. Data collected on identified outcomes is reviewed by the IEP team to assist with determining present levels of academic achievement and functional performance and is reported during the required annual review.

Section 504/Americans with Disabilities Act

Section 504 of the Rehabilitation Act prohibits discrimination on the basis of disability for any program receiving federal funds, including schools, early intervention, and Head Start programs. The Americans with Disabilities Act also prohibits discrimination on the basis of disability in education, employment, transportation, health care, and a host of other services and activities of state and local governments, including child care. Students with disabilities who are not eligible for services under IDEA may be eligible under Section 504 or the ADA if the disability is such that it significantly limits "one or more major life activities." Examples include students who have HIV/AIDS, asthma, arthritis, attention deficit disorder/attention deficit hyperactivity disorder, traumatic brain disorder, conduct disorder, or depression.

Occupational therapists may be asked to help local school district teams determine student eligibility under Section 504 and to assist in the identification of services and development of the 504 plan. If the 504 committee determines that an educational need for occupational therapy exists, services may be provided directly to a child or as a necessary accommodation. While no additional federal funds are available for services under Section 504 or the ADA, compliance with the requirements are mandatory for early childhood and school settings.

Response to Intervention and Early Intervening Services

Two provisions in the 2004 reauthorization of IDEA provide additional opportunities for occupational therapy practitioners to contribute to the success of general education students who are struggling with learning or behavior. The first of these provisions, *Early Intervening Services (EIS)*, provides supports for students in kindergarten through 12th grade who are struggling with learning or behavior. School districts can use a portion of their IDEA funds to provide professional development for teachers and other staff and to provide direct services such as educational and behavioral evaluations, behavioral interventions, small group instruction, and instruction in the use of adaptive and instructional software for students who "need additional academic and behavioral supports to succeed in the general education environment" (see §613(f)(1)).

The second provision, *Response to Intervention (RtI)*, is a systematic process that closely monitors how students respond to different types of services and instruction. In the RtI process, increasingly intense levels of support are provided. Decisions about which supports to provide and at what level of intensity are made through progress monitoring and data analysis. At each step of the process, monitoring and record keeping provide critical information about the student's ongoing instruction and intervention needs.

Both EIS and RtI are preventative, proactive strategies aimed at minimizing the occurrence of behavior and learning problems as early as possible, thereby reducing the need for more intensive services later. When these approaches are used, occupational therapy practitioners implement strategies that can be used throughout a school. For example, suggestions might include the use of wide-lined paper or a pencil grip to support improvements in handwriting, modification of the classroom environment to increase accessibility, use of elastic-waist pants for a child unable to fasten clothing after toileting, strategies to deal with a child who hits others on the playground when he or she becomes frustrated, or general strategies for breaking down steps for jumping rope so that a child struggling with this skill can be successful in physical education. In addition, occupational therapy practitioners may collaborate with other professionals to design school-wide positive mental health programs, positive behavioral support services, and anti-bullying campaigns.

The occupational therapy role in EIS and RtI will vary from state to state and from district to district depending on how these provisions are implemented. Because both initiatives are targeted toward general education, school-based practitioners may need to educate student support teams on how occupational therapy helps meet student's learning and behavioral needs in those environments. In addition, practitioners should participate in state and district professional development activities related to EIS and RtI and become full participants on the local teams considering interventions and supports students need to succeed in school (Clark, 2008; Clark & Polichino, 2008; Jackson, 2007).

OT and OTA Partnerships

Occupational therapists and occupational therapy assistants work together in early childhood and school settings to deliver needed services. Occupational therapists are responsible for formal evaluation and also are accountable for the safety and effectiveness of the service delivery process, including intervention planning, implementation, outcome review, and dismissal/discharge. The occupational therapy assistant implements the intervention plan under the supervision of and in partnership with the therapist. State occupational therapy regulatory agencies determine supervision frequency, methods, and documentation.

Supervision of Other Personnel

Many early intervention programs, schools, or community agencies employ paraprofessionals to assist in the classroom or to provide direct support to some students. The occupational therapist may utilize these individuals, as allowed by state law and regulation, to carry out selected aspects of a service. Paraprofessionals must be properly trained and carefully supervised at all times to assist with the provision of selected activities or programming that will enhance the student's ability to achieve his or her IEP goals or IFSP outcomes. Paraprofessionals do not provide skilled occupational therapy, nor are they substitutes for the occupational therapist. Paraprofessionals perform only those tasks that can be safely performed within the child's routine and do not require the expertise of an occupational therapist or occupational therapy assistant.

The tasks delegated to a paraprofessional should be documented. A plan to train and supervise the paraprofessional must be developed by the occupational therapist. An occupational therapy assistant may train and supervise a paraprofessional in specifically delegated tasks; however, the occupational therapist is ultimately responsible for monitoring programs carried out by paraprofessionals and occupational therapy assistants.

Conclusion

Occupational therapists and occupational therapy assistants provide services to children and youth, families, caregivers, and educational staff within a variety of programs and settings. The ultimate outcome of occupational therapy services in early childhood and school programs is to enable the child to participate in ADLs, education, work, play, leisure, and social interactions.

References

American Occupational Therapy Association. (2006). Policy 1.44: Categories of occupational therapy personnel. In *Policy manual* (2009 ed., pp. 33–34). Bethesda, MD: Author.

American Occupational Therapy Association. (2008). Occupational therapy practice framework: Domain and process (2nd ed.). *American Journal of Occupational Therapy, 62*, 625–683.

American Occupational Therapy Association. (2009). Guidelines for supervision, roles, and responsibilities during the delivery of occupational therapy. *American Journal of Occupational Therapy, 63*(6), 797–803.

American Occupational Therapy Association. (2010a). Occupational therapy code of ethics and ethics standards (2010). *American Journal of Occupational Therapy, 64*(Suppl.), S17–S26.

American Occupational Therapy Association. (2010b). Standards of practice for occupational therapy. *American Journal of Occupational Therapy, 64*(Suppl.), S106–S111.

Americans with Disabilities Act of 1990, Pub. L. 101-336, 104 Stat. 327.

Americans with Disabilities Act Amendments Act of 2008, Pub. L. 110-325, 122 Stat. 3553.

Assistive Technology Act of 2004, Pub. L. 108-364, 118 Stat. 1707.

Brannen, S. J., Cooper, E. B., Dellegrotto, J. T., Disney, S. T., Eger, D. L., Ehren, B. J, et al. (2002). *Developing educationally relevant IEPs: A technical assistance document for speech–language pathologists*. Reston, VA: Council for Exceptional Children.

CAST. (2008). *Universal design for learning guidelines, version 1.0*. Wakefield, MA: Author.

Clark, G. F. (2008). Getting into a collaborative school routine. In B. Hanft & J. Shepherd (Eds.), *Collaborating for student success: A guide for school-based occupational therapy* (pp. 105–137). Bethesda, MD: AOTA Press.

Clark, G. F., & Polichino, J. (2008). *FAQ on response to intervention for school-based occupational therapists and occupational therapy assistants.* Bethesda, MD: American Occupational Therapy Association.

Hanft, B., & Shepherd, J. (2008). *Collaborating for student success: A guide for school-based occupational therapy.* Bethesda, MD: AOTA Press.

Improving Head Start for School Readiness Act of 2007, Pub. L. 110-134, 121 Stat. 1363, 42 U.S.C. 9801 *et seq.*

Individuals with Disabilities Education Improvement Act of 2004, Pub. L. 108-446, 20 U.S.C. §1400 *et seq.*

Jackson, L. (Ed.). (2007). *Occupational therapy services for children and youth under IDEA* (3rd ed.). Bethesda, MD: AOTA Press.

Law, M., Polatajko, H., Baptiste, W., & Townsend E. (1997). Core concepts of occupational therapy. In E. Townsend (Ed.), *Enabling occupation: An occupational therapy perspective* (pp. 29–56). Ottawa, ON: Canadian Association of Occupational Therapists.

No Child Left Behind Act of 2001, Pub. L. 107-110, 116 Stat. 3071.

Nolet, V., & McLaughlin, M. J. (2005). *Accessing the general curriculum: Including students with disabilities in standards-based reform* (2nd ed.). Thousand Oaks, CA: Corwin Press.

Rehabilitation Act Amendments of 2004, 29 U.S.C. §794.

Social Security Act of 1965, Pub. L. 89-97, 79 Stat. 286, Title XIX.

U.S. Department of Agriculture Food and Nutrition Service. (2001). *Accommodating children with special dietary needs in the school nutrition programs: Guidance for school food service staff.* Washington, DC: Author.

Authors

Gloria Frolek Clark, MS, OTR/L, BCP, FAOTA
Leslie Jackson, MEd, OT, FAOTA
Jean Polichino, MS, OTR, FAOTA

for

The Commission on Practice
Janet V. DeLany, DEd, MSA, OTR/L, FAOTA, *Chairperson*

Adopted by the Representative Assembly Coordinating Council (RACC) for the Representative Assembly.

Revised by the Commission on Practice 2011.

This revision replaces the 2004 document *Occupational Therapy Services in Early Childhood and School-Based Settings* (previously published and copyrighted in 2004 by the American Occupational Therapy Association in the *American Journal of Occupational Therapy, 58,* 681–685).

Occupational Therapy Services in Facilitating Work Performance

The purpose of this statement is to describe for external audiences the role of occupational therapists and occupational therapy assistants[1] in facilitating successful engagement of people in their chosen work activities and in meaningful work roles. The overarching goal of occupational therapy is to support people's "health and participation in life through engagement in occupation" (American Occupational Therapy Association [AOTA], 2008, p. 626). Work is one of eight areas of occupation[2] categorized with the domain of occupational therapy practice (AOTA, 2008). The *Occupational Therapy Practice Framework: Domain and Process, 2nd Edition* defines *work* as "activities needed for engaging in remunerative employment or volunteer activities . . . [and includes] identifying and selecting work opportunities, employment seeking and acquisition tasks, job performance issues, retirement preparation and adjustment, volunteer exploration and volunteer participation" (AOTA, 2008, p. 632). Work performance supports meaningful participation and attainable productivity, which are essential for people's health and well-being.

Occupational therapy practitioners[3] provide services to clients at the individual, organizational, and population level who are experiencing problems or who have concerns for potential problems for engaging in work-related occupations. Difficulties or potential difficulties in work performance may arise from challenges the client is experiencing related to motor, sensory–perceptual, emotional regulation, cognitive, or communication and social performance skills or from those associated with performance patterns, the activity demands, or the context and environment. Occupational therapy practitioners provide work-related services in a variety of settings, including, but not limited to, business and industrial environments, acute care and rehabilitation facilities, psychiatric centers, sheltered workshops, schools, and community settings. Within these settings occupational therapy practitioners provide services that address work hardening/conditioning, pre-work screening, functional capacity assessment and ergonomics, pre-vocational assessment and training, sheltered employment, supported employment, and transition from school to work. The occupational therapy process includes evaluation; intervention planning, implementation, and review; and outcome monitoring. The key services include wellness and prevention services, restorative and compensatory interventions, consultation, education, advocacy, and case management.

Occupational Therapy Evaluation in Work Programs

Using a client-centered approach, the occupational therapist develops an occupational profile to understand the client's occupational history and reasons for seeking services. As part of the process, the occupational therapist gathers information about the client's capacities and needs, values and interests, priorities, and desired outcomes. The occupational therapist then analyzes information about the client's occupa-

---

[1]*Occupational therapists* are responsible for all aspects of occupational therapy service delivery and are accountable for the safety and effectiveness of the occupational therapy service delivery process. *Occupational therapy assistants* deliver occupational therapy services under the supervision of and in partnership with an occupational therapist (AOTA, 2009).

[2]Areas of occupation include "Activities of daily living, instrumental activities of daily living, rest and sleep, education, work, play, leisure, and social participation (AOTA, 2008, p. 630).

[3]When the term *occupational therapy practitioner* is used in this document, it refers to both occupational therapists and occupational therapy assistants (AOTA, 2006).

tional performance gathered through formal evaluation, record review, interview, and observations related to the client's body functions, performance skills, performance patterns, the demands of the work activity, and the context and environment of the work occupation (AOTA, 2008). The occupational therapy evaluation may include data collection in the following areas:

- Job analysis to identify the required activity demands of the work tasks and possibilities for assistive technologies, job adaptations, or work accommodations;

- Evaluation of work and productive tasks, including work routines, tools and equipment, ergonomic considerations, and accessibility;

- Evaluation of work organizational culture, including psychological and social factors, and productivity expectations and job requirements both internal and external to the organization, including regulatory issues (Gupta & Sabata, 2010);

- The client's social and communication skills; functional abilities; potential for improvement; and need for adaptation, compensation, or occupational change; and

- The client's vocational aptitudes and interests necessary for development of transition plan from school to work preparation.

This information is synthesized to develop a plan of intervention that addresses the client's work participation needs, desired outcomes, and performance goals.

Occupational Therapy Intervention in Work Programs

Occupational therapy practitioners provide services to develop or increase the ability of the client to participate in and manage productive work, maintain health, adhere to safe work practices, and prevent work-related disability. Using the information gathered in the evaluation process, the occupational therapy practitioner collaborates with the client and other team members (e.g., employers, case managers, family members) or agencies (e.g., educational, local/state, vocational rehabilitation and social services departments and programs) to plan and implement intervention strategies. When developing these intervention strategies, occupational therapy practitioners consider the client's age, interests, values, beliefs, culture, skills and abilities, motivation, and psychological and social status. They address issues of worker role, task demands, work context, and work culture, as well as identify available resources. Intervention strategies are designed to identify, explore, and expand work options; enhance or develop work-related abilities (e.g., improve physical capacities, improve health and safety performance, develop skills and ability to participate); and obtain or retain employment. The following are some examples of occupational therapy interventions aimed at improving work performance and facilitating safe participation in work activities:

- Education related to health, safety and injury prevention, proper body mechanics, postural awareness, joint protection, ergonomic considerations, symptom awareness, and stress and pain management strategies applicable to work and productive activities;

- Adaptations to work activities, the work environment, and work demands and the use of assistive technologies that support the client's participation in the desired work activities;

- Strategies to improve social, communication, emotional regulation, and coping skills;

- Strategies to improve foundational work behaviors and work skills;

- Development of programs that incorporate graded activity, simulated activity, and work activity trials to allow for the gradual return to full work activity after illness or injury;

- Development of occupational activities to develop, increase, or improve productive work behaviors and skills;

- Development of work transition programs, job modifications, or job adaptations to facilitate successful work performance;

- Development of individualized plans for the transition of individuals with disabilities from school to work;

- Consultation and collaboration with clients about adaptations of work tasks, tools, equipment, and the work environment;

- Consultation with clients regarding injury management and prevention to reduce the incidence of disability-related injury;

- Collaboration with other team members, employers, services, and agencies to coordinate restorative and prevention services provided to the worker; and

- Case management services to assist in the coordination and planning for beginning or returning to work.

Table 1 provides examples of how performance related to work may be compromised and how occupational therapy practitioners may assist clients in participating in meaningful and productive work activities.

Funding Sources

Reimbursement for services related to occupational performance is dependent upon the type of services provided, the beneficiary of the services, and the setting where services are provided. Reimbursement may include, but may not be limited to,

- Direct reimbursement by employers or agencies for services to individuals or populations such as job analysis for a population; development of pre-work screens; ergonomic assessment of work, worker, and workplace; and educational programs for health, safety, and injury prevention.

- Local, state, or federally related program including workers' compensation, special education, Social Security Disability Insurance, and Medicare or medical assistance (see Appendix A for an overview of relevant legislation affecting rehabilitation services for the worker).

- Community agency resources using funds secured through federal or state monies, community or private grants, or other philanthropic donations. This often includes services provided to sheltered workshops, supported employment programs, and programs supporting individuals who are at a socioeconomic disadvantage (see Appendix B).

Table 1. Selected Case Examples

Descriptions of Client Work Performance	Occupational Therapy Evaluation	Occupational Therapy Intervention

Industrial Site—Strains and Sprains
 	
An employer in a heavy equipment manufacturing plant has recently noted a decrease in productivity and an increase in workers' compensation claims in the maintenance department. Further investigation revealed a high incidence of upper-extremity and low-back muscle strains and sprains among the maintenance crew.
 	
The employer contacts an occupational therapist for consultation to help address the problem.
 	
The employer's goals are to reduce strains and sprains, lost days of work, and costs associated with workers' compensation claims. He also is interested in promoting a safer workplace and improving employee job satisfaction and security.
	• Conduct preliminary onsite inspection of department to identify triggers such as makeshift changes to equipment and signs of worker movement and positional discomfort that could be contributing to upper-extremity and back complaints.
	• Interview employees to gain their perspective on incidence of injuries, probable causes, and suggested remedies.
	• Perform a functional job task analysis, including identification of the physical job demands and ergonomic considerations for the different maintenance activities, including
	  o Materials handling, equipment operations, and tools usage;
	  o Postural considerations;
	  o Work environment;
	  o Stress factors such as force, repetition, hold time/rest time, angle/twist/body mechanics, impact, vibration, acceleration, and work time duration.
	• Analyze the data from the work site.
	• Determine areas requiring intervention.
	• Evaluate potential modifications to job, environment, tools, or client functions.
		• Collaborate with the employer to identify and implement ergonomic changes in specific work areas to minimize risk factors associated with equipment, required body positions, and the environment (Chiarello, 2003).
		• Develop an in-service education program for the maintenance department to address risk factor reduction strategies and body mechanics.
		• Develop a wellness program that includes daily flexibility and stretching sessions in addition to worker-centered lifestyle choice classes (e.g., smoking cessation, weight control, stress reduction; Gupta, 2008).
		• Cross-train workers to ensure adequate staffing coverage in the event of absenteeism as well as job rotation to allow a variety of positions, physical exertions, and equipment usage.
		• Institute an annual onsite evaluation to monitor modifications and programs.

Repetitive Strain Injury—Factory Worker
 	
Carla is a 43-year-old woman working as a sewing machine operator and fabric cutter in a garment factory. For the past several months, she has worked 8 hours per day, 5 days per week, plus 4 hours of overtime 2–3 days per week.
 	
She recently was diagnosed with right-dominant-hand deQuervain's tenosynovitis and has been off work for 2 months. Her case manager reports that she has experienced improvement in her wrist and hand function since undergoing treatment but is reluctant to return to work due to concerns she will have a relapse and not be able to do her job.
 	
The employer is willing to consider a transitional return-to-work option. The physician refers the employee to an occupational therapist to determine her functional abilities and potential for successful return to work.
	• Conduct a functional capacity evaluation to determine the physical and functional abilities of the client, including upper-extremity strength and overall endurance to perform work task.
	• Assess worksite, and offer employer suggestions to reduce risk to client.
	• Assess body mechanics and risk for repeated injury associated with
	  o Repetitive cutting through several layers of fabric and
	  o Static positioning of wrists and fingers when guiding material through an industrial sewing machine.
		• Instruct client with incorporating proper body mechanics and use of ergonomic scissors when cutting layers of fabric.
		• Provide employer with strategies regarding institution of job rotation program and incorporation of improved positioning and work techniques for all employees (Jaegers, 2008).
		• Implement a work conditioning program that includes education, flexibility and stretching, work simulation, and strengthening activities.
		• Collaborate with client and employer to identify ergonomic changes and accurate job placement for safe, productive, functional work performance (Sandqvist & Henriksson, 2004).

Developmental Disabilities **Mark is an 18-year-old high school senior with Down Syndrome** resulting in mild intellectual disability. Mark lives with his parents, who drive him to and from school. He wants to seek employment after graduation. Mark received occupational therapy services during his elementary and middle school years. The focus of occupational therapy was on	• Review Mark's records and interview Mark and his parents to learn about his occupational performance related to work, and identify his perceived needs as he moves forward (Sabata & Endicott, 2005). • Determine a work transition plan that addresses work behaviors, communication skills, and social interaction skills.	• Educate Mark and his family about pertinent laws, community agencies, and resources available to assist him in seeking gainful employment (Sabata & Endicott, 2007; Vogtle & Brooks, 2005). • Collaborate with speech–language pathologist to incorporate peer buddy system to strengthen social and communication skills.

Table 1. Selected Case Examples *(cont.)*

Descriptions of Client Work Performance	Occupational Therapy Evaluation	Occupational Therapy Intervention
Developmental Disabilities *(cont.)* independence in daily living skills and the development of appropriate social behaviors. The goal was to maximize classroom learning and interaction with his classmates, ultimately affording Mark the skills to participate in his community (AOTA, 2008). Mark has not worked outside the home and has not had the opportunity to develop work skills or work behaviors. He has difficulty with time management, attention span, and sustained focus on a task.	• Assess the level of difficulty he has with time management, especially with his morning routine. • Assess his pre-work skills, including concentration span, attention to task, and organizational skills; ability to follow written and verbal directions; and ability to communicate his ideas to others. • Determine performance skills in the area of community mobility and transportation usage (AOTA, 2008).	• Instruct Mark on the use of a visual calendar to help him stay focused and complete his morning routines in a timely manner. • Assist Mark in mastering the steps necessary to ride the city bus as a means to travel to and from a job.
Mental Health—Schizophrenia **Natalie, a 27-year-old woman** with a history of schizophrenia, is a consumer at a community support day program. She lives in a subsidized apartment with two other individuals who also have been diagnosed with a mental illness. In the past Natalie has not been able to secure a job due to disorganized thinking, which affected her concentration and follow-through. Based on recent positive response to antipsychotic medication and success in volunteer work at the day program, Natalie has identified a goal of acquiring part-time office work and getting an apartment of her own. Natalie states that she lacks self-confidence related to working and that she is afraid she will not remember how to use a computer or be able to keep up with everyone else at a job. Her case worker has sought the services of an occupational therapist to assist in the work transition process.	Administer an occupational profile to determine Natalie's occupational history, work experiences, interests, patterns of daily living, and meaningful occupations (AOTA, 2008). Assess Natalie's abilities in the following areas: • Problem-solving skills • Independence in daily living activities • Use of public transportation • Medication management • Seeking help and advocating for her needs. Determine her work readiness skills development in task organization and time management.	• Collaborate with Natalie to locate and select appropriate resources and support systems to help her seek, obtain, and sustain gainful part-time employment (Liu, Hollis, Warren, & Williamson, 2007). • Assist Natalie with experiential exploration of potential jobs of interest. • Collaborate with a vocational counselor to set up a supported employment program (Liu et al., 2007). • Work with employer on reasonable accommodations per Natalie's ability to perform the essential functions of a given job (Americans with Disabilities Act, 1990). • Meet with job coach and Natalie to provide specific strategies for work skills development while building on her current skills and strengths (Sabata & Endicott, 2007).
Rheumatoid Arthritis **Sarah, a 45-year-old woman** with rheumatoid arthritis, is employed as a housekeeper at a hotel. She is unable to perform her work tasks due to exacerbation of her rheumatoid symptoms. She presents with decreased gross grasp, decreased pinch strength, difficulty reaching above shoulder height, and poor endurance for continuous work activity over 4 hours.	The occupational therapist observes performance and analyzes activities to determine points of difficulty. In collaboration with Sarah, the therapist concludes that dusting and washing pictures, mirrors, and door frames above shoulder level are no longer possible without adaptation of the equipment used to perform these tasks. Grasp of smaller items (e.g., dusters with ½" handles and mops with 1" handles) is particularly difficult for Sarah in her work. She demonstrates difficulty changing toilet paper roles that require lateral and three-point pinch. Sarah uses her arms to lift bed linens and has difficulty grasping the material as she makes beds. She requires a rest period after cleaning each room.	• Work with Sarah and her employer to identify and prioritize work activities. • Recommend adaptations and modifications in processes, approaches, and the contexts of required housekeeping tasks to support improved performance. • Recommend ergonomic changes to the tools and materials needed to do her job. • Train Sarah in work simplification and adapted techniques. • Work with Sarah to identify alternate work options, including training at a local community college in a career that requires less physical effort and stress upon the body.

(Continued)

Table 1. Selected Case Examples *(cont.)*

Descriptions of Client Work Performance	Occupational Therapy Evaluation	Occupational Therapy Intervention
Older adults seeking volunteer activities **A group of senior citizens** who attend a weekly "Dine and Learn" lunch program at a local senior center were discussing their interest in volunteering in their community. They are interested in volunteerism as a way to stay physically and mentally active. The seniors have not had previous volunteer experience and are not certain where to begin to find a suitable venue and offer their services.	The occupational therapist uses a leisure activity check list to begin identifying areas of potential interest, such as woodworking, home repairs, working with adolescents, and financial consultation. As a result of an Internet search, the seniors identify local organizations and programs in need of volunteers that could benefit from their expertise. Settings include a Boys Club program teaching inner-city youth to make small furniture and decorative items, a service run by an area church to assist elders completing complex tax returns, and the local chapter of Habitat for Humanity.	• Establish a data bank and referral system that matches interests of group members with related volunteer opportunities. • Organize a volunteer fair for the seniors to connect with and learn about the community organizations volunteer needs. • Develop a training program within the senior center to prepare the seniors to match their skills with the specific needs and interests of the organizations.

References

American Occupational Therapy Association. (2006). Policy 1.44: Categories of occupational therapy personnel. In *Policy manual* (2007 ed., pp. 33–34). Bethesda, MD: Author.

American Occupational Therapy Association. (2008). Occupational therapy practice framework: Domain and process (2nd ed.). *American Journal of Occupational Therapy, 62,* 625–683.

American Occupational Therapy Association. (2009). Guidelines for supervision, roles, and responsibilities during the delivery of occupational therapy services. *American Journal of Occupational Therapy, 63,* 797–803.

Americans with Disabilities Act of 1990, P. L. 101-336, 104 Stat. 327.

Chiarello, B. (2003). Does ergonomics improve productivity? An evidenced–based review. *Work Programs Special Interest Section Quarterly, 17*(4), 1–4.

Gupta, J. (2008). Promoting wellness at the workplace. *Work and Industry Special Interest Section Quarterly, 22*(2), 1–4.

Gupta, J., & Sabata, D. (2010). Older workers: Maintaining a worker role and returning to the workplace. In B. Braveman & J. J. Page (Eds.), *Work: Occupational therapy intervention to promote participation and productivity.* Philadelphia: F. A. Davis.

Jaegers, L. (2008). Ergonomics, health, and wellness in industry. A holistic approach. *Work Programs Special Interest Section Quarterly, 22*(3), 4.

Liu, K. W. D., Hollis, V., Warren, S., & Williamson, D. L. (2007). Supported-employment program processes and outcomes: Experiences of people with schizophrenia. *American Journal of Occupational Therapy, 61,* 543–554.

Sabata, D., & Endicott, S. (2007). Workplace changes: Seizing opportunities for persons with disabilities in the workplace. *Work Programs Special Interest Section Quarterly, 21*(2), 1–3.

Sandqvist, J. L., & Henriksson, C. M. (2004). Work functioning: A conceptual framework. *Work: A Journal of Prevention, Assessment, and Rehabilitation, 23,* 147–157.

Vogtle, L. K., & Brooks, B. (2005). Common issues for adults with DD. *OT Practice, 10,* 8–12.

Additional Readings

Aja, D. (2004, March). Using a functional capacity evaluation as a successful benchmark in the life care plan process. *Work Programs Special Interest Section Quarterly, 18*(1), 1–4.

American Medical Association. (2008). *International classification of diseases* (9th rev., Clinical Modification, Hospital, Vols. 1–3). Chicago: Author.

Gibson, L., Strong, L., & Wallace, B. (2005). Functional capacity evaluation as a performance measure: Evidence for a new approach for clients with chronic back pain. *Clinical Journal of Pain, 21*, 207–215

Glass, L. S. (Ed.). (2004). *Occupational medicine practice guidelines* (2nd ed.). Beverly Farms, MA: OEM Press.

Gross, D. P., & Battie, M. C. (2003). Construct validity of a kinesiophysical functional capacity evaluation administered within a worker's compensation environment. *Journal of Occupational Rehabilitation, 13*, 287–295.

Gross, D. P., Battie, M. C., & Cassidy, D. (2004). The prognostic value of functional capacity evaluation in patients with chronic low back pain: Part 1. Timely return to work. *Spine, 29*, 914–919.

Haldorsen, E. M., Grasdal, A. L., Skouen,. S., Risa, A. E., Skronholm, K., & Ursin, H. (2002). Is there a right treatment for a particular patient group? Comparison of ordinary treatment, light multidisciplinary treatment, and extensive multidisciplinary treatment for long-term sick-listed employees with musculoskeletal pain. *Pain, 95*, 49–63.

Hayden, J., van Tulder, M., Malmivaara, A., & Koes, B. (2005). Meta-analysis: Exercise therapy for nonspecific low back pain. *Annals of Internal Medicine, 142*, 765–775.

Heymans, M., van Tulder, M., Esmail, R., Bombardier, C., & Koes, B. (2004). Back schools for non-specific low-back pain. *Cochrane Database of Systematic Reviews, 3*, CD000261.

Howard, N., Spielholz, P., Bao, S., Silverstein, B., & Fan, Z. (2009). Reliability of an observational tool to assess the organization of work. *International Journal of Industrial Ergonomics, 39*, 260–266.

Innes, E. (2006). Reliability and validity of functional capacity evaluations: An update. *International Journal of Disability Management Research, 135*, 135–148.

Innes, E., & Straker, L. (2003). Attributes of excellence in work-related assessment. *Work: A Journal of Prevention, Assessment and Rehabilitation, 20*(1), 63–76.

Jacobs, K. (2008). *Ergonomics for therapists* (3rd ed.). St. Louis, MO: Mosby.

Kaskustas, V., & Snodgrass, J. (2009). *Occupational therapy practice guidelines for individuals with work-related injuries and illnesses.* Bethesda, MD: AOTA Press.

Larson, B. A., & Ellexson, M. T. (2000). Blueprint for ergonomics. *Work: A Journal of Prevention, Assessment, and Rehabilitation, 15*, 107–112.

Larson, B. A., & Ellexson, M. T. (2009). Industrial rehabilitation and work injury prevention. In I. Söderback (Ed.), *International handbook of occupational therapy interventions.* New York: Springer.

Maher, C., & Bear-Lehman, J. (2008). Orthopaedic conditions. In M. V. Radomski & C. A. Trombly Latham (Eds.), *Occupational therapy for physical dysfunction* (6th ed., pp. 1106–1130). Baltimore: Lippincott Williams & Wilkins.

Maloney, C. C. (2003, September). Work simulation strategies in work programs. *Work Programs Special Interest Section Quarterly, 17*(3), 1–3.

Matheson, L. (2003). Functional capacity evaluation. In G. Andersson, S. Demeter, & G. Smith (Eds.), *Disability evaluation* (2nd ed.). Chicago: Mosby.

Meyer, K., Fransen, J., Huwiler, J., Uebelhart, T., & Klipstein, A. (2005). Feasibility and results of a randomized pilot-study of a work rehabilitation programme. *Journal of Back and Musculoskeletal Rehabilitation, 18*, 67–78.

Miller, D. M. (2004, February 9). Psychosocial issues and the return-to-work process. *OT Practice, 9*(3), 16–20.

Moyers, P. A., & Dale, L. M. (2007). *The guide to occupational therapy practice* (2nd ed.). Bethesda, MD: AOTA Press.

Musich, S., Napier, D., & Edington, D. W (2001). The association of health risks with workers' compensation costs. *Journal of Occupational and Environmental Medicine, 43*(6), 534–541.

National Committee on Vital and Health Statistics. (2002). *Classifying and reporting functional status* (Report of the Subcommittee on Population). Retrieved February 8, 2009, from http://ncvhs.hhs.gov/020211mn.htm

Sanders, M. J. (Ed.). (2003). *Management of musculoskeletal disorders*. Newton, MA: Butterworth Heinemann.

Siporin, S., & Lysack, C. (2004). Quality of life and supported employment: A case study of three women with developmental disabilities. *American Journal of Occupational Therapy, 58*, 455–465.

Soer, R., van der Scnans, C., Groornoff, J. W. Ceenzen, J. H., & Reneman, M. E. (2008). Towards consensus in operational definitions in functional capacity evaluation: A Delphi survey. *Journal of Occupational Rehabilitation, 18*, 389–400.

Stutzman, L. (2001, August). Evidence-based return to work guidelines. *CWCE Magazine*, pp. 36–38.

U.S. Bureau of Labor Statistics. (2008). *Nonfatal occupational injuries and illnesses requiring days away from work, 2007* [Press release from the U.S. Department of Labor, No. 08-1716]. Washington, DC: Author.

World Health Organization. (2003). *The burden of musculoskeletal conditions at the start of the new millennium* (WHO Technical Report Series). Geneva, Switzerland: Author.

Authors

Melanie Ellexson, MBA, OTR/L, FAOTA
Barbara Larson, MA, OTR, FAOTA

for

The Commission on Practice
Janet V. DeLany, DEd, OTR/L, FAOTA, *Chairperson*

Adopted by the Representative Assembly Coordinating Council (RACC) for the Representative Assembly.

Revised by the Commission on Practice 2011.

This revision replaces the 2005 document *Occupational Therapy Services in Facilitating Work Performance* (previously published and copyrighted in 2005 by the American Occupational Therapy Association in the *American Journal of Occupational Therapy, 59*, 676–679).

Appendix A. Selected Work Legislation

Legislation	Scope
Federal Employees Liability (FELA) Act, 1908 (45 U.S.C. 51 et seq.)	Established the no-fault insurance system that pays benefits to employees for accidental injuries or diseases that are work related.
Vocational Rehabilitation Act Amendments of 1943 (P.L. 78–113)	Changed the original provision of the Vocational Rehabilitation Act of 1920 (P.L. 66–236). Added people with physical disabilities, blindness, developmental delays, and psychiatric disabilities to those served. Established the Office of Vocational Rehabilitation. Put a new emphasis on activities of daily living and adaptation. Removed ceiling on appropriation.
Vocational Rehabilitation Act Amendments (Hill–Burton Act) of 1954 (P.L. 86–565)	Authorized greater financial support, research and demonstration grants, professional preparation grants, state agency expansion and improvements grants, and grants to expand rehabilitation facilities.
Vocational Rehabilitation Act Amendments of 1965 (P.L. 89–333)	Increased services for several types of people with disabilities and social handicaps. Made construction money available for rehabilitation centers and workshops.
Architectural Barriers Act of 1968 (P.L. 90–48)	Led the way to changes in access for people with disabilities.
Developmental Disabilities Services and Facilities Construction Act of 1970 (P.L. 91–517)	Gave states broad responsibility for planning and implementing a comprehensive program of services to people with developmental delays, epilepsy, cerebral palsy, and other neurological impairments.
Occupational Safety and Health Act of 1970 (P.L. 91–596)	Mandated that the employer provide employment free from recognized hazards that are likely to cause death or serious harm to workers.
Rehabilitation Act of 1973 (P.L. 93–112)	Expanded services to people with more severe disabilities. Provided for affirmative action in employment (Section 503) and nondiscrimination in facilities (Section 504) by federal contractors and grantees.
Rehabilitation Act Amendments of 1986 (P.L. 99–506)	Clarifications included that in evaluating rehabilitation potential, one must consider recreation, employability, and rehabilitation engineering needs.
Education of the Deaf Act (EDA) of 1986 (P.L. 99–371)	Extended statutory authority of the National Technical Institute of the Deaf to provide technical training and education to prepare deaf people for employment.
Omnibus Budget Reconciliation Act of 1987 (P.L. 100–203)	Permitted states to offer prevocational, educational, and supported employment services to people deinstitutionalized at any time before the waiver program.
Americans with Disabilities Act (ADA) of 1990 (P.L. 101–336)	Prevented discrimination against individuals with disabilities. Guaranteed equal protection for individuals with disabilities in employment, public accommodations, transportation, state and local government, and telecommunications.
Ticket-to-Work and Work Incentives Improvement Act of 1999 (P.L. 106–170)	Established to increase opportunities and choices for Social Security disability beneficiaries to obtain employment, vocational rehabilitation, and other support services from public and private providers, employers, and other organizations.
Americans with Disabilities Act Amendments Act (ADAAA) of 2008 (P.L. 110-325)	Focuses on the discrimination at issue instead of the individual's disability. Makes important changes to the definition of the term *disability* by rejecting the holdings in several Supreme Court decisions and portions of Equal Employment Opportunity Commission's (EEOC) ADA regulations. Retains the ADA's basic disability definition as an impairment that substantially limits one or more major life activities, a record of such an impairment, or being regarded as having such an impairment.

Appendix B. Internet Resources

American National Standards Institute	www.ansi.org
Board of Certification in Professional Ergonomics	www.bcpe.org
California Code of Regulations, Title 8, § 5110. Repetitive Motion Injuries	www.dir.ca.gov/title8/5110.html
California Department of Industrial Relations	www.dir.ca.gov
Canadian Centre for Occupational Health and Safety	www.ccohs.ca
Centers for Disease Control and Prevention	www.cdc.gov
Ergoweb	www.ergoweb.com
Foundation for Professional Ergonomics	www.ergofoundation.org
Health calculator page	www.halls.md/index.htm
Human Factors and Ergonomics Society	www.hfes.org
IIEE Applied Ergonomics Community	www.appliedergo.org
Institute for Work and Health	www.iwh.on.ca
International Ergonomics Association	www.iea.cc
International Society for Occupational Ergonomics and Safety	www.isoes.info
National Safety Council	www.nsc.org/Pages/Home.aspx
National Institute for Occupational Safety and Health	www.cdc.gov/niosh/homepage.html
Occupational Safety and Health Administration	www.osha.gov
The (Ontario, Canada) Workplace Safety and Insurance Board	w.wsib.on.ca/wsib/wsibsite.nsf/public/homepage
U.S. Department of Labor	www.dol.gov

The Philosophical Base of Occupational Therapy

Occupations are activities that bring meaning to the daily lives of individuals, families, and communities and enable them to participate in society. All individuals have an innate need and right to engage in meaningful occupations throughout their lives. Participation in these occupations influences their development, health, and well-being across the lifespan. As such, participation in meaningful occupation is a determinant of health.

Occupations occur within diverse social, physical, cultural, personal, temporal, or virtual contexts. The quality of occupational performance and the experience of each occupation are unique in each situation due to the dynamic relationship between factors intrinsic to the individual, the contexts in which the occupation occurs, and the characteristics of the activity.

The focus and outcome of occupational therapy are individuals' engagement in meaningful occupations that support their participation in life situations. Occupational therapy practitioners conceptualize occupations as both a means and an end to therapy. That is, there is therapeutic value in occupational engagement as a change agent, and engagement in occupations is also the ultimate goal of therapy.

Occupational therapy is based on the belief that occupations may be used for health promotion and wellness, remediation or restoration, health maintenance, disease and injury prevention, and compensation/adaptation. The use of occupation to promote individual, community, and population health is the core of occupational therapy practice, education, research, and advocacy.

Authors

The Commission on Education:

Jyothi Gupta, PhD, OTR/L, OT(C), *Chairperson*
Andrea R. Bilics, PhD, OTR/L, FAOTA
Donna M. Costa, DHS, OTR/L, FAOTA
Debra J. Hanson, PhD, OTR
Mallory Duncan, *ASD Liaison* (ASD)
Susan M. Higgins, MA, OTR/L
Linda Orr, MPA, OTR/L
Diane Parham, PhD, OTR/L, FAOTA
Jeff Snodgrass, PhD, MPH, OTR, CWCE
Neil Harvison, PhD, OTR/L, FAOTA, *AOTA Staff Liaison*

Adopted by the Representative Assembly

Revised by the Commission on Education, 2011

This revision replaces the 1979 *The Philosophical Base of Occupational Therapy* (previously published and copyrighted in 1995 by the American Occupational Therapy Association in the *American Journal of Occupational Therapy*, 49, 1026). Reviewed by COE and COP in 2004.

Philosophy of Occupational Therapy Education

Occupational therapy education is grounded in the belief that humans are complex beings engaged in a dynamic process of interaction with the physical, social, temporal, cultural, psychological, spiritual, and virtual environments. Through active engagement within the internal and external environments, humans evolve, change, and adapt. Occupational therapy educators advocate the use of occupation to facilitate health promoting growth, change, and/or adaptation with the goal of participation in meaningful occupation that supports survival, self-actualization, occupational balance, and quality of life.

The profession of occupational therapy is unique and dynamic, grounded in core principles of occupation, and is influenced by emerging knowledge and technologies. Thus, the education of future occupational therapists and occupational therapy assistants must consistently reinforce the development of new knowledge supporting the use of occupation, the application of clinical reasoning based on evidence, the necessity for lifelong learning, and the improvement of professional knowledge and skills.

Occupational therapy education promotes competence through educational experiences that foster the occupational therapists' and occupational therapy assistants' practice potential and scholarship development. Occupational therapy educators use active learning that engages the learner in a collaborative process that builds on prior knowledge and experience and integrates professional academic knowledge, experiential learning, clinical reasoning, and self-reflection. Occupational therapy education promotes integration of philosophical and theoretical knowledge, values, beliefs, ethics, and technical skills for broad application to practice in order to improve human participation and quality of life for those individuals with and without impairments and limitations.

The occupational therapy education process emphasizes continuing critical inquiry in order that occupational therapists and occupational therapy assistants be well prepared to function and thrive in the dynamic environments of a diverse and multicultural society, using the power of occupation as the primary method of evaluation, intervention, and health promotion.

Authors
The Commission on Education:
David A. Haynes, MBA, OTR/L, OTA, *Program Director*
Terrianne Jones, MA, OTR/L, OTA, *Academic Educator*

for

The Commission on Education
Linda S. Fazio, PhD, OTR/L, FAOTA, *Chairperson*

Adopted by the Representative Assembly 2007C9

Note: This document replaces the 2003 *Philosophy of Professional Education* (previously published and copyrighted in 2003 by the American Occupational Therapy Association in the *American Journal of Occupational Therapy, 57,* 640).

Providing Occupational Therapy Using Sensory Integration Theory and Methods in School-Based Practice

The American Occupational Therapy Association (AOTA) recognizes sensory integration (SI) as one of several theories and methods used by occupational therapists and occupational therapy assistants[1] working with children in public and private schools to improve a child's ability to access the general education curriculum and to participate in school-related activities. These methods are used to achieve the overarching goal of occupational therapy to improve the client's health and participation through engagement in everyday activities or "occupations" (AOTA, 2008). SI methods are used within occupational therapy when sensory-related issues are suspected to affect a child's ability to access the general and special education curriculum, behave adaptively, and participate in activities at school. It is estimated that, within the general population, approximately 5–10 percent of children may have SI dysfunction (Ahn, Miller, Milberger, & McIntosh, 2004).

Operating Within State and Federal Mandates in Public and Private Education

According to AOTA's (2009b) *Scope of Practice*,

> Occupational therapists and occupational therapy assistants are required to abide by statutes and regulations when providing occupational therapy services. State laws and other regulatory requirements typically include statements about educational requirements to practice occupational therapy, procedures to practice occupational therapy legally within the defined area of jurisdiction, the definition and scope of occupational therapy practice, and supervision requirements. (p. 283)

Specific to public schools are parameters established by federal law such as the Individuals with Disabilities Education Improvement Act (IDEA, 2004), No Child Left Behind (NCLB) of 2001, and Section 504 of the Rehabilitation Act of 1973 mandating a child's right to a free, appropriate public education that includes occupational therapy as a related service. General education initiatives such as early intervening services and special education criteria for eligibility and related services are determined by each state on the basis of federal code. Local education agencies must provide, at a minimum, services mandated by federal and state levels and are able to provide a creative range of services at their own discretion.

Occupational therapists and occupational therapy assistants working in public schools may provide intervention to students in general education under early intervening services (e.g., using a response-to-intervention approach) and to students who are eligible under IDEA or Section 504 of the Rehabilitation Act of 1973. A child determined by the educational team to have a disability under IDEA must have an individualized education program (IEP). This includes a statement of the child's present level of functioning and the impact of the disability on the child's involvement and progress in the general education curriculum (§300.320(a)(1)(i)). The IEP must contain "a statement of the special education and related services...based on peer-reviewed research to the extent practicable, to be provided to the child, or on behalf of the child"

---

[1] *Occupational therapists* are responsible for all aspects of occupational therapy service delivery and are accountable for the safety and effectiveness of the occupational therapy service delivery process. *Occupational therapy assistants* deliver occupational therapy services under the supervision of and in partnership with an occupational therapist (AOTA, 2009a). When the term *occupational therapy practitioner* is used in this document, it refers to both occupational therapists and occupational therapy assistants (AOTA, 2006).

(§300.320(4)) in order for the child to progress on annual IEP goals, to be involved and make progress in the general education curriculum, and to be educated and participate with other children. A child determined by the school district to be a "qualified student with a disability" under Section 504 must have a 504 Plan that identifies the accommodations, modifications, and services needed. Occupational therapists and occupational therapy assistants may be participants in the development of the 504 Plan.

Application of SI Theory and Methods in Schools

Clinical and Professional Reasoning

Clinical reasoning based on professional training, evidence, and expertise guides the occupational therapist's selection of the use of one or more frames of reference such as SI (Burke, 2001; Parham, 1987; Schaaf & Smith Roley, 2006; Schell & Schell, 2008). While concepts of SI theory are included in the entry-level education of occupational therapists (Jacobs, Koomar, Mailloux, & Smith Roley, 1999), comprehensive assessment and intervention focused on SI is considered advanced-level practice (Smith Roley & Jacobs, 2008). Opportunities for additional knowledge and skills are available to therapists through workshops, publications, mentoring, and post-graduate certification in SI, including administering and interpreting the Sensory Integration and Praxis Tests (SIPT).[2]

SI theory describes information processing as a neurobiological process requiring the detection, assimilation, organization, interpretation, and use of sensory information that allows an individual to interact adaptively within the environment in daily activities at home, at school, and in other settings (Ayres, 1972b). The theory of SI is grounded on research in neuroscience (Ayres, 1972a; Bundy, Lane, & Murray, 2002; Smith Roley, Blanche, & Schaaf, 2001) and occupational science (Blanche & Parham, 2001; Parham, 2002; Smith Roley & Jacobs, 2008). Occupational therapy provides evaluation and interventions designed to identify, prevent, and remediate deficits related to the child's sensory sensitivities, sensory–perceptual skills, motor and praxis skills, and related patterns of performance (Ayres, 1972b, 1975; Bundy et al., 2002; Dunn, 2001; Mulligan, 1998a, 1998b, 2000; Schaaf & Smith Roley, 2006; Smith Roley et al., 2001; Smith Roley, Mailloux, Miller-Kuhaneck, & Glennon, 2007). The outcome of occupational therapy using SI theory is to improve function in various daily occupations (Ayres, 1979; Bundy et al., 2002; Dunn, 2001; Parham & Mailloux, 2004; Roley, Blanche, & Schaaf, 2001; Spitzer, Roley, Clark, & Parham, 1996).

Evaluations

Occupational therapy practitioners working in schools consider existing academic and nonacademic expectations when determining the child's academic, adaptive, and functional needs. Services are recommended as a result of the findings to support success in reaching positive yearly and long-term outcomes in education. Evaluations in the educational setting must include a review of educational information including (1) information and evaluation results provided by the parents, (2) assessment or observation results related to performance in the current classroom or on local or state assessments, and (3) teacher and other service provider observations (§300.305). In addition, therapists may review pertinent medical information; interview teachers, parents, and the student; observe in natural settings to observe performance; and use various assessments, including standardized tests (Clark & Coster, 1998). Multiple sources of information must

---

[2]It is important to note occupational therapy's use of the term *sensory integration*. A. Jean Ayres developed her sensory integration theory originating from the work of Sherrington (1906, cited in Ayres, 1972a). Using supportive evidence from neuroscience and applied science, this theoretical model supports its application in occupational therapy practice. The trademarked term *Ayres Sensory Integration*™ is used to describe the use of sensory processing and sensory-related methods as guided by Ayres's sensory integration theory. Occupational therapy practitioners are the key professionals using this sensory integration therapy founded on principles of neuroscience (Reeves, 2007).

be used when determining educational disabilities. The occupational therapist selects a variety of measures that include developmental and skill-based observations in addition to those that identify occupational and sensory strengths and weaknesses. The occupational therapist interprets the test findings relative to the child's performance skills, patterns of engagement, and ability to participate.

The evaluation specific to SI includes performance measures of the child's ability to adapt, organize, and integrate sensory information in the environment that affects participation in academic and nonacademic activities at school. Sensory deficits are complex and include various patterns of perceptual, motor, and praxis difficulties (Parham & Mailloux, 2004) affecting the speed and accuracy of learning as well as variations in sensory responsiveness (Ayres & Tickle, 1980; Dunn, 1999) affecting emotional well-being (Ayres, 1979) and social competencies, including play (Mailloux & Burke, 2008).

Structured and unstructured assessments of sensory responsiveness, sensory perception, motor skills, and praxis are essential features of the evaluation (Windsor, Smith Roley, & Szklut, 2001). Multiple data sources should be used when evaluating skills and performance in SI.

Several structured screenings and assessments have been developed for children:

- *DeGangi Berk Test of Sensory Integration* (DeGangi & Berk, 1983) is a preschool screening focused on sensory-based postural and motor functions.

- *Sensory Integration and Praxis Tests (SIPT)* (Ayres, 1989, 1998) is a standardized performance measure used to diagnose sensory integrative dysfunction related to learning and behavior. Professionals using this tool must complete postgraduate training leading to certification in the administration and interpretation of the SIPT and related measures. The SIPT (Ayres, 1989, 1998) is a series of 17 individual tests that provide information on visual perception, visual–motor and fine-motor performance, construction, tactile discrimination, tactile sensitivity, kinesthesia, vestibular functions including post-rotary nystagmus and balance, bilateral motor control, and praxis, including following verbal instructions, sequencing, oral–facial imitation, and imitation of body gestures. This test is predictive of academic function especially math and reading abilities (Parham, 1998).

- *Sensory Processing Measure (SPM)* (Miller-Kuhaneck, Henry, Glennon, Parham, & Ecker, 2007), for home and school, is an integrated system of rating scales that enables assessment based on parent and educational staff report of sensory processing issues, planning and ideas, and social participation in elementary school-age children.

- *Sensory Profile* (Dunn, 1999), *Infant/Toddler Sensory Profile* (Dunn, 2002), and the *Sensory Profile School Companion* (Dunn, 2006) are standardized questionnaires that focus on the student's sensory processing performance patterns within the natural context.

Unstructured assessments may include direct observation of the child's performance in a variety of tasks to analyze the sensory–motor and cognitive demands of the activities, the social and physical characteristics of the environment(s), the effectiveness of the student's performance skills and patterns in those activities and environments, and assessments of neuromotor functions via clinical observations (Blanche, 2002; Wilson, Pollock, Kaplan, & Law, 1994) and play performance (Knox, 2008; Skard & Bundy, 2008).

Intervention and Service Delivery

The team determines services necessary for the child to access general education and benefit from special education on the basis of the child's educationally related needs. Guided by the identified needs and IEP goals of the child, the occupational therapist working in collaboration with the student and the IEP team determines the most appropriate and effective interventions and service delivery models to address the goals. By definition, occupational therapy services are a collaborative process used for the benefit of individuals, populations, and organizations (AOTA, 2008). Related to a child's classroom placement, IDEA requires that "removal of children with disabilities from the regular educational environment occurs only if the nature or severity of the disability is such that education in regular classes…cannot be achieved satisfactorily" (34 C.F.R. 300.114(a)(i)).

Occupational therapy interventions can occur in a variety of settings to support the child's success within the least restrictive environment (LRE). The context of service delivery can include locations at the school such as the classroom, playground, lunchroom, bathroom, or therapy room and off-site locations within the community. Interventions may include one or more of the following types of occupational therapy interventions, preparatory methods, purposeful activities, and occupation-based interventions, depending on the needs of the child and identified outcomes.

Occupational therapy services in schools include the application of specialized knowledge and skills to facilitate adaptive responses the children need to support their learning and behavior. Consultation and direct intervention are both aspects of the service. As related to the use of SI interventions, this may include education that reframes the understanding of the sensory-related concerns; recommendations that incorporate sensory–motor activities throughout the day such as before, during, and after school; and environmental modifications that assist the student's school-related performance. Sensory activities directed by the occupational therapist can be embedded into the classroom routine that can be carried out by the teacher, instructional aides, or parent volunteers. It also may include direct intervention that address the underlying sensory, motor, and praxis concerns through therapeutic use of environment affordances such as mats and swings that provide opportunities for moving through space; climbing in, over, and under large equipment; falling safely onto matted areas; and rearranging the equipment.

Characteristics of the SI approach are outlined in the work conducted by several researchers on adherence to fidelity to the intervention (Parham et al., 2007). Table 1 provides examples of OT intervention approaches using a SI frame of reference. Table 2 provides case examples. The choice of interventions is guided by research regarding the effectiveness of the intervention related to the identified goals for the child.

Outcomes

The federal NCLB and IDEA are two of the most important federal laws relating to the outcomes of education for children with and without disabilities. NCLB seeks to improve accountability for the outcomes of education for all children, and IDEA ensures that children with disabilities will have individualized services to meet unique needs in order to benefit from and appreciate positive outcomes of public education. Both NCLB and IDEA endorse the need for an evidence-based education approach. NCLB stresses accountability as measured by the "use of effective methods and instructional strategies that are based on evidence-based practice" (Sec. 1114 (b)(1)(B)(ii)). IDEA 2004 states that the child's IEP will provide "a statement of the special education and related services and supplementary aids and services, based on peer-reviewed research to the extent practicable" (Sec. 614(d)(1)(A)(i)(IV)).

Occupational therapy using SI theory and methods is designed to improve a person's ability to interact adaptively in the environment, learn, behave, and to prevent future adaptive difficulties and thus improve quality of life. The efficacy of occupational therapy's use of SI has been investigated by several researchers over the past 35 years. Critical review of the literature has provided evidence of efficacy as well as limitations in the design of several studies. Examples of studies supporting occupational therapy using SI theory and methods are provided in Table 3.

Through accurate functional baseline data, measurable student goals, and data collection to monitor a child's successful participation in the natural environment, occupational therapists provide accountability for a child's progress in occupational therapy intervention as it relates to education. Goal attainment scal-

Table 1. Approaches and Sensory Strategies for Occupational Therapy Intervention

Occupational Therapy Approaches	Examples of Sensory-Related Strategies
Create, Promote Health and Participation	• Create a class for parents and/or educational staff to teach the relationships among sensory processing, learning, and behavior • Promote increased physical activity for students to improve physical and mental health and cognitive and social performance • Support installment of a variety of equipment available at schools and public playgrounds to promote a diversity of sensory play experiences • Design sensory-enriched classrooms with a variety of seating options, as well as opportunity for tactile, movement, and proprioceptive experiences throughout the day
Establish/Restore Performance Skills and Performance Patterns	• Design activities rich in tactile, vestibular, and proprioceptive information that increase body awareness needed during activities of daily living • Facilitate the development of appropriate SI and motor-planning skills needed for organizing materials, completing tasks within an appropriate time frame, and adapting to transitions • Establish/restore mobility needed for social and object play • Provide controlled sensory input through activities that require increasingly more complex adaptive responses to novel activity to support ability to engage in group activities with peers
Maintain Student Ability to Engage in and Cope With School-Related Activities	• Structure sensory environment to meet the student's needs such as reducing distractions and improving attention to salient auditory and visual information • Teach sensory strategies for emotional, physiological, behavioral, motor, and social self-regulation • Maintain ability to organize behavior by providing scheduled sensory breaks and sensory accommodations such as changing the size, texture, and location of the desk • Maintain peer relationships by supporting and compensating for motor planning needs in age-appropriate games and sports • Maintain student productivity by providing compensation techniques for sensory and motor-planning deficits using study carrels, visual timers, weighted vests, alternate seating arrangements, modified writing tools, paper, and other assistive technology
Modify Activity to Help Student Compensate for Sensory, Motor, and Praxis Deficits	• Through collaborative consultation with education staff and parents, develop strategies for modifying the sensory, motor, or praxis demands of assignments to increase student productivity • Support student participation in general curriculum by modifying sensory and motor-planning (praxis) demands of activity • Structure or modify the environment to support the student's sensory, motor, motor-planning, and self-regulatory capacities and needs
Prevent Barriers to Participation and Improve Safety	• Prevent inattention, poor posture, and restlessness when sitting for prolonged periods by modifying seating options, allowing sensory breaks, and allowing student to work in various positions • Prevent social isolation by providing motor-planning and social strategies to participate with peers • Prevent socially inappropriate behaviors and behavioral distress or disruption by detecting and meeting sensory and self-regulatory needs • Prevent injury by providing ergonomic seating and safety strategies for students whose nervous systems fail to register sensory information • Prevent barriers to child participation by increasing the understanding of the school district staff regarding of the role that SI and praxis play in influencing learning and behavior

Note. SI = sensory integration.

Table 2. Case Examples

The following vignettes are outlined relative to the *Occupational Therapy Practice Framework: Domain and Process,* 2nd Edition (AOTA, 2008) to illustrate occupational therapy using sensory integrative theory and methods in schools.

Case No. 1 Natasha: Preschool-Age Child

Evaluation

Referral: Natasha is a 3-year-old child enrolled in a special education preschool. The IEP team recommended an OT evaluation because Natasha has difficulty with classroom transitions and social interactions.

Occupational Profile

Natasha's family and educational team are seeking OT services due to her difficulty with transitioning and coping in the classroom. Natasha is sensitive to noise, cries, and clings to the aide in the classroom. She performs well at skilled tasks. Additional information was gathered from her medical, developmental, educational, and occupational histories. The priorities listed by the teacher and parents include social interactions (friendships) and performance within the flow of the classroom (transitioning).

Evaluation and Analysis of Occupational Performance

Interview data:
- *Speech and language therapist report:* Receptive language is below average and decreases when there is noise in the room.
- *Teacher report:* Natasha has difficulty adapting to the flow of classroom activities. She needs an exceptional amount of attention from adults in order to stay calm. Natasha is able to cognitively perform the tasks but is overwhelmed with the noise and movement in the room.
- *Parent report:* Natasha's mother is concerned about her unhappiness at school and her inability to play and make friends.

Observation data:
- Natasha prefers to sit alone or next to an adult.
- Natasha needs extra cues to pay attention. Although physically capable, she does not complete the fine-motor preschool activity without adult direction.
- She does not initiate social interaction with other children and becomes irritable when children come near her.
- She cries when entering the lunchroom or when a group of noisy children run past her during recess.
- She does not like to go to lunch and refuses to eat anything but chips.

Test data:
- Infant/Toddler Sensory Profile demonstrates inefficient sensory self-regulation and sensory modulation, poor tactile discrimination, poor motor planning, and increased auditory sensitivity.
- Beery Visual Motor Integration suggests poor visual–motor integration.
- Knox Preschool Play Scale shows immature play patterns.
- Adequate cognitive performance (from IQ measures).
- Adequate fine-motor performance.
- Miller Function and Participation Scales demonstrates delays in gross-motor and visual–motor skills.

Intervention (includes, but not limited to, the following ideas)

IEP Goals:
Natasha:
- Will transition between classroom activities independently 4 out of 5 transitions for 3 days.
- Will sustain adult-facilitated interaction with her peers during free play for 5 minutes during a 15-minute observation 4 out of 5 free play periods.
- Will carry out verbal instructions with visual cues 4 out of 5 opportunities with 80% accuracy.

OT Intervention Plan Includes the Following Goals:
OT is provided within the classroom setting during routine activities. Natasha's response to intervention in relation to learning, behavior, and adjustment to preschool will be monitored closely for progress and signs of a disorder in SI. Changes to the service delivery may be recommended, as needed, to the IEP team.
Natasha:
- Will regulate her responses to environmental stimuli to remain calm during routine class transitions.

OT Intervention Process and Strategies:
The OT practitioner will facilitate and enhance performance through these interventions:
Client Level:
- Increase sensory modulation through the use of heavy work activities.
- Improve vestibular spatial body awareness through moving on swings and locating visual and auditory targets.
- Improve adaptive responses and motor planning to increase competence when faced with dynamic activities and overall repertoire of play skills.

Table 2. Case Examples *(cont.)*

Case No. 1 Natasha: Preschool-Age Child *(cont.)*

Intervention (includes, but not limited to, the following ideas) *(cont.)*

- Will self-regulate her responses to tactile stimuli to sit next to several peers and focus on the activity during playground and eating activities.
- Will motor plan her body movements to engage in preschool play.
- Will improve spatial location of sound relative to the position of her body in the classroom with and without background noise.

Activity Level:
- Increase texture and weight of materials used during class activities.
- Use visual cues for improved independence during familiar sequences and routines.

Environmental Level:
- Before class, Natasha will arrive early and will enter classroom prior to other children to gradually adjust to the increased noise and pace of the day.
- Natasha will receive visual cues and tangible transition prompts such as a visual schedule to provide advanced notice of classroom activity changes.
- Natasha will be provided with a variety of seating options during circle time such as a bean bag chair, rocking chair, ball chair, or cube seat.
- Seating will be arranged near an adult.

Natasha:
- Will regulate her responses to environmental stimuli to remain calm during routine class transitions.
- Will self-regulate her responses to tactile stimuli to sit next to several peers and focus on the activity during playground and eating activities.
- Will motor plan her body movements to engage in preschool play.
- Will improve spatial location of sound relative to the position of her body in the classroom with and without background noise.

Outcomes

Outcomes were reported by members of the IEP team:

Performance Skills:
- Improvement noted in all skill areas: sensory–perceptual skills, motor and praxis skills, emotional regulation skills, cognitive skills, and social communication skills.

Performance Patterns:
- Easier transitions.
- Increased attention.
- Developed friendships.
- Sustained participation during classroom activities without withdrawing.
- Teacher and parent are pleased that Natasha is able to participate in her preschool program and appears happier at school.

Adaptation:
- Improved self-regulation and adaptation in the preschool routine.

(Continued)

Table 2. Case Examples *(cont.)*

Case No. 2 Billy: Elementary School-Age Student

Evaluation

Referral: Billy is a 7-year-old student in a general education classroom environment. An OT evaluation was requested due to Billy's extremely poor handwriting.

Occupational Profile

Billy's guardians and educational team requested an OT evaluation due to his difficulty with writing, attention, and peer relationships. Information was obtained from the medical, developmental, educational, and occupational histories. Priorities include improving Billy's ability to meet state standards in Language Arts, that is, complete written work legibly, and to adapt to the social and prevocational expectations in first grade by engaging with peers and staying on task at school.

Evaluation and Analysis of Occupational Performance

Interview data:

Teacher report:

- Billy has above-average academic ability but completes less than half of his assignments in the proper amount of time.
- Billy does not interact with his peers.
- He expressed concerns that as the demands of school increased, Billy was going to fall further and further behind.
- Billy has poor use of his hands for tasks, such as opening his lunch containers and managing classroom tools.
- Billy's writing is illegible.

Parent report:

- He has no friends.
- He has difficulty comprehending simple verbal instructions.
- He has unusual habits and rituals.
- He has poorly established patterns of daily activities, such as getting ready to go to bed or mealtimes.

Test data:

Sensory Integration and Praxis Tests and clinical observations results:

- Visual–perception tests within normal limits.
- Visual–motor tests fall 1–2 standard deviations below the mean.
- Visual construction test scores fall in the high average range.
- Poor bilateral motor control.
- Poor oral praxis and postural praxis.
- Poor tactile discrimination.
- Poor posture and eye control.
- Decreased prone extension and supine flexion.

Sensory Processing Measure–Home Form (Miller-Kuhaneck et al., 2007) revealed definite differences in social participation, movement, tactile functions, body awareness, and ideas and planning.

Sensory Processing Measure–Main Classroom Form revealed definite differences in response to movement and body awareness; he is easily overwhelmed with auditory and visual activity in the environment.

Classroom handwriting portfolio was compared with peers to determine discrepancy.

Intervention (includes, but not limited to, the following ideas)

IEP Goals:

Billy:

- Will be able to write 3 legible sentences in his journal during a 20-minute writing period 4 out of 5 opportunities.
- Will stay on topic and remain in his seat for the duration of a 15-minute social studies lesson 4 out of 5 opportunities.
- Will participate appropriately in a structured playground activity with one other child without leaving the activity or arguing with the child for 10 minutes during

OT Intervention Plan Includes the Following Goals:

OT was recommended to improve visual–motor control and improve overall attention.

OT to be provided to student in a specially equipped environment, and consultation to be provided to the IEP team members

Billy:

- Will organize visual–motor information in order to write legible words.

OT Intervention Process and Strategies:

The OT will facilitate adaptive responses through provision of sensory and motor challenges through the following interventions:

Client Level:

- Use weight-bearing and heavy work activities to increase strength of Billy's trunk and upper extremities.
- Increase exploration of multiple textures, sizes, and shapes to improve sensitivity and stereognosis in his hands.

Table 2. Case Examples *(cont.)*

Case No. 2 Billy: Elementary School-Age Student *(cont.)*

Intervention (includes, but not limited to, the following ideas) *(continued)*

the recess or lunch break 2 out of 3 opportunities.

- Will organize somatosensory input from his body to imitate and follow visual directions during structured playground activities.
- Will remain comfortably seated and regulate his attention during instruction so that he remains focused and on task during social studies.
- Will confidently access playground equipment and perform in recess and physical education games with peers.

Activity Level:
- Instruct teacher in kinesthetic and visual support method to re-teach fundamentals of handwriting.
- Use weighted pencils, pencil grips, and paper with highlighted areas.
- Allow Billy to do some of his work while standing, ball-sitting, or lying on his stomach.

Environmental Level:
- Provide written text to copy rather than copying from blackboard.
- Provide written instructions and pictures of daily sequences of activities, with times and locations.
- Allow structured time for movement throughout the day as needed.

Outcomes

Outcomes that were reported by IEP team members:

Occupational Performance:
- Improved penmanship and Language Arts skills.
- Increased attention to topic.
- Increased amount of time spent focused and ready to learn, sitting still and upright in the chair.
- Increased self-determination and independent engagement in structured activities.
- Improved participation and organization of behavior in daily routines.
- Increased spontaneous peer interaction during academic tasks, lunchtime, and playground activities.

(Continued)

Table 2. Case Examples *(cont.)*

Case No. 3 John: Middle-School Student

Evaluation

Referral: John is 12 years old and entering middle school. The IEP team requested an OT evaluation because he cannot organize his belongings and schedule or find his way around the middle school campus and is experiencing high anxiety, refusing to go to his new school. While psycho-educational assessments reveal adequate cognitive abilities, the IEP team members report escalating concerns related to his ability to keep up with his peers academically and physically.

Occupational Profile

John's family and the educational team requested an OT evaluation due to his difficulty finding his way around his school and his resulting in anxiety and depression. Additional information from medical, developmental, educational, and occupational histories was reviewed. Team priorities include increasing John's confidence and independence in performing school curriculum activities and ability to navigate around school without getting lost.

Evaluation and Analysis of Occupational Performance

Interview Data:

Parent reports that John:

1. Gets lost easily.
2. Works best in a self-contained classroom with group transitions; however, the middle school is not structured this way.
3. Demonstrates poor spatial abilities such as when aligning numbers in math.
4. Talks his way out of anything he finds difficult.

John reports that he:

- Has anxiety attacks.
- Feels sick during rides in the car.
- Feels stupid.
- Wants to be home-schooled.
- Spends most of his day in sedentary activities.
- Cannot tolerate backward movement of his head.
- Cannot play desired team sports at the skill level of his peers and as a result feels rejected and humiliated by other children.

Data From Record Review:

The elementary school file indicates that John is good in academics but rarely finishes written work on time in a legible or organized manner. He is well behaved and liked by peers.

- Teacher noted that John did not volunteer for classroom errands on the school grounds unless he could go with a peer.
- John often lost his completed assignments in the classroom, later to be found lost in his messy desk or in unlikely places in the classroom.

Observation Data:

- Below-age level on Beery Visual Motor Integration and Visual Perception Within normal limits on Beery (fine) Motor Coordination in tracing precision.
- Poor 2- and 3-dimensional construction ability.
- Poor balance with eyes closed.
- Self-reports of dizziness on playground swings.
- Poor disassociation of his head, neck, and body.
- Excessive talking to avoid performing during the evaluation observation.
- Inability to locate familiar landmarks such as office.

Intervention (includes, but not limited to, the following ideas)

IEP Goals:

John:

- Will arrive at all of his classes independently and on time, for 2 weeks.
- Will attend school and for 8 of 10 days with low levels of anxiety as noted by self-report.
- Will show increased tolerance for bus rides as reported by child, guardian, and bus driver 4 of 5 days.

OT was recommended for this student in his school setting.

OT Intervention Plan Includes the Following Goals:

John:

- Will identify a strategy out of 3 options (map, written sequence, or self-instruction) that works best for him to get to familiar places.

OT Intervention Process and Strategies:

The OT will facilitate and enhance performance through these interventions:

Client:

- Practice various strategies developed by the OT to improve awareness of the geography of the campus.
- Provide strategies to help John

Table 2. Case Examples *(cont.)*

Case No. 3 John: Middle-School Student *(cont.)*

Intervention (includes, but not limited to, the following ideas) *(cont.)*		
• Will identify age-appropriate leisure time options that are within his ability and interest level such as individually oriented community sports and lessons (e.g., karate, yoga, swimming, chess, arts and crafts). • Will explore junior high extracurricular activities and clubs	• Will identify, select, and participate in leisure and extracurricular physical activities. • Will learn to identify antecedents to the periods of his increased anxiety and utilize relaxation techniques to remain calm when transitioning from home to school and between classes.	become aware of and identify his own sensory strengths, sensitivities, and preferences. • Increase proprioceptive "heavy work" activities to improve sense of body in space. • Avoid intense vestibular activities. *Activity Level:* • Provide cues, landmarks, and signs that John can record as he walks to his class. • Enroll John in extracurricular activities such as karate, yoga, swimming, or rock climbing *Environmental Level:* • Pair John initially with a peer to walk to class. • Make a list of visual details as landmarks, take pictures, or put room numbers on an index card color-coded for each of John's classes to enable him to get to different classes.

Outcomes

Outcomes that were reported by IEP team members:

Participation:
- *Self-confidence in his own ability to adapt to and meet the everyday spatial demands of school activities, greatly reducing stress at school.*
- *Self-awareness and self-determination to seek advice in devising strategies to compensate for things that are uncomfortable or intimidating.*
- *Arrives at class on time.*
- *Able to finish and find 75% of his assignments independently.*
- *No longer resists going to school.*
- *Initiates participation in leisure activities with peers, such as school clubs.*

Client Satisfaction:
- *John is confident that he can travel between classes without assistance.*
- *Parents report that John is much happier at home and at school.*
- *There are no further reports of depression or anxiety.*

Note. IEP = individualized education program; OT = occupational therapy; SI = sensory integration.

Table 3. Occupational Therapy Service Continuum and Curriculum-Related Outcomes

The following table provides samples of studies supporting various SI-related methods and outcomes in school-based practice. It is not an exhaustive list of the available evidence.

Examples of OT Focus Areas Using SI Theory in School-Based Practice	Projected Educational Outcomes	Examples of Resources and Evidence
Participation in education Emotional regulation, sensory–perceptual, motor, praxis, and cognitive skills	Students will access general education curriculum and attend to classroom instruction for longer periods of time prior to identification for special education eligibility and formal OT evaluation.	Schilling, D. L., Washington, K., Billingsley, F. F., & Deitz, J. (2003). Classroom seating for children with attention deficit hyperactivity disorder: Therapy balls versus chairs. *American Journal of Occupational Therapy, 57,* 534–541.
School readiness for education participation Play and leisure Communication and social skills	Students access general education standards and learn adaptive behavior and social skills.	Jarrett, O. S., & Maxwell, D. M. (2000). What research says about the need for recess. In R. Clements (Ed.), *Elementary school recess: Selected readings, games, and activities for teachers and parents* (pp. 12–23). Lake Charles, LA: American Press. Pellegrini, A. D., & Smith, P. K. (1993). School recess: Implications for education and development. *Review of Educational Research, 63,* 51–67. Pellegrini, A. D., & Smith, P. K. (1998). Physical activity play: The nature and function of a neglected aspect of play. *Child Development, 69,* 577–598.
Self-regulation, including the development of emotional regulation, cognitive, and sensory–perceptual skills	Students build sensory self-awareness and self-regulatory strategies to increase focus of attention and completion of school work.	Williams, M. S., & Shellenberger, S. (1994). *How does your engine run? A leader's guide to the Alert Program for Self-regulation.* Albuquerque, NM: TherapyWorks.
Attention/on-task behavior to improve participation in education	Students increase on-task behavior through sensory strategies, sensory breaks, and sensory diets integrated into the school routine.	VandenBerg, N. L. (2001). The use of a weighted vest to increase on-task behavior in children with attention difficulties. *American Journal of Occupational Therapy, 55,* 621–628.
Cognitive, sensory–perceptual, and motor and praxis skills that enhance academic learning	Academic scores are improved through SI methods focusing on eliciting adaptive responses during OT.	Ayres, A. J. (1972a). Improving academic scores through sensory integration. *Journal of Learning Disabilities, 5,* 338–343.
Cognitive, sensory–perceptual, and motor and praxis skills that enhance academic learning	Gains in language comprehension and on expressive language measures are noted after OT using SI methods.	Ayres, J., & Mailloux, Z. (1981). Influence of sensory integration procedures on language development. *American Journal of Occupational Therapy, 35,* 383–390.

Table 3. Occupational Therapy Service Continuum and Curriculum-Related Outcomes *(cont.)*

Examples of OT Focus Areas Using SI Theory in School-Based Practice	Projected Educational Outcomes	Examples of Resources and Evidence
Sensory functions and sensory–perceptual skills influencing the readiness to learn Adaptation	This study analyzed which sensory test variable predicted response to therapy. Participants with hyper-responsiveness such as tactile defensiveness and gravitational insecurity and orienting to an air puff responded better than those with under-responsiveness or who failed to orient to sensory input.	Ayres, A. J., & Tickle, L. S. (1980). Hyper-responsivity to touch and vestibular stimuli as a predictor of positive response to sensory integration procedures by autistic children. *American Journal of Occupational Therapy, 34,* 375–381.
Cognitive, sensory–perceptual, and motor and praxis skills that enhance academic learning and communication and social skills	Following sensory-based intervention, children with decreased cognitive function showed improved spontaneous language, indicating that vestibular activities are effective nonverbal strategies for increasing spontaneous language.	Magrun, W. M., Ottenbacher, S. M., & Keefe, R. (1981). Effects of vestibular stimulation on spontaneous use of verbal language in developmentally delayed children. *American Journal of Occupational Therapy, 35,* 101–104.
Participation in activities of daily living and availability to engage in a variety of functional activities	Group who received SI intervention showed reduced self-stimulating behaviors that interfere with participation in functional activities. Study compared an SI approach with tabletop activities in children with pervasive developmental disorder and mental retardation.	Smith, S. A., Press, B., Koenig, K. P., & Kinnealey M. (2005). Effects of sensory integration intervention on self-stimulating and self-injurious behaviors. *American Journal of Occupational Therapy, 59,* 418–425.
Sensory–perceptual and fine-motor skills affecting penmanship and handwriting	Implementing interventions related to sensory processing improved visual–motor skills, which support penmanship, and writing skills using sensory strategies via classroom consultation and direct intervention.	Hall, L., & Case-Smith, J. (2007). The effect of sound-based intervention on children with sensory processing disorder and visual–motor delays. *American Journal of Occupational Therapy, 61,* 209–215.
Participation in play and leisure, including curiosity and independent learning	SI approaches improved play and interactions with others and with toys and other objects, as well as tolerance for vestibular and proprioceptive sensations, and led to greater sensory exploration of the environment. Sensory exploration improves as a key feature of independent learning intervention when OT with a SI approach was used to address symptoms related to learning disorders.	Schaaf, R., Merrill, S., & Kinsella, N. (1987). Sensory integration and play behavior: A case study of the effectiveness of occupational therapy using sensory integrative techniques. *Occupational Therapy in Health Care, 4*(2), 61–75.

(Continued)

Table 3. Occupational Therapy Service Continuum and Curriculum-Related Outcomes *(cont.)*

Examples of OT Focus Areas Using SI Theory in School-Based Practice	Projected Educational Outcomes	Examples of Resources and Evidence
Reading	Smooth eye pursuits, which are important in developing reading skills, improved in this study, which demonstrated a reduction in the number of saccades for the intervention cohort and reduced time necessary to accomplish smooth pursuits.	Horowitz, L. J., Oosterveld, W. J., & Adrichem, R. (1993). Effectiveness of sensory integration therapy on smooth pursuits and organization time in children. *Pediatrie und Grenzgebiet, 31,* 331–344.
Academic skills Motor skills	SI intervention methods proved equally as effective as tutoring in improving academic and motor skills with maintenance of gains in motor-skills development. This randomized clinical trial compared OT using SI with tutoring to improve academic and motor skills. Although the SI group did not make greater gains in the initial study, at follow-up 2 years later only the SI group maintained their gross-motor skills.	Wilson, B., Kaplan, B., Fellowes, S., Gruchy, C., & Faris, P. (1992). The efficacy of sensory integration intervention compared to tutoring. *Physical and Occupational Therapy in Pediatrics, 12,* 1–37.
Emotional regulation skills resulting in positive behavior Health and wellness Quality of life	A decrease in disruptive behaviors was noted with improved speech, play, attention, and social dialogue. This single-case study of 2 children demonstrated improvements in social interaction, approach to novel activities, response to affection, and response to movement.	Linderman, T. M., & Stewart, K. B. (1999). Sensory integrative–based occupational therapy and functional outcomes in young children with pervasive developmental disorders: A single-subject study. *American Journal of Occupational Therapy, 53,* 207–213.
Self-advocacy and parent advocacy Quality of life	Parents reported increased ability to advocate for their child based on improved understanding of their child's behavior and validation of their parenting efforts. At the clinic site, waiting room interactions allowed parents time to share experiences and resources with others and expand their understanding of their children.	Cohn, E. S. (2001). Parent perspectives of occupational therapy using a sensory integration approach. *American Journal of Occupational Therapy, 55,* 285–294. Cohn, E. S., Miller, L. J., & Tickle-Degnan, L. (2000). Parental hopes for therapy outcomes: Children with sensory modulation disorders. *American Journal of Occupational Therapy, 54,* 36–43.
Positive behavior Increased engagement Independent work	Supporting behavior in preschool-age child, including increased engagement, decreased aggression, less need for intense teacher direction, and decreased mouthing of objects. Using a single-case-study design, the researchers found that the child benefited from classic Ayres Sensory Integration, affecting his preschool performance.	Roberts, J. E., King-Thomas, L., & Boccia, M. L. (2007). Behavioral indices of the efficacy of sensory integration. *American Journal of Occupational Therapy, 61,* 555–562.

Table 3. Occupational Therapy Service Continuum and Curriculum-Related Outcomes *(cont.)*

Examples of OT Focus Areas Using SI Theory in School-Based Practice	Projected Educational Outcomes	Examples of Resources and Evidence
Participation at school	Supporting occupational performance and behavior in a school-age child, improving participation at school, at home, and in the community. Using a single-case-study design, the researchers found that the child benefited from classic Ayres Sensory Integration, affecting his occupational performance and behavior.	Schaaf, R. C., & Nightlinger, K. M. (2007). Occupational therapy using a sensory integrative approach: A case study of effectiveness. *American Journal of Occupational Therapy, 61,* 239–246.
Play Learning	Research suggests that learning is enhanced by emotion, spontaneity, and play, which are the essential ingredients in a SI approach used within OT. Physiological data shows increased cortical blood volume during performance of novel integration activities in a spontaneous, playful manner.	Peyton, J. L., Bass, W. T., Burke, B. L., & Frank, M. (2005). Novel motor and somatosensory activity is associated with increased cerebral cortical blood volume measured by near-infrared optical topography. *Journal of Child Neurology, 20,* 817–821.
Occupational performance in educational settings observed via academic achievement	Measures of SI in elementary students are significantly related to school achievement both concurrently and predicatively over a 4-year period, even when controlling for intelligence. A particularly strong link between praxis and math achievement is evident.	Parham, L. D. (1998). The relationship of sensory integrative development to achievement in elementary students: Four-year longitudinal patterns. *Occupational Therapy Journal of Research, 18,* 105–127.

Note. OT = occupational therapy; SI = sensory integration.

ing is a promising method providing therapists the possibility to measure achievement towards customized goals (Mailloux et al., 2007).

Summary

AOTA recognizes SI as one of several theories and methods used by occupational therapists and occupational therapy assistants working with children in public and private schools. Regardless of the theories and methods utilized, occupational therapy practitioners work within the framework of occupational therapy toward the desired outcome of health and participation through engagement in occupations that allow participation in a child's daily life (AOTA, 2008). When children demonstrate sensory-related deficits that interfere with their ability to access the general education curriculum, occupational therapy using a sensory integrative approach is appropriate.

References

Ahn, R. R., Miller, L. J., Milberger, S., & McIntosh, D. N. (2004). Prevalence of parents' perception of sensory processing disorders among kindergarten children. *American Journal of Occupational Therapy, 58,* 287–293.

American Occupational Therapy Association. (2006). Policy 1.44: Categories of occupational therapy personnel. In *Policy manual* (2008 ed., p. 10). Bethesda, MD: Author

American Occupational Therapy Association. (2008). Occupational therapy practice framework: Domain and process (2nd ed.). *American Journal of Occupational Therapy, 62,* 625–683.

American Occupational Therapy Association. (2009a). Guidelines for supervision, roles, and responsibilities during the delivery of occupational therapy services. *American Journal of Occupational Therapy, 63.*

American Occupational Therapy Association. (2009b). Scope of practice. *American Journal of Occupational Therapy, 63.*

Ayres, A. J. (1972a). Improving academic scores through sensory integration. *Journal of Learning Disabilities, 5,* 336–343.

Ayres, A. J. (1972b). Types of sensory integrative dysfunction among disabled learners. *American Journal of Occupational Therapy, 26,* 13–18.

Ayres, A. J. (1975). Sensorimotor foundations of academic ability. In W. M. Cruickshank & D. P. Hallahan (Eds.), *Perceptual and learning disabilities in children* (Vol. 2, pp. 301–358). Syracuse, NY: Syracuse University Press.

Ayres, A. J. (1979). *Sensory integration and the child.* Los Angeles: Western Psychological Services.

Ayres, A. J. (1989). *Sensory integration and praxis tests manual.* Los Angeles: Western Psychological Services.

Ayres, A. J. (1998). *Sensory integration and praxis tests manual* (rev. ed.). Los Angeles: Western Psychological Services.

Ayres, A. J., & Mailloux, Z. (1981). Influence of sensory integration procedures on language development. *American Journal of Occupational Therapy, 35,* 383–390.

Ayres, A. J., & Tickle, L. S. (1980). Hyper-responsivity to touch and vestibular stimuli as a predictor of positive response to sensory integration procedures by autistic children. *American Journal of Occupational Therapy, 34,* 375–381.

Blanche, E. I. (2002). *Observations based on sensory integration theory.* Torrance, CA: Pediatric Therapy Network.

Blanche, E. I., & Parham, L. D. (2001). Praxis and organization of behavior in time and space. In S. Smith Roley, E. I. Blanche, & R. Schaaf (Eds.), *Understanding the nature of sensory integration with diverse populations* (pp. 183–200). San Antonio, TX: Therapy Skill Builders.

Bundy, A. C., Lane, S. J., & Murray, E. A. (2002). *Sensory integration: Theory and practice* (2nd ed.). Philadelphia: F. A. Davis.

Burke, J. (2001). Clinical reasoning and the use of narrative in sensory integration assessment and intervention. In S. Roley, E. Blanche, & R. Schaaf (Eds.), *Understanding the nature of sensory integration with diverse populations* (pp. 203–214). San Antonio, TX: Therapy Skill Builders.

Clark, G. F., & Coster, W. (1998). Evaluation/problem solving and program evaluation. In J. Case-Smith (Ed.), *Making a difference in school practice* (pp. 1–36). Bethesda, MD: American Occupational Therapy Association.

Cohn, E. S. (2001). Parent perspectives of occupational therapy using a sensory integration approach. *American Journal of Occupational Therapy, 55,* 285–294.

Cohn, E. S., Miller, L. J., & Tickle-Degnan, L. (2000). Parental hopes for therapy outcomes: Children with sensory modulation disorders. *American Journal of Occupational Therapy, 54,* 36–43.

DeGangi, G. A., & Berk, R. A. (1983). *DeGangi–Berk Test of Sensory Integration manual.* Los Angeles: Western Psychological Services.

Dunn, W. (1999). *The Sensory Profile.* San Antonio, TX: Psychological Corporation.

Dunn, W. (2001). The sensations of everyday life: Empirical, theoretical, and pragmatic considerations. *American Journal of Occupational Therapy, 55,* 608–620.

Dunn, W. (2002). *Infant/Toddler Sensory Profile.* San Antonio, TX: Psychological Corporation.

Dunn, W. (2006). *The Sensory Profile School Companion.* San Antonio, TX: Psychological Corporation.

Hall, L., & Case-Smith, J. (2007). The effect of sound-based intervention on children with sensory processing disorder and visual–motor delays. *American Journal of Occupational Therapy, 61,* 209–215.

Horowitz, L. J., Oosterveld, W. J., & Adrichem, R. (1993). Effectiveness of sensory integration therapy on smooth pursuits and organization time in children. *Pediatrie und Grenzgebiet, 31,* 331–344.

Individuals with Disabilities Education Improvement Act, P.L. 108–446, 118 Stat. 2647 (2004).

Jacobs, S. E., Koomar, J., Mailloux, Z., & Smith Roley, S. S. (1999). Entry-level curriculum content for sensory integration: Survey results and proposed teaching modules. *Sensory Integration Special Interest Section Quarterly, 2*(3), 1–3.

Jarrett, O. S., & Maxwell, D. M. (2000). What research says about the need for recess. In R. Clements (Ed.), *Elementary school recess: Selected readings, games, and activities for teachers and parents* (pp. 12–23). Lake Charles, LA: American Press.

Linderman, T. M., & Stewart, K. B. (1999). Sensory integrative–based occupational therapy and functional outcomes in young children with pervasive developmental disorders: A single-subject study. *American Journal of Occupational Therapy, 53,* 207–213.

Knox, S. (2008). Development and current use of the revised Knox Preschool Play Scale. In L. D. Parham & L. S. Fazio (Eds.), *Play in occupational therapy for children* (2nd ed., pp. 55–70). St. Louis, MO: Mosby/Elsevier.

Magrun, W. M., Ottenbacher, S. M., & Keefe, R. (1981). Effects of vestibular stimulation on spontaneous use of verbal language in developmentally delayed children. *American Journal of Occupational Therapy, 35,* 101–104.

Mailloux, Z., & Burke, J. P. (2008). Play and the sensory integrative approach. In L. D. Parham & L. S. Fazio (Eds.), *Play in occupational therapy for children* (2nd ed., pp. 263–278). St. Louis, MO: Mosby/Elsevier.

Mailloux, Z. K., May-Benson, T. A., Summers, C. A., Miller, L. J., Burke, J. P., Brett-Green, B., et al. (2007). Goal attainment scaling as a measure of meaningful outcomes for children with sensory integration disorders. *American Journal of Occupational Therapy, 61,* 254–259.

Miller-Kuhaneck, H., Henry, D., Glennon, T., Parham, D., & Ecker, C. (2007). *Sensory Processing Measure: Home form, main classroom form, and school environments form.* Los Angeles: Western Psychological Services.

Mulligan, S. (1998a). Application of structural equation modeling in occupational therapy research. *American Journal of Occupational Therapy, 52,* 829–834.

Mulligan, S. (1998b). Patterns of sensory integration dysfunction: A confirmatory factor analysis. *American Journal of Occupational Therapy, 52,* 819–828.

Mulligan, S. (2000). Cluster analysis of scores of children on the Sensory Integration and Praxis Tests. *Occupational Therapy Journal of Research, 20,* 256–262.

No Child Left Behind Act of 2001, P.L. 107–110, [20, USC §6301].

Parham, L. D. (1987). Toward professionalism: The reflective therapist. *American Journal of Occupational Therapy, 41,* 555–561.

Parham, L. D. (1998). The relationship of sensory integrative development to achievement in elementary students: Four-year longitudinal patterns. *Occupational Therapy Journal of Research, 18,* 105–127.

Parham, L. D. (2002). Sensory integration and occupation. In A. C. Bundy, S. J. Lane, & E. A. Murray (Eds.), *Sensory integration theory and practice* (2nd ed., pp. 413–434). Philadelphia: F. A. Davis.

Parham, L. D., Cohn, E. S., Spitzer, S., Koomar, J. A., Miller, L. J., Burke, J. P., et al. (2007). Fidelity in sensory integration intervention research. *American Journal of Occupational Therapy, 61,* 216–227.

Parham, L. D., Ecker, C., Miller- Kuhaneck, H., Henry, D. A., & Glennon, T. J. (2007). *Sensory Processing Measure.* Los Angeles: Western Psychological Services.

Parham, L. D., & Mailloux, A. (2004). Sensory integration. In. J. Case- Smith (Ed.), *Occupational therapy for children* (5th ed., pp. 356–411). St. Louis, MO: Mosby.

Pellegrini, A. D., & Smith, P. K. (1993). School recess: Implications for education and development. *Review of Educational Research, 63,* 51–67.

Pellegrini, A. D., & Smith, P. K. (1998). Physical activity play: The nature and function of a neglected aspect of play. *Child Development, 69,* 577–598.

Peyton, J. L., Bass, W. T., Burke, B. L., & Frank, M. (2005). Novel motor and somatosensory activity is associated with increased cerebral cortical blood volume measured by near-infrared optical topography. *Journal of Child Neurology, 20*(1), 817–821.

Reeves, G. (2007). Looking back on 30 years of the Sensory Integration Special Interest Section. *Sensory Integration Special Interest Section Quarterly 30*(4), 1–4.

Roberts, J. E., King-Thomas, L., & Boccia, M. L. (2007). Behavioral indices of the efficacy of sensory integration. *American Journal of Occupational Therapy, 61,* 555–562.

Roley, S., Blanche, E., & Schaaf, R. (Eds.). (2001). *Understanding the nature of sensory integration with diverse populations.* San Antonio, TX: Therapy Skill Builders.

Schaaf, R. C., Merrill, S., & Kinsella, N. (1987). Sensory integration and play behavior: A case study of the effectiveness of occupational therapy using sensory integrative techniques. *Occupational Therapy in Health Care, 4*(2), 61–75.

Schaaf, R., & Smith Roley, S. (2006). *Sensory integration: Applying clinical reasoning to practice with diverse populations.* San Antonio, TX: ProEd.

Schaaf, R. C., & Nightlinger, K. M. (2007). Occupational therapy using a sensory integrative approach: A case study of effectiveness. *American Journal of Occupational Therapy, 61,* 239–246.

Schell, B. A. B., & Schell, J. W. (2008). *Clinical and professional reasoning in occupational therapy.* Baltimore: Lippincott Williams & Wilkins.

Schilling, D. L., Washington, K., Billingsley, F. F., & Deitz, J. (2003). Classroom seating for children with attention deficit hyperactivity disorder: Therapy balls versus chairs. *American Journal of Occupational Therapy, 57,* 534–541.

Section 504 of the Rehabilitation Act of 1973, 29 U.S.C. 706(8) and 794.

Skard, G., & Bundy, A.C. (2008). Test of playfulness. In L. D. Parham & L. Fazio (Eds.), *Play in occupational therapy for children* (2nd ed., pp. 71–93). St. Louis, MO: Mosby/Elsevier.

Smith, S. A., Press, B., Koenig, K. P., & Kinnealey, M. (2005). Effects of sensory integration intervention on self-stimulating and self-injurious behaviors. *American Journal of Occupational Therapy, 59,* 418–425.

Smith Roley, S., Blanche, E. I., & Schaaf, R. C. (Eds.). (2001). *Understanding the nature of sensory integration with diverse populations.* San Antonio, TX: Therapy Skill Builders.

Smith Roley, S., & Jacobs, S. (2008). Sensory integration. In E. B. Crepeau, E. S. Cohn, & B. A. B. Schell (Eds.), *Willard and Spackman's occupational therapy* (11th ed., pp. 792–817). Philadelphia: Lippincott Williams & Wilkins.

Smith Roley, S., Mailloux, Z., Miller-Kuhaneck, H., & Glennon, T. (2007). Understanding Ayres Sensory Integration.® *OT Practice, 12*(17), CE1–CE8.

Spitzer, S., Roley, S. S., Clark, F., & Parham, D. (1996). Sensory integration: Current trends in the United States. *Scandinavian Journal of Occupational Therapy, 3,* 123–138.

VandenBerg, N. L. (2001). The use of a weighted vest to increase on-task behavior in children with attention difficulties. *American Journal of Occupational Therapy, 55,* 621–628.

Williams, M. S., & Shellenberger, S. (1994). *How does your engine run? A leader's guide to the Alert Program for Self-Regulation.* Albuquerque, NM: TherapyWorks.

Wilson, B., Kaplan, B., Fellowes, S., Gruchy, C., & Faris, P. (1992). The efficacy of sensory integration intervention compared to tutoring. *Physical and Occupational Therapy in Pediatrics, 12,* 1–37.

Wilson, B. N., Pollock, N., Kaplan, B. J., & Law, M. (1994). *Clinical observations of motor and postural skills.* Tucson, AZ: Therapy Skill Builders.

Windsor, M., Smith Roley, S., & Szklut, S. (2001). Assessment of Sensory Integration and Praxis. In S. Roley, E. Blanche, & R. Schaaf. (Eds.), *Understanding the nature of sensory integration with diverse populations* (pp. 215–245). San Antonio, TX: Therapy Skill Builders.

Authors

Susanne Smith Roley, MS, OTR/L, FAOTA
Julie Bissell, MA, OTR/L
Gloria Frolek Clark, MS, OTR/L, FAOTA

for

The Commission on Practice
Janet V. DeLany, DEd, OTR/L, FAOTA, *Chairperson*

Adopted by the Representative Assembly 2009FebCS110

Note: This document replaces the 1997 *Sensory Integration Evaluation and Intervention in School-Based Occupational Therapy* and the 2003 *Applying Sensory Integration Framework in Educationally Related Occupational Therapy Practice* (previously published and copyrighted by the American Occupational Therapy Association in 2003 in the *American Journal of Occupational Therapy, 57,* 652–659.

The Role of Occupational Therapy in End-of-Life Care

The purpose of this statement is to describe the role of occupational therapists and occupational therapy assistants in providing services to clients who are living with chronic or terminal conditions and are at the end of life. It also serves as a resource for occupational therapy practitioners,[1] hospice and palliative care programs, policymakers, funding sources, and clients and caregivers who receive hospice and palliative care services. Occupational therapy practitioners provide skilled intervention to improve quality of life by facilitating engagement in daily life occupations throughout the entire life course. Participation in meaningful life occupations continues to be as important at the end of life as it is at earlier stages. The term *end-of life care* has replaced the term *terminal care* and encompasses both hospice and palliative care that can occur during the final stages of life.

Hospice

The contemporary definition of *hospice* encompasses a philosophy of care for individuals of any age with life-limiting illnesses for whom further curative measures are no longer desired or appropriate. Hospice referrals require that the client have a life expectancy of 6 months or less with the usual course of the diagnosis (Centers for Medicare and Medicaid Services, 2010). Hospice care focuses on symptom control and meeting the emotional, social, spiritual, and functional needs of the client and family. As an example, the *Medicare Benefit Policy Manual* states that "Physical therapy, occupational therapy, and speech–language pathology services may be provided for purposes of symptom control or to enable the individual to maintain activities of daily living and basic functional skills."

Reimbursement for hospice care may be provided by a variety of medical insurers, including Medicare, Medicaid, and private insurance. Some hospice organizations receive funds from grants and private donations that are used to cover services. Local civic, charitable, or religious organizations also may provide funding to help patients and their families with hospice expenses.

The basic philosophy of hospice is described in the *Standards of Practice for Hospice Programs* (National Hospice and Palliative Care Organization, 2002):

> Hospice provides support and care for persons in the last phases of incurable disease so that they may live as fully and as comfortably as possible. Hospice recognizes that the dying process is a part of the normal process of living and focuses on enhancing the quality of remaining life. Hospice affirms life and neither hastens nor postpones death. Hospice exists in the hope and belief that, through appropriate care and the promotion of a caring community sensitive to their needs, individuals and their families may be free to attain a degree of satisfaction in preparation for death. Hospice recognizes that human growth and development can be a lifelong process. Hospice seeks to preserve and promote the inherent potential for growth within individuals and families without regard to age, gender, nationality, race, creed, sexual orientation, disability, diagnosis, availability of a primary caregiver, or ability to pay. (p. ii)

---

[1]When the term *occupational therapy practitioner* is used in this document, it refers to both occupational therapists and occupational therapy assistants (AOTA, 2006). *Occupational therapists* are responsible for all aspects of occupational therapy service delivery and are accountable for the safety and effectiveness of the occupational therapy service delivery process. *Occupational therapy assistants* deliver occupational therapy services under the supervision of and in partnership with an occupational therapist (AOTA, 2009).

Palliative Care

Hospice and palliative care are closely related. Both approaches are directed toward providing intervention services to those with life-threatening illnesses. Palliative care differs from hospice care in that it can be initiated at any point in the course of the client's illness. Curative care interventions also may be used within the context of palliative approach, whereas curative services are not provided when a client is receiving hospice care. A client receiving palliative and curative services simultaneously may transition to a hospice service when curative therapies are no longer appropriate or desired and the end of life is more imminent. The World Health Organization (2002) defines *palliative care* as

> An approach that improves the quality of life of patients and their families facing the problem associated with life-threatening illness, through the prevention and relief of suffering by means of early identification and impeccable assessment and treatment of pain and other problems, physical, psychosocial, and spiritual.

Care Settings

End-of-life care may take place in a variety of settings, depending on the client's need and situation. Many individuals served by hospice organizations are seen in their homes (Marrelli, 2005). Hospice care also may be provided in freestanding community in-patient facilities and in specified units or beds within a skilled nursing facility or hospital. Some home health care agencies also provide hospice services staffed by designated hospice care providers.

Hospice teams are interdisciplinary. In addition to occupational therapy practitioners, teams include counselors, clergypersons, and volunteers, as well as physicians, nurses, social workers, dieticians, physical therapists, and speech–language pathologists.

Role of Occupational Therapy

Individuals with life-threatening and life-limiting illness often have difficulty participating in daily occupations because of decline in their motor, sensory, emotional, cognitive, or communication skills. Occupational therapy practitioners help clients find relief from pain and suffering and improve their quality of life by supporting their engagement in daily life occupations that clients find meaningful and purposeful. The occupational therapy practitioner considers environmental and contextual factors (e.g., caregiver training, accessibility of objects or places in the environment, social contacts available to prevent isolation), as well as personal factors (e.g., decreased endurance, increased anxiety) that may be limiting a client's abilities and satisfaction when performing desired occupations. The occupational therapy practitioner collaborates with the client and family members throughout the occupational therapy process to identify occupations that are especially meaningful and to incorporate strategies that support occupational engagement. As Kaye (2006) points out in *Notes on Symptom Control in Hospice and Palliative Care*, "Loss of independence and role can result in social death prior to biological death. Occupational therapy can help a person to adopt new and appropriate functions and roles and to maintain self-esteem" (p. 214).

Quality of Life at the End of Life

Improved quality of life is a primary outcome of all occupational therapy interventions (AOTA, 2008). Occupational therapy practitioners believe that engaging in occupations underlies health and quality of life. At the end of life when clients often face loss of previously established occupational roles, occupations, and performance abilities, their need to identify and sustain meaningful engagement is heightened. Family members and professionals alike may find it difficult to comprehend the diminution of life quality when illness interferes with abilities to carry out familiar occupations. The pleasure and sense of self-worth inherent in participating in familiar occupations, even those as basic as making a cup of coffee at the time one wants to have a cup of coffee, is immeasurable. The value lies not so much in the cup of coffee, which can be provided by someone else, but in having control over choosing when to have the coffee and perhaps making the coffee when desired.

Numerous researchers have examined how persons at the end of life view their quality of life and quality of care. Many of these research studies have identified factors that affect quality of life and quality of care that are similar to the factors that occupational therapy practitioners address during their interventions (see Table 1).

Research to Support Practice

Although occupational therapy practice with clients at the end of life is not new, evidence that supports this area of practice is less well developed. Since the 1970s, occupational therapists have investigated and described how occupational therapy practitioners provide services to clients at this life stage (Bye, 1998; Picard & Magno, 1982; Pizzi, 1984; Pizzi & Briggs, 2004; Rahman, 2000; Tiggs & Sherman, 1983). These studies have pointed out occupational therapy's role in supporting the individual's quality of life by facilitating role performance and function in desired occupations, competence, control, and coping to

Table 1. Factors Influencing Quality of Life and Quality of Care at the End of Life

Factor	Relationship to Occupational Therapy	References
Maintaining functioning and involvement in desired life activities contributes to quality of life.	Occupational therapy practitioners believe that continuing to engage in occupations allows a person to continue his or her life—and is central to health and quality of life. Modifying previous occupations so that they can still be performed and adding new occupations to replace lost ones prevents isolation, a common experience at the end of life, and contributes to the sustainment of self-worth.	Arnold, Artin, Griffith, Person, & Graham, 2006; Egan & DeLaat, 1997; Gourdjii, McVey, & Purden, 2009; Jacques & Hasselkus, 2004; Lyons, Orozovic, Davis, & Newman, 2002; Ryan, 2005
Maintaining a sense of control contributes to quality of life.	By participating in daily life occupations that they value as purposeful and meaningful, individuals make choices that give them a sense of control, identity, and competence.	Christiansen, 1999; Egan & DeLaat, 1997; Singer, Martin, & Kelner, 1999; Vrkljan & Miller-Polgar, 2001
Continuing to contribute to others and staying connected to important relationships contributes to quality of life.	Engaging individuals in tasks and activities is a central focus of the occupational therapy intervention process. Completing tasks such as writing letters to grandchildren or recording favorite recipes within an individual's social context allows a person to feel productive and to strengthen social relationships.	Enes, 2003; Gourdji et al., 2009; Hunter, 2008; Lyons et al., 2002; Singer et al., 1999; Steinhauser et al., 2000
Continuing to search for meaning and purpose in life and one's relationship to a higher being also is referred to as *spirituality*.	Occupational therapy practitioners recognize spirituality as an important client factor. They believe that the process of engaging in occupations helps the person connect to the meaning and purpose in life, which enhances spiritual well-being, quality of life, and ability to cope. Engaging in occupations can counteract feelings of hopelessness, helplessness, and uselessness that may develop during the end of life. Occupational therapy practitioners help individuals identify meaningful occupations in which they want to engage and teach coping strategies that allow continued participation.	AOTA, 2008; Chochinov & Cann, 2005; Egan & DeLaat, 1997; Lin & Bauer-Wu, 2003; Pizzi & Briggs, 2004; Prince-Paul, 2008; Unruh, Smith, & Scammell, 2000

589

assist the person in bringing closure to his or her life. Several phenomenological studies conducted by occupational therapists have elucidated how occupations contribute to living at the end of life and how individuals at the end of life describe the benefits of engaging in daily life occupations (Lyons et al., 2002; Unruh et al., 2000).

The validity of specific interventions that occupational therapy practitioners may use is beginning to be investigated. La Cour, Josephsson, and Luborsky (2005) and La Cour, Josephsson, Tishelman, and Nygård (2007) have explored the effects of using creative activities with clients who have life-threatening illnesses. In both studies, the researchers found that participation in creative activities allowed clients to cope with declining abilities and to create connections to life. Clients reported an improved existential awareness of their past, their present, and possible future.

Hunter (2008) further explored the ideas of existential meaning, which people at the end of life confront. She explored the responses of 38 women to understand how they defined legacy and its importance in their lives. She found that legacy is closely related to transmitting one's sense of who they are to others. Legacy transmission can be effected by transmitting actions (behaviors) as well as artifacts (concrete items). In either case, these legacies are closely connected to the occupations and occupational identities that people develop throughout their life. Occupational therapy practitioners who are sensitive to the client's occupational profile and identity can facilitate the client's ability to identify and transmit purposeful legacies.

Effectiveness of palliative care programs also is beginning to be documented. Several studies have reported on how outpatient palliative rehabilitation programs, palliative day care programs, and inpatient palliative care units have improved patient satisfaction, functional performance, emotional well-being, and symptoms (Cohen, Boston, Mount, & Porterfield, 2001; Hospital Case Management, 2003; Strasser et al., 2004; Svidòn, Fürst, von Koch, & Borell, 2009). In two of these studies (Hospital Case Management, 2003; Strasser et al., 2004), an occupational therapist was specifically mentioned as a member of the team.

Saarik and Hartley (2010) reported on a 4-week fatigue management program in Britain carried out by an occupational therapist and a physiotherapist specializing in palliative care. The program was delivered in a hospice day care program with patients with cancer. Clients who completed the program reported decreased fatigue levels, overall improved functioning, and enhanced ability to cope.

Occupational therapy practitioners have recognized the need to provide evidence that supports the profession's contribution to quality of life at the end of life. Pearson, Todd, and Futcher (2007) have proposed that occupational therapy practitioners use a quality of life measure during their evaluations to measure the effectiveness of occupational therapy interventions in palliative care practice. They identified 24 possible tools and plan to evaluate them further for application by occupational therapists.

Occupational Therapy Process

Evaluation

A client may be referred for occupational therapy at any point during the end-of-life process. Any health care provider may identify the need for occupational therapy.

The occupational therapist begins the evaluation process by conducting an occupational profile. The occupational therapist gathers information for the profile by talking to the client to gain an understanding of meaningful and relevant occupations, daily routines, interests, values, and priorities, as well as the client's view of life and expectations of dying. Interviewing caregivers, including family or significant others, to determine their priorities and concerns is important, especially when the client is unable to express his or her desires and wishes pertaining to end-of-life care. The interview also examines cultural, spiritual, and social factors that influence a client's expectations for the end of life.

This client-centered approach enables the occupational therapy practitioner to establish a relationship that facilitates discussion of important occupational areas. For example, the client may prefer to be dressed by the caregiver to save energy to tape stories to share with his or her grandchild.

On the basis of these priorities and concerns, the occupational therapist may specifically assess and analyze the client's or caregivers' performance skills in the desired activities and roles. Although clients receiving hospice or palliative care services may have declining performance skills, the occupational therapist assesses strengths and capacities that can support continued performance of desired occupations. The occupational therapist analyzes the demands of activities important to the client and the supports and barriers of the context or environment as they affect outcomes. The evaluation also may include assessment of caregivers' skills and need for skill training and support, as well as identification of the adaptive or compensatory strategies needed to carry out task performance and/or the environmental modifications that need to be implemented to support the client's skills and capabilities. Identification of the client's needs and wishes, combined with analysis of the client's performance capacities, allows the occupational therapist to identify effective and client-centered occupational therapy interventions, which are then incorporated into the interdisciplinary plan of care.

Intervention

The occupational therapist develops an intervention plan in collaboration with the client and the caregivers. The intervention plan identifies the outcomes of intervention and the approaches to be used. Occupational therapy interventions are targeted toward creating a fit between the client's and caregivers' capabilities and the demands of the activities that are important to the client and caregivers. Intervention may be provided directly to the client or the caregivers or family members. Intervention directed toward caregivers frequently consists of education and consultation to support efficacy and satisfaction with the care they provide. Interventions chosen will depend on the client's needs and desires and medical status at the time of referral. For example, a client with cancer who is alert and aware of his or her surroundings but dealing with issues of pain management, symptom control, and loss of occupational roles and relationships will face different challenges than a client who is referred in the later stages of Alzheimer's disease who is cognitively disoriented but is experiencing little pain. In the latter situation, intervention may more appropriately be directed at numerous challenges facing caregivers, such as instruction in managing behaviors and safety precautions.

Interventions for the client may focus on relieving symptoms that interfere with function. For example, if pain or shortness of breath is limiting function, repositioning to a supported sitting position in bed may relieve pain and improve breathing, enabling the client to write letters. Engaging in meaningful occupations not only improves quality of life but also can serve as an important tool for symptom management. Clients whose attention is focused on meaningful occupations pay less attention to physical symptoms.

Approaches most commonly used by occupational therapy at the end of life are compensation, adaptation, and preservation of existing capacities. Occupational therapy practitioners focus on modifying the demands of activities or the habits and routines associated with the occupations to match the client's or caregiver's performance skills, tolerances, and capacities. Occupational therapy practitioners also use interventions targeted toward minimizing barriers to performance.

Ongoing review of occupational therapy interventions is critical in evaluating effectiveness and progress toward targeted outcomes. Because clients may experience sudden and sometimes unexpected changes, interventions may have to be modified significantly as the client's status changes. Progress also is defined by the nature of care. Acceptance and improved quality of life is progress, even as a client's body systems and performance skills decline. Occupational therapy services may be appropriate at different points during the course of hospice and palliative care for a given client as that client's needs, priorities, and abilities change over time.

Outcomes

The ultimate outcome of end-of-life care is supporting or improving the client's and family's quality of life. The following case examples (Table 2) illustrate how occupational therapy intervention may be provided to address different needs and priorities for clients, caregivers, and families that contribute to quality of life.

Table 2. Case Examples

Case Description	Occupational Therapy Interventions	Outcomes
Gertrude, an 80-year-old grandmother with 11 supportive grandchildren, moved into a hospice facility after a significant decline in her physical status. The hospice team was concerned about her refusal to follow the pain medication regime and requested an occupational therapy referral to address strategies for pain management.	After talking to Gertrude, the occupational therapist determined that Gertrude avoided taking her pain medication because she was afraid of having slurred speech and being confused and lethargic, symptoms that might frighten her grandchildren when they visited. Although without pain medications she was alert when her grandchildren visited, her pain limited her ability to enjoy these visits or to participate in other activities that were important to her. The occupational therapist recommended changes in Gertrude's daily routines to accommodate her desired roles, meaningful occupations, and pain management needs. The occupational therapist facilitated the collaboration of the hospice team. Together, they worked with Gertrude and her family to develop a modified visitation and medication schedule so that family visits were not occurring at times when the medication's effects on Gertrude's alertness were most intense.	With her anxiety about frightening her grandchildren lessened, Gertrude was more agreeable to taking her medications regularly. The resulting effective management of her pain allowed her to increase involvement in valued occupations and to maintain her role as a loving grandmother.
Gustavo, a man in his 50s, had several metastatic tumors, including one recently removed from his right shoulder. Gustavo was ambulatory, and although he did not have any active right shoulder movement, he was able to complete basic self-care and was to be discharged to his home with hospice care. Gustavo expressed discouragement at his inability to complete two meaningful projects at home: a mural on the living room wall and a wooden boat he was building.	The occupational therapist worked with Gustavo on fatigue management, ergonomics, pacing, and setting priorities for activities. Strategies included positioning his right arm on a leaning pole to act as a support while completing the mural. Adaptive techniques for building the boat included having his nephew work as an apprentice to help with the heavy tasks while Gustavo passed on his boat-building skills.	Gustavo now looked forward to going home, "because I'm not going home to die, I'm going back to my art."
Asuka, a 60-year-old woman from Japan, had difficulty expressing her desires even with the support of an interpreter. She appeared depressed and usually stayed in her room sleeping with the lights off rather than visiting with her daughters when they arrived at the facility.	The occupational therapist met with Asuka's daughters to identify any meaningful activities that she had done in the past. Her daughters identified origami as a valued family activity that their mother used to enjoy. The occupational therapist encouraged the daughters to bring in origami supplies and to work on this activity even though their mother did not respond. As the daughters struggled to remember how to fold the paper to look like a crane, they began laughing. Their laughter woke Asuka, who sat up, asked to have the lights turned on, took the paper from them, and demonstrated how to create an origami crane.	Engagement in this activity allowed Asuka to resume the role of mother and teacher of activities that she valued as culturally significant. She went on to draw each child's name in Japanese calligraphy. This generated increased family interactions and provided meaningful time together.

Table 2. Case Examples *(cont.)*

Case Description	Occupational Therapy Interventions	Outcomes
Dmitri resided in an assisted living facility (ALF) with his wife of 52 years. When Dmitri's health condition was considered terminal, he elected to receive hospice care. Dmitri, his wife, and the hospice team were concerned that, as his abilities declined, his need for assistance might exceed the level permitted for him to remain in the ALF. Care provided by professionals or paraprofessionals was limited to a specific number of hours per week for Dmitri to remain in the ALF, but care provided by his wife was not included in this limit. During the initial occupational therapy encounter, it became evident that Dmitri's concern was not to burden his wife with his increasing needs for assistance.	The occupational therapy practitioner implemented an intervention plan that involved both Dmitri and his wife. Instructions were provided regarding techniques for completing activities of daily living—bathing, dressing, and toileting—as well as assuring both Dmitri and his wife's safety. Planning with his family to address his continued physical decline included introducing adaptive equipment and modifications to the home, which reduced the demands of important activities and made them manageable for Dmitri and his wife. His environment was adapted to allow him to continue to participate in his long-standing weekly poker party and to maintain his role as a vital and active member in the ALF.	Dmitri was able to stay in his ALF home environment without the need of additional staff time. His wife was able to care for him effectively, and he was able to maintain his roles as husband and community member during his last days as a result of these interventions.
Fatima wanted to maintain her role as a mother despite being diagnosed with terminal cancer. Because Fatima had two small children, a referral was made to occupational therapy to identify strategies for her to participate in caring for her children and engaging in other occupations related to being a mother.	The occupational therapist provided services to both Fatima and her husband. The occupational therapist recommended positioning techniques to allow Fatima to hold and feed her toddler. Other interventions focused on strategies so that she could bathe her toddler, assist her older daughter with picking out clothes for school, and participate in family outings. The occupational therapy assistant worked with Fatima to write letters and make video recordings and other remembrances so that she would be able to leave something for each of her children as they went through milestones of life, such as high school graduation, entering college, marriage, and the birth of a child.	This occupational therapy intervention supported Fatima's desire to maintain her role as mother until her death and then to leave something behind so that she would still be a presence in the lives of her children.
Peter was a 5-year-old boy who received hospice care. Both of his parents and two older siblings lived with Peter and were involved in his care. Occupational therapy was included in the hospice plan of care to maintain Peter's ability to play and engage socially with his family despite declining physical and cognitive abilities.	The occupational therapy practitioner involved both Peter and his family in interventions, which included modifications for current games and activities that Peter enjoyed and appropriate positioning strategies to support his participation.	Peter was able to successfully maintain his ability to engage in play and family interaction even as his condition deteriorated.
Ethel, an older woman with cancer, lived with her husband. When her cancer metastasized, Ethel made the decision to terminate planned interventions and to elect hospice care. Initially, Ethel's ability to engage in daily routines and roles was unchanged, but she gradually experienced significant fatigue and had difficulty performing valued activities, such as cooking and cleaning her house.	The occupational therapy practitioner taught Ethel how to use energy conservation strategies to reduce fatigue and accommodate her limited tolerance while continuing to perform household tasks. As Ethel's disease progressed and her ability to perform these occupations declined, interventions focused on interdependence by using modifications to activities that she and her husband could do together.	Ethel still could participate actively in valued activities such as planning meals and helping her husband prepare a grocery list, while her husband completed components of the activities to reduce stress and fatigue. At all stages the occupational therapist worked with Ethel to help her to begin to plan for her death. Occupational therapy interventions involved occupations such as passing on recipes to family members, teaching family members how to make specific foods and recipes, and bequeathing a favorite cooking utensil to a particular family member.

Summary

Occupational therapy practitioners are an important part of hospice and palliative care teams as direct care providers and consultants. Occupational therapy practitioners educate other team members on the meaning and importance of occupation in a person's life and in the dying process. An occupational therapy practitioner's deep understanding of the meaning of occupation makes a powerful contribution to the process of caring for the dying person.

To this end, occupational therapy practitioners function across the continuum of end-of-life care to help support the roles of the client with terminal illness. Although a client's body systems and skills may deteriorate, occupational therapy interventions can support the client's ability to maintain important roles and relationships and to engage in the occupations related to those roles. Having choices and being able to participate in daily activities of self-care can support a sense of self-efficacy and control during the dying process. Continuation of important rituals of everyday activity can support meaningfulness in the dying person's final days (Thompson, 1991).

References

American Occupational Therapy Association. (2006). Policy 1.44: Categories of occupational therapy personnel. In *Policy manual* (2009 ed.). Bethesda, MD: Author.

American Occupational Therapy Association. (2008). Occupational therapy practice framework: Domain and process (2nd ed.). *American Journal of Occupational Therapy, 62*(6), 625–683.

American Occupational Therapy Association. (2009). Guidelines for supervision, roles, and responsibilities during the delivery of occupational therapy services. *American Journal of Occupational Therapy, 63*(6), 797–803.

Arnold, E. M., Artin, K. A., Griffith, D., Person, J. L., & Graham, K. G. (2006). Unmet needs at the end of life: Perceptions of hospice social workers. *Journal of Social Work End-of-Life Palliative Care, 2*(4), 61–83.

Bye, R. A. (1998). When clients are dying: Occupational therapists' perspectives. *Occupational Therapy Journal of Research, 18*(1), 3–24.

Centers for Medicare and Medicaid Services. (2010). Coverage of hospice services under hospital insurance. *Medicare benefit policy manual* (rev. 121). Available online at https://www.cms.gov/manuals/Downloads/bp102c09.pdf

Chochinov, H. M., & Cann, B. J. (2005). Intervention to enhance the spiritual aspects of dying. *Journal of Palliative Medicine, 8*(Suppl. 1), 103–115.

Christiansen, C. H. (1999). Defining lives: Occupation as identity: An essay on competence, coherence, and the creation of meaning (1999 Eleanor Clarke Slagle). *American Journal of Occupational Therapy, 53*(6), 547–558.

Cohen, S. R., Boston, P., Mount, B. M., & Porterfield, P. (2001). Changes in quality of life following admission to palliative care units. *Palliative Medicine, 15*(5), 363–371.

Egan, M., & DeLaat, M. D. (1997). The implicit spirituality of occupational therapy practice. *Canadian Journal of Occupational Therapy, 64*(3), 115–121.

Enes, S. P. (2003). An exploration of dignity in palliative care. *Palliative Medicine, 17,* 263–269.

Gourdji, I., McVey, L., & Purden, M. (2009). A quality end of life from a palliative care patient's perspective. *Journal of Palliative Care, 25*(1), 40–50.

Hospital Case Management. (2003, October). Critical path network—Cancer rehab improves function, quality of life. *Hospital Case Management,* pp. 151–152.

Hunter, E. G. (2008). Legacy: The occupational transmission of self through actions and artifacts. *Journal of Occupational Science, 15*(1), 48–54.

Jacques, N. D., & Hasselkus, B. R. (2004). The nature of occupation surrounding dying and death. *OTJR: Occupation, Participation and Health, 24,* 44–53.

Kaye, P. (2006). *Notes on symptom control in hospice and palliative care.* Machiasport, ME: Hospice Education Institute.

La Cour, K., Josephsson, S., & Luborsky, M. (2005). Creating connections to life during life-threatening illness: Creative activity experienced by elderly people and occupational therapists. *Scandinavian Journal of Occupational Therapy, 12,* 98–109.

La Cour, K., Josephsson, S., Tishelman, C., & Nygård, L. (2007). Experiences of engagement in creative activity at a palliative care facility. *Palliative and Supportive Care, 5*(3), 241–250.

Lin, H. R., & Bauer-Wu, S. M. (2003). Psycho-spiritual well-being in patients with advanced cancer: An integrative review of the literature. *Journal of Advanced Nursing, 44*(1), 69–80.

Lyons, M., Orozovic, N., Davis, J., & Newman, J. (2002). Doing–being–becoming: Occupational experiences of persons with life-threatening illnesses. *American Journal of Occupational Therapy, 56*(3), 285–295.

Marrelli, T. M. (2005). *Hospice and palliative care handbook: Quality, compliance, and reimbursement* (2nd ed.). St. Louis, MO: Elsevier/Mosby.

National Hospice and Palliative Care Organization. (2002). *Standards of practice for hospice programs.* Arlington, VA: Author.

Pearson, E. J., Todd, J. G., & Futcher, J. M. (2007). How can occupational therapists measure outcomes in palliative care? *Palliative Medicine, 21*(6), 477–485.

Picard, H., & Magno, J. (1982). The role of occupational therapy in hospice care. *American Journal of Occupational Therapy, 36*(9), 597–598.

Pizzi, M. (1984). Occupational therapy in hospice care. *American Journal of Occupational Therapy, 38*(4), 252–257.

Pizzi, M., & Briggs, R. (2004). Occupational and physical therapy in hospice—The facilitation of meaning, quality of life, and well-being. *Topics in Geriatric Rehabilitation, 29*(2), 120–130.

Prince-Paul, M. (2008). Relationship among communicative acts, social well-being, and spiritual well-being on the quality of life at the end of life in patients with cancer enrolled in hospice. *Journal of Palliative Medicine, 11*(1), 20–25.

Rahman, H. (2000). Journey of providing care in hospice: Perspectives of occupational therapists. *Qualitative Health Research, 10,* 806–818.

Ryan, P. Y. (2005). Approaching death: A phenomenologic study of five older adults with advanced cancer. *Oncology Nursing Forum, 32*(6), 1101–1108.

Saarik, J., & Hartley, J. (2010). Living with cancer-related fatigue: Developing an effective management programme. *International Journal of Palliative Nursing, 16*(1), 8–12.

Singer, P. A., Martin, D. K., & Kelner, M. (1999). Quality end-of-life care: Patient's perspective. *Journal of the American Medical Association, 13*(2), 163–168.

Steinhauser, K. E., Clipp, E. C., McNeilly, M., Christakis, N. A., Mcintyre, L. M., & Tulsky, J. A. (2000). In search of a good death: Observations of patients, families, and providers. *Annals of Internal Medicine, 132*(10), 825–832.

Strasser, F., Sweeney, C., Willey J., Benisch-Tolley, S., Palmer, J. L., & Bruera, E. (2004). Impact of a half-day multidisciplinary symptoms control and palliative care outpatient clinic in a comprehensive cancer center on recommendations, symptoms intensity, and patient satisfactions: A retrospective descriptive study. *Journal of Pain Symptom Management, 27*(6), 481–491.

Svidòn, G. A., Fürst, C. J., von Koch, L., & Borell, L. (2009). Palliative day care—A study of well-being and health-related quality of life. *Palliative Medicine, 23*(5), 441–447.

Tiggs, K., & Sherman, L. (1983). The treatment of the hospice patient: From occupational history to occupational role. *American Journal of Occupational Therapy, 37*(4), 235–238.

Thompson, B. (1991). Occupational therapy with the terminally ill. In J. Kiernat (Ed.), *Occupational therapy and the older adult* (pp. 324–337). Gaithersburg, MD: Aspen.

Unruh, A. M., Smith N., & Scammell, C. (2000). The occupation of gardening in a life-threatening illness: A qualitative pilot project. *Canadian Journal of Occupational Therapy, 67*(1), 70–77.

Vrkljan, B. H., & Miller-Polgar, J. (2001). Meaning of occupational engagement in life-threatening illness: A qualitative pilot project. *Canadian Journal of Occupational Therapy, 68*(4), 237–246.

World Health Organization. (2002). *National cancer control programmes: Polices and managerial guidelines* (2nd ed.). Geneva: Author.

Related Readings

Albom, M. (1997). *Tuesdays with Morrie*. New York: Doubleday.

Byock, I. (1997). *Dying well: The prospect for growth at the end of life*. New York: Riverhead.

Callahan, M., & Kelley, P. (1992). *Final gifts*. New York: Bantam.

Jacques, N. D., & Thompson, B. (2001). Occupational therapy. In *Complementary therapies in end-of-life care* (pp. 69–82). Arlington, VA: National Hospice and Palliative Care Organization.

Levine, S. (1982). *Who dies?* Garden City, NY: Anchor Press/Doubleday.

Nuland, S. (1993). *How we die*. New York: Random.

Trump, S. M. (2000). The role of occupational therapy in hospice. *Home and Community Health Special Interest Section Quarterly, 7*(2), 1–4.

Trump, S. M. (2001). Occupational therapy and hospice: A natural fit. *OT Practice, 6*(20).

Authors

Ann Burkhardt, OTD, OTR/L, BCN, FAOTA
Mack Ivy, MOT, OTR
Kathleen R. Kannenberg, MS, OTR/L, CCN
Jaclyn F. Low, PhD, LOT
James Marc-Aurele, MBA, OTR/L
Mary Jane Youngstrom, MS, OTR, FAOTA

for

The Commission on Practice
Janet DeLany, DEd, OTR/L, FAOTA, *Chairperson*

Adopted by the Representative Assembly 2011AprC14.

Note. This replaces the 2004 document *Occupational Therapy and Hospice* (previously published and copyrighted in 2005 by the American Occupational Therapy Association in the *American Journal of Occupational Therapy, 59,* 671–675).

The Scope of Occupational Therapy Services for Individuals With an Autism Spectrum Disorder Across the Life Course

The primary purpose of this paper is to define the role of occupational therapy and the scope of occupational therapy services available for individuals with an autism spectrum disorder (ASD) to persons outside of the occupational therapy profession. In addition, this document is intended to clarify the role of occupational therapy with this population for occupational therapists and occupational therapy assistants.[1] "The American Occupational Therapy Association (AOTA) asserts that occupational therapy services are grounded in the belief that persons with an ASD are integral members of their families and communities and have the right to fully participate in the educational, social, cultural, political, and economic life of society" (AOTA, 2009a, p. 843). Occupational therapy practitioners work collaboratively with individuals on the autism spectrum, their families, other professionals, organizations, and community members in multiple contexts to advocate for and provide a range of needed resources and services that support the individuals' ability to participate fully in life (Case-Smith & Arbesman, 2008). According to a study conducted by the Interactive Autism Network (2009), occupational therapy ranks second to speech and language as the most frequently provided services for people with autism throughout the United States.

Prevalence data suggest that autism currently affects approximately 1 in 100 children (Centers for Disease Control and Prevention, 2009), with the same rate being reported in adults (Brugha et al., 2009). Other estimates of ASD diagnoses in the United States have suggested that these rates might be higher, with as many as 1 in 91 children ages 3–17 having a parent-reported diagnosis on the autism spectrum (Kogan et al., 2009). These figures reflect a dramatic increase in the number of individuals living with an ASD in the United States over the past 15 years.

Pervasive developmental disorder (PDD) is the diagnosis used in the *Diagnostic and Statistical Manual of Mental Disorders, 4th edition, text revision* (DSM-IV-TR; American Psychiatric Association [APA], 2000) and in the *International Classification of Functioning, Disability and Health* (ICF; World Health Organization [WHO], 2001) to describe the cluster of symptoms that range in type and severity and include (1) qualitative impairment in social interaction; (2) communication disorders; and (3) stereotyped, repetitive patterns of behaviors or a restricted range of interests. Depending on the level and distribution of symptoms across these categories, a child can be diagnosed with autistic disorder, Asperger disorder, or pervasive developmental disorder–not otherwise specified (PDD–NOS). At present, this range of disorders often is referred to as the *autism spectrum disorders (ASD)* rather than the PDDs. This shift in terminology reflects better awareness on the part of researchers and clinicians that services often appropriate for individuals with autism are suitable for other individuals on the spectrum (Johnson, Myers, & Council on Children With Disabilities, 2007; Lord & Risi, 2000). It reflects general agreement that individuals with lesser impairments should also be considered part of the spectrum.

Rather than using the term *ASD*, the Individuals with Disabilities Education Improvement Act of 2004 (IDEA; P. L. 108–446) uses the term *autism* as a disability category under which children might be eligible

---

[1] When the term *occupational therapy practitioner* is used in this document, it refers to both occupational therapists and occupational therapy assistants (AOTA, 2006). *Occupational therapists* are responsible for all aspects of occupational therapy service delivery and are accountable for the safety and effectiveness of the occupational therapy service delivery process. *Occupational therapy assistants* deliver occupational therapy services under the supervision of and in partnership with an occupational therapist (AOTA, 2009b).

for special education and related services. The IDEA regulations define *autism* as a developmental disability significantly affecting verbal and non-verbal communication and social interaction generally evident before age 3 that adversely affects a child's educational performance. Other characteristics often associated with autism are engagement in repetitive activities and stereotyped movements, resistance to environmental change or change in daily routines, and unusual responses to sensory experiences. (IDEA, 2004, §300.8[c][1][i])

Under Part B of IDEA, occupational therapy is a related service; under Part C, occupational therapy is a primary service. Thus, occupational therapy must be provided to students with autism if those services will help the student to benefit from special education (IDEA, 2004, §602[26][A]). Because educational classification and identification criteria vary considerably from state to state, readers are referred to the specific state policies and requirements.

Occupational Therapy Domain and Process

The aim of occupational therapy is to support individuals' health and participation in life through engagement in occupations (AOTA, 2008). Occupations are activities that are meaningful to individuals and that support their health, well-being, and development (AOTA, 2008). Occupational therapy services focus on enhancing participation in and performance of activities of daily living (ADLs), instrumental activities of daily living (IADLs), rest and sleep, education, work, play, leisure, and social participation within their natural and daily contexts. Consistent with all occupational therapy intervention, the focus of services for individuals with an ASD is determined by their specific goals and priorities for participation. Given that individuals with an ASD may experience complex challenges including social–communication difficulties, the collaboration with key people such as family members, caregivers, and educators is important for determining goals and priorities. Some examples of occupations (ADLs) that may be challenging for people with an ASD and that can be addressed by the occupational therapy practitioner are included in Table 1.

Table 1. Potentially Challenging Areas of Occupation

Areas of Occupation	Examples of Occupations (Daily Life Activities) That May Be Challenging for People With an ASD
Activities of daily living (ADLs)	Bathing, showering, dressing, eating, toilet hygiene, personal hygiene and grooming, sexual activity
Instrumental activities of daily living (IADLs)	Communication management, community mobility, meal preparation, fiscal management, health management and maintenance, home establishment and management, meal preparation and cleanup, safety and emergency maintenance, shopping
Rest and sleep	Achieving a calm state, sleep preparation, developing routines that support sleep, sleep participation
Education	Formal and informal education participation; written language skills; computer use; assistive technology; skills needed to access the curriculum; participation and transition within school environments such as classroom, cafeteria, playground, hallways, auditorium; and other school activities
Work	Employment interests and pursuits, employment seeking and acquisition, job performance, retirement preparation and adjustment, volunteer exploration, volunteer participation
Play and leisure	Play and leisure, exploration and participation
Social participation	Appropriate interactions with others (e.g., family, peers and friends, community), social competencies and management of novel situations, behavior management

The process of occupational therapy service delivery includes evaluation, intervention, and assessment of outcomes. Services can be provided to the client at the individual, organizational, and population levels and may include direct service, consultation, education, and advocacy to support the individual, family members, health professionals, educational staff, and community agencies. At the individual level, collaboration with family, caregivers, educators, and other team members is essential for understanding the daily life experiences of individuals with an ASD and those with whom they interact. At the organizational level, services may focus on educating staff and designing programs and environments that are more socially inclusive for persons on the autism spectrum. At the population level, occupational therapy practitioners may engage in education, consultation, and advocacy initiatives with ASD consumer groups.

The evaluation process is designed to gain an understanding of the client's occupational profile and occupational performance. This process includes an analysis of the client's strengths and challenges related to occupations, performance skills, performance patterns, body functions and body structures, and activity demands. The evaluation process is comprehensive and tailored to the concerns of the specific client, organization, or population. Evaluation information collected through interviews, structured observations, and standardized assessments guides occupational therapy services. Because the literature shows that individuals with an ASD may have difficulties in areas of occupation such as self-care; IADLs; sleep; functional and pretend play; leisure pursuits; social participation; education and work performance; and performance skills such as sensory modulation, self-regulation, praxis, and motor imitation, occupational therapy evaluations conducted at the individual level should assess these areas (Baranek, 2002; Case-Smith & Bryan, 1999; Dawson & Watling, 2000; Kientz & Dunn, 1997; Libby, Powell, Messer, & Jordan, 1998; Rutherford & Rogers, 2003; Shattuck et al., 2007; Watson, Baranek, & DiLavore, 2003; Zaks, 2006). At the organizational level the evaluation process may focus on analyzing the program structure, resources, and services that support persons on the autism spectrum to engage in desired occupations. At the population level the evaluation process may focus on collaborating with ASD consumer groups to identify their capacities and needs to support societal participation. Recent textbook chapters and practice guidelines have been developed to inform the practice of occupational therapy related to ASD and include comprehensive chapters on the evaluation process (Frolek Clark, Miller-Kuhanek, & Watling, 2004; Tomchek, 2001; Tomchek & Case-Smith, 2009; Watling, 2010).

Occupational therapy intervention is based on the results of the evaluation and is implemented to foster occupational engagement and social participation by attending to the transaction among the client, the activity, and the environment. The goal of intervention is to promote engagement in and performance of daily activities, personal satisfaction, adaptation, health and wellness, role competence, quality of life, and occupational justice for people with an ASD within the contexts of their families and communities. At the individual level the intervention may emphasize social engagement and participation, include strategies to improve adaptive behaviors and occupational performance, and support family priorities. Some research has demonstrated the effectiveness of occupational therapy interventions for children and adolescents with an ASD that lead to improvement in self-care and play and that include the use of activities that promote social interaction, problem solving, and pivotal behaviors (e.g., joint attention, initiative, persistence, executive functioning, cooperation) in addition to addressing specific skill acquisition (Case-Smith & Arbesman, 2008). Effective interventions also address contextual factors such as structure, consistency of routine, sensory environments that optimize attention and arousal, and caregiver skills that contribute to occupational performance. Research evidence indicates that the occupational therapy intervention process should be individualized, intensive, and comprehensive; include the family; and facilitate active engagement of the individual (Tomchek & Case-Smith, 2009). There is additional support in the literature for the use of developmental and behavioral approaches to intervention for individuals with an ASD, in particular, for young children (Callahan, Henson, & Cowan, 2008; Dawson et al., 2009; Rogers & Vismara, 2008). Environmental modification to address problem behaviors also has been shown to be effective (Horner, Carr, Strain, Todd, & Reed, 2002).

At the organizational level, interventions could include recommendations for educational and policy initiatives, provision of staff education, and development of new programs. At the population level, emphasis may be on inclusion and advocacy initiatives.

Assessing the outcomes of service is an integral part of the occupational therapy process and is important for determining future actions and for evaluating occupational therapy services provided for the individual, organization, or population. This assessment involves monitoring the client's responses to intervention, reevaluating and modifying the intervention plan, and measuring intervention success through outcomes that are important to the client within the dynamic physical and social environments and cultural contexts where functioning occurs. Progress is noted through improvement in the client's occupational performance, adaptation, participation in desired activities, satisfaction, role competence, health and wellness, and quality of life and through prevention of further difficulties and facilitation of effective transitions. Occupational therapy practice for individuals with an ASD is consistent with the WHO's 2001 *ICF* and the National Research Council's 2001 recommended practices for educating individuals with an ASD. Table 2 provides case examples that reflect a range of occupational therapy evaluation and intervention services for people with an ASD at the individual, organizational, and population levels across the lifespan.

Table 2. Case Studies of Occupational Therapy Evaluation and Intervention Services for People With an ASD

Client and Background	Evaluation	Intervention
• **Kamau** is a 2½ -year-old boy with autism. His language consists of single-word utterances. He has an intense interest in a few objects such as wheels and mobiles. • His mother's primary concerns are his limited social interaction, delayed pretend play, hyperactive behaviors, and picky eating. • Kamau also is receiving speech therapy services and an applied behavioral analysis program at home through the state early intervention program.	• Develop occupational profile of play behaviors, family interactions, and food preferences through parent interview. • Gather clinical observations of behavior, self-regulation, and parent–child interaction during free play and interactive parent–child play. • Conduct structured observation of parent–child interaction during play and while Kamau is eating. • Administer Infant/Toddler Sensory Profile (Dunn, 2002), Bayley Scales of Infant and Toddler Development (Bayley, 2006), and Pediatric Evaluation of Disability Inventory, Self-Care Scale (Haley et al., 1992).	• Provide weekly occupational therapy in the home setting with mother present to facilitate Kamau to establish self-regulation, social engagement, and pretend-play skills (Greenspan & Wieder, 1997; Kasari, Freeman, & Paparella, 2006; Mahoney & Perales, 2005; Salt et al., 2001). • Utilize sensory integration methods; behavioral strategies, including positive reinforcement; and reciprocal play to improve social interaction. • Collaborate with the speech–language pathologist regarding Kamau's intervention program, and arrange co-treatment sessions to promote social interaction. • Collaborate with the behavioral therapist (Cohen, Amerine-Dickens, & Smith, 2006; Smith, Groen, & Wynn, 2000) to integrate sensory and behavioral strategies helpful in modulating Kamau's behavior. • Provide parent training related to sensory processing and behavior management strategies and social participation. • Provide parent consultation to improve the family's mealtime routine and the variety of foods Kamau eats (Horner et al., 2002; Ledford & Gast, 2006).

Table 2. Case Studies of Occupational Therapy Evaluation and Intervention Services for People With an ASD *(cont.)*

Client and Background	Evaluation	Intervention
• **Heang** is a 4-year-old girl with autism and attends an inclusive preschool through her school district. • Her parents have sought individualized occupational therapy services from an outpatient clinic. • She uses only a few basic gestures to communicate. • She primarily engages in solitary sensory–motor exploration of her environment and does not yet spontaneously play beside other children or with toys. • She has frequent tantrums and screams particularly when there are changes in the environment or when being directed toward a specific task.	• Develop an occupational profile of behavior and self-regulation in play through parent and teacher interview. • Conduct clinical observations of behavior, self-regulation, parent–child and teacher–child interaction, and play skills. • Administer the Sensory Profile (Dunn, 1999) and the First STEp Developmental Screening (Miller, 1993).	• Provide weekly occupational therapy in a clinical setting with the parent present. • Consult with preschool team, including teacher and speech–language pathologist. • Provide interventions to improve self-regulation to allow for socially appropriate behavior (Greenspan & Wieder, 1997; Kasari et al., 2006; Mahoney & Perales, 2005; Salt et al., 2001, 2002). • Incorporate sensory integration techniques (Baranek, 2002); visual supports for structure (Ozonoff & Cathcart, 1998) and communication; and behavioral strategies, including positive reinforcement, redirection, elimination of antecedents to her tantrums, and reinforcement of her positive behaviors (Horner et al., 2002; Rogers & Vismara, 2008). • Educate parents on how to recognize when Heang is becoming over-aroused, and implement both positive behavior (Horner et al., 2002) and sensory-based strategies to help her modulate her arousal (Baranek, 2002).
• **Jorge** is a 6-year-old kindergarten boy with a diagnosis of PDD–NOS. • He demonstrates minimal social initiation with peers, although he interacts better with adults. • When peers initiate interaction, he withdraws or responds aggressively. • He needs direct adult supervision to manage his school materials and complete school tasks.	• Develop an occupational profile of play, work/reward routine, and behavior regulation through parent and teacher interview. • Conduct structured clinical observations of classroom behavior, social–communication, parent–child interaction, and play skills. • Administer Short Sensory Profile (McIntosh, Miller, & Shyu, 1999) and School Function Assessment (Cognitive/Behavior Scales; Coster, Deeney, Haltiwanger, & Haley, 1998). • Conduct formal functional behavior analysis of aggressive behaviors.	• Provide occupational therapy services within the school setting. • Collaborate with teacher to implement structured teaching methods based on TEACCH (Ozonoff & Cathcart, 1998; Panerai, Ferrante, & Zingale, 2002) and a visual schedule in the classroom (Ganz, 2007). • Implement positive behavior supports (Horner et al., 2002) and a sensory diet, including strategies for self-regulation based on the functional analysis of aggressive behaviors (Borrero & Borrero, 2008) • Develop and implement social stories (Reynhout & Carter, 2006) prior to challenging school situations (e.g., standing in line, assemblies, fire drills) to encourage appropriate behavior. • Develop peer buddies and modeling program to build social–communica-tion skills during naturally occurring play activities (Harper, Symon, & Frea, 2008). • Consult with the classroom teacher and family to promote generalization of strategies across home and school settings.

(Continued)

Table 2. Case Studies of Occupational Therapy Evaluation and Intervention Services for People With an ASD *(cont.)*

Client and Background	Evaluation	Intervention
• The **local museum of science** is interested in making the museum more accessible to people with an ASD. • The museum hosts school classes on a daily basis and specialized weekend learning programs.	• Develop an occupational profile of supports and inhibitors to engagement in museum activities through observation of museum patrons of various ages interacting with museum exhibits. • Complete structured observation of behavioral, sensory, and social demands of the museum, including structure, timing, and transitions of docent-led groups, signage, "way-finding" materials, and universal design features of physical space. • Conduct focus groups at the museum with parents who have children with an ASD to elicit their recommendations for improving accessibility.	• Provide an educational presentation to museum education staff about the characteristics associated with an ASD and strategies for supporting informal learning. • Consult with museum staff to develop a Social Story to be placed on museum Web site for families to use before visiting the museum. • Consult with museum staff to develop an after-school program for adolescents with an ASD.
• **T. J.** is a 21-year-old young man with Asperger syndrome. T. J. currently is enrolled in a junior college and is having, difficulty finding a needed part-time job. • He lives independently in an apartment. • He presents with poor grooming and hygiene skills and pragmatic language deficits. • He has several interests but spends most of his free time reading about antique cars. • His interest in cars has led to distractibility during driving and resulted in a minor auto accident and a traffic citation for failing to stop at a stop sign.	• Develop an occupational profile of ADL and IADL performance, leisure activities, and driving behaviors through personal interview about his concerns and his interests. • Conduct structured observation of role playing a job interview. • Administer the Scales of Independent Behavior–Revised (SIB–R; Bruininks, Woodcock, Weatherman, & Hill, 1997) and Occupational Self Assessment (Baron, Kielhofner, Iyenger, Goldhammer, & Wolenski, 2006).	• Initially provide occupational therapy on a weekly basis in the clinic, then in the community. • Provide direct intervention to address grooming and hygiene needs through the use of a specific step-by-step self-monitoring system. • Consult with the Division of Vocational Rehabilitation to assist in the employment search. • Use role playing, video self-modeling, and collaborative problem solving to address social communication/pragmatic language needs related to the interview process and interaction with coworkers. • Initiate job coaching to allow T. J. to learn and master job functions and to problem solve when needed. • Refer to an occupational therapy driving rehabilitation specialist to assess driving safety and provide interventions to improve executive functioning and focused attention during driving occupations (Stav, Hunt, & Arbesman, 2006).

Table 2. Case Studies of Occupational Therapy Evaluation and Intervention Services for People With an ASD *(cont.)*

Client and Background	Evaluation	Intervention
T.J. *(cont.)*	• Develop an occupational profile regarding behavior regulation and interpersonal relatedness through interview.	• Facilitate T. J.'s enrollment in an existing on campus support group of other college students with Asperger disorder.
• **Sanjaya** is a 34-year-old man diagnosed with Asperger disorder. • He lives in an apartment with his wife and contributes to the family income through an online business. • Sanjaya has challenges with arousal regulation and coping skills, difficulty with body space awareness, and difficulty reading and sending body language signals that affect his social participation. • Sanjaya has tactile defensiveness, which leads to difficulties with intimacy.	• Administer the Adolescent/Adult Sensory Profile (Brown & Dunn, 2002) and the Canadian Occupational Performance Measure (Law et al., 1998).	• Initially provide occupational therapy services in the therapist's office to address Sanjaya's poor processing of tactile, vestibular, and proprioceptive input. • Develop a sensory diet for Sanjaya to implement on a daily basis in his natural environment. • Consult with and train Sanjaya and his wife in the Alert Program (Williams & Shellenberger, 1996) to recognize when his arousal level is high and to provide a language to aid in their communication. • Perform video analysis (Bellini & Akullian, 2007) and role playing to help develop an awareness of non-verbal communication through facial expression and body language as well as practice pragmatic skills. • Train Sanjaya and his wife in the use of deep tactile pressure and proprioceptive input to diminish tactile defensiveness.
• **Martina** is a 47-year-old woman with high-functioning autism who has recently transitioned from her parent's home to a group home with 24-hour supervision due to her parents' declining ability to care for her. • She works at a local bookstore where she shelves books and organizes incoming orders. • She has funding for services through the Department of Developmental Disabilities and a small amount of private resources. • Martina becomes anxious when her routine is disturbed, demands are placed on her, or her desires are not granted.	• Develop an occupational profile of ADL and IADL routines through interview with Martina and her parents. • Administer the Canadian Occupational Performance Measure (Law et al., 1998), Adolescent/Adult Sensory Profile (Brown & Dunn, 2002), and Test of Grocery Shopping Skills (Brown, Rempfer, & Hamera, 2009). • Conduct clinical observations of behavior during self-care, cooking activities, laundry, and cleaning tasks, as well as path finding and skills for using public transportation.	• Provide occupational therapy services in the group home to help Martina organize her belongings; establish a routine for daily self-care and weekly household tasks; and ensure her success in using the available stove, washer, dryer, and vacuum. • Coach Martina to access online bus schedules, match the bus schedule to her work schedule, walk from the house to the bus stop, board the bus, pay the fare, watch for her stop, exit the bus, and walk to work, as well as learn the steps necessary to return home after her work day.

(Continued)

Table 2. Case Studies of Occupational Therapy Evaluation and Intervention Services for People With an ASD *(cont.)*

Client and Background	Evaluation	Intervention
Martina *(cont.)* • Her parents arranged for contract occupational therapy services to facilitate her transition to the group home, with a focus on establishing routines for self-care and household chores, understanding and using transportation services to and from work, and regulatory difficulties that are known to affect her sleep cycles when substantial transitions occur.		• Teach residential program staff to implement educational strategies, such as forward and backward chaining, visual supports, and environmental structure to support success during intervention (Horner et al., 2002; Hwang & Hughes, 2000) and during everyday activities. • Conduct staff training regarding environmental accommodations and environmental supports. • Collaborate with Martina to develop an evening routine that includes making a phone call or sending email to her parents, preparing for the next day's activities, and enjoying soothing music in preparation for sleep (Reed et al., 2009). Martina will use a sleep chart each morning to record which strategies she used the night before, whether she felt anxious or relaxed at bedtime, and how late she remembers being awake. The occupational therapist monitors the sleep chart weekly and makes needed adjustments to her evening routine until it reflects a successful return to a regular and effective sleep cycle.

References

American Occupational Therapy Association. (2006). Policy 1.44: Categories of occupational therapy personnel. In *Policy manual* (2009 ed.). Bethesda, MD: Author.

American Occupational Therapy Association. (2008). Occupational therapy practice framework: Domain and process (2nd ed.). *American Journal of Occupational Therapy, 62,* 625–688.

American Occupational Therapy Association. (2009a). AOTA's societal statement on autism spectrum disorders. *American Journal of Occupational Therapy, 63*(6), 843–844.

American Occupational Therapy Association. (2009b). Guidelines for supervision, roles, and responsibilities during the delivery of occupational therapy services. *American Journal of Occupational Therapy, 63,* 796–803.

American Psychiatric Association. (2000). *Diagnostic and statistical manual of mental disorders* (4th ed., text rev.). Washington, DC: Author.

Baranek, G. T. (2002). Efficacy of sensory and motor interventions in children with autism. *Journal of Autism and Developmental Disorders, 32*(5), 397–422.

Baron, K., Kielhofner, G., Iyenger, A., Goldhammer, V., & Wolcnski, J. (2006). *Occupational Self Assessment (OSA)* (version 2.2). Chicago: MOHO Clearinghouse.

Bayley, N. (2006). *Bayley Scales of Infant and Toddler Development* (3rd ed.). San Antonio, TX: Psychological Corporation.

Bellini, S., & Akullian, J. (2007). A meta-analysis of video modeling and video self-modeling interventions for children and adolescents with autism spectrum disorders. *Exceptional Children, 73*(3), 264–287.

Borrero, C. S., & Borrero, J. C. (2008). Descriptive and experimental analyses of potential precursors to problem behavior. *Journal of Applied Behavior Analysis, 41,* 83–96.

Brown, C., & Dunn, W. (2002). *Adolescent/Adult Sensory Profile.* San Antonio, TX: Pearson.

Brown, C., Rempfer, M., & Hamera, E. (2009). *Test of Grocery Shopping Skills.* Bethesda, MD: AOTA Press.

Brugha, T., McManus, S., Meltzer, H., Smith, J., Scott, F. J., Purdon, S., et al. (2009). *Autism spectrum disorders in adults living in households throughout England: Report from the Adult Psychiatric Morbidity Survey 2007.* Leeds, England: Health and Social Care Information Centre, Social Care Statistics. Retrieved January 11, 2010, from http://www.ic.nhs.uk/statistics-and-data-collections/mental-health/mental-health-surveys/autism-spectrum-disorders-in-adults-living-in-households-throughout-england--report-from-the-adult-psychiatric-morbidity-survey-2007

Bruininks, R. H., Woodcock, R. W., Weatherman, R. F., & Hill, B. K. (1997). *Scales of Independent Behavior–Revised.* Rolling Meadows, IL: Riverside.

Callahan, K., Henson, R. K., & Cowan, A. K. (2008). Social validation of evidence-based practices in autism by parents, teachers, and administrators. *Journal of Autism and Developmental Disorders, 38,* 678–692.

Case-Smith, J., & Arbesman, M. (2008). Evidence-based review of interventions for autism used in or of relevance to occupational therapy. *American Journal of Occupational Therapy, 62,* 416–429.

Case-Smith, J., & Bryan, T. (1999). The effects of occupational therapy with sensory integration emphasis on preschool-age children with autism. *American Journal of Occupational Therapy, 53,* 489–497.

Centers for Disease Control and Prevention. (2009, December 18). Prevalence of autism spectrum disorders—Autism and Developmental Disabilities Monitoring Network, United States, 2006. *Morbidity and Mortality Weekly Report, 58,* SS-10.

Cohen, H., Amerine-Dickens, M., & Smith, T. (2006). Early intensive behavioral treatment: Replication of the UCLA model in a community setting. *Development and Behavioral Pediatrics, 27,* S145–S155.

Coster, W., Deeney, T., Haltiwanger, J., & Haley, S. (1998). *School Function Assessment.* San Antonio, TX: Psychological Corporation.

Dawson, G., Rogers, S., Munson, J., Smith, M., Winter, J., Greenson, J., et al. (2009). Randomized, controlled trial of an intervention for toddlers with autism: The Early Start Denver Model. *Pediatrics, 121*(1), 17–23.

Dawson, G., & Watling, R. (2000). Interventions to facilitate auditory, visual, and motor integration in autism: A review of the evidence. *Journal of Autism and Developmental Disorders, 30,* 415–421.

Dunn, W. (1999). *Sensory Profile.* San Antonio, TX: Psychological Corporation.

Dunn, W. (2002). *Infant/Toddler Sensory Profile.* San Antonio, TX: Psychological Corporation.

Frolek Clark, G., Millcr Kuhancck, H., & Watling, R. (2004). Evaluation of the child with an autism spectrum disorder. In H. Miller-Kuhaneck (Ed.), *Autism: A comprehensive occupational therapy approach* (2nd ed., pp. 107–153). Bethesda, MD: AOTA Press.

Ganz, J. B. (2007). Classroom structuring methods and strategies for children and youth with autism spectrum disorders. *Exceptionality, 15,* 249–260.

Greenspan, S. I., & Wieder, S. (1997). Developmental patterns and outcomes in infants and children with disorders in relating and communicating: A chart review of 200 cases of children with autistic spectrum diagnoses. *Journal of Developmental and Learning Disorders, 1,* 87–142.

Haley, S. M., Coster, W. J., Ludlow, L. H., Haltiwanger, J. T., & Andrellos, P. J. (1992). *Pediatric Evaluation of Disability Inventory.* San Antonio, TX: Psychological Corporation.

Harper, C. B., Symon, J. B., & Frea, W. D. (2008). Recess is time-in: Using peers to improve social skills of children with autism. *Journal of Autism and Developmental Disorders, 38,* 815–826.

Horner, R., Carr, E., Strain, P., Todd, A., & Reed, H. (2002). Problem behavior interventions for young children. *Journal of Autism and Developmental Disorders, 32,* 423–446.

Hwang, B., & Hughes, C. (2000). The effects of social interactive training on early social communicative skills of children with autism. *Journal of Autism and Developmental Disorders, 30,* 331–343.

Individuals with Disabilities Education Improvement Act of 2004, Pub. Law 108–446, 20 U.S.C.

Interactive Autism Network. (2009). Most popular treatments. *IAN Treatment Reports.* Retrieved from http://www.iancommunity.org/cs/therapies_treatments/

Johnson, C. P., Myers, S. M., & Council on Children With Disabilities. (2007). Identification and evaluation of children with autism spectrum disorders. *Pediatrics, 5,* 1183–1215.

Kasari, C., Freeman, S., & Paparella, T. (2006). Joint attention and symbolic play in young children with autism: A randomized controlled intervention study. *Journal of Child Psychology and Psychiatry and Allied Disciplines, 4,* 611–620.

Kientz, M. A., & Dunn, W. (1997). A comparison of the performance of children with and without autism on the Sensory Profile. *American Journal of Occupational Therapy, 51,* 530–537.

Kogan, M. D., Perrin, M., Ghandour, R. M., Singh, G. K., Strickland, B. B., Trevathan, E., et al. (2009). Prevalence of parent-reported diagnosis of autism spectrum disorder among children in the US, 2007. *Pediatrics, 124,* 1–9.

Law, M., Baptiste, S., Carswell, A., McColl, M., Polatajko, H., & Pollack, N. (1998). *Canadian Occupational Performance Measure* (3rd ed.). Ottawa, ON: CAOT Publications.

Ledford, J. R., & Gast, D. L. (2006). Feeding problems in children with autism spectrum disorders: A review. *Focus on Autism and Other Developmental Disabilities, 21*(3), 153–166.

Libby, S., Powell, S., Messer, D., & Jordan, R. (1998). Spontaneous play in children with autism: A reappraisal. *Journal of Autism and Developmental Disorders, 28,* 487–497.

Lord, C., & Risi, S. (2000). Diagnosis of autism spectrum disorders in young children. In A. M. Wetherby & B. M. Prizant (Eds.), *Autism spectrum disorders: A transactional developmental perspective* (pp. 167–190). Baltimore: Brookes.

Mahoney, G., & Perales, F. (2005). Relationship-focused early intervention with children with pervasive developmental disorders and other disabilities: A comparative study. *Developmental and Behavioral Pediatrics, 26,* 77–85.

McIntosh, D. N., Miller L. J., & Shyu, V. (1999). *Short Sensory Profile.* San Antonio, TX: Psychological Corporation.

Miller, L. J. (1993). *First STEp screening tool.* San Antonio, TX: Psychological Corporation.

National Research Council. (2001). *Educating children with autism.* Washington, DC: National Academy Press.

Ozonoff, S., & Cathcart, K. (1998). Effectiveness of a home program intervention for young children with autism. *Journal of Autism and Developmental Disorders, 28,* 25–32.

Panerai, S., Ferrante, L., & Zingale, M. (2002). Benefits of the treatment and education of autistic and communication handicapped children (TEACCH) programme as compared with a non-specific approach. *Journal of Intellectual Disability Research, 46,* 318–327.

Parham, D., & Ecker, C. J. (2007). *Sensory Processing Measure–Home form.* Los Angeles: Western Psychological Services.

Reed, H. E., McGrew, S. G., Artibee, K., Surdkya, K., Goldman, S. E., Frank, K., et al. (2009). Parent-based sleep education workshops in autism. *Journal of Child Neurology, 24*(8), 936–945.

Reynhout, G., & Carter, M. (2006). Social Stories for children with disabilities. *Journal of Autism and Developmental Disorders, 36,* 445–469.

Rogers, S. J., & Vismara, L. A. (2008). Evidence-based comprehensive treatments for early autism. *Journal of Clinical Child and Adolescent Psychology, 37,* 8–38.

Rutherford, M. D., & Rogers, S. J. (2003). Cognitive underpinnings of pretend play in autism. *Journal of Autism and Developmental Disorders, 33,* 289–302.

Salt, J., Shemilt, J., Sellars, V., Boyd, S., Coulson, T., & McCool, S. (2001). The Scottish Centre for Autism preschool treatment programme. I: A developmental approach to early intervention. *Autism, 5*(4), 362–373.

Salt, J., Shemilt, J., Sellars, V., Boyd, S., Coulson, T., & McCool, S. (2002). The Scottish Centre for Autism preschool treatment programme. II: The results of a controlled treatment outcome study. *Autism, 6*(1), 34–46.

Shattuck, P. T., Seltzer, M. M., Greenberg, J. S., Orzmond, G. I., Lounds, J., Kring, S., et al. (2007). Changes in autism symptoms and maladaptive behaviors in adolescents and adults with autism spectrum disorders. *Journal of Autism and Developmental Disorders, 37,* 1735–1747.

Smith, T., Groen, A. D., & Wynn, J. W. (2000). Randomized trial of intensive early intervention for children with pervasive developmental disorder. *American Journal on Mental Retardation, 105*(4), 269–285.

Sparrow, S. S., Cichetti, D. V., & Balla, D. A. (2005). *Vineland Adaptive Behavior Scales* (2nd ed.). Circle Pines, MN: American Guidance Services.

Stav, W. B., Hunt, L. A., & Arbesman, M. A (2006). *Occupational therapy practice guidelines for driving and community mobility for older adults.* Bethesda, MD: AOTA Press.

Tomchek, S. D. (2001). Sensorimotor assessment of individuals with autism spectrum disorders. In R. Huebner (Ed.), *Autism and related disorders: A sensorimotor approach to management* (pp. 103–138). Gaithersburg, MD: Aspen.

Tomchek, S. D., & Case-Smith, J. (2009). *Occupational therapy practice guidelines for children and adolescents with autism.* Bethesda, MD: AOTA Press.

Watling, R. (2010). Occupational therapy evaluation for individuals with an autism spectrum disorder. In H. Miller Kuhanek & R. Watling (Eds.), *Autism: A comprehensive occupational therapy approach* (3rd ed., pp. 285–303). Bethesda, MD: AOTA Press.

Watson, L. R., Baranek, G. T., & DiLavore, P. C. (2003). Toddlers with autism: Developmental perspectives. *Infants and Young Children, 16,* 201–214.

Williams, M. S., & Shellenberger, S. (1996). *How does your engine run? A leader's guide to the Alert Program for Self-Regulation.* Albuquerque, NM: Therapy Works.

World Health Organization. (2001). *International classification of functioning, disability and health (ICF).* Geneva, Switzerland: Author.

Zaks, Z. (2006). *Life and love: Positive strategies for autistic adults.* Shawnee Mission, KS: Autism Asperger Publishing.

Authors

Scott Tomchek, PhD, OTR/L, FAOTA
Patti LaVesser, PhD, OTR/L
Renee Watling, PhD, OTR/L

for

The Commission on Practice
Janet DeLany, DEd, OTR/L, FAOTA, *Chairperson*

Adopted by the Representative Assembly Coordinating Council (RACC) for the Representative Assembly.

Revised by the Commission on Practice 2010

Note: This document replaces the 2005 *The Scope of Occupational Therapy Service for Individuals With Autism Spectrum Disorders Across the Life Span* (previously published and copyrighted in 2005 by the American Occupational Therapy Association in the *American Journal of Occupational Therapy, 59,* 680-683).

PART II

Societal Statements

AOTA's Societal Statement on Combat-Related Posttraumatic Stress

Self-report of symptoms of post-traumatic stress disorder (PTSD) have tripled among combat-exposed military personnel, compared to those who have not deployed, since 2001 (Smith et al., 2008). Tanielian and Jaycox (2008) have estimated that approximately 300,000 military personnel previously deployed to Iraq or Afghanistan currently experience PTSD or major depression. Military personnel are returning home and demonstrating signs and symptoms of combat-related PTSD, such as nightmares, flashbacks, memory loss, insomnia, depression, avoidance of social interaction, fear, decreased energy, drug and alcohol use, and the inability to concentrate. These signs and symptoms could affect these individuals' ability to effectively negotiate their personal lives and work roles. Specifically during work, the avoidance of social interactions and avoidance of situations that resemble the traumatic event may interfere with coworker relationships or may be perceived as the lack of motivation or ability to be successful in a work setting (Penk, Drebing, & Schutt, 2002).

Combat-related PTSD not only affects military personnel but also the family and the community in which military personnel interact. If unidentified and untreated, the effects of combat-related PTSD may have a delayed onset and cause problems such as depression, social alienation, marital communication problems, difficulty with parenting, and alcohol and drug abuse, and each can cause a disruption in military personnel's personal lives, professional abilities, and overall physical and mental health (Baum, 2008). It is vital for military personnel and health care providers to be educated on these signs and symptoms and detect them early to ensure that military personnel receive adequate opportunities for prompt intervention services and to access support. This is something that occupational therapists and occupational therapy assistants can do.

The overarching goal of occupational therapy for military personnel coping with combat-related PTSD is to use strategies to help them recover, compensate, or adapt so they can reengage with activities that are necessary for their daily life. Occupational therapists and occupational therapy assistants also help military personnel coping with combated-related PTSD to develop strategies to self-manage the long-term consequences of the condition. These strategies are important to promote their health and participation in family, community, and military life because these strategies support their ability to engage or re-engage in daily life activities and occupations that are necessary and meaningful to them. Because of their knowledge and skills in addressing the physical, cognitive, and psychosocial factors associated with combat-related PTSD, occupational therapists and occupational therapy assistants bring broad expertise to help personnel identify the barriers that are limiting their recovery and participation in meaningful activities (American Occupational Therapy Association [AOTA], 2005). AOTA supports recognition of and intervention services for military personnel coping with combat-related PTSD, including research, advocacy, education, and resource allocation consistent with professional standards and ethics.

References

American Occupational Therapy Association. (2005). Occupational therapy code of ethics (2005). *American Journal of Occupational Therapy, 59*, 639–642.

Baum, C. M. (2008, April 1). *Post traumatic stress disorder treatment and research: Moving ahead toward recovery.* Statement of Carolyn M. Baum, PhD, OTR/L, FAOTA, before the House Committee on Veterans' Affairs. Available online at http://veterans.house.gov/hearings/Testimony.aspx?TID=26235& Newsid=188 &Name=%20Carolyn%20M.%20Baum,%20Ph.D,%20OTR/L,%20FAOTA

Penk, W., Drebing, C., & Schutt, R. (2002). PTSD in the workplace. In J. C. Thomas & M. Hersen (Eds.), *Handbook of mental health in the workplace* (pp. 215–248). Thousand Oaks, CA: Sage.

Smith, T. C., Ryan, M. A., Wingard, D. L., Slymen, D. J., Sallis, J. F., & Kritz-Sivlerstein, D. (2008). New onset and persistent symptoms of post-traumatic stress disorder self-reported after deployment and combat exposures: prospective population-based US military cohort study. *British Medical Journal, 336,* 336–371.

Tanielian, T. L., & Jaycox, L. H. (Eds. 2008). *Invisible wounds of war: Psychological and cognitive injuries, their consequences, and services to assist recovery.* Santa Monica, CA: Rand Corporation. Available online at http://www.rand.org/pubs/monographs/2008/RAND_MG720.pdf

Authors

Robinette J., Amaker, PhD, OTR/L, CHT, FAOTA
Yvette Woods, PhD, OTR/L
Steven M. Gerardi, MS, OTR/L, CHT

The views expressed in this article are those of the authors and do not reflect the official policy or position of the Department of the Army, Department of Defense, or the U.S. Government.

for

The Representative Assembly Coordinating Council (RACC):
Deborah Murphy-Fischer, MBA, OTR, BCP, IMT, *Chairperson*
Brent Braveman, PhD, OTR/L, FAOTA
Coralie Glantz, OTR/L, BCG, FAOTA
René Padilla, PhD, OTR/L, FAOTA
Kathlyn Reed, PhD, OTR, FAOTA, MLIS
Barbara Schell, PhD, OTR/L, FAOTA
Pam Toto, MS, OTR/L, BCG, FAOTA
Carol H. Gwin, OT/L, *AOTA Staff Liaison*

Adopted by the Representative Assembly 2008CS84

AOTA's Societal Statement on Health Disparities

It is widely recognized that disparities in health status and the availability of or access to health and social services exist in the United States. The Trans–National Institutes of Health (NIH) Work Group on Health Disparities defined the term *health disparities* as "differences in incidence, prevalence, morbidity, mortality, and burden of diseases and other adverse health conditions that exist among specific population groups" (NIH, 2002).

Health disparities result from the complex interactions among biological factors (e.g., genetics, family history), the environment (e.g., social discrimination; availability, access, and quality of health care), and specific health behaviors (e.g., smoking, alcohol abuse). Health disparities can affect population groups on the basis of gender, age, ethnicity, socioeconomic and educational status, geography, sexual orientation, and disability. Inequities in health exist when the disparities in factors are avoidable and unfair (United Nations Committee for Development Policy, 2009). Groups who have persistently experienced historical trauma, social disadvantage, or discrimination systematically experience worse health or greater health risks than more advantaged social groups (Williams, 2010).

Occupational therapy practitioners have the responsibility to intervene with individuals and communities to limit the effects of inequities that result in health disparities. Practitioners have knowledge and skills in evaluating and intervening with individuals and groups who face physical, social, emotional, or cultural challenges to participation. Further, the American Occupational Therapy Association (AOTA) supports advocacy to increase access to health services for persons in need, and efforts to lessen or eliminate health disparities are consistent with the *Occupational Therapy Code of Ethics and Ethics Standards (2010)* (AOTA, 2010).

References

American Occupational Therapy Association. (2010). Occupational therapy code of ethics and ethics standards (2010). *American Journal of Occupational Therapy, 64*(6 Suppl.), S17–S26. http://dx.doi.org/10.5014/ajot.2010.64S17

National Institutes of Health. (2002). *Strategic research plan and budget to reduce and ultimately eliminate health disparities, Vol. 1, Fiscal years 2000–2006.* Washington, DC: U.S. Department of Health and Human Services. Retrieved June 23, 2011, from www.nimhd.nih.gov/our_programs/strategic/pubs/VolumeI_031003EDrev.pdf

United Nations Committee for Development Policy. (2009). *Policy note: Implementing the Millenium Development Goals: Health inequality and the role of global health partnerships.* New York: Author. Retrieved January 14, 2011, from www.un.org/esa/policy/devplan/cdppublications/2009cdp_mdg health.pdf

Williams, R. A. (2010). Historical perspectives on healthcare disparities: Is the past prologue? In R. A. Williams (Ed.), *Eliminating healthcare disparities in America: Beyond the IOM report* (pp. 3–20). Totowa, NJ: Humana Press.

Authors

Brent Braveman, PhD, OTR/L, FAOTA
Jyothi Gupta, PhD, OTR/L
René Padilla, PhD, OTR/L, FAOTA

The Representative Assembly Coordinating Council (RACC):
Denise Chisholm, PhD, OTR/L, FAOTA, *Chairperson*
Yvonne Randall, EdD, OTR/L, FAOTA
Jyothi Gupta, PhD, OTR/L
Andrea Bilics, PhD, OTR/L
Barbara Hemphill, DMin, OTR, FAOTA, FMOTA
Yvette Hachtel, JD, MEd, OTR/L
Debbie Amini, EdD, OTR/L, CHT
Mary Kay Currie, OT, BCPR
Kimberly Hartmann, PhD, OTR/L, FAOTA
Laurel Cargill Radley, MS, OTR/L, *AOTA Staff Liaison*

Adopted by the Representative Assembly 2006C360; revised 2011 by the RACC; revised 2013 by the RACC.

To be published and copyrighted in 2013 by the American Occupational Therapy Association in the *American Journal of Occupational Therapy, 67*(Suppl.).

AOTA's Societal Statement on Health Literacy

Health literacy, or the ability of individuals to gather, interpret, and use information to make suitable health-related decisions (Institute of Medicine, 2004), promotes participation, empowerment, and control over daily life (Nutbeam, 2008). Persons with inadequate health literacy are more likely to experience adverse health outcomes (DeWalt, Berkman, Sheridan, Lohr, & Pignone, 2004). Although those who possess adequate health literacy achieve better health outcomes, an estimated 90 million people in the United States have limited reading literacy, which also affects their ability to access services and achieve optimal health (Kirsch, Jungeblut, Jenkins, & Kolstat, 2002). Inadequate health literacy disproportionately affects people living at or below the poverty level, limiting their ability to sufficiently participate in health-related activities (Greenfield, Sugarman, Nargiso, & Weiss, 2005).

Occupational therapy can promote health through the development and use of health education approaches and materials that are understandable, accessible, and usable by the full spectrum of consumers. Occupational therapy practitioners can assist in ensuring that all health-related information and education provided to recipients of occupational therapy or other health related services match that person's literacy abilities; cultural sensitivities; and verbal, cognitive, and social skills.

In line with the health communication objectives (U.S. Department of Health and Human Services, 2010), the American Occupational Therapy Association strives to ensure that occupational therapy practitioners possess appropriate communication and education skills that can help enable all people to gain access to, understand, and use occupational therapy and other health-related services, information, and education to promote self-management for optimum health and participation.

References

DeWalt, D. A., Berkman, N. D., Sheridan, S., Lohr, K. N., & Pignone, M. P. (2004). Literacy and health outcomes: A systematic review of the literature. *Journal of General Internal Medicine, 19,* 1228–1239.

Greenfield, S., Sugarman, D., Nargiso, J., & Weiss, R. (2005). Readability of patient handout materials in a nationwide sample of alcohol and drug abuse treatment programs. *American Journal on Addictions, 14,* 339–345.

Institute of Medicine. (2004). *Health literacy: A prescription to end confusion.* Washington, DC: National Academies Press.

Kirsch, I., Jungeblut, A., Jenkins, L., & Kolstat, A. (2002). *Adult literacy in America: A first look at the findings of the National Adult Literacy Survey* (3rd ed.). Washington, DC: National Center for Education, U.S. Department of Education.

Nutbeam, D. (2008). The evolving concept of health literacy. *Social Science and Medicine, 67,* 2072–2078.

U.S. Department of Health and Human Services. (2010). *Public comment on healthy people 2020.* Retrieved November 16, 2010, from http://www.healthypeople.gov/HP2020/Objectives/TopicArea.aspx?id=25&TopicArea=Health+Communication+and+Health+IT

Authors

Kris Pizur-Barnekow, PhD, OTR/L
Amy Darragh, PhD, OTR/L

for

The Representative Assembly Coordinating Council (RACC):
Mary F. Baxter, PhD, LOT, FAOTA, *Chairperson*
Janet V. DeLany, DEd, OTR/L, FAOTA
Barbara Hemphill, DMin, OTR, FAOTA, FMOTA
Yvonne Randall, EdD, OTR/L, FAOTA
Barbara Schell, PhD, OT/L, FAOTA
Pam Toto, PhD, OTR/L, BCG, FAOTA
Laurel Cargill Radley, MS, OTR/L, *AOTA Staff Liaison*

Adopted by the Representative Assembly 2011AprC21.

AOTA's Societal Statement on Livable Communities

The demographic profile of the United States is rapidly changing, with an increasing number of older adults and persons with disabilities who desire to remain in their homes and communities as they grow older, a concept referred to as *aging-in-place*. According to the United Nations (2007), persons with disabilities have the same right as all other members of society to live in the community with opportunities to choose their place of residence and to have equal access to support services that promote full participation in all aspects of community living. To support these rights, society must create communities that enable all residents to live, work, play, and participate in locations of their choice (AARP, 2005; National Council on Disability, 2004). "A livable community is one that has affordable and appropriate housing, supportive community features and services, and adequate mobility options, which together facilitate personal independence and engagement of the residents in civic and social life" (AARP, 2005, p. 4).

The American Occupational Therapy Association's (AOTA's) *Core Values and Attitudes of Occupational Therapy Practice* (AOTA, 1993) and *Occupational Therapy Code of Ethics* (AOTA, 2005) support equality for all individuals, and are congruent with the goals of livable communities. Occupational therapy practitioners plan and implement strategies that promote their client's participation in community life by creating opportunities to establish, restore, or maintain the skills used in activities of daily living and other meaningful occupations and by supporting clients' who are advocating for their own and others' rights. Further, occupational therapy practitioners advocate for universal design and environmental modifications that remove barriers in homes and communities to ensure access to supportive community services, including transportation, personal care, health care, education, employment, and other services, and to facilitate engagement in social and civic activities. Occupational therapy promotes public health and civic engagement by advocating for and assisting in the creation of more livable communities through effective partnerships with individuals, private organizations, and government agencies. Supporting health and participation through active engagement in meaningful activities in the home and community contributes to health, wellness, and quality of life for all individuals (AOTA, 2006).

References

AARP Public Policy Institute. (2005). *Beyond 50.05—A report to the nation on livable communities: Creating environments for successful aging.* Washington, DC: Author.

American Occupational Therapy Association. (1993). Core values and attitudes of occupational therapy practice. *American Journal of Occupational Therapy, 47,* 1085–1086.

American Occupational Therapy Association. (2005). Occupational therapy code of ethics (2005). *American Journal of Occupational Therapy, 59,* 639–642.

American Occupational Therapy Association. (2006). *AOTA Board Task Force on Health and Wellness: Report to the Executive Board.* Retrieved February 4, 2008, from www.atoa.org/News/Centennial/AdHoc/2006/40407.aspx

National Council on Disability. (2004, December). *Livable communities for adults with disabilities: The 2004 report, executive summary.* Available online at http://www.ncd.gov/newsroom/publications/2004/pdf/livablecommunities.pdf

United Nations. (2007). *Rights and dignity of persons with disabilities, Article 19.* Retrieved May 11, 2008, from http://www.un.org/disabilities/documents/convention/convoptprot-e.pdf

Authors
Lisa Ann Fagan, MS, OTR/L
Cheri Cabrera, OTR

for

The Representative Assembly Coordinating Council (RACC):
Deborah Murphy-Fischer, MBA, OTR, BCP, IMT, *Chairperson*
Brent Braveman, PhD, OTR/L, FAOTA
René Padilla, PhD, OTR/L, FAOTA
Kathlyn Reed, PhD, OTR, FAOTA, MLIS
Janet V. DeLany, DEd, OTR/L, FAOTA
Pam Toto, MS, OTR/L, BCG, FAOTA
Barbara Schell, PhD, OTR/L, FAOTA
Carol H. Gwin, OT/L, *AOTA Staff Liaison*

Adopted by the Representative Assembly 2008CS85

AOTA's Societal Statement on Stress and Stress Disorders

Stress is a pervasive societal challenge that affects the social participation of people of varying ages, ethnicity, gender, and socioeconomic status (U.S. Department of Health and Human Services [USDHHS], 2000). It is a significant risk factor in a number of health problems, including mental illness, cognitive decline, cardiovascular disease, musculoskeletal disorders, and workplace injuries. Individuals with disabilities are disproportionately affected, with 49 percent of these people reporting adverse health effects from stress, compared with 34 percent of the general population (USDHHS, 2000).

Individuals, families, organizations, and communities differ significantly in their perceptions of and vulnerability to stressful events, as well as in their coping strategies. Organizational stressors, such as relocation or restructuring, may result in financial strain and loss of personnel. Community or population catastrophes, such as natural disasters or wars, result in stress from overwhelming personal loss, forced displacement, and a disruption of massive proportions in familiar daily routines and occupations (Wein, 2000).

The occupational therapy profession promotes the establishment of healthy habit patterns; familiar, predictable routines; and increased engagement in meaningful occupations that serve both as protective and healing factors in combating the negative effects of stress. Occupational therapy practitioners[1] develop evidence-based interventions based on this philosophy, and conduct research to establish their efficacy for coping with stress (Jackson, Carlson, Mandel, Zemke, & Clark, 1998; Nelson, 1996; Oaten & Chen, 2006; Wein, 2000).

References

American Occupational Therapy Association. (2006). Policy 1.44: Categories of occupational therapy personnel. *American Journal of Occupational Therapy, 60,* 683–684.

Hinojosa, J., & Kramer, P. (1997). Statement—Fundamental concepts of occupational therapy: Occupation, purposeful activity, and function. *American Journal of Occupational Therapy, 51,* 864–866.

Jackson, J., Carlson, M., Mandel, D., Zemke, R., & Clark, F. (1998). Occupation in lifestyle redesign: The Well Elderly Study Occupational Therapy Program. *American Journal of Occupational Therapy, 52,* 326–336.

Nelson, D. L. (1996). Therapeutic occupation: A definition. *American Journal of Occupational Therapy, 50,* 775–782.

Oaten, M., & Chen, K. (2006). Longitudinal gains in self-regulation from regular physical exercise. *British Journal of Health Psychology, 11,* 717–733.

U.S. Department of Health and Human Services. (2000). *Healthy people 2010: Understanding and improving health* (2nd ed.). Washington, DC: U.S. Government Printing Office.

---

[1]When the term *occupational therapy practitioner* is used in this document, it refers to both occupational therapists and occupational therapy assistants (AOTA, 2006).

Wein, H. (2000). *Stress and disease: New perspectives* [NIH Word on Health]. Retrieved October 20, 2006, from http://www.nih.gov/news/WordonHealth/oct2000/story01.htm

Related Reading

Selye, H. (1975). Stress and distress. *Comprehensive Therapy, 1*(8), 9–13.

Author
Susan Stallings-Sahler, PhD, OTR/L, FAOTA

for

The Representative Assembly Coordinating Council (RACC):
Deborah Murphy-Fischer, MBA, OTR, BCP, IMT, *Chairperson*
Brent Braveman, PhD, OTR/L, FAOTA
Linda Fazio, PhD, OTR/L, LPC, FAOTA
Coralie Glantz, OTR/L, BCG, FAOTA
Wendy C. Hildenbrand, MPH, OTR/L, FAOTA
Kathlyn L. Reed, PhD, OTR, FAOTA, MLIS
S. Maggie Reitz, PhD, OTR/L, FAOTA
Susanne Smith Roley, MS, OTR/L, FAOTA
Carol H. Gwin, OT/L, *AOTA Staff Liaison*

Adopted by the Representative Assembly 2007C82

AOTA's Societal Statement on Youth Violence

A nationwide crisis related to youth violence has resulted in this being the second-leading cause of death among all youth aged 15 to 24 years and the leading cause of death among African American youth of the same age (U.S. Department of Health and Human Services, 2000). Acts of violence include bullying, verbal threats, physical assault, domestic abuse, and gunfire. Premature death, disability, and academic failure occur due to violent activity that surrounds youth. Risk factors that lead to youth violence include history of being abused or abusing others, school truancy, poor time use, exposure to crime, mental illness, drug and alcohol use, gang involvement, access to guns, and absence of familial and social support structures. Rising health care costs, decreased property values, and social services disruption are indicators of the impact that violence has on the health of communities, as well as on individual participation in society (Centers for Disease Control & Prevention, 2006). Individual participation can be limited by reduced access to services, fear of harm to self or others, and the inability to perform valued roles. The severity of this issue has forced policymakers, health care providers, teachers, parents, and students to recognize, examine, and alter social conditions, cultural influences, and relationships.

The profession of occupational therapy has the societal duty and expertise to respond to youth violence by promoting overall health and well-being among youth (American Occupational Therapy Association, 2006). Occupational therapy practitioners work toward understanding the occupational nature of violence, researching effective interventions, creating collaborations, and advocating for public health and social services for youth. Violence and its antecedents can deprive this growing segment of youth of necessary and meaningful occupations (Whiteford, 2000), leaving them insufficiently prepared for their future. Positive change can occur by providing youth with opportunities to replace poor occupational choices with healthy, safe, productive, and socially acceptable activities (Snyder, Clark, Masunaka-Noriego, & Young, 1998). Ultimately, occupational therapy practitioners provide services that support a vision of social justice, dignity, and social action throughout the life span by addressing the engagement patterns and lifestyle choices of at-risk youth through methods such as effective transition services and life skills remediation.

References

American Occupational Therapy Association. (2006). *Centennial Vision: Ad hoc report on children and youth.* Retrieved August 7, 2007, from http://www.aota.org/News/Centennial/Updates/AdHoc.aspx

Centers for Disease Control and Prevention. (2006). *Understanding youth violence* [Fact Sheet]. Retrieved August 9, 2007, from http://www.cdc.gov/ncipc/pub-res/YVFactSheet.pdf

Snyder, C., Clark, F., Masunaka-Noriega, M., & Young, B. (1998). Los Angeles street kids: New occupations for life program. *Journal of Occupational Science, 5,* 133–139.

U.S. Department of Health and Human Services. (2000). *Healthy People 2010: Injury and violence prevention.* Retrieved November 17, 2006, from http://www.healthypeople.gov/docuament/html/volume1/07ed.htm

Whiteford, G. (2000). Occupational deprivation: Global challenge in the new millennium. *British Journal of Occupational Therapy, 63,* 200–204.

Author
Heather D. Goertz, OTD, OTR/L

Author
Creighton University Class of 2007 occupational therapy doctoral students:
  Bryan Benedict, Oanh Bui, Stacy Peitz, Rose Ryba
Susan Cahill, MAEA, OTR/L, Clinical Instructor, University of Illinois at Chicago

for

The Representative Assembly Coordinating Council (RACC):
Deborah Murphy-Fischer, MBA, OTR, BCP, IMT, *Chairperson*
Brent Braveman, PhD, OTR/L, FAOTA
Janet V. Delany, DEd, OTR/L, FAOTA
Coralie Glantz, OTR/L, BCG, FAOTA
René Padilla, PhD, OTR/L, FAOTA
Kathlyn L. Reed, PhD, OTR, FAOTA, MLIS
Barbara Schell, PhD, OTR/L, FAOTA
Susanne Smith Roley, MS, OTR/L, FAOTA
Carol H. Gwin, OT/L, *AOTA Staff Liaison*

Adopted by the Representative Assembly 2007CO144

PART III

The American Occupational Therapy Foundation, Inc.

Bylaws:
The American Occupational Therapy Foundation, Inc. (Delaware)

Revised March 26, 1998
Amended March 25, 2006
Amended June 27, 2006
Amended September 4, 2006

ARTICLE I: NAME

The name of this corporation shall be The American Occupational Therapy Foundation, Inc. (hereinafter called the Foundation).

ARTICLE II: PURPOSE

The Foundation is organized exclusively for the charitable, scientific, literary, or educational purposes within the meaning of Section 501(C)(3) of the Internal Revenue Service Code of 1954, or corresponding Section of any future federal tax code as stated in its Certificate of Incorporation.

The particular business and objects of the corporation shall be to advance the science of occupational therapy and increase the public knowledge and understanding thereof by the encouragement of the study of occupational therapy (1) through the provision of scholarships and fellowships, (2) by engaging in studies, surveys and research, and (3) by all other proper means.

ARTICLE III: OFFICES

Section 1. Principal Office. The principal office of the Foundation in the State of Delaware shall be at No. 1209 Orange Street, City of Wilmington, County of New Castle, and the resident agent in charge thereof shall be The Corporation Trust Company.

Section 2. Other Offices. The Foundation may have offices either within or without the State of Delaware and at such place or places as may from time to time be designated by the Board of Directors. Until further action by the Board of Directors, the principal office of the Foundation shall be designated by the Board of Directors.

ARTICLE IV: MEMBERSHIP

The members of the Foundation shall be the voting members of the Board of Directors, including officers and directors.

ARTICLE V: BOARD OF DIRECTORS

Section 1. Responsibilities and Powers.

A. The Board of Directors may exercise all such powers of the corporation required to govern the organization with prudence and ethics within the laws of the State of Delaware, including but not limited to: consent to the appointment of members of all committees and their chairmen; elect individuals to fill vacancies on the Board of Directors including officers; adopt standing rules consistent with the Bylaws to regulate matters; and select a certified public accountant to audit the financial statements and accounts.

B. The Board of Directors shall operate with integrity. The Board of Directors shall assure that there is no discrimination on the basis of creed, religion, race, age, gender, sexual orientation, disability or national origin.

C. Notwithstanding any other provision of these articles, the Foundation shall not conduct any activities not permitted by (I) an organization exempt from federal income tax under the IRS Code, (ii) an organization whose contributions are deductible under Section 170. (C). (2) of the IRS Code (or corresponding provision of any future United States Internal Revenue

Law), and (iii) an organization recognized as tax-exempt under the laws of the State of Delaware.

D. The Board of Directors shall employ, monitor and remove an Executive Director upon such terms and conditions as shall be determined by the Board to carry out the operations of the organization. The policies of the Board will be communicated to the Executive Director on a regular basis.

Section 2. Composition. The organization will be governed by a Board of eleven voting members, including officers and directors who shall be elected at the annual meeting. A majority of the voting members of the Board of Directors shall be occupational therapy practitioners and members of the American Occupational Therapy Association.

Non-voting members shall be the Honorary President Emerita of the Foundation who shall serve in perpetuity, the Chair of the Research Advisory Council, the Executive Director of the Foundation and a liaison from the American Occupational Therapy Association (AOTA) to be appointed annually by the AOTA President.

Honorary life members of the Board of Directors may be elected from time to time, at the discretion of the Board of Directors, in recognition of exemplary service as defined in Board policies. Honorary life members of the Board of Directors shall serve without vote, may speak, but may not make motions.

Section 3. Election and Term of Office. The directors shall be elected to serve for three years or until their successors are elected, and their term of office shall begin at the close of the meeting at which they are elected. No director shall be eligible to serve more than two consecutive terms in office unless the term of office is extended one year, for purposes of continuity, by a two-thirds vote of the members of the board.

Section 4. Resignation. Any director may resign at any time by written notice to the President. Any resignation shall take effect at the time specified, or if not specified, shall take effect immediately upon its receipt by the President.

Section 5. Removal. For cause outlined in Board policies, the Board of Directors may by a two-thirds vote remove a director and declare the office vacant.

Section 6. Vacancies. Any vacancy on the Board of Directors caused by death, resignation or removal of a director shall be filled by a majority vote of the remaining members of the Board.

A person elected to a vacancy shall serve the unexpired term of the director. If a director whose office has become vacant has served more than half of a three-year term, his successor shall be eligible to be re-elected to two successive three-year terms. If the director whose office has become vacant has served less than one half of his term, then the replacement director shall be eligible to be re-elected to one three-year term and thereafter, may not serve an additional successive term.

Section 7. Compensation. Members of the Board of Directors shall not be entitled to any compensation for their services, but voting members of the Board of Directors shall be reimbursed for expenses related to Board service. No salaried staff member of the Foundation shall serve as a director of the Foundation.

ARTICLE VI: MEETINGS

Section 1. Regular Meetings. There shall be at least one regular meeting each year, held in conjunction with the Annual Meeting of the Board of Directors, for the purpose of conducting business. Additional regular meetings may be held at any time and place on the direction of the President with written notice.

Section 2. Annual Meeting. The Annual Meeting for the purpose of electing officers and directors and for any other business that may arise shall be held on the first Sunday in November. The President, upon thirty days prior notice in writing, may change the time, date and place for this meeting.

Section 3. Special Meetings. Special meetings of the Board of Directors, for the purpose of considering one or more items of business specified in the call for the meeting, can be called by the President or by the Executive Committee and shall be called upon the written request of five of the members of the Board. Except in an emergency, written notice of such meetings of the Board of Directors shall be sent to each director and officer at least two days before the day upon which the meeting is to be held. Each such notice shall state the time, place, and purpose(s) of the meeting being called.

Section 4. Quorum. A majority of the voting members of the Board of Directors, including directors and officers present shall constitute a quorum for the transaction of business at any meeting of the Board of Directors. The act of a majority of such members of the Board of Directors present at any meeting, at which a quorum is present, shall be the act of the Board of Directors, except as may be otherwise specifically provided by statute, or by the Certificate of Incorporation, or by these Bylaws.

Section 5. Members of the Board of Directors, or any committee of the Board of Directors, may participate in and act at any meeting of such Board or committee through the use of a conference telephone or other communications equipment by means of which all persons participating in the meeting can communicate with each other. Participation in such a meeting shall constitute attendance and presence in person at the meeting of the person or persons so participating.

Section 6. Any action required to be taken at a meeting of the Board of Directors, or of any committee thereof, may be taken without a meeting if a consent in writing, setting forth the action so taken, shall be signed by all members of the Board of Directors entitled to vote with respect to the subject matter thereof, or by all the members of such committee, as the case may be. Any such consent signed by all voting members of the Board of Directors, or all the members of the committee shall have the same effect as a unanimous vote at a meeting of the Board of Directors at which a quorum was present, and may be stated as such in any document to be filed with the Secretary of State, or with anyone else.

ARTICLE VII: OFFICERS

Section 1. The President and Vice President of the American Occupational Therapy Foundation shall be occupational therapists and a current or previous member of the Board of Directors of the Foundation. The Secretary and Treasurer shall also be a current or previous member of the Board of Directors of the Foundation. Officers shall be voting members of the Board of Directors and shall have all powers and duties generally assigned their respective positions by Roberts Rules of Order Newly Revised and as specifically stated in Board Policies. The President is an ex-officio member of all committees except the Nominating Committee. The President shall vote only when his or her vote is required to break a tie vote of the members of the Board of Directors.

Honorary officers may be elected from time to time, at the discretion of the Board of Directors, in recognition of exemplary service as defined in Board policies. Honorary officers shall serve without vote, may speak but may not make motions.

Section 2. Election, Term of Office. The officers shall be elected to serve for three years or until their successors are elected, and their term of office shall begin at the close of the meeting at which they are elected. No officer shall be eligible to serve more than two consecutive terms in the same office or more than twelve successive years on the board without a three-year leave of absence unless the term of office is extended one year, for purposes of continuity, by a two-thirds vote of the members of the board.

Section 3. Resignation. Any officer may resign at any time by written notice to the President. Any resignation shall take effect at the time specified, or if not specified, shall take effect immediately upon its receipt by the President. In the event of the resignation of the President, such shall be submitted in writing to the Secretary, acting as the representative of the Board of Directors.

Section 4. Removal. For cause, outlined in Board Policies, the Board of Directors by a two-thirds vote shall remove any officer and declare the office vacant.

Section 5. Vacancies. Any vacancy in any office caused by death, resignation or removal of an officer shall be filled by majority vote of the remaining members of the Board at the Annual Meeting or a special meeting held for that purpose.

A person elected to a vacant office shall serve the unexpired term of the officer. If the officer whose office has become vacant has served more than one half of a three-year term, his successor shall be eligible to be re-elected to serve two three-year terms. If the officer whose office has become vacant has served less than one half of a three-year term, then the replacement officer shall be eligible to be re-elected to one three-year term and thereafter, may not serve an additional successive term.

Section 6. Compensation of Officers. Officers shall not be entitled to any compensation for their services as officers, but may be reimbursed for expenses related to their service as officers. No salaried staff member of the Foundation shall serve as an officer of the Foundation.

ARTICLE VIII: COUNCILS

Research Advisory Council. The purpose of the Research Advisory Council shall be to promote research in occupational therapy, anticipate the research needs for the profession and coordinate research activities within the profession. The Chairman of the Council shall be appointed by the President of the Foundation in consultation with the President of AOTA, and shall be accountable to the President of the Foundation. The Chairman shall serve on the Foundation Board of Directors without vote for a term of three years, and may be appointed to serve an additional three-year term. The membership of the Council shall be defined by the Standard Operating Procedures for this group.

ARTICLE IX: COMMITTEES

Section 1. Nominating Committee. Annually, at least sixty days in advance of the scheduled Annual Meeting, the President shall appoint a Chairman of the Nominating Committee who must be a voting member of the Board of Directors. The Chairman shall appoint two committee members who must also be voting members of the Board of Directors. The Board of Directors shall confirm the Chairman and the members of the Nominating Committee. The Nominating Committee shall prepare a slate of candidates for the election of officers and directors to be mailed to members of the Board of Directors at least thirty days prior to the Annual Meeting and elected by ballot by a quorum of the members of the Board of Directors present at the Annual Meeting.

Section 2. The Executive Committee. The Executive Committee shall consist of elected officers of the Board including the President, Vice-President, Secretary, and Treasurer. Meetings of the Executive Committee may be called by the President at such times as are necessary to take action on items of business which shall be binding until ratified by the Board of Directors at its next meeting.

Section 3. Standing Committees.

    A. The Standing Committees of the Foundation shall be the Bylaws, Policies and Procedures, the Awards of Recognition Committee, and the Investment Committee.

    B. The President shall nominate, and the Board of Directors shall confirm the appointment of all committee chairmen and the President shall serve as ex-officio member of all standing committees.

C. Chairmen of Standing Committees must be voting members or previous members of the Board of Directors. The membership of these Committees need not be restricted to members of the Board of Directors.

D. Committees shall report to the Board of Directors and shall assume such duties as shall be assigned by the Board of Directors.

E. A committee chairman shall appoint the members of the committee with the advice and consent of the President acting on behalf of the Board of Directors. A majority of the members of any committee shall constitute a quorum.

Section 4. Special Committees. If the Board of Directors shall create committees for special purposes, the chairs and membership need not be restricted to members of the Board of Directors. Committees shall report to the Board of Directors and shall assume such duties as shall be assigned by the Board of Directors. A committee chairman shall appoint the members of the committee with the advice and consent of the President acting on behalf of the Board of Directors. A majority of the members of any committee shall constitute a quorum.

ARTICLE X: INDEMNIFICATION

The Foundation shall indemnify (a) any person who was or is a party or is threatened to be made a party to any threatened, pending or completed action or suit by or in the right of the Foundation to procure a judgment in its favor by reason of the fact that such person is or was a director, officer, employee or agent of the Foundation or is or was serving at the request of the Foundation as a director, officer, employee or agent of another corporation, partnership, joint venture, trust or other enterprise, against expenses (including attorney's fees) actually and reasonably incurred by such person in connection with the defense or settlement of such action or suit, and by any person who was or is a party or is threatened to be made a party to any threatened, pending, or completed action, suit or proceeding, whether civil, criminal, administrative or investigative (other than an action by or in the right of the Foundation) by reason of the fact that he is or was a director, officer, employee or agent of the Foundation, or who was serving at the request of the Foundation as a director, officer, employee, or agent of another corporation, partnership, joint venture, trust or other enterprise, against expenses (including attorney's fees), judgements, fines and amounts paid in settlement actually and reasonably incurred by him in connection with any such action, suit or proceeding, in each case to the fullest extent permissible under applicable laws, as amended from time to time, or in the indemnification provision of any successor statute.

ARTICLE XI: DISSOLUTION CLAUSE

In the event the Foundation should be dissolved for any reason, any remaining assets shall be distributed for purposes within the scope of the Internal Revenue Service Code 501(c) 3, or any amendment thereto and according to the Eleventh Article of the Certificate of Incorporation of the American Occupational Therapy Foundation, Inc.

ARTICLE XII: SEAL

The corporate seal shall bear the name of the Foundation, the year of its organization and the words "Corporate Seal, Delaware."

ARTICLE XIII: PARLIAMENTARY AUTHORITY

The rules contained in Robert's Rules of Order Newly Revised shall govern the Foundation in all cases to which they are applicable and in which they are not inconsistent with these Bylaws and/or the Foundation's Articles of Incorporation.

ARTICLE XIV: AMENDMENTS

The Foundation shall make and from time to time alter and amend these Bylaws as may be necessary to carry into effect any of the purposes of the Foundation, or which may be needful in its governance, or in the conduct of its business. Such Bylaws may be made or amended at any regular or special meeting of the Foundation, provided, however, that any proposed Bylaw change shall be made available to all voting members of the Board of Directors no less than twenty days prior to the meeting at which such proposed Bylaw change shall be considered for adoption.

Certificate of Incorporation

CERTIFICATE OF INCORPORATION

OF

THE AMERICAN OCCUPATIONAL THERAPY FOUNDATION, INC.

FIRST. The name of the corporation is The American Occupational Therapy Foundation, Inc.

SECOND. Its principal office in the State of Delaware is located at No. 100 West Tenth Street, in the City of Wilmington, County of New Castle. The name and address of its resident agent is The Corporation Trust Company, No. 100 West Tenth Street, Wilmington 99, Delaware.

THIRD. The corporation is organized exclusively for charitable, scientific, literary, and educational purposes, including, for such purposes, the making of distributions to organizations that qualify as exempt organizations under Section 501(c)(3) of the Internal Revenue Code of 1954. The particular business and objects of the corporation shall be to advance the science of occupational therapy and increase the public knowledge and understanding thereof by the encouragement of the study of occupational therapy (1) through the provision of scholarships and fellowships, (2) by engaging in studies, surveys and research, and (3) by all other proper means. No

REC C 85 PAGE 692

activities shall be pursued by the corporation for a profit, to such an extent as to constitute such activities a trade or business, but solely for the purposes hereinabove set forth; and no part of the net earnings of the corporation shall inure to the benefit of any member, director, officer or employee of the corporation or any other individual, except reasonable compensation for services actually rendered in effecting one or more of the corporation's purposes set forth hereinabove. The corporation shall not in any way, directly or indirectly, carry on propaganda, or otherwise attempt to influence legislation, or participate in, or intervene in (including the publishing or distributing of statements), any political campaign on behalf of any candidate for public office; nor shall any of its funds, property or income be used for such purpose.

In pursuance of and not in limitation of the general powers conferred by law, and the objects and purposes herein set forth, it is expressly provided that the corporation shall also have the following powers:

To do all such acts as are necessary or convenient to attain the objects and purposes herein set forth, to the same extent and as fully as any natural person could or might do, and as are not forbidden by law or by this certificate of incorporation or by the by-laws of this corporation;

To purchase, lease, receive by gift, devise or bequest, or otherwise acquire, either absolutely or in trust,

2

REC C 85 PAGE 693

hold, sell, mortgage, or otherwise dispose of real, personal or mixed property; and to invest the principal thereof, to accumulate, administer, expend and distribute any such property or the income therefrom in the form of gifts, grants, and endowments for and to institutions and organizations primarily engaged in charitable, scientific, literary or educational purposes, or gifts, grants and endowments to individuals for educational or scientific purposes or research;

To enter into, make, perform and carry out contracts of every kind with any person, firm, corporation, or association; to do any acts necessary or expedient for carrying on any and all of the activities and pursuing any and all of the objects and purposes set forth in this certificate of incorporation and not forbidden by the laws of the State of Delaware.

To have offices and promote and carry on its objects and purposes within or without the State of Delaware, in other states, the District of Columbia, the territories or colonies of the United States.

In general, to have all powers conferred upon a corporation by the laws of the State of Delaware, except as herein prohibited, or forbidden by the by-laws of this corporation.

3

REC C 85 PAGE 694

FOURTH: The corporation shall not have authority to issue capital stock. The conditions of membership of the corporation shall be stated in the by-laws.

FIFTH: The names and places of residence of the incorporators are as follows:

NAMES	RESIDENCES
Ruth W. Brunyate, OTR	306 South Wind Road Ruxton 4, Maryland
Alice C. Jantzen, OTR	2711 N.W. 2nd Avenue Gainesville, Florida
Mary Frances Heormans, OTR	429 West Prospect Appleton, Wisconsin
Ethel E. Huebner, OTR	13 Pennwood Drive Trenton, New Jersey 08638
Marion W. Crampton, OTR	109 Bartlett Avenue Arlington, Massachusetts 02174
Janet C. Stone, OTR	4435 East Ocean Blvd., Apt. 12, Long Beach, California 90803
Sister Miriam Joseph, OTR	Chairman, Dept. of OT, College of St. Catherine 2004 Randolph St. Paul, Minn. 55116
Florence Cromwell, OTR	1179 Yocum Street Pasadena, California
Dean R. Tyndall, OTR	444 Campbell Avenue Kalamazoo, Michigan
Mary Van Gorden, OTR	401 East 2nd Street Duluth, Minnesota 55805

4

REC C 85 PAGE 695

SIXTH. The corporation shall have perpetual existence.

SEVENTH. The private property of the members shall not be subject to the payment of corporate debts to any extent whatever.

EIGHTH. The activities and affairs of the corporation shall be managed by a board of directors. The number of directors which shall constitute the whole board shall be such as from time to time shall be fixed by or in the manner provided in the by-laws, but in no case shall the number be less than three. The incorporators shall act as the members and first Board of Directors until the adoption of by-laws and the first election of directors.

The corporation may in its by-laws confer powers upon the Board of Directors in addition to the foregoing, and in addition to the powers and authority expressly conferred upon them by statute, provided that the Board of Directors shall not exercise any power or authority reserved herein or by statute to the members.

NINTH. Meetings of members may be held without the State of Delaware, if the by-laws so provide. The books of the corporation may be kept (subject to any provision contained in the statutes), outside of the State of Delaware at such place or places as may be from time to time

5

REC C 85 PAGE 696

designated by the Board of Directors. Election of directors
need not be by ballot unless the by-laws of the corporation
shall so provide.

TENTH. The corporation reserves the right to
amend, alter, change or repeal any provision contained in
this certificate of incorporation, in the manner now or
hereafter prescribed by statute, and all rights conferred
upon members herein are granted subject to this reservation.

ELEVENTH. No dividends of any nature whatsoever
nor any other distribution of earnings or surplus shall be
declared or paid to the members of the corporation; and no
part of the net earnings of the corporation shall enure to
the benefit of any member or individual. All profits or
surplus shall be used by the corporation to further its
purposes. Upon any dissolution of the corporation no
member or any other private individual shall be entitled
to any distribution or division of its remaining assets,
but the net assets of the corporation, after the payment of
debts and necessary expenses, shall be distributed to or
among one or more other organizations organized and
operated exclusively for charitable, religious, scientific,
literary and/or educational purposes.

WE, THE UNDERSIGNED, being each of the incorporators
hereinbefore named, for the purpose of forming a corporation
pursuant to the General Corporation Law of the State of

6

REC C 85 PAGE 697

Delaware, do make this certificate, hereby declaring and
certifying that the facts herein stated are true, and
accordingly have hereunto set our hands and seals this
5ᵗʰ day of April, A. D. 1965.

Ruth W. Brunyate, OTR _____ (Seal)

Alice C. Jantzen, OTR _____ (Seal)

Mary Frances Heermans, OTR (Seal)

Ethel E. Huebner, OTR _____ (Seal)

Marion W. Crampton, OTR _____ (Seal)

Elizabeth Wagner, OTR   W.D.B. _____ (Seal)

Janet C. Stone, OTR _____ (Seal)

Sister Miriam Joseph, OTR _____ (Seal)

Florence Cromwell, OTR _____ (Seal)

Dean R. Tyndall, OTR _____ (Seal)

Mary Van Gorden, OTR _____ (Seal)

REC C 85 PAGE 698

STATE OF IOWA)
: ss.:
COUNTY OF POLK)

      BE IT REMEMBERED that on this 5 day of April
A. D. 1965, personally came before me, a Notary Public for
the State of Iowa, Ruth W. Brunyate, OTR, Alice C. Jantzen,
OTR, Mary Frances Heermans, OTR, Ethel K. Huebner, OTR,
                             W.D.B.
Marion W. Crampton, OTR, ~~Elizabeth Wagner, OTR,~~ Janet C.
Stone, OTR, Sister Miriam Joseph, OTR, Florence Cromwell,
OTR, Dean R. Tyndall, OTR, and Mary Van Gorden, OTR, all of
the parties to the foregoing certificate of incorporation,
known to me personally to be such, and severally acknowledged
the said certificate to be the act and deed of the signers
respectively and that the facts therein stated are truly
set forth.

      GIVEN under my hand and seal of office the day
and year aforesaid.

~~[NOTARIAL~~
~~SEAL]x~~   WILLARD D. BRITTIN
                                 Notary Public

WILLARD D. BRITTIN
NOTARIAL SEAL
IOWA

8

PART IV

Rescissions, Revisions, and Changes

Rescissions, Revisions, and Changes

The following rescissions, revisions, and changes have been made since the publication of previous editions of the *Reference Manual of the Official Documents of the American Occupational Therapy Association, Inc.*

Bylaws

Incorporation Papers and Bylaws (1991, 1996, 1999, 2002, 2003, 2005). Bylaws and Glossary Sections **revised** and **replaced** 2007. Bylaws, Glossary, and Incorporation Sections **revised** and **replaced** 2010. Incorporation papers and Bylaws **revised** and **replaced** 2013.

Accreditation

Accreditation Standards for a Doctoral-Degree-Level Educational Program for the Occupational Therapist (2007), Accreditation Standards for a Master's-Degree-Level Educational Program for the Occupational Therapist (2007), and Accreditation Standards for an Educational Program for the Occupational Therapy Assistant (2007). **Replaced** by 2011 Accreditation Council for Occupational Therapy Education (ACOTE®) Standards (2012).

Essentials and Guidelines for an Accredited Educational Program for the Occupational Therapist (1935, 1943, 1949, 1965, 1973, 1983, 1991, 1995, 1998). **Rescinded** 2007. **Replaced** by Accreditation Standards for a Doctoral-Degree-Level Educational Program for the Occupational Therapist (2007) and Accreditation Standards for a Master's-Degree-Level Educational Program for the Occupational Therapist (2007). **Replaced** by 2011 Accreditation Council for Occupational Therapy Education (ACOTE®) Standards (2012).

Essentials and Guidelines for an Accredited Educational Program for the Occupational Therapy Assistant (1958, 1962, 1967, 1970, 1975, 1983, 1991, 1995, 1998). **Rescinded** 2007. **Replaced** by Accreditation Standards for an Educational Program for the Occupational Therapy Assistant (2007). **Replaced** by 2011 Accreditation Council for Occupational Therapy Education (ACOTE®) Standards (2012).

Concept Papers

Cross-Training Concept Paper (1997). **Rescinded** 2002.

The Role of Occupational Therapy in Disaster Preparedness, Response, and Recovery: A Concept Paper (2011). **Revised** 2011.

Scholarship and Occupational Therapy (2003). **Revised** 2009.

Service Delivery in Occupational Therapy (1995). **Rescinded** 2004.

Education

Academic Terminal Degree (2003). **Replaced** by Academic Terminal Degree (2008).

Philosophy of Professional Education (1997, 2003). **Replaced** by Philosophy of Occupational Therapy Education (2007).

Purpose and Value of Occupational Therapy Fieldwork Education (1996). **Replaced** by The Purpose and Value of Occupational Therapy Fieldwork Education (2003). **Replaced** by Occupational Therapy Fieldwork Value and Purpose (2009).

Standards and Guidelines for an Occupational Therapy Affiliation Program (1970). **Rescinded** 1983.

The Viability of Occupational Therapy Assistant Education (2002). **Replaced** by the Importance of Occupational Therapy Assistant Education (2008).

Ethics

Core Values and Attitudes of Occupational Therapy Practice (1993). **Rescinded** 2010.

Enforcement Procedures for Occupational Therapy Code of Ethics (1994, 1996, 1998, 2000, 2002, 2004, 2005, **edited** 2006). **Replaced** by Enforcement Procedures for Occupational Therapy Code of Ethics (2007). **Replaced** by Enforcement Procedures for Occupational Therapy Code of Ethics and Ethics Standards (2010).

Guidelines to the Occupational Therapy Code of Ethics (1998). **Replaced** by the Guidelines to the Occupational Therapy Code of Ethics (2006). **Rescinded** (2010).

Occupational Therapy Code of Ethics (1988, 1994, 2000). **Replaced** by Occupational Therapy Code of Ethics (2005, **edited** 2006). **Replaced** by Occupational Therapy Code of Ethics and Ethics Standards (2010).

Guidelines

Elements of Clinical Documentation (1994). **Rescinded** 2003. **Replaced** by Guidelines for Documentation of Occupational Therapy (2003, **edited** 2007).

Guide for Supervision of Occupational Therapy Personnel (1994). **Rescinded** 1999. **Replaced** by Guide for Supervision of Occupational Therapy Personnel in the Delivery of Occupational Therapy Services (1999, *AJOT*, *53*(6):592–594 [correction, *54*(2):235]).

Guide for Supervision of Occupational Therapy Personnel in the Delivery of Occupational Therapy Services (1994, 1999). **Rescinded** 2004. **Replaced** by Guidelines for Supervision, Roles, and Responsibilities During the Delivery of Occupational Therapy Services (2004, **edited** 2009).

Guide to Classification of Occupational Therapy Personnel (1987). **Rescinded** 1991. **Replaced** by Occupational Therapy Roles (1993) and Companion Guide (1994).

Guidelines for Documentation of Occupational Therapy (2008). **Edited** 2013.

Guidelines for an Occupational Therapist Providing Services as a Supervisor (1974). **Replaced** by Guide for Supervision of Occupational Therapy Personnel (1981, 1994).

Guidelines for Occupational Therapy Documentation (1986). **Replaced** by Elements of Clinical Documentation (1994).

Guidelines for the Use of Aides in Occupational Therapy Practice (1996, 1999). **Rescinded** 2004. **Replaced** by Guidelines for Supervision, Roles, and Responsibilities During the Delivery of Occupational Therapy Services (2004, **edited** 2009).

Hierarchy of Competencies Relating to the Use of Standardized Instruments and Evaluation Techniques by Occupational Therapists (1984). **Rescinded** 1992.

Minimal Occupational Therapy Classification Standards (1971). **Revised** 1997. Replaced by Guide to Classi-fication of Occupational Therapy Personnel (1985, **edited** 1987). **Replaced** by Occupational Therapy Roles (1993) and Companion Guide (1994).

Occupational Therapy Practice Framework. **Replaced** by Occupational Therapy Practice Framework: Domain and Process, 2nd Edition (2008).

Occupational Therapy Product Output Reporting System (1979). **Rescinded** 1994.

Supervision Guidelines (1986). **Rescinded** 1992. **Replaced** by Guidelines for Supervision, Roles, and Responsibilities during the Delivery of Occupational Therapy Services (2004, **edited** 2009).

Supervision Guidelines for Certified Occupational Therapy Assistants (1990). **Rescinded** 1993.

Uniform Occupational Therapy Evaluation Checklist (1981). **Rescinded** 1994.

Uniform Terminology for Reporting Occupational Therapy Services—First Edition (1979). **Replaced** by Uniform Terminology for Occupational Therapy (Second Edition) and the Application of Uniform Termi-nology to Practice (1989). **Replaced** by Uniform Terminology for Occupational Therapy (Third Edition) and Application to Practice (1994). **Rescinded** 2002.

Work Hardening Guidelines (1986). **Replaced** by Statement: Occupational Therapy Services in Work Practice (1992).

Specialized Knowledge and Skills Papers

Specialized Knowledge and Skills for Occupational Therapy Practice in the Neonatal Intensive Care Unit (1993, 2000). **Replaced** by Specialized Knowledge and Skills for Occupational Therapy Practice in the Neonatal Intensive Care Unit (2006).

Specialized Knowledge and Skills in Adult Vestibular Rehabilitation for Occupational Therapy Practice (2000). **Replaced** by Specialized Knowledge and Skills in Adult Vestibular Rehabilitation for Occupational Therapy Practice (2006).

Specialized Knowledge and Skills in Eating and Feeding in Occupational Therapy Practice (2000). **Replaced** by Specialized Knowledge and Skills in Feeding, Eating, and Swallowing for Occupational Therapy Practice (2007).

Position Papers

AOTA Position Paper on Early Childhood Intervention (1986). **Replaced** by Occupational Therapy Services in Early Intervention and Preschool Services (1988). **Rescinded** 2002.

Broadening the Construct of Independence (1995, 2002). **Rescinded** 2007.

Complimentary and Alternative Medicine Position Paper (CAM) (2011). **Revised** 2011.

Human Immunodeficiency Virus (1984). **Replaced** by Providing Services for Persons with HIV/AIDS and Their Caregivers (1996). **Rescinded** 2002.

Obesity and Occupational Therapy (2007). **Revised** 2013.

Occupation: A Position Paper (1995). **Rescinded** 2004.

Occupational Performance: Occupational Therapy's Definition of Function (1995). **Rescinded** 2002.

Occupational Therapy: A Profession in Support of Full Inclusion (1995) with White Paper: The Role of the Occupational Therapy Practitioner in the Implementation of Full Inclusion (1996). Position Paper and

White Paper **rescinded** 1999. **Replaced** by Position Paper, Occupational Therapy's Commitment to Non-discrimination and Inclusion (1999, *AJOT*, *53*(6):598 [correction, *54*(2):235]).

Occupational Therapy and Assistive Technology (1991). **Replaced** by The Use of General Information and Assistive Technology Within Occupational Therapy Practice (1998).

Occupational Therapy and Eating Dysfunction (1989). **Replaced** by Eating Dysfunction Position Paper (1996). **Replaced** by Specialized Knowledge and Skills for Eating and Feeding in Occupational Therapy Practice (2000).

Occupational Therapy and Hospice (1986,1991). **Replaced** by Statement, Occupational Therapy and Hospice (1998).

Occupational Therapy and Long-Term Services and Supports (1994). **Rescinded** 2002.

Occupational Therapy and The Americans With Disabilities Act (ADA) (1993, 2000). **Rescinded** 2005.

Occupational Therapy as an Education-Related Service (1981). **Rescinded** 1987.

Occupational Therapy for Sensory Integrative Dysfunction (1982). **Rescinded** 1991.

Occupational Therapy in Adult Day-Care (1986). **Rescinded** 1992.

Occupational Therapy in the Promotion of Health and the Prevention of Disease and Disability (1989). **Rescinded** 2000. **Replaced** by Statement: Occupational Therapy in the Promotion of Health and the Prevention of Disease and Disability (2000).

Occupational Therapy Services for Alzheimer's Disease and Related Disorders Position Paper (1986). **Replaced** by Occupational Therapy Services for Persons with Alzheimer's Disease and Other Dementias (Statement [1994]). **Rescinded** 2000.

Occupational Therapy's Commitment to Nondiscrimination and Inclusion (1999). **Replaced** by Occupational Therapy's Commitment to Nondiscrimination and Inclusion (2004, **edited** 2009).

Physical Agent Modalities: A Position Paper (1992). **Replaced** by Physical Agent Modalities Position Paper (**edited** 1997). **Rescinded** 2003. **Replaced** by Physical Agent Modalities: A Position Paper (2003, **edited** 2007). **Replaced** by Physical Agent Modalities: A Position Paper. **Revised** (2012).

Purposeful Activities (1983). **Replaced** by Position Paper: Purposeful Activity (1993). **Rescinded** 2002.

The Psychosocial Core of Occupational Therapy (1995, **edited** 1997). **Rescinded** 2004. **Replaced** by Psychosocial Aspects of Occupational Therapy (2004).

Psychosocial Aspects of Occupational Therapy (2004). **Replaced** by Occupational Therapy Services in the Promotion of Psychological and Social Aspects of Mental Health (2010).

Scope of Practice (2005). **Replaced** by Scope of Practice (2009).

Telerehabilitation (2005). **Revised** (2010). **Replaced** by Telehealth (2013).

Use of Occupational Therapy Aides in Occupational Therapy Practice (1995, **edited** 1996). **Rescinded** 1999. **Replaced** by Guidelines for the Use of Aides in Occupational Therapy Practice—Guidelines (1999, *AJOT*, *53*(6):595–597 [correction, *54*(2):235]).

The Use of General Information and Assistive Technology Within Occupational Therapy Practice (1991, 1998). **Rescinded** 2004. **Replaced** by Assistive Technology Within Occupational Therapy Practice (2004, **Rescinded** 2009).

Roles Papers

Entry-Level Role Delineation for OTRs and COTAs (1981). **Revised** 1990. **Rescinded** 1994. **Replaced** by Occupational Therapy Roles (1993) and Companion Guide (1994).

Occupational Therapy: Its Definitions and Functions (1972). **Replaced** by Definitions (1981). **Rescinded** 1992.

Occupational Therapy Roles (1993) and Career Exploration and Development: A Companion Guide to the Occupational Therapy Roles Document (1994). **Rescinded** 2004. **Replaced** by Guidelines for Supervision, Roles, and Responsibilities During the Delivery of Occupational Therapy Services (2004, **edited** 2009) and Scope of Practice (2004, **edited** 2009).

Occupational Therapy's Role in Independent or Alternative Living Situations (1981). **Rescinded** 1991. **Replaced** by The Role of Occupational Therapy in the Independent Living Movement (Statement [1993]). **Rescinded** 1999.

Role Competencies for An Academic Fieldwork Coordinator (2003). **Rescinded** 2009. **Replaced** by Specialized Knowledge and Skills of Occupational Therapy Educators of the Future (2009).

Role Competencies for a Faculty Member in an OTA Academic Setting (2005). **Rescinded** 2009. **Replaced** by Specialized Knowledge and Skills of Occupational Therapy Educators of the Future (2009).

Role Competencies for a Fieldwork Educator (2005). **Rescinded** 2009. **Replaced** by Specialized Knowledge and Skills of Occupational Therapy Educators of the Future (2009).

Role Competencies for a Professional-Level OT Faculty memeber in an Academic Setting (2005). **Rescinded** 2009. **Replaced** by Specialized Knowledge and Skills of Occupational Therapy Educators of the Future (2009).

Role Competencies for a Professional-Level Program Director in an Academic Setting (2009). **Rescinded** 2009. **Replaced** by Specialized Knowledge and Skills of Occupational Therapy Educators of the Future (2009).

Role Competencies for a Program Director in an OTA Academic Setting (2003). **Rescinded** 2009. **Replaced** by Specialized Knowledge and Skills of Occupational Therapy Educators of the Future (2009).

Roles and Functions of Occupational Therapy in Adult Day-Care (1986). **Rescinded** 1992.

Roles and Functions of Occupational Therapy in Burn Care Delivery (1985). **Rescinded** 1991.

Roles and Functions of Occupational Therapy in Hand Rehabilitation (1985). **Rescinded** 1991.

Roles and Functions of Occupational Therapy in Long-Term Care: Occupational Therapy and Activity Programs (1983). **Rescinded** 1992. **Replaced** by Occupational Therapy and Long-Term Services and Supports (Position Paper [1994]).

Roles and Functions of Occupational Therapy in the Management of Patients with Rheumatic Diseases (1986). **Rescinded** 1992.

Roles and Functions of Occupational Therapy in Mental Health (1986). **Rescinded** 1991.

Roles and Functions of Occupational Therapy Services for the Severely Disabled (1983). **Rescinded** 1992.

Roles and Functions of the Occupational Therapist in the Treatment of Sensory Integrative Dysfunction (1982). **Rescinded** 1991.

Roles of Occupational Therapists and Occupational Therapy Assistants in Schools (1987). **Rescinded** 1997.

The Role of the Occupational Therapist in Home Health Care (1981). **Rescinded** 1991.

The Role of the Occupational Therapist in the Promotion of Health and Prevention of Disabilities (1976). **Replaced** by Occupational Therapy in the Promotion of Health and the Prevention of Disease and Disabilities (1976). **Replaced** by Occupational Therapy in the Promotion of Health and the Prevention of Disease and Disability (Position Paper [1989]).

The Role of Occupational Therapy in the Vocational Rehabilitation Process (1980). **Rescinded** 1991.

The Scope of Occupational Therapy Services for Individuals With an Autism Spectrum Disorder Across the Life Span (2005). **Replaced** by The Scope of Occupational Therapy Services for Individuals With an Autism Spectrum Disorder Across the Life Course (2010).

Standards

Glossary of Terms Used in the Standards of Practice (1985). **Rescinded** 1991.

Standards for Continuing Competence (1999). **Replaced** by Standards for Continuing Competence (2005). **Revised** (2010).

Standards of Practice for Occupational Therapy (1983, 1992, 1994, 1998). **Replaced** by Standards of Practice for Occupational Therapy (2005). **Revised** (2010).

Standards of Practice: Developmental Disabilities (1979, 1988). **Rescinded** 1991.

Standards of Practice: Home Health (1979, 1988). **Rescinded** 1991.

Standards of Practice: Mental Health (1979, 1988). **Rescinded** 1991.

Standards of Practice: Physical Disabilities (1979, 1988). **Rescinded** 1991.

Standards of Practice for Occupational Therapy Services in Schools (1987). **Rescinded** 1994.

Statements

Applying Sensory Integration Framework in Educationally Related Occupational Therapy Practice (2003). **Rescinded** 2009. **Replaced** by *Providing Occupational Therapy Using Sensory Integration Therapy and Methods in School-Based Practice* (2009).

Assistive Technology Within Occupational Therapy Practice (2004). **Rescinded** 2009. **Replaced** by *Specialized Knowledge and Skills in Technology and Environmental Interventions for Occupational Therapy Practice* (2009).

AOTA Statement of Physical Agent Modalities (1991). **Rescinded** 1997.

Driving and Community Mobility (2005). **Replaced** 2010.

Fundamental Concepts of Occupational Therapy: Occupation, Purposeful Activity, Function (1997). **Rescinded** 2005.

Management of Occupational Therapy Services for Persons with Cognitive Impairments (1999). **Rescinded** 2003.

Nondiscrimination and Inclusion Regarding Members of the Occupational Therapy Professional Community (1995). **Rescinded** 2005.

Ocupational Therapy and Hospice (1998). **Replaced** by Occupational Therapy and Hospice (2004). **Replaced** by The Role of Occupational Therapy in End-of-Life Care (2011).

Occupational Therapy for Individuals with Learning Disabilities (1991, 1998). **Rescinded** 2004. **Replaced** by Occupational Therapy Services in Early Intervention and School-Based Programs (2004). **Replaced** by Occupational Therapy Services in Early Childhood and School-Based Settings (2011).

Occupational Therapy in the Promotion of Health and the Prevention of Disease and Disability (2000). **Replaced** by Occupational Therapy in the Promotion of Health and the Prevention of Disease and Disability 2007).

Occupational Therapy Provision for Children with Learning Disabilities and/or Mild to Moderate Perceptual and Motor Deficits (1991). **Replaced** by Occupational Therapy for Individuals with Learning Disabilities (1998).

Occupational Therapy Services for Individuals Who Have Experienced Domestice Violence (2006). **Revised** 2011.

Occupational Therapy Services for Persons with Alzheimer's Disease and Other Dementias (1994). **Rescinded** 2000.

Occupational Therapy Services in Work Practice (1992). **Replaced** by Statement, Occupational Therapy Services in Facilitating Work Performance (2000). **Replaced** by Occupational Therapy Services in Facilitating Work Performance (2005). **Revised** 2011.

Occupational Therapy Services Management of Persons With Cognitive Impairments (1991). **Rescinded** 1999. **Replaced** by Management of Occupational Therapy Services for Persons With Cognitive Impairments (1999).

Psychosocial Concerns Within Occupational Therapy Practice (1995). **Rescinded** 2004.

The Occupational Therapist as Case Manager (1991). **Rescinded** 2002.

The Philosophical Base of Occupational Therapy (1979). **Revised** 2011.

The Role of Occupational Therapy in the Independent Living Movement (1993). **Rescinded** 1999.

Sensory Integration Evaluation and Intervention in School-Based Occupational Therapy (1997). **Rescinded** 2003. **Replaced** by Applying Sensory Integration Framework in Educationally Related Occupational Therapy Practice (2003).

Statement of Occupational Therapy Referral (1969, 1980, 1994). **Rescinded** 2004. **Replaced** by the Guidelines for Supervision, Roles, and Responsibilities During the Delivery of Occupational Therapy Services (2004, **edited** 2009) and Scope of Practice (2004, **edited** 2005).

Societal Statements

AOTA's Societal Statement on Autism Spectrum Disorders (2009). **Rescinded** 2013.

AOTA's Societal Statement on Family Caregivers (2007). **Rescinded** 2013.

AOTA's Societal Statement on Health Disparities (2011). **Revised** 2013.

AOTA's Societal Statement on Obesity (2006). **Revised** 2012. **Rescinded** 2013.

AOTA's Societal Statement on Play (2007). **Rescinded** 2013.

Certification Document Changes

The following certification documents have been removed from earlier editions of this manual:

AOTA Certification Requirements. **Rendered moot** by the formation of the American Occupational Therapy Certification Board.

Requirements for Graduates from Foreign Schools to Become OTRs. **Rendered moot** by the formation of the American Occupational Therapy Certification Board.

Policy Governing Lapsed Certification of Occupational Therapists and Occupational Therapy Assistants. **Rescinded** 1986.

Index

Note: Page references in *italic* refer to figures and tables.